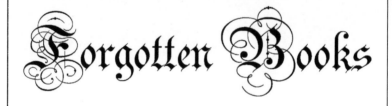

ISBN 978-1-5278-2942-8
PIBN 10013298

Forgotten Books is a registered trademark of FB &c Ltd.
Copyright © 2018 FB &c Ltd.
FB &c Ltd, Dalton House, 60 Windsor Avenue, London, SW19 2RR.
Company number 08720141. Registered in England and Wales.

For support please visit www.forgottenbooks.com

1 MONTH OF
FREE
READING

at
www.ForgottenBooks.com

English
Français
Deutsche
Italiano
Español
Português

www.forgottenbooks.com

Mythology Photography **Fiction**
Fishing Christianity **Art** Cooking
Essays Buddhism Freemasonry
Medicine **Biology** Music **Ancient**
Egypt Evolution Carpentry Physics
Dance Geology **Mathematics** Fitness
Shakespeare **Folklore** Yoga Marketing
Confidence Immortality Biographies
Poetry **Psychology** Witchcraft
Electronics Chemistry History **Law**
Accounting **Philosophy** Anthropology
Alchemy Drama Quantum Mechanics
Atheism Sexual Health **Ancient History**
Entrepreneurship Languages Sport
Paleontology Needlework Islam
Metaphysics Investment Archaeology
Parenting Statistics Criminology
Motivational

UNIVERSAL EXPOSITION, ST. LOUIS, U.S.A.

DAVID R. FRANCIS,
President of Exposition.

1904.

HOWARD J. ROGERS,
Director of Congresses.

TRANSACTIONS

OF THE

Fourth International Dental Congress

HELD AT

ST. LOUIS, MO., U.S.A.,

August 29 to September 3, 1904.

*EDITED FOR THE COMMITTEE OF ORGANIZATION
BY EDWARD C. KIRK, WILBUR F. LITCH,
AND JULIO ENDELMAN.*

IN THREE VOLUMES.

VOL. III.

Philadelphia:
PRESS OF THE "DENTAL COSMOS,"
The S. S. White Dental Mfg. Co.
1905.

CONTENTS OF VOL. III.

Section VII.

OPERATIVE DENTISTRY.

144368

Section VIII.

PROSTHESIS.

Section IX.

EDUCATION, NOMENCLATURE, LITERATURE, AND HISTORY.

Section X.

LEGISLATION.

—— — —— —

THE CLINICS.

Fourth International Dental Congress.

— — — —

SECTION VII.

SECTION VII:

Operative Dentistry.

Chairman—C. N. JOHNSON, Chicago, Ill.
Secretary—GEO. E. HUNT, Indianapolis, Ind.

FIRST DAY—Monday, August 29th.

Dr. C. N. JOHNSON, the chairman, called the section to order at 2 o'clock P.M., and after a few preliminary remarks delivered his address to the section, as follows:

Chairman's Address.

It is not my intention to make any extended remarks at the opening of the sessions of this section. I merely wish to call attention to the great possibilities of the work to be accomplished during the coming week in our deliberations on the various topics presented for consideration. These topics embrace a wide range of subject-matter from the broad question of "Operative Dentistry" itself—a paper which seemed to your chairman to be of such a character as to preclude the necessity for a lengthy chairman's address—to the more specific subjects of filling pulp-canals, the specific gravity of gold fillings, inlay work—considered in a somewhat new light—the enamel in cavity preparation, filling materials of various kinds, matrices, pressure anesthesia, etc.

Operative dentistry is extending year by year in its scope to a degree which keeps even its most earnest devotees constantly on the alert to encompass its varying phases of development. New ideas spring up in rapid succession to be advocated more or less strenuously by those who introduce them, then to be digested by the profession, and if found available to be finally assimilated into our professional knowledge.

In this process there is frequently much which of necessity must be cast aside as waste material, and it is to this sifting procedure that we are now about to devote our energies. In deliberations such as these it is well to have the contact of minds not only of different individuals but also of different groups of thinkers as represented by those coming

3

from different sections or different countries. And so today we are most fortunately situated in having with us representative men from all parts of the world assembled together with the sole object of getting at the truth of many of the perplexing problems which confront us in our service to the human race. Above all things it is the truth we are seeking, and in our deliberations let us at all times consider only the essentials of the subject and eliminate so far as possible our preconceived and personal predilections, to the end that we may accomplish the greatest good to the greatest number.

Remember that the saving of the human teeth, the placing of them in a condition of comfort, usefulness, and beauty is the true function of operative dentistry. Just so long as we approach our discussions with this end in view —so long will our meeting together be profitable, but if we allow ulterior or irrelevant ideas to bias us and carry us away from this main purpose, then shall we dissipate our energies and go away from the meeting little better than we came.

I now most cordially invite you to the work of the session with the earnest hope that every member of the section may feel himself impressed with the idea that our time is precious, and that every moment of it should be occupied to the best advantage.

The CHAIRMAN. On account of a very serious surgical operation Dr. E. A. BOGUE of New York city is prevented from being with us today. I know that every member of this section extends his sympathy to Dr. Bogue and regrets that he is not able to be with us. He has, however, sent his paper to me with the request that it be read by a gentleman who has a voice—a voice that will reach every individual in the audience. It therefore gives me great pleasure to introduce to you Dr. E. K. Wedelstaedt, who will read the paper by Dr. Bogue upon the subject of "Operative Dentistry."

Dr. E. K. Wedelstaedt then read the paper by Dr. E. A. BOGUE, New York, upon the subject of

Operative Dentistry.

By E. A. BOGUE, D.D.S., New York, N. Y.

OPERATIVE dentistry, as I understand it, is such a combination of science and art as enables the operator to so repair defective human teeth as to preserve the dental arches for the longest possible period of time and in the best possible condition. To that end it behooves us to understand the meaning and the use of the positions, shapes, sizes, texture, and color of the normal human teeth.

The enamel of the teeth begins to form on the summit of the cusps and extends downward toward the center of the grinding surface. On the sides it forms downward from the apex of the cusps toward the cervix of the tooth at the gum. If the vigor of the individual is sufficient to perfectly form that enamel, completely to bridge over the sulci and to leave no crevices between the different plates of enamel as they approach each other, then the tooth will have a perfect coat of mail, so to speak—a perfect coating of enamel, polished on the surface and hard. In all those cases where this degree of strength has existed in the formative processes, the teeth will be found rounded and not flat, rather short, and if not interfered with in their development, they will be regularly arranged in the two antagonizing arches, upper and lower, in such fashion that the very act of mastication is preservative, in that it tends toward cleansing those teeth through the processes of mastication and insalivation.

Superadd to this plenty of water and coarse and fibrous food and we shall have a dental apparatus that has no need of dentists nor of tooth-brushes or silk. Antiseptic mouth-washes would be uncalled for, and all the paraphernalia of modern dentistry would be a superfluity. By just so much as we lack of these conditions, decay and calculus enter in and become the antagonists of health and comfort.

By just so much therefore as we can take the cases presented for our care and restore them to the conditions just described as normal, by just so much have we put the patient upon the road to retain his teeth in comfort for the longest possible time.

At whatever point we have failed in restoring normal conditions and normal function we have left a weak point for the attack of one or other of the two diseases that we combat. These two diseases are decay and calcic deposit—the former of these arising from an acid condition existing somewhere in contact with the tooth; the latter—calculus—being most rapidly deposited when the conditions surrounding the tooth are alkaline. But both conditions involve the presence of some foreign substance or substances upon the tooth which do not belong there, and which, were the highest normal conditions always present, would never be there for any length of time.

But how is operative dentistry to control either or both of these conditions? It is to do it indirectly by placing the teeth into such a normal condition that they may be kept clean, and then by instructing all patients not only that the teeth need to be kept clean, but by showing them how to do it.

Operative dentistry does not consist in extracting teeth and replacing them with artificial substitutes, nor even in relieving pain, nor in filling up a few cavities in teeth presented by a patient for operation. It is the province of the true dentist to carefully examine each tooth and all the teeth in the mouth, mentally segregating each one from all the others, to carefully note all points where the enamel is deficient, indicating these conditions on an appropriate chart and indicating also all variations, of whatever nature, from normality, and then to explain to the patient what is required and why it is best to restore the teeth in that mouth to a normal condition as far as is practicable.

Perhaps the first thing to be done will be to see to it that all defects in the enamel covering are remedied by substituting an indestructible substance for the defects, so that the enamel may present a smooth and unbroken surface over the whole tooth, a surface upon which food will not be prone to lodge, because both shape and polish are opposed to such lodgment. Next it may be best to see to it that there is absolute and rounded contact between all the teeth of each of the arches, so that they may support each other laterally and so be able to sustain the force of mastication. Finally it may be necessary to replace into their normal position teeth that have gone astray and antagonize improperly.

If I can truthfully say that no child who has been put into my hands during the past twenty years and left there, and of whom I have had oversight regularly, has ever had the toothache or lost a tooth, I am claiming a great deal for operative dentistry. Among the children that I know there is one child whose teeth when erupted had from six to eight cavities of decay in every tooth, and although she is now twenty-five or twenty-six years of age, and the mother of a little family, she has never had a toothache and never lost a tooth. This proves the effectiveness of the treatment and the correctness of the theory on which that treatment is based; and although our absolute knowledge is very limited, enough is known to enable us, in most cases, to preserve the natural organs in comfort to extreme old age, providing we have the intelligent co-operation of the patient.

In 1877 a lady came to me with her lower incisors biting into the gum above in such way as to cause continual soreness and inability to masticate, or even to close the teeth without pain. There were apparently two ways of overcoming the difficulty. One, the empirical way of grinding off a portion of the cutting ends of the lower incisors, and so giving relief for a time. The other way involved building up the ends of the grinding teeth, and so opening the bite. Neither of these expedients seemed to me satisfactory, and I began then to inquire what had caused the difficulty, and

to seek as far as circumstances would permit to remove the cause and so to restore the teeth to comfort and utility in the hope of preserving them while life should last. I concluded that the extraction of the principal molars was the main cause of the difficulty, as the approximation of the other teeth in the mouth had greatly shortened the bite. Superadded to that were a number of places where the teeth having approximal cavities of decay had been filled, or had been decayed so deeply as to cause a falling together of the various members of the arches.

I concluded finally to wedge apart all teeth which were decayed approximally and to make contour fillings which would restore the teeth at least to their original size and shape, if indeed the fillings did not somewhat exaggerate the original size of the teeth. This was done with all the molars, and now for twenty-seven years these fillings have stood, with only one marked breakdown, in the lower left molars, which called for a replacement of the fillings at that point. The bite has been kept open so that the incisor teeth have never again wounded the gums. Incidentally the doctrine recently promulgated of extension for prevention has received a hearty indorsement from the behavior of these fillings during these twenty-seven years, and again, incidentally, it has been proved that the dental arches when supported by thorough contact of each member with its adjoining members are susceptible of standing firmly during many years without a break, while had these molars been capped or built down, or extended in any way to lengthen them without their having been formed into their proper occlusal arches with lateral contact, the teeth so extended would have been driven into their sockets to their former level.

I have upon a number of occasions spoken of a man fifty-two years of age, who told me he had never had a tooth-brush in his mouth. Yet that man's teeth were clean and in good condition, and his gums hard, pink, and healthful. The dental apparatus was so admirably arranged for the purposes of mastication that it not only did that part of the work thoroughly, but in the very act of mastication the teeth were cleansed by the flow of the saliva and by the friction of the food taken in. It is true he lived on plain food, often cooked out-of-doors —where his life was mostly passed, he being a railroad contractor on the Trans-Siberian Railroad. When civilization came and gave us soft food instead of hard, cooked food instead of fibrous and raw food, it did us a great damage.

Civilization indulges in soft food, cooked until it is still softer. It is therefore already in the best possible condition to be driven into crevices, there to remain lodged until fermentation shall have produced the acids and bacteria which lead to decay.

This is my reason for thinking that all operative dentists should study with the utmost accuracy the position, size, shape, and arrangement of the teeth in the skulls that are now exposed for our study in the museums, until they know what those forms and positions are that have endured the longest, surviving the vicissitudes of life. Then, and not till then, will we learn that any interference with normal conditions, whether by natural or artificial and mechanical processes, tends toward early destruction. Then, and then only, can we understand what the survival of the fittest means, and only

by such study can we know what is that fittest which survives.

Discussion.

The CHAIRMAN. I assure you we all appreciate Dr. Bogue's paper. Dr. Wedelstaedt has our cordial thanks for reading it. The discussion will be opened by a gentleman from abroad who has been associated to a considerable extent with Dr. Bogue. It gives me great pleasure to introduce to you Dr. I. B. Davenport of Paris.

Dr. I. B. DAVENPORT, Paris, France. In opening the discussion of Dr. Bogue's paper I find myself in the embarrassing position of complete accord—a condition, I fear, not compatible with proper discussion.

The predominating thought in the paper is prevention. Repair defects and prevent recurrence of disease by bringing about normal conditions of form and occlusion as far as possible, before decay, and pyorrhea, and kindred manifestations make their appearance. We should early determine the defective arrangement of occlusion, and orthodontia becomes an important factor in operative dentistry. At the same time Dr. Bogue recognizes the fact that perfect occlusion is not always possible to secure, and that mastication, as a normal cleanser of the teeth is, owing to modern civilization, usually insufficient. Dr. Bogue insists upon special care, giving special instruction to our patients in all the known methods of insuring cleanliness of the teeth and health of the gums. That Dr. Bogue has faithfully practiced what he preaches, in that he has most successfully preserved the teeth of those

brought up under his care, I can personally vouch for by the large number of
cases that have come under my direct
observation.

In his closing remarks Dr. Bogue
pleads "that operative dentists should
study with the utmost accuracy the position, size, shape, and arrangement of the
teeth of skulls in museums, until they
know what those forms and positions are
that have endured the longest and sur-
vived the vicissitudes of life, and learn
to understand that interference with normal conditions, whether by natural, artificial, or mechanical processes, tends toward early destruction."

These remarks afford me the satisfaction and comfort which only those familiar with dental literature of fifteen
to twenty years ago can realize, for not
only has the position I then took been
proved and accentuated in my daily practice, but Dr. Bogue has proved it true
in his own experience.

The CHAIRMAN. It was also Dr.
Bogue's desire that this discussion be
continued by Dr. E. K. Wedelstaedt. It
gives me pleasure, therefore, to call upon
Dr. Wedelstaedt to further discuss the
paper.

Dr. E. K. WEDELSTAEDT, St. Paul,
Minn. I am placed in rather an embarrassing position. I have just read this
essay and now I am called upon to discuss the ideas which it contains. Each
day cases present themselves to us, some
of which are the same as those to which
Dr. Bogue has called our attention. As
Dr. Bogue says, it behooves us to study
these different cases with more than ordinary care. The object in making dental operations is the same as is the object
in making surgical operations, i.e. to
eradicate the abnormal conditions, stamp
out the disease, and then return the parts

to as near a condition of normality as lies
in our power. Can we do this in the face
of the strenuous life which so many of us
are living? Will our patients permit of
it being done? I can answer this by saying, that it is being done by every intelligent practitioner who has at heart the
welfare of his patients, the dental profession, and humanity.

Where we ignore conditions and do
not make a restoration of the parts to
that degree of normality which the case
demands, we are not doing the best for
the patient. We are culpable in bringing
discomfort to the patient, in setting a
bad example to others, and in not doing
the best which can be done. The essayist fully illustrates this point in calling
our attention to the case where the patient was annoyed by having the lower
incisors continually striking into the
gum in the lingual surface of the maxilla.
This condition he corrected, and the
changes he made brought comfort to that
patient by returning the parts to a condition of normality. This is well illustrated by taking a typical case. Suppose a patient twenty-six years of age
consults us concerning a cavity of decay
in the distal surface of an upper right
second bicuspid. A cavity of decay also
exists in the mesial surface of the adjacent molar. Let us suppose that on account of neglecting this condition the
molar has moved forward, causing the
teeth to come into contact from the occlusal surface to the gingival margin. The
interproximal space has been completely
obliterated. What is our duty in this
case? Is it to at once fill those cavities,
ignoring entirely the conditions which
surround the case? Or is it our duty
to gain such separation as will upon
completion of the operation restore the
parts to a condition of normality? All

thinking practitioners follow the latter course with the full knowledge that it is the only method which can bring comfort to the patient, the only method which does away with a condition of faulty environment, the only method which returns the teeth to their normal positions and permits the parts to return to their normal conditions. The men who carry out their operations with these things in view are the professional men in dentistry.

Dr. J. E. ROSE, Vinton, Ia. I do not feel that I can add anything in the way of information to this paper that has not already been presented, but there is just one thought I would like to leave with this congress, which has helped me, and it is this: When we proceed to restore a tooth to its normal condition we should go about it with this thought in mind, that we perform the operation but once.

Dr. W. R. CLACK, Clear Lake, Ia. I wish that such a paper might be read every week before every dentist in the world. I do not believe there is any danger of too often calling attention to the points brought out in this paper, and I wish to leave a thought for those who are not already practicing what I wish to recommend. Where the approximal surfaces of the teeth have been lost through decay or otherwise, the first operation after cleansing that mouth is to take an impression of those teeth and of all the adjacent parts. It only takes a very few moments to get the modeling composition ready and to obtain the impression, and then lay that impression away. If there are any fillings to be removed that are defective or otherwise, probably lacking in contour, remove those fillings carefully, place them in their proper positions in the cast, thus

obtaining a facsimile of the patient's mouth for comparison at a future date. Now place the teeth as nearly as is possible in their normal condition, probably not in the original condition, for it is possible that the normal condition did not obtain originally. It is the dentist's duty to obtain this separation that Dr. Wedelstaedt speaks of. The operation may be hastened by the use of a mechanical separator, plugging those spaces with gutta-percha and insisting that the patient masticate his food on the gutta-percha fillings. In a few months it will be found that the teeth have become sufficiently separated without any inconvenience to the patient. Then, after restoration has been made, insist on seeing the patient every few months, and take a number of impressions of the mouth at those different periods to show the change for the better in the environment of the teeth and the surrounding gum tissue.

The CHAIRMAN. This section is honored by the presence of a gentleman who has just taken his seat in the rear of the hall, and I do not feel that we can continue the session with so distinguished a man sitting in the audience. I must ask him to take a seat upon the platform. I refer to our honored *confrère*, Dr. Charles Godon. (Applause.) It is a very high compliment that Dr. Godon should visit the section of Operative Dentistry.

Dr. CHARLES GODON, Paris, France. I thank you, gentlemen, for this compliment which you have bestowed upon me.

Dr. G. R. WARNER, Grand Junction, Colo. After the mouth is placed in a normal condition, as Dr. Bogue has described, it behooves us to keep it in that condition, and we cannot do it alone with our perfect contact points. We cannot do it alone with tooth-brushes, mouth-washes, etc., we have also the food to consider, as Dr. Bogue has said. So many people ask us why Indians do not have tooth troubles. They use the proper foods. The aborigines had no tooth troubles to speak of. If we should examine the cliff-dwellers' skulls we will find comparatively perfect mouths. But the people of today, as Dr. Bogue has said, live on soft cooked foods—foods that by the exertion of mastication do not cleanse the teeth, do not strengthen the gums, and do not nourish the body. If we would instruct our patients to use the proper food we would not only help their teeth but we would also help the teeth of the coming generation. I simply want to emphasize this question of food; let us study it for the benefit of our patients.

Dr. F. L. FOSSUME, New York, N. Y. I recently had two cases, one a boy about twelve years of age, and the other a girl about nine. In both cases the first molars, upper and lower, were so badly decayed and broken down that they had elongated and were occluding into one another so as to make it impossible to restore the contour without opening the bite. I treated the boy first, and inserted amalgam fillings in the molars on the right side, removing the pulps from the lower one. I contoured the fillings so as to restore the cusps and original form of the teeth, using a quick-setting amalgam. When the operations were completed it was too late to carve the fillings to relieve the bite, and I therefore requested him to return early the next morning. He did not show up for a week, and when he came I found to my surprise that the two teeth had adjusted themselves and the occlusion was perfect. The amalgam fillings were not broken, not worn, and had probably set perfectly before he

had masticated on them. I did the same thing on the left side, with the same result.

The little girl's teeth were also treated in this way and in a few days the teeth were in normal position. Had I carved the first two fillings the same day they were constructed I would not have discovered this point, which I consider most valuable.

Dr. R. C. TURNER, Caldwell, Kan. I think Dr. Merriman has touched the keynote of the whole business. A few years ago I took a trip down the Canadian river and went among three thousand Indians. I examined the teeth of those Indians as far as they would allow me to examine them, and I did not find a single carious tooth among all those Indians. They were meat-eating people. This dietary subject is a very important one in dentistry; that we all know. Here is the idea: these milling men that grind our wheat make it into white flour, taking away all the bone-forming substance. I think the question of diet is a very important one for dentists to consider.

Dr. J. H. RIGGLE, Port Washington, O. A very interesting case has been described in the course of this discussion. I refer to the building up of those first molars. I would like to know first whether those teeth were driven into their sockets, or did the readjustment within the glenoid fossa bring the articulation to that point? Did the anterior teeth move down to their proper occlusion, or was that accomplished by the lengthening of the hinge of the jaw?

Dr. FOSSUME. The change took place in the position of the teeth, for when I examined these teeth I found that instead of being so much longer they were in their normal positions in the alveoli. I believe the change that had taken place was simply a thickening of the pericementum, which was quickly reduced by the pressure of the occluding teeth, after being restored to their natural shape and size by the amalgam fillings.

Dr. C. H. LAND, Detroit, Mich. I have had considerable experience with irregularities in various ways, and believe the case referred to was one of malocclusion. My impression is that in many instances when in attempting to change the position of an individual tooth that has not quite reached its correct position we cement metal caps on one or more of the adjacent teeth it forces them down a little and the other short teeth will correct themselves. In this way I have regulated teeth for patients ranging in age from ten or twelve years to thirty-six. I find that even at the age of thirty-six years it is possible to force teeth into their alveoli. They give way in that direction as well as in any other by exercising sufficient pressure on a few individual teeth. I have a case now, that of a child of ten or twelve years of age, which will take me six months to correct, waiting for the incisors, canines, and bicuspids to extend.

Dr. J. A. TODD, St. Louis, Mo. As the question of the aborigines was brought up, I can say that I have had some experience with the Utah Indians. They live on white bread, cooked potatoes, and other food of the same nature, and they have the same troubles with their teeth as the civilized people. They suffer from pyorrhea alveolaris and have their teeth extracted, for as it is they have nothing else done for the relief of their dental troubles. It is not because they are or are not Indians, but because they live in the manner of civilized people and eat the same kind of food that they have "civilized" diseases.

Dr. J. H. NICHOLSON, Ardmore, I. T. I wish to corroborate the statement made by the previous speaker, that the teeth of the Indians are subject to the same troubles and diseases as the teeth of white or civilized people when they eat the same kind of food and do not take care of them.

Dr. R. C. TURNER, Caldwell, Kan. Those were semi-civilized Indians I had reference to; they lived on meat. It was in 1893 that I saw them and they were in a semi-civilized state. But they were not living on potatoes, wheat, sugar, etc. The government issued meat rations each week, and they lived entirely on meat. They did not want flour or anything of that kind; they threw it away.

Dr. C. H. WORBOYS, Albion, Mich. The problem of taking care of the teeth is a considerable one. In regard to taking care of children's teeth I will tell you what I do with my own little ones. I have a boy and a girl. They still have their deciduous teeth. I feed those children nuts, and they must crack them with their teeth if they can. I believe the very best permanent set will result only from a thorough use of the deciduous teeth. I know of no better way of stimulating the organs concerned in the development of the permanent teeth than by a thorough use of the deciduous teeth. When their food is cut into little pieces and the children are not allowed to make use of their teeth the very best for the future health of their teeth is not being done. In the case of the permanent teeth I do not believe there is a dentist practicing who is not familiar with the natural forms of those teeth. It is not only our duty to repair them by filling or any other method that we know of, but we are likewise bound to see that the teeth grow perfectly, and the best method I believe is to advocate the thorough use of the deciduous organs.

Dr. J. I. HART, New York, N. Y. I think we all concur with what the last speaker has said as to the *proper* use of the teeth, but his suggestion as to permitting children or adults to crack the shells of nuts with their teeth I think is not good practice. If the teeth are used sufficiently we induce proper salivation and we get sufficient blood to the parts to secure healthy peridental membranes. But the crushing with the teeth of such hard substances as the last speaker has suggested, would be found to fracture the enamel, ultimately producing decay. I fully agree with the suggestion to use them moderately; but in putting the deciduous teeth to such use as has been mentioned there is great danger of forcing them out of their sockets and losing them before the proper time.

Dr. WORBOYS. In reference to what the last speaker said as to the danger of using those hard substances, permit me to state that any baby or little one will use no more force than is necessary to crack a nut, and if they have not muscle enough they cannot crack the nut, and any tooth in healthy condition will stand anything the muscles of the jaws will stand. If those muscles are strong enough to bring the jaws together I warrant you the teeth will stand it. If the tooth is decayed or filled it is not wise to use it, of course, but the exercise those deciduous teeth get in using them in that way aids the development of the coming teeth and strengthens the muscles, and it gets the young one into the habit of grinding the food instead of bolting it.

Dr. R. OTTOLENGUI, New York, N. Y.

I would like Dr. Worboys to reply to that criticism that the deciduous roots might be loosened by this process. When do they begin to lose their stability?

Dr. WORBOYS. As I said before, if a tooth is weak or tender the child will not attempt to bite hard on it, no more than any of us will try to lift a heavy weight if the arm is rheumatic or if the muscles are weak. You cannot make them overdo it. I do not think it is possible to get a child to use a tooth when the roots have begun to absorb to such an extent that they are likely to be a little bit loose. So far as getting the other teeth out of line from use when the roots have become absorbed, I do not think that is possible. The permanent teeth as a rule follow directly after them. In nearly all cases I have found that the bicuspids are developing almost in the center between the roots of the deciduous molars, and the support is greatest over them. It is not distributed on both sides. I do not believe you can force a growing permanent tooth out of line by the use of the deciduous teeth. I am so fully convinced of the advantages accruing from the active use of the first teeth that I teach my little ones to use them just as hard as they can, and when I find a good hard hazelnut they cannot crack with their teeth the rest of us will have to take a hammer. It produces a thorough development of the muscles of mastication. I do not know of any better way of getting blood to those parts than by just such a thorough use of the teeth as I have described.

Dr. RIGGLE. There is one thing in this discussion that has not been brought out, namely, when the roots of the deciduous teeth are being absorbed the other teeth are coming into place. The first permanent molar is already in evidence before the roots of the first or second molar begin to be absorbed. I heartily indorse what Dr. Worboys said. That is nature's way of keeping the teeth clean, firm, and healthy.

Dr. J. L. HOWELL, Creede, Colo. In the main I agree with Dr. Worboys, but there are one or two exceptions. We all know that the things we are taught when we are young stay with us when we become old. I would not teach a patient of mine to crack nuts with his deciduous teeth or his permanent teeth, but I would teach him to keep up a healthy circulation by the proper use of a proper tooth-brush. I would advise his parents to feed him the proper kind of food, hard toast and tough beefsteak. A child uses his deciduous teeth in cracking nuts, which the gentleman says is the proper way to stimulate a flow of blood around the roots of the teeth, but if you allow him to do that when he is a child he will do it when he gets his permanent set of teeth. I have such patients come to my office; they tell me they have destroyed the enamel by cracking nuts and things of that kind. I tell them they must stop trying to do things with their teeth that nature clearly never intended. The Great Architect built our teeth for the proper mastication of food. He never intended us to crack nuts with our teeth, but did intend that we should use them in a proper manner in the mastication of our food. I will tell you a little incident. An expert happened into my college. He was a Malay with the finest set of teeth I ever saw in a human being. He had a masticating strength of 458 pounds. He would take a piece of the hardest granite and for a small compensation would show us what he could do with his teeth. He would crush it between his teeth. One of the molars

was entirely gone. He said he would not crush harder than his teeth could stand. Those teeth were small but they were magnificent. However, he had ruined one of them. I would advise the proper use of the teeth in masticating food and the use of a good, hard tooth-brush, brushing the teeth downward, and to the child I would give brittle toast and food of that nature to eat.

Dr. OTTOLENGUI. Dr. Worboys reported that he had his babies crack nuts with their teeth, another gentleman indorsed the same habit for his babies, and I hope before we adjourn we may get all the testimony possible on that subject. I hope the stenographer has got the statement down made by the gentleman in regard to the case of the Malay who could use 458 pounds pressure, and had only one tooth broken. It seems to me, that the real solution of this question of what food to eat, is to inquire to what class of animals we belong, and study the kind of food used by that genus. I would suggest to Dr. Worboys that nut-eating animals, such as the squirrel, have a totally different kind of tooth-structure from that of man. The gnawing animals have teeth which wear out at the incisive ends but grow out from the bottom. The identical tooth continues to grow just as our fingernails grow, and as the teeth of human beings are not constructed on that principle I do not believe we should allow children to crack nuts with their teeth.

Dr. ROBIN ADAIR, Atlanta, Ga. Inasmuch as we have digressed from the subject I will say a few words on "foods." I do not believe that the importance which dentists give to food is really necessary. When we consider the chemical analysis of our simplest food we know that from any of it we can take more building material than the human body can assimilate. I might refer to the Boer, who eats the coarsest food. The Boers have the poorest teeth of any civilized or semi-civilized nation of the earth. The tooth-brush is unknown to them. On the other hand, some of the savage races in the same country carry about with them a powder with which they scrub their teeth after every meal, and they have the best teeth in South Africa. It does not lie so much in the dentist telling us what kind of food to eat as it lies in the influence of the dentist to show us how under our present supply of food and condition of food to keep our teeth in the best condition possible. There are people who do not eat solid food and they have as good teeth as the aborigines ever had. I think the main idea is to show people the benefit of prophylaxis. I think the gentleman who read the paper had that same idea in his mind. The points so nicely brought out by the essayist are ideal and we should all strive to put them into practice.

Dr. WEDELSTAEDT, representing essayist (closing the discussion). There is but one speaker to answer and, if I have understood him correctly, I desire to say that for many years I have been of the opinion that we as a profession were too enlightened to hear a man again say that in making operations in the approximal surfaces of teeth it was not necessary to gain separation. I made some remarks regarding this subject and I am here to defend my position. I do not consider it good practice for any man to make fillings in the approximal surfaces unless he has sufficient room in which to operate and to return the parts to a condition of normality. It is a poor practice for a surgeon to operate on unclean parts, and he does not do so. If he does operate on parts that are not clean, he knows what the results will be, and we also know what the results will be if operations are not made as they should be. The essayist fully set forth the irreparable harm which so often follows where no attention is given a study of conditions, and operations are made irrespective of them. I believe in making operations which will be a comfort to the patient and which will not invite disease. If operations cannot be made with this idea in view, it is better that they be not made.

The CHAIRMAN. The next paper on the program is one by Dr. E. K. WEDELSTAEDT, St. Paul, Minn., entitled "Gold and Tin."

The paper was then read, as follows:

Gold and Tin.

By E. K. WEDELSTAEDT, D.D.S., St. Paul, Minn.

IN 1884 my attention was called to the use of tin and gold. It was asserted that where the gingival portion of cavities in the approximal surfaces were filled with tin, and gold was used to complete the operation, recurrence of decay would not take place. Fig. 1 illustrates the method used in cavities which were filled in the approximal surfaces of incisors and canines. Fig. 2 illustrates the method used when dealing with similarly situated cavities in bicuspids and molars.

For four or five years this method was closely adhered to.

In 1889 my attention was called to gold and tin in combination. It was alleged at the time that greatest benefit resulted from the use of this combination. Gold and tin in combination were used in the same place as the tin.

In 1891 the use of tin, and gold and tin in combination, was discontinued in my office. For seven years prior to this time the gingival third of practically every cavity in the approximal surface which I had filled with gold contained some tin or gold and tin in combination.

say in its favor, I say what I do on account of the bitter experience which I have had by making use of these materials.

ARGUMENT.

Where the gingival portion of a cavity in the approximal surface is filled with tin and the operation completed with gold, what results? First, we have a movement in the tin. The tin moves toward the gold and away from the cavo-surface angle of the cavity. (Figs. 2 and 3.) Secondly, with this movement

FIG. 1.

FIG. 2.

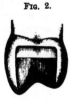

FIG. 3.

For the past ten years so many of my patients have been returning with cavities of decay around the gingival margin, which it was supposed was protected by the tin or the gold and tin in combination, that I felt much trouble might be saved others if attention were called to this subject.

In so far as they relate to the preservation of the human teeth, there is absolutely no virtue in tin or in gold and tin in combination, provided they are used in conjunction with gold as is illustrated in Figs. 1 and 2. On the other hand there is no filling material that has done so much harm and been the direct cause of destroying the life of the pulp and destroying the dentin, in proportion to its use, as tin or gold and tin in combination. I cannot help what others may

in the tin we have an opening between it and the cavo-surface angle. The moisture enters between the cavo-surface angle and the tin, and an oxidation of the tin takes place. Thirdly, with the oxidation of the tin we have an infiltration of stannic acid into the tissues of the tooth which surround it. This causes the tooth to have the appearance of Fig. 4. Wherever that blackened condition exists, we have dead tissue. Fourthly, if the condition as illustrated in Fig. 4 is left to itself it is but a question of time before the oxidation penetrates to such an extent as to impair the vitality of the tooth. The dentinal fibrils are destroyed. This is followed by the death of the pulp, and the tooth is on this account degenerated; it is then in a fit condition to invite caries. In fact, the moment there is the slightest movement in the tin, causing it to draw away from the cavo-surface angle, small particles of food and micro-organisms occupy the space between the filling material and the cavo-surface angle. The greater the movement of the tin, the larger is the ditch which exists along the gingival margin. We all know that wherever there are ditches of this kind we have a condition which invites caries. In my studies of these conditions where tin, or gold and tin in combination, have been

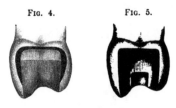

Fig. 4.   Fig. 5.

used, as is illustrated in Figs. 1 and 2, I have seen all kinds of caries around the gingival margins and in the cavity itself. Indeed, I have seen not only the whole axial wall between the gold and the pulp a mass of softened black decay, but I have seen many cases where the gingival seat and the axial wall had the appearance of Fig. 5.

If this much can be said of the results which follow the use of tin in connection with gold, what can be said of the results which follow the use of gold and tin in combination? All writers who have advanced the use of gold and tin in combination agree on one point, which it is asserted is in its favor, and that is, its remarkable change of character. In other words, when we first place mats or cylinders of gold and tin into cavities they are very soft. Later on, there is a change in the materials; they become

very hard. What is this change? It is purely and simply a crystallization. In the process of crystallization the molecules are drawn more closely together and we have as a result a change of form as well as a change in the character of the material. Wherever there is a crystallization we know that there must be either an expansion or a contraction in the mass. All scientists recognize this as a fact, for it is one of the fundamental principles of chemistry. We know definitely that in the crystallization of gold and tin we have exactly the same conditions existing around the gingival margin as where tin is used in connection with gold. What are some of these conditions? We have an open ditch around the gingival margin, absorption of the gum in the interproximal space, destruction of that portion of the pericementum which is adjacent to that tin or gold and tin in combination—a condition which invites disease, a faulty environment which if left to itself will naturally lead to the destruction of the tooth, etc. The use of materials which bring about such results is not to be considered an aid to the preservation, much less to the salvation, of the human teeth.

We know definitely a number of things, and among these things are two of much importance which are directly connected with the subject under discussion. What results where we take a sheet of No. 4 gold foil and over its surface sprinkle an imperceptible amount of tin? If we lay this sheet of gold between two pieces of paper we shall, on examining it at a later period, find that we have nothing left but a black powder which is a metallic oxid. (I am indebted to Dr. G. V. Black of Chicago for this experiment). The contact of the tin with the gold causes a chemical action to take place which results in our having nothing left but a black powder. This black powder has been called a black oxid of gold. Does any thinking practitioner mean to say that we, as intelligent men in a progressive calling, are justified in using materials which, when placed in cavities in the human teeth, undergo a distinct chemical change? I have answered this question for myself and I leave it for others to do likewise.

The second fact is this. Suppose that the distal surfaces of two upper bicuspids were decayed. It will be supposed that both teeth are normally situated. Suppose when the cavities are ready for the filling material it is found that both are of about the same size. Suppose that there is an equal chance for making a permanent operation in both teeth. Suppose, however, that one of the cavities is filled with gold, and the other has the gingival third of the cavity filled with tin, or gold and tin in combination, as is illustrated in Fig. 2. Suppose that both operations were made by the same man, and an equal amount of skill was used in making both operations. What would be the natural outcome? The operation illustrated in Fig. 2 would later on require attention, for this would be necessary on account of the change of character and form of the tin, or gold and tin in combination, which had been placed in the gingival portion of that cavity. This condition would make it necessary to refill that cavity; not to repair the filling, but to take out the whole filling, remove the decay around the axial wall and gingival seat and refill the cavity with gold. This operation is likely to stand for all eternity. Gold does not undergo a change of character of form.

The best results are always obtained where but one metal is used in a given cavity.

CONCLUSIONS.

First, if we believe in the results of the researches of Black and Williams regarding the cause of the decay of the human teeth, then the use of a combination of two metals which in crystallizing contract should under no circumstances ever receive any consideration from intelligent practitioners. Secondly, the use of any material which causes the dentin to oxidize, thereby destroying the life in the fibrils and the pulp, this in turn leading to the degeneracy of the tooth, cannot be indorsed. The use of such materials is to be absolutely condemned. Thirdly, it is to be deplored that so many men are making the claim that beneficial results can follow the use of combinations of metals of the kind to which attention has been called in this essay. Poorer results than those which have taken place in my own practice no man could possibly have.

I do not believe that the patients for whom I have operated have secretions in their oral cavity which are in any manner different from those of the people who live in other parts of the world. It is also impossible for me to believe that others can obtain results differing from those which I have observed to follow the use of these materials and which have been so fully outlined in this essay. Those who in the past have so strenuously advocated the use of such combinations as I have called attention to are requested to read a short essay in *Current Literature* for August 1903, page 151, the title of which essay is "Are Metals Alive?"

Discussion.

Dr. H. L. AMBLER, Cleveland, O. As long as the essayist has seen fit to criticize the use of tin, and tin and gold in combination, as a filling material, it seems to me that it would be fair to consider the properties of tin where it is used entirely for a filling.

Tin foil has been used for about one hundred years in the United States, and one of our distinguished operators said a few years ago, when he was about seventy-two years of age, that if all other filling materials were blotted out of existence and only tin foil was left more teeth would be saved than ever had been in the past.

Where teeth have been filled with tin it has been continually demonstrated that after a time in most cases where the tin was removed the dentin of the tooth had solidified. One of our teachers in a dental college, an expert microscopist, who had observed that fact several times, has termed it "progressive calcification," because, under the filling, especially where it had been placed in a tooth of rather soft structure, the dentin became further calcified and was harder than when the tin filling was placed there. I can show you specimens of teeth filled with tin foil that have been worn in the mouth for years, illustrating this phenomenon. Dr. Chase of St. Louis was one of the prominent men who recommended tin foil for filling sensitive cavities, and with no successful methods of obtunding the sensitive dentin it was too painful for the patient to have them thoroughly excavated; he therefore excavated the cavities as well as he could and filled them with tin. After some months, or perhaps a year or two in some cases, the tin was removed and he was able to cut retaining grooves or pits, or make a dovetail form, whichever he chose, in the cavity without excessive pain. According to his testimony on record, corroborated by the testimony of others, it was found that those cavities had lost most if not all of their sensitiveness, so that they could be prepared for a permanent filling. That is rather different testimony than is given to us in the essay.

I have been using tin foil for filling teeth for over thirty years. At the outset I made no record of my cases, as in those days very few dentists kept any, but in 1883 I commenced keeping a record of cases where the cavities had been filled with tin, and also of those where the gingival third or half of the cavity was filled with tin, and the remainder with cohesive gold. My discussion of this paper is based upon the supposition that the essayist used cohesive gold.

Dr. WEDELSTAEDT. That is correct.

Dr. AMBLER. That is what I thought, and that is the material I myself use. In 1882 I filled on the buccal surface of the lower left second molar a cavity embracing about two-thirds of the surface. Beginning at the gingival portion I covered the nearly exposed pulp with tin, continuing it for about one-third of the way occlusally, then completed the filling with cohesive gold. Two weeks ago I examined that tooth and there was no sign of decay around the tin or gold.

In 1889 I filled for a patient a disto-occlusal cavity in a bicuspid and a mesio-occlusal cavity in a molar. Ten days ago I examined them and no decay was perceivable around the tin or the gold.

Now, if there is any danger of pulps dying under the tin, why not cover the thin portion of the dentinal wall with some cavity lining? Wherein do we derive protection from the use of gold in preference to tin? Gold is four times as good a conductor of heat, and six times as good a conductor of electricity as tin, so under which metal will the pulp be likely to die the quicker owing to thermal and galvanic action, tin or gold?

I have found since 1882, at the time I commenced using tin for about one-third and sometimes one-half of the gingival portion of the cavity, that one filling in a disto-occlusal cavity in a lower right second molar failed around the gold, the gingival half of the cavity being filled with tin and the rest with gold; the wearing down of the tooth-structure and the gold on the occlusal surface had fractured the enamel so that it broke away, and the filling began to leak around the gold. The patient allowed it to go so long that the gold was forced nearly out of the cavity. I also found that three fillings failed for about one-third the distance across the cervical margin; one filling failed at the cervical margin after it had been in six years, and another after it had been in seven years. That makes seven failures, some total and some partial, of those cases which I have been able to watch.

The essayist tells you that he has used tin in the cervical portion of the cavity for four or five years, but it seems to me that thirty years is a better test than four or five.

Now it may be possible that good tin foil was not used in those cases where the essayist failed. I do not know what kind of tin the essayist used, nor does he describe his method of using it, so I must conclude from what I know about this matter that either the tin foil was poor material or else the method of manipulation was faulty. Now I know that his method of manipulation of gold is com-

plete, and no doubt the same may be said of tin, so the factor of manipulation will have to be eliminated. Then again it might happen that the preparation of the cavity was faulty, yet I think that in the cases he cited that cannot be true, because the essayist is thorough in the preparation of cavities. We are therefore compelled to fall back upon the first premise, that it was poor material. A great deal of the tin foil put on the market for filling purposes is not fit to put in a cavity.

The essayist says that tin destroys the dentin and kills the pulp. The facts, according to my experience, are these: After the tin is placed in the cavity at the cervical margin, filling the remainder of the cavity with cohesive gold, a galvanic action takes place between the tin and gold, the tin being the positive element and the gold the negative; this galvanic action ceases after the tin filling becomes oxidized, and no further galvanic action occurs. In some instances I have found that this oxid does penetrate a slight distance into the dentinal tubuli. I take the ground that if it does so penetrate it helps protect the ends of the tubuli, acting as a barrier to the further progress of decay.

I know that this is true, and if you gentlemen will take the trouble to examine a display which will be found in the educational department in this building you will be convinced by an ocular demonstration of the facts I am stating. You will find in this exhibit a disto-occlusal filling where tin was used at the cervical part of the cavity, the balance being gold, that remained intact in the mouth for twenty-six years, the tooth for some reason or other having been lost. There are teeth in that exhibit, filled by different operators, that have been worn in the mouth all the way from seven to twenty-six years, filled with tin at the base and the rest of the filling gold, and there is no decay around the tin or the gold.

I can show you in my own mouth an upper lateral that has been filled twice with cohesive gold in the last twenty years by one of the best operators I know, and both of those fillings failed. Ten years ago that tooth was refilled, using tin at the cervical portion and the rest with cohesive gold, and today there is no decay around either the tin or the gold.

I have also a lower left lateral incisor which was filled with cohesive gold and proved a failure. I had it refilled seven years ago at the lingual and also the cervical margin with tin, and there is no decay; the remainder of the filling, being of gold, is also intact.

I have a disto-occlusal cavity in the upper left first molar that was filled with cohesive gold, which was a failure, and six years ago I had it filled with tin foil across the cervical margin, completing the filling with gold, and that is in perfect condition today.

On the right side I have a disto-occlusal cavity in the second bicuspid, a mesio-occlusal cavity in the first molar, filled with gold and tin, the gold being on the occlusal surface; these have been in use three years.

I use tin foil of Nos. 5, 10, or 20—any of those numbers; it does not make so much difference about the gage of the tin. If an operator is accustomed to use thin gold foil he had better have thin tin; if accustomed to the use of heavier gold foil, use heavy tin. Any of those numbers can be manipulated so as to make tight margins. There is another advantage in the use of tin at the cervical margin; it is inserted more quickly and easily than gold, and one cannot fail to cut off the projecting portion, as might happen when using cohesive gold.

I do not say that you cannot make a tight cervical margin with cohesive gold, or with non-cohesive. The question is, does tin make a tight margin? Of course, if there is leakage around a filling the tooth generally begins to decay. But does it not do the same thing around gold and amalgam? Why should tin bear the burden of tooth decay? Do not place the entire blame on the tin alone. Amalgam fillings, cement fillings, and gold fillings all fail at the cervical margins at times.

The essayist says that the tin oxidizes and stannic acid is formed which penetrates the tubuli of the dentin, destroys the dentinal fibrillæ, and kills the pulp. He does not say this occurs every time, and I do not suppose he means to imply that it always occurs. I would be very glad to know how it is done, and how stannic acid is formed from a piece of tin foil upon a solid mass of tin foil well malleted. I want him to explain for my information how it can be that stannic acid is formed from a solid mass of tin in the tooth? I say that as far as my chemistry goes, which is corroborated by two dental chemists, that cannot be possible. Stannic acid is a white substance, and here we have a black substance, the essayist says, penetrating the fibrillæ and killing the pulp.

The essayist also says, whenever a tooth becomes black from the use of tin the dentin becomes soft and you can scoop it out. In those cases where the decay extends along the buccal or lingual wall, the tooth softens. Would it not soften with gold, or anything else? The tin is not to blame.

I think that the drawings the doctor has given us are fair so far as I can judge.

About one-third of the cervical portion is shown filled with tin, the rest with gold. Nor do I find any fault with the form of the cavities.

I never have seen a dead pulp under a tin-foil filling. If pulps die under tin, why is this operation advocated by Dr. Herbst of Germany, who says that he amputates the coronal portion of exposed pulps, applies creasote, burnishes a mat of tin foil into the pulp-cavity, and fills the rest with any desirable material.

Now take up the matter of tin and gold in alternate layers in equal parts. If you use a sheet of No. 4 tin, also use a sheet of No. 4 gold. It can be used in any proportion, but equal portions of tin and gold, in alternate layers, either No. 5 or No. 10, folded as thick as desired and condensed with a mallet, will produce the best results. I always fold it into a tape, folding the tin and the gold over and over, so as to make No. 20, 30, or 40, and if the materials be used in equal proportions it will stay right where placed. Most of my experience with this method has been in the occlusal surfaces of molars and bicuspids in large cavities, and I have never seen a failure in a filling made with equal parts in alternate layers folded back and forth in the cavity and malleted down with the hand mallet the same as with cohesive gold.

In 1838 Dr. McBride of Pittsburg, Pa., used tin and gold by rolling the tin and gold together, keeping the tin on the inside and the gold on the outside, wedging it in the cavity in the old manner of wedging fillings. If this method had been a failure, would it not have been ascertained long ago? He is the first man that has gone on record as using tin and gold in that way. Dr. John S. Clark of St. Louis, in 1851, was probably the first man to make cylinders of tin and gold in alternate layers.

I can show you specimens where equal parts of tin and gold were used in the cervical third of the cavity, the rest being filled with cohesive gold, and no decay ensued; but my experience in that only extends back for six years, and that is a comparatively short time. I do not use it very often in the above location, because I know that pure tin alone at the cervical margin will answer every purpose.

Just a word about the action that takes place between tin and gold. After electrolysis takes place the joint between the tin and gold cannot be separated with a chisel. The two metals cannot be forced apart exactly at the joint, because electrolysis has caused them to cohere so firmly. When galvanic action takes place in the mouth the tin is discolored and the galvanic action stops. The under surface of the tin filling will generally be black, because there is just enough moisture in the tubuli to oxidize the tin, and this oxidation fills up the ends of the dentinal tubuli and is a bar to the ingress of bacteria, if any happen to be present.

One reason why fillings fail where tin is used at the cervical margin is because the operator did not put in enough tin. If a man thinks he can take one thickness of tin foil No. 10, lay it over the cervical margin in approximal cavities, then go on and complete with cohesive gold and have a tight, lasting filling, he is mistaken. Put in one-third or one-half tin, and very seldom will any of the fillings fail.

The essayist refers to using tin and gold in alternate layers for four or five years. Others have been doing it for forty or fifty years, and have not found out what he has. He refers to an experiment made by Dr. Black, who is known to be a scientific man and nearly always right. In this experiment he says Dr. Black placed an "imperceptible" amount of tin powder upon a sheet of No. 4 gold and laid it away for a time between two leaves of a book, and when he examined it the tin and gold were oxidized and crumbled up fine.

After conferring with Dr. Black I find that the experiment which he made does not bear any resemblance to the one quoted. It was made years ago and probably the essayist had forgotten just what it was.

Since I had the doctor's paper, some four days ago, I have endeavored to procure this "imperceptible" amount of tin. I took a piece of tin and lightly scraped it with a knife blade, removing the very smallest specks that I could and placed those particles upon a piece of No. 4 gold foil, exposed it to the atmosphere in my cabinet, and for the four days that it remained there no change had taken place in the tin or gold. One month has now elapsed and still there is no change.

Five years ago I was informed that if a sheet of gold were placed between two sheets of tin and laid away in a book, in a little while the tin would become oxidized, and that you could blow it away. I tried the experiment, beginning three years ago, but the result referred to did not happen. A few days ago I looked at it, and no more change in that gold can be seen than if it had been placed in contact with the tin yesterday, and there was no cohesion between the leaves of gold and tin, and no oxidation.

So I claim that all thinking practitioners are justified in using tin at the cervical margin. The essayist says gold will last to all eternity. Gold fillings of 24-karat gold do not last to all eternity in the mouth. If you will look at the *Cosmos* for March 1904, p. 178, you will see an account by Dr. W. D. Miller of a tooth filled with gold, malleted into the buccal surface of a bicuspid, where grooves had been cut in the gold by erosion; so that gold will not last forever in the mouth. And we have seen a case of a gold crown on an incisor, made of 23-karat gold, where nearly all of the labial surface of the gold had disappeared, leaving an opening in the shape of a letter U; this shows that gold does not last forever in the mouth.

Dr. D. J. McMILLEN, Kansas City, Mo. I am not an advocate of tin and gold as a filling material. There is no question in my mind that for some purposes a tin filling is one of the best fillings to put in the tooth, although it is not a proper material for every tooth. The fact that one tooth decays under a certain kind of filling is no reason for discontinuing the use of that filling material. If we should discontinue the use of fillings for the reason that teeth decay under them we should have to discontinue the filling of teeth altogether.

There are many things to think of beside the material with which we fill a tooth. The preparation of your cavity has a great deal more to do with the preservation of the tooth than the use of the material, whether tin, or tin and gold, or gold, or amalgam.

If I were allowed to criticize those cavities illustrated by the essayist I should like to do so, although the matter of preparation is not touched upon in the paper. In filling teeth with tin and gold we must not forget two things: (1) That there must not be any square corners; (2) at the point of juncture between the two filling materials, unless extreme care is used a condition will result at that point very apt to lead to decay, as Fig. 5 would demonstrate to my mind in presenting a corner there that is exceedingly difficult to fill.

One reason why I have not advocated the use of tin as a base for filling is that it discolors the cervical wall and makes an unsightly filling. It does not absolutely fill that portion of the tooth if you use tin cylinders; using all gold, and non-cohesive gold, there is no question in my mind but that it adapts itself better to the walls of the tooth than any tin that can be made. I would not be in favor of using thick tin. In adapting a filling of any description, whether it be tin or non-cohesive gold, if I were to undertake to fill the cervical wall with either material, I would not expect to make a tight filling if I used a thick foil. In using this kind of filling it should be a thin sheet of gold or tin. I think tin if properly handled, used either in combination or by itself, has a virtue in saving teeth.

Dr. N. S. JENKINS, Dresden, Germany. Permit me, gentlemen, to say that where perhaps any member here present has seen one filling of tin and gold, I have seen a thousand. Tin and gold had its origin in Europe for practical uses. It was before the age of the rubber dam; it was an expedient designed to overcome the great difficulties of preserving teeth, before the rubber dam or cohesive gold had been dreamed of. It serves two purposes: It immediately stops decay and it continues to improve in its beneficent action. I have seen innumerable teeth which have been in their partially erupted condition exposed to the ravages of decay and which have been filled under water with tin and gold to the preservation of those teeth for thirty years without recurrence of decay.

Now you will naturally inquire, How did that happen? Gentlemen, it is my belief that it occurred only through perfect mechanical adaptation and not through any chemical action, or at least the chemical action being only subsidiary. When tin and gold united in proper proportion is packed into a cavity by lateral pressure, the only way in which it can be judiciously applied, it is almost immediately subjected to electrical influence, and as Dr. Miller has so exactly explained to us, an oxid of tin is formed, the filling becomes distinctly greater in bulk and possessed of a crystallization which makes it resistant to the force of mastication. That is the reason that teeth are preserved by tin and gold, because the filling by expansion improves after it is made, and tin and gold, so far as I know, is the only material with the exception of porcelain which exercises a continual progressive protective power against the ravages of decay.

Dr. W. R. CLACK, Clear Lake, Iowa. I was taught to use tin foil and a combination of tin foil and gold between 1876 and 1878. Undoubtedly, owing to the imperfect manner in which I had used it, I am obliged to stand here and tell you gentlemen that every filling that I have had the opportunity of watching and observing has failed. Be it understood I was a young practitioner, and also be it understood that a great many of the fillings that I made with cohesive gold and with amalgam also, at that time, have since failed. So that that is not conclusive proof that it was all on account of tin.

The idea of the oxidization of tin or any metal preserving the tooth-structure, has always been to me a queer proposition. It seems to me as if it were an argument that it was necessary to partially destroy the substance in order to bring out its best qualities. I know that it has been a custom to use silver nitrate for the prevention of decay. If you could have been in Dr. Wedelstaedt's office last winter and seen a set of teeth that had been treated by an advocate of silver nitrate for the prevention of caries in the human teeth, I do not believe you would have been guilty of again using it. It did undoubtedly prevent decay for the time being; but the after effects of that application were a great deal worse than the first condition. I am not able to give you just the chemical reasons why this result occurred.

That those fillings have failed where cohesive gold has been used in the gingival third of cavities in approximal surfaces of bicuspids and molars is nothing to be wondered at. Gentlemen, a man is an expert who can make a perfectly absolute adaptation of annealed gold at the gingival margin of those cavities every time; there are very few such men alive today. In place of cohesive gold I use unannealed gold, because I believe it is as easy of adaptation as tin foil and I believe that it is as lasting and can be just as evenly placed.

Right here let me say that the criticism of those fillings as failing because of the overhang at the gingival margin is not a criticism necessarily against gold any more than any other material. Any man who leaves an overhanging margin invites the recurrence of decay.

I have not been in practice quite as long as Dr. Ambler, and I have not been as close an observer for as many years as he has, but I can show you a patient in the city now who has nearly every approximal surface of the bicuspids and

molars filled with unannealed gold for the gingival third; and there is no recurrence of decay.

The last speaker told us of fillings made for him with gold that have failed. Granted. He tells us on the other hand of fillings that have been made with a combination of gold and tin that are in perfect condition today. We believe there is such a thing as immunity. I have cavities that decayed in my central incisors twenty-seven years ago, and I cannot see by the closest examination that they have progressed a particle in all that time.

Dr. AMBLER. Have they been filled?

Dr. CLACK. No, sir; they are open cavities. I have seen in Dr. Wedelstaedt's office a patient who has also upper central incisors slightly decayed, where there has been a total cessation of that decay and the patient is absolutely immune to the ravages of decay, those cavities still being unfilled.

Unless those cavities mentioned by the last speaker had been filled by the most expert operators, a recurrence of decay would likely have ensued; but in certain other cavities a man can make a filling with almost any material and there will be no recurrence of decay. These cavities were filled for Dr. Ambler when he was young; he has been confined to an indoor life, and I would judge his teeth are subject to decay from the number of cavities he has spoken of, and no doubt a great many of those fillings had that overhang.

As for the preservation of any particular tooth for any length of time by the use of any one material, it does not prove anything. Several years ago I was out hunting near Clear Lake, Iowa, with an old soldier who had a great habit of chewing bird-shot. He had a cavity, decayed, in the buccal surface of the lower right first molar which he had often intended to have filled but had never done so. One day he came up into my office and said, "I was going to have a filling put in that tooth, but I have one there already." On examining it I found the cavity to be closed with one of those birdshot. This spring he came in again, and I extracted that molar with that birdshot in the cavity, seemingly just as absolutely perfect a filling as any that could have been made for him of other material. So that it does not do to tie up to any one thing in the way of filling material; and I believe that these cavities in Dr. Ambler's teeth, which he refers to as having been in for only the last three years, were inserted at a period of immunity to caries; and I believe that a gold filling, properly placed there, would undoubtedly have been there today.

Dr. WEDELSTAEDT (closing the discussion). I have called your attention to such conditions as I have found to exist where tin, and a combination of gold and tin, have been used in the gingival third of cavities in the approximal surfaces and gold has been·used to complete the operation. I have called your attention to the exact conditions as I have found them to exist.

One speaker stated that gold and tin in combination is the best material to use for filling cavities in the human teeth. He alleges that there is no material any better except the porcelain inlay. And yet experimental research proves beyond a doubt that it requires more pounds pressure to crush cement than it does to crush similarly sized pieces of some porcelain inlay material which is at present being made considerable use of. Porcelain inlays have but a limited use and are temporary fillings, which

sooner or later must be replaced with something more permanent. As Dr. Southwell so truly says, "Porcelain inlays are but plastic operations."

Another speaker said that he made nine combination fillings in cavities in approximal surfaces. The gingival third of these cavities he filled with gold and tin in combination, and then completed the operation with gold. He alleges that seven of these nine operations failed. His statement merely proves the contention which I made. The same speaker said that for years it has been the habit of many practitioners, when dealing with unusually sensitive dentin, to fill the cavities with tin. The tin is then allowed to remain in the cavities for six or eight months. At the end of this time, when the tin is removed, it will be found that sensitivity has entirely disappeared and the cavity can be prepared without the patient suffering any pain. His statement also proves my contention as to the ability of the tin to destroy the life in the fibrillæ. And yet, again, he asserts that he has in his exhibit many extracted filled teeth which have been filled according to the method which I condemn, and that not one of the operations shows any sign of failure. I have been requested to ask where these teeth were obtained and why they were extracted. If they were extracted from the mouths of people who are dead, his evidence is of little value. If they were extracted from the mouths of those suffering from pyorrhea alveolaris, why then I can say that where this condition exists decay does not readily take place.

The present condition of affairs as it ·relates to our profession is very singular. I read an essay for your consideration, embodying therein my ideas of certain conditions as I have found them to exist after making combination fillings in the cavities. You are told that such conditions cannot possibly exist. Yet for the past eight or ten years I have been, and am still, meeting with just such conditions as described in my essay. If others have not sufficient ability to recognize the existence of these conditions, it surely is no fault of mine. The conditions spoken of are there and they can readily be found. I have come to you calling attention to these conditions, not for my own glory but for the good of those whom we serve. This is not only for our own advancement at the present time, but that those who may come after us and who will make the experiments—thus proving the truth of my ideas—may say that all were not so ignorant at that time and age.

I believe in a man standing by his convictions, provided that they are based on experience which he has gained either at the chair or in proving experimental research. Where a man has such evidence he has a just cause and a good fighting foundation. Where, however, a man has convictions which are based upon "say so," and makes contentions for the wrong, that man has no right to be a dentist, and further he has no place in our profession. By continually dwelling upon the importance of following something the truth of which he cannot prove he becomes an enemy of mankind. This continual clash of ideas between those who know and know why they know, and those who think that they know and know not, should long since have come to an end.

Let us try to do good and be kind, in preference to doing some things about which the less said the better. Let us discuss these matters from a foundation which rests upon knowledge and experimental research, which will prove the truth of our results. Nothing is ever gained by making contentions where there is not a vestige of truth to prove the contention. Let us rather work for the future of our profession, its advancement and progress, than to be forever dwelling upon its past history.

It is a self-evident fact that this is about the time and place to use a saying of the brainy Prof. Lewis. In a discussion very similar to the one which has taken place here today he was called upon to close the discussion. He arose and said, "Vell, all I have to say is this, Some mens have nothing to learn and nothing to forget." I am very thankful to say that I still have very much to learn and consequently will have something to forget.

Adjourned until Tuesday, August 30th, at 2.30 P.M.

SECTION VII—Continued.

SECOND DAY—Tuesday, August 30th.

THE section was called to order promptly at 2.30 P.M. by the chairman, Dr. C. N. Johnson.

The CHAIRMAN. We have with us on the platform Dr. John I. Hart, a member of the Section of Operative Dentistry, and from whom I expect a great deal of help in the conduct of this section. It gives me pleasure to introduce to you Dr. Hart.

Dr. J. I. HART, New York, N. Y. I am very glad to meet you, and I wish to take this opportunity of congratulating you upon the program that has been prepared through the efforts of your chairman and secretary. The work of the congress after all depends upon the sections, and it would be very unfortunate if the Section of Operative Dentistry of the Fourth International Dental Congress should fall below the standard created by this country in operative work. So far this section has maintained the position which this branch of our specialty should stand for.

The CHAIRMAN. The first paper on the program is by Dr. JAMES M. MAGEE of St. John, N. B., and is entitled "The Instrumentation and Filling of Crooked Root-Canals."

Dr. Magee then read his paper, as follows:

Instrumentation and Filling of Crooked Root-Canals.

By Dr. JAMES M. MAGEE, St. John, N. B.

LET me state at the outset that while a large measure of success has attended the practice of opening and filling root-canals as I have followed it, my practice is not intended to be an infallible method, because there are root-canals which no man living can successfully open with instruments. The few cases I show will demonstrate the idea, and perhaps help to prove the claim I make, that 90 per cent. of all root-canals we attempt to fill can be filled completely to their apical openings, and it may here be remarked that the apical opening is not always at the apex of the root. (Fig. 1.)

With a desire to make this paper as

brief as possible I have confined myself
to the subject of instrumentation and
the filling of the canals in crooked roots,
and since molars more frequently than

FIG. 1.

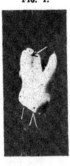

any other teeth have curved and crooked
roots a description of the procedure of
opening and closing the canals of these
teeth will serve as an illustration for all.

The treatment for fistulæ and putrescent canals opens up too large a field for
discussion, therefore I shall not suggest
anything in that connection, except to
say that once the canal is opened its
treatment, if any be needed, will be simplified.

Of course, no one can say positively
that the roots of any unextracted tooth
are crooked unless he is possessed of an
X-ray apparatus, so the ordinary operator is obliged to depend upon his sense
of touch to enable him to see, in his
mind's eye, the shape of the root he is
working in. Nevertheless, with few exceptions quite as satisfactory results can
be obtained without the X ray as with
it. Before we begin opening the pulp-
canals we examine for the possibilities
of an easy or difficult operation. Youth
is a factor in favor of easy access to the
apical openings, since the canals are
larger in early than in mature life. A

perfectly regular arch will rarely contain
teeth having badly curved roots, while
contracted arches will usually contain
teeth of this class; however, the only certainty we have of being able to reach the
apical opening is a knowledge of the fact
that we have once done so.

Many of the difficulties encountered
may be entirely overcome if at the beginning free access be obtained to all the
canals. Free access does not simply
mean that condition which will permit
reaching the orifice of the canal. It
means that so much of the tooth-structure must be cut away as to permit the
passing of an instrument directly to the
end of the canal, if it be at all nearly
straight.

Let us first consider a lower molar.
(See Figs. 2, 3, 4, 5.) Should the opening into the pulp-chamber be through
a cavity in the distal surface we must
cut forward through the morsal surface
sufficiently far for at least a perpendicu-

FIG. 2.

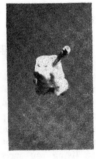

lar entrance to the anterior canals.
(Figs. 3 and 4.)

It is no economy of either time or
tooth-structure to abstain from cutting
for fear of weakening the crown, since
the crown will be of little service unless

the roots are healthy and comfortable, and even if the ultimate result was likely to be as good (which it is not) the time

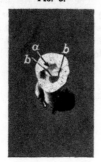

FIG. 3.

consumed would be infinitely greater. However, the question of saving time must never be considered when the real issue is saving the tooth.

When the carious cavity through which the pulp-chamber is perforated is in the mesial surface, it is not necessary to cut away quite so much of the morsal surface, since the posterior canal may be easily reached without cutting to a per-

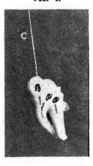

FIG. 4.

pendicular with the posterior wall of the pulp-chamber. (Fig. 2.)

The roots of the lower molars almost always slant backward, and are often-

times curved, particularly the anterior. (Fig. 4.) The anterior roots of lower first molars always have two canals, and usually two are found in the anterior roots of the second and third molars also. It is quite easy to open the posterior canal, since it is large, the posterior root being rarely found with two canals. Those in the anterior root often diverge and then converge again (Fig. 5) sometimes to a common apical opening, and an explorer to enter the canal would have to be pointed decidedly forward. (Fig. 5, d.) So in order to ap-

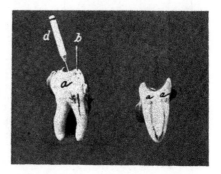

FIG. 5.

proach the extremity of the canals we must enlarge the orifices laterally and anteriorly; that is, we enlarge the orifice of the lingual one toward the tongue, and a little forward, and the buccal we enlarge toward the cheek and a little forward. Two bristles stuck in these canals now would stand diverging, pointing outward and slightly forward. (Fig. 5, b.)

A Gates-Glidden drill is one of the best instruments suitable for this enlargement, though a round bur must often be used also. While revolving in the engine the drill should be moved up and down, cutting widest at the entrance, though it should never be pushed as far into the canal as it will go. This cutting of course tends to straighten the canal. Having enlarged the orifice, we now pass an exploring instrument down the canal to determine whether we can open it successfully with instruments alone, or if we must use acid to facilitate its opening. The instruments I find best suited for the work in root-canals

in the engine, but be worked with the fingers, because opening a root-canal is too important a thing to trust to the haphazard results of a drill driven by engine power. The right-angle Beutelrock drills may be used even in the molars, the short stem affording a firm grip for the fingers. The smallest size will frequently follow and open up a fine

FIG. 6.

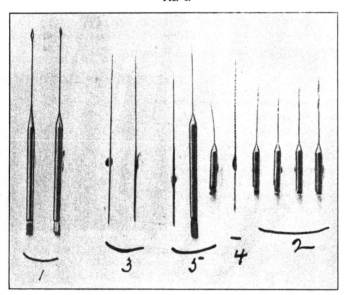

are Gates-Glidden drills of large size, for enlarging the orifices, the four smaller sizes of Beutelrock drills for the right-angle, as well as those for the ordinary engine handpiece, the two smaller sizes of Donaldson canal cleansers, and fine Ivory broaches. (Fig. 6.)

The Gates-Glidden drills should be used in the engine and only for enlarging the orifices of the canals.

The other drills should *never* be used

canal, even to its extremity, which the smallest size Donaldson cleanser will fail to open.

To make an instrument which will follow almost any canal, and almost any curve, take the smallest Beutelrock drill and grind it down to a hairlike tapering point by pressing it with the fingers against the side of a fine corundum wheel, and rotating it while the wheel is revolving. Then partially draw the temper. The finest Donalson cleanser, with the barbs all ground away, and having the temper drawn, will also serve; but I like the material of which the Beutelrock drills are made, as it is especially tough. In addition to that, the shank of the engine point serves admirably for a handle, while the other instruments must be fastended in a broach-holder. (Fig. 6, 5.)

Having enlarged the orifices of all the canals and determined that the case in hand demands the use of acid, we dip the points of our foil-carriers in the

FIG. 7.

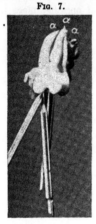

acid (I prefer sulfuric, at least 50 per cent.), carry a drop to the canal, when it will run in, and insert our fine instrument. Carefully feeling our way we find it sticks at the bend of the root; we withdraw it, and again return with a gentle pressure. We repeat this a few times and then use either the smallest drill or cleanser, as may be preferred, to enlarge a little. A saturated solution of sodium bicarbonate pumped in with an Ivory broach having a wisp of cotton around it will boil out any débris remaining in the canal. We mop out the soda solu-

tion, apply more acid, and repeat the procedure until sensation is experience l. (Figs. 7 and 8. *a a a*.) Then, being thor-

FIG. 8.

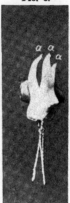

oughly washed out and dried, the canal is ready for filling.

The same necessity exists regarding room for opening the canals of upper mo-

FIG. 9.

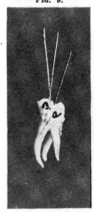

lars, though as a rule there is difficulty with only one, the anterior buccal. As the curve in this root, when it is present,

is always backward, the enlargement of
the orifice must be outward and forward.
(Fig. 9.)

FIG. 10.

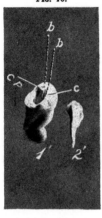

Except in the molars of the quite
youthful it is almost always necessary to
enlarge the canals, and they are best
treated by using different sized instruments, the largest at the orifice, and the

FIG. 11.

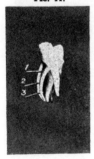

smallest toward the apical opening. It
is well to have the canals tapering, so
that after the canal filling is inserted it
may not be possible by making pressure
upon the superimposed filling to force

the point through the apical opening.
(Fig. 11, *1, 2, 3.*) Given a large orifice
and a canal graduated as regards enlargement, with three or four sizes of instruments, and we have an almost ideal condition for filling.

Having our canals now ready for filling, we decide whether we shall fill with
gutta-percha or zinc oxychlorid. My
choice for a canal which has been difficult
to open is gutta-percha, since I feel sure
I can reach the apical opening with it.
Select a canal point longer than the
tooth, and which cannot be pushed quite
to the apical opening, place it in the

FIG. 12.

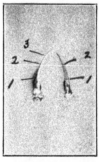

canal (Fig. 10), dip the foil-carriers in
oil of cajuput and carry the drop which
they will hold to the orifice of the canal.
It will instantly run in. Catch the projecting gutta-percha and move it up and
down. Friction on the sides of the canal,
aided by the solvent action of the oil of
cajuput, will make the gutta-percha fit
the canal accurately. Should the patient
warn us that sensation is experienced before the gutta-percha is felt to stick on
being withdrawn, remove it, and snip
a tiny piece off the end. When repeated
trials have satisfied us that it can just
be felt, that it sticks on withdrawal, and
that further pressure does not cause pain,

we may rest assured that we have as perfect a filling as can be inserted in that canal. (Figs, 10 2' and 11.) The only objection that can be offered against the use of oil of cajuput is in case the tooth is subsequently to be bleached.

Should the canal be sufficiently large to admit the passage of an ordinary canal probe directly to the end, the filling may be done with zinc oxychlorid almost as quickly and quite as satisfactorily as with gutta-percha. Measure the canal length with a tiny piece of rubber dam on the probe. Make a mix of zinc oxychlorid of a creamy consistence, and carry what clings to the probe when passed through it, to the canal. Push the probe to the end of the canal, and then carefully work it backward and forward, pushing a little of the oxychlorid before it. In nearly every instance pain will be experienced when the filling reaches the end of the canal. After a few movements of the probe it will be noticed that the little piece of dam does not touch the tooth when the probe is pushed in as far as it will go. Then we know that the upper end of the canal is plugged. Carry a little more of the mix to place on the probe, and repeat the procedure until the canal is full.

Until the success of some method of electric sterilization of root-canals, which is now being worked out by men such as Zieler of Wurzburg, Brauer of Vienna, and Hoffendahl and Miller of Berlin, is demonstrated to be absolutely accurate, and this to be followed by the insertion of some imperishable canal filling which will run like melted wax to the apical opening, hermetically sealing the canal, we shall have to continue doing the best we can from our manipulative standpoint.

As consolation for the operator who has hitherto not been very successful in opening root-canals, let me add that if he follows the plan I have been endeavoring to explain and gives earnest conscientious effort to every operation, his failures will decrease and he will be surprised to find how few are the canal fillings that he does not dismiss with an easy conscience.

Discussion.

Dr. J. I. HART, New York, N. Y. I was delighted at two features brought out by the essayist. One was where he laid stress upon the importance of cutting away sufficient tooth-structure to properly reach the root-canals. In attempting to save tooth-structure of the crown, reaching the canals can only be accomplished by instruments bent at sharp angles, which weakens the force which can safely be applied to those instruments. It increases the danger of breaking the instruments in the root-canals.

I was delighted where the essayist laid importance upon enlarging the canal towards the pulp-chamber by the use of an instrument, but he distinctly warned us against the use of those instruments in the engine to penetrate farther into the canal. An instrument may be revolved in the engine, but as we bear up toward the apex it is apt to crowd at some point, bend, and create a false opening in the side of the root. Too many roots have been lost in this manner. In my own practice, rather than carry the acid in enlarging a root-canal on the side or point of the instrument, I prefer using a minim dropper fitted with a platinum tube which will convey a droplet of acid into the root-canal opening, and can be more readily carried into the root-canal than from the slab on the instrument point to the root-canal.

Dr. GEO. E. HUNT, Indianapolis, Ind. The section is indebted to Dr. Magee for his excellent paper. There was one statement, however, that I cannot altogether indorse, and that was in regard to the stage at which he uses his Gates-Glidden drill. He says he uses the acid, then the drill, and then the sodium bicarbonate to froth out the débris. My experience with the Gates-Glidden drill is that in wet root-canals especially, they are more apt to be broken off than when the canals are dry. Wet dentin is a good deal like a wet plank; it is difficult to bore an auger through a wet plank, and it is difficult to get a drill through wet dentin. I prefer to use the sodium bicarbonate first and then dry out the root-canal before using the drill, so as to take less chances of breaking it.

Dr. A. C. SEARL, Owatonna, Minn. I would like to ask the essayist the question as to the time at which he inserts the filling. As I understood him he made it at the first sitting.

Dr. W. K. KASSAB, Chester, Pa. I enjoyed very much listening to the essay and approve of it in almost every detail. I follow Dr. Magee's method a great deal, still I am not afraid of perforating with my canal drill. I am not afraid to use the canal drill in most cases, for they are of such shape that they can be removed if they should break. There is something that has helped me a great deal, and that is the Kerr broach, which is screw-shaped. I have discarded entirely the use of sulfuric acid. I mention this special broach because I have found it very useful.

Dr. R. C. TURNER, Caldwell, Kans. The essayist and the rest of the gentlemen have not stated whether they put on the rubber dam or whether they open the root-canals without the rubber dam. My method is always to apply the rubber dam, remove all the débris with the broach; and then always with my Glidden drill I open up the canals and work out the débris the best I can. After the first sitting I fill the root-canals with gutta-percha.

Dr. G. R. WARNER, Grand Junction, Colo. I enjoyed this paper very much. I also indorse what Dr. Hart said about the Gates-Glidden drill for opening the canals. In some canals they are safe, but in others they are not. They may penetrate the side of the root or they may break off. They may break off near the shank or they may not, but if they break off near the head they are in there for all time. I want to mention a little expedient for the cleansing of the canals of the lower molars, particularly anterior canals. You may not always have a right-angled cleanser, but you almost always have a straight cleanser. Cut off the stiffened part of the straight cleanser, turn the end over and roll a little dental lac or modeling compound around the curl, which makes a nice handle. A broach so shaped can be introduced into an anterior canal very easily and withdraws the contents of the canal without trouble.

Dr. W. I. BRIGHAM, South Framingham, Mass. I am interested in the paper and very much interested in the matter of drilling out pulp-canals. When I first started out in the practice of dentistry I used the Gates-Glidden drill, but since then I have discarded it entirely, for in my experience a canal that cannot be reached without a Gates-Glidden drill can seldom be reached with one. It is not the best drill to use. The little broach that has been spoken of is valuable in preparing the smaller canals, and the larger canals do not need enlargement. They can be thoroughly cleaned and sterilized without enlargement. In the matter of handling short broaches I wish to say that it is of the utmost importance. Instead of putting on a handle made of shellac or modeling compound I always use a Donaldson drill or broach, cut a groove across it with a broach, take a piece of metal and cut out a piece about ½ x 1/16 inch and wrap it around to make a handle. It is an instrument so delicate that you can tell in a moment whether there is any débris there or not, and the canal that is so small that the smallest broach will not enter seldom gives any trouble. The advantage of a metal handle over one made of shellac or modeling compound lies in that it can be sterilized; the handle does not have to be removed.

Dr. B. Q. STEVENS, Hannibal, Mo. I have used drills for opening pulp-canals, but have abandoned them long ago; I use barbed or smooth broaches, and prefer the Donaldson broach. The drill is liable to leave the canal and perforate the side of the root. If the canal is so obstructed that it cannot be followed as far as the broach ought to penetrate, put in a little oil of cassia and seal the canal up for a few days, when it will be possible to penetrate it as far as necessary. If there is a sensitive branch and all remedies fail to anesthetize it, cover it with a small piece of cotton saturated in wood creasote, and seal it tight for a week or two. I fill every root as soon as the pulp is removed, unless I know it is septic—sometimes one root in a three- or four-rooted molar, sometimes all but one. I do not think chloro-percha is the proper material to fill root-canals with, as it will shrink and become porous.

After the canal is ready to fill I select a smooth broach that will reach to the end of the root, I slip on to this broach a small disk that I punch out of my rubber dam and pass the broach into the canal to obtain the exact length of the root I wish to fill. I then mark this length with chloro-percha on a correspondingly small peg made of orange-wood or silver wire, to the extremity of which I apply a small amount of the chloro-percha.

I then have prepared some small wafers of sheet gutta-percha about ¼ inch square; this I wrap tightly around my wooden peg, by holding them over a small lamp and warming the gutta-percha! At this point the canal may be lubricated with chloro-percha. The prepared wood point is then warmed and pushed up into the canal as far as the mark. If the patient flinches, draw the peg out a little and then force it to the end of the root.

To prepare these gutta-percha wafers, pour rather thin chloro-percha on a clean piece of glass previously moistened with glycerin. In about an hour it can be taken off and cut into little squares of suitable size.

In filling root-canals in this way it is not necessary to have the canal dry, but it must be in an antiseptic condition. The majority of root-canals I fill are not dry, and I would not continue the practice if it were a failure.

Dr. C. M. BORDNER, Shenandoah, Pa. There seems to be a great deal of opposition to the use of the Gates-Glidden drill. The gentleman who has just preceded me states that he does not want to use the drill, but wants to use broaches. How many break the broaches? It is very seldom I use a broach, except in the anterior teeth. I use the Gates-Glidden drill entirely for molars. I have them made to order. Those we get ordinarily are too long. I have them made slightly shorter. It is very seldom I break a Gates-Glidden drill. As they are made at the present time it is not often that they cannot be taken out after breaking in the canal. I have been using the Gates-Glidden drill in the posterior part of the mouth for the past sixteen years with a great deal of success. I start with the smallest Gates-Glidden drill and end with the third largest; but as I have before stated I have them made slightly shorter than the ones kept in stock ordinarily.

Dr. J. FREMONT BURKET, Kingman, Kans. I was pleased with Dr. Magee's paper, and I think his method of opening the canal is ideal. We should never attempt to fill a root-canal unless we can obtain direct access to it. The idea of firing around a corner to fill a root-canal is absurd. In regard to drills, I had my lesson in my life practice, and my advice is never to use a Glidden drill in connection with the engine. I usually open up the canal, sterilize the parts, and then with a Donaldson broach, the smallest to be had, clean out the canal. If the canal is small, with time and care it can be gradually drilled out. To open up a root-canal with a bur is something I seldom do. As to the filling, after the canal is opened I use hydrogen dioxid. In the case of abscesses with fistula inject hydrogen dioxid until it comes out through the fistula, it is then ready for filling. I place a little iodoform in the canal, then I put a gutta-percha point in the canal, one that is small enough and will reach the apex. As soon as it is introduced into the canal I drop in with a drop-tube a drop of chloroform which will instantly go to the end of the cone in the root. It will follow that cone to the end and will soon dissolve it. Then I apply another drop and another gutta-percha cone to force the liquid to the sides of the canal if not round. It will obliterate all space, which is exactly what we have to accomplish in filling a root-canal. Keep this up until the canal is completely filled. The chloroform soon evaporates and the root-canal will be filled to the apex. If a little goes beyond the apex it never gives me any concern.

Dr. OTTO HOLLINGER, Chicago, Ill. I disagree with the essayist on the use of drills inside of root-canals. I use them occasionally at the mouth of the canal after having softened the dentin in that locality with sulfuric acid. My procedure is as follows:

(1) Open the pulp-chamber with a bur (round) and clean out the pulp-chamber with broaches and round bur.

(2) Enlarge mouth of canal with sulfuric acid by means of a gold or platinum broach.

(3) Neutralize sulfuric acid with an alkali (sodium carbonate).

(4) Wash pulp-chamber with hydrogen dioxid.

(5) Clean out débris from mouth of canal with drill, usually using a small round bur.

(6) After cleaning out débris apply one of the digesters such as pepsin or carica papaya, using a solvent of 2/10 of 1 per cent. acid solution (because they only act in solution acidulated to the degree found in the stomach) and force as much into the canals as possible. Leave in for forty-eight hours, and if necessary apply again, and repeat until pulp is digested, requiring two to three treatments.

Before re-applying the digester wash out the old with hydrogen dioxid and dry the cavity well. After the last treatment an essential oil dressing is placed in the cavity and left there for two days. Then fill the roots in usual way

Dr. EMIL SCHREIER, Vienna, Austria. I often wonder that the question whether in treating root-canals drills ought to be used or not, is always discussed and never decided. There are many men who tell us that they always use drills for this purpose and never break one, and still there are many others who seldom use drills and always break them. No doubt very good results can be obtained by drilling root-canals, still it must be admitted that a great many teeth have been lost under this treatment in the hands of the most careful operators. Those who recommend the use of drills claim that their results are the best. They ought to know that the same results can be obtained by other methods without any risk. Some of the best men in the profession did wonderfully good work in dentistry without the use of the rubber dam, yet not one of them could tell us in the present time to follow their line of practice and drop the use of the rubber dam in order to come up to their standard. It seems to me that using the drill in the treatment of root-canals, now that better methods exist, is not good advice. The time for this instrument is gone, and it should be discarded.

Dr. J. L. SWEETMAN, Manistee, Mich. Since people are taking sides I have a very decided opinion to express in this matter. Every man who does his work thoroughly uses the Gates-Glidden drill. It is a bad instrument in unskilled hands. There are places where it is indispensable. It is a most particular kind of work to open up the canals of the roots of teeth. When a man starts in he must remember that he is entering upon a del-

icate piece of work, and in the ability to work in those roots there is nothing to take the place of the Gates-Glidden drill. Other instruments are only auxiliaries.

Dr. PITT S. TURNER, Belton, Tex. There is no question that confronts the dentist more frequently in every-day work than the one which is now under discussion. Various methods have been presented here and success is claimed for all of them. I have not wholly discarded the Gates-Glidden drill, but in the majority of cases I use a bud-shaped drill for opening up the orifices to the dental canal. I know there is no danger of breaking it off, and if the root cannot be entered with the broach I do not try to open it up to the end. I go on the theory that if it is left in as nearly its normal or natural condition as possible the better it will be. There are many canals that we cannot easily cleanse, treat, and fill by such methods as we use, and it is only in special cases where I use the Gates-Glidden drill. I do not advocate the cutting away of the inside of the canal, believing that the natural construction is better than after it has been cut away. I have followed this course for nearly twenty years. Now and then I fail, just as we all have failures, but where there is no abnormal condition of the roots it is unnecessary, in my opinion, to enlarge the canals. But there are conditions where it is necessary to try to enlarge them, then I adopt such methods as the case calls for.

Dr. L. P. HALL, Ann Arbor, Mich. I just want to say a word about the use of the Gates-Glidden drill. In the first place those canals do not always need to be opened so much if we have access to them. I would not suggest sacrificing the tooth-substance unnecessarily, but cut away just enough to obtain access to

the canals, especially in the anterior canals of the lower molars and the anterior
buccal canal of the upper molars.   In
regard to the use of the Gates-Glidden
drill, if the largest drill be used first
and be followed successively with the
smaller as far as it seems necessary to
go, there is less danger of breaking them.
In the first place the portion of the root-
canal nearest the pulp-chamber is the
largest part, therefore a larger portion
can be cut out than where they are finer.
For myself I have been using the Kerr
broach much more than the Gates-Glidden drill, and find that by using the large
first and following with the smaller secure
very good results.

Dr. A. M. LEWIS, Austin, Minn. A
number of my friends here have told us
how easy it is to properly open the root-
canal, cleanse, and fill it.   I wish now
somebody would tell me how hard it is
to properly open up, cleanse, and fill a
root-canal. Perhaps I am making a very
bold statement, but I do not believe that
fifty per cent. of root-canals are perfectly sealed.   I have made tests in my
own office and I have seen tests made by
others, and I think I am quite safe in
saying that fifty per cent. of root-canals
are not properly filled.   I think it would
surprise members of the congress if they
were to make such tests in their own
laboratories, taking extracted teeth, filling the root-canals and then breaking
them to find out for themselves whether
they are perfectly filled or not.   I think
they would find that less than fifty per
cent. were hermetically sealed.

Dr. L. D. MITCHELL, Arkansas City,
Kans. This is certainly a very important subject, and has been discussed in
almost every manner within reason. One
man uses nothing but the Gates-Glidden
drill, while another uses only the broach,

but our more conservative practitioners
use both.   It is my opinion that there is
a place for both, with the places for drills
much in the minority.   The drill, I
think, can generally be used to advantage only directly from the pulp-chamber
for a short distance.   One gentleman
made the statement to the effect that it
is very necessary that this part of the
work be done thoroughly. If that is so,
the Gates-Glidden drill is a very dangerous instrument to use when it is desired
to reach the apex.   If a man starts for
the apex with a Gates-Glidden drill, and
strikes a turn in the root, he is not liable
to know when he strikes it. But if he
takes a very small broach there is no danger of perforation, and the broach will
frequently conform itself to considerable
of a turn.   If the canal is so small that
the broach stops, in all probability the
root will give no trouble if left alone.
One gentleman spoke of performing experimental operations in the laboratory.
Such operations cannot be compared to
those performed in the mouth.   In my
judgment we should depend almost entirely upon the response of the patient to
determine whether the root is filled perfectly or not.   Always endeavor to open
the root to such an extent that the patient may feel the broach, then to fill
until complete, hesitate a moment, and
try again.   In case compressed air causes
the response, the second push after a
moment's hesitation will force it out and
fill the root perfectly, or more nearly so.
If pushed too far it is likely to cause
trouble; however, this must be controlled
by the individual judgment.

Dr. J. L. HOWELL, Creede, Colo. The
two things I would like to know are
these: When the smallest Downey
broach will not penetrate up to the apex
in small canals, will they abscess? My

experience has been from observation that in those small, tortuous canals my *confrères* have been more fortunate in filling to the apex, as they claim, than I have been. I have not been so fortunate as to pat myself on the back and make myself believe that I have been so thorough. Time and time again I have spent day in and day out, working three sittings, trying to open up those tortuous canals, and when they were finished I was not satisfied with my work. I have often so informed the patients, and told them if they ever had trouble with that canal they must not blame me, because I did the very best I could. My experience from observation of teeth the seat of abscesses, which I have extracted, is that the canals had no abscess at the end of the apex where the smallest Downey broach could not penetrate, but the abscess was invariably located upon the root of the tooth which was large enough to admit the broach clear through to the apex of that root. I did at one time use the Gates-Glidden drill, but I discarded it because I got more satisfaction with the Downey, the Kerr, and the Donaldson broaches. I have not used them exclusively. I would like to know from the author of this good paper whether it has been his experience that the tortuous roots become the seat of abscesses.

The second question is in regard to the use of sulfuric acid. I never use it for the reason that I do not know where its action is going to cease. Is it not better to take a fine Donaldson broach and then a size larger until all the débris is removed? These are two points I would like to know about. I would like to have the author answer these points.

Dr. F. L. Fossume, New York, N. Y. I do not believe the Gates-Glidden drill is as good an instrument in tortuous and small clogged root-canals as is the Beutelrock excavator. These excavators or drills are so finely tempered that they can be tied into a knot and are exceedingly tough. They are indispensable in lower central incisors, the anterior root of lower first molars and in upper first bicuspids. There are times when these canals ought to be opened, as when the infection has penetrated through the apex, and where the tooth is so tender that vent must be given either through the alveolus or the root-canal. In such cases the excavator will clean the root and open it better than anything I have yet tried.

After having mechanically cleaned the root-canal I use the sodium and potassium paste to chemically cleanse and sterilize, neutralizing with mercury bichlorid and hydrogen dioxid; by this cleansing process the dentin becomes almost white and all odor disappears except a peculiar smell just like Castile soap, due to the saponification and disorganization of the organic matter in the root-canal. I believe this a most efficacious method for cleaning putrescent root-canals.

Dr. C. F. Shoop, Central City, Colo. We know that by pressure we can force an anesthetic through the tubuli of the dentin and into the pulp itself. Now, to fill small root-canals, pump in chloropercha with a broach; then use pressure, as in pressure anesthesia, to force the chloro-percha to the apex. If you wish, put in a gutta-percha point. This method can be tested in the laboratory, using extracted teeth bedded in plaster.

Dr. Jas. M. Magee (closing the discussion). In regard to Dr. Hart's remarks about using a platinum point or tube for carrying the acid, the idea is a good one, yet that is a matter of detail, for it really make no difference so long as the material goes where it is required.

Replying to Dr. Hunt's question, I do not advocate the Gates-Glidden drill after using sulfuric acid. I use a very fine Beutelrock drill.

Dr. Searl asked, when do I insert the filling? I did not make mention of that point, as every operator must decide that question for himself. Sometimes a root is ready for filling at the first sitting, and sometimes not until a later sitting.

Dr. Kassab mentioned the use of the Kerr drill in opening fine canals. The canals I refer to are those which even the finest instrument will either enter with difficulty or not at all. The Beutelrock drills I mentioned will oftentimes open a canal which a Kerr instrument cannot even be felt to catch in. They should never be used in the engine, but held in the fingers and worked forward with a movement similar to that given to a brad-awl.

I thought that all good operators used the rubber dam for this work, and that will be an answer to Dr. Turner.

Dr. Brigham and Dr. Warner advocate improvised handles for the fine canal cleaners, and they are worthy of consideration, but I have found them unnecessary in my practice, since the Beutelrock drills will accomplish all that they can.

The question was asked, how do I open those difficult canals in roots abruptly bent? I wish I might read the paper again as an answer to this question. I used the word "almost"—"almost any canal, and almost any curve"—and it was a desire to eliminate the "almost" as far as possible that prompted me to write the paper.

Dr. Stevens says: "You push your canal point until you think you have it right up to the end." It should be the aim of every operator to be positive about that. Having reached the end of your canal—there is not the least difficulty in measuring its length—then, as I stated in the paper, you take a canal point a little longer than the tooth, mark on it the length of the canal (just a little pinch with the finger nails) and you can be absolutely certain when it reaches the end of the canal.

The use of hydrogen dioxid comes under the head of treatment, which I feel does not come within the scope of the paper, but I will just say in reply to the question that after even a liberal use the canal is not necessarily rendered ready for filling.

Chloroform and chloro-percha have been mentioned by several as being used in canals. I do not think I can emphasize the point too strongly that chloroform should never be used in pulp-canals as an aid to filling with gutta-percha. I formerly used it, but have abandoned it for very good cause. I have never yet opened or drilled into a canal filled with chloro-percha of gutta-percha alone which did not have an abominable odor. If you experiment, you will find that that is always the case. I now use oil of cajuput, and I use it for no other purpose. Since it is used at no other time than when the canal is filled, if I get that odor when working on a tooth which I myself have cared for, I know what has been done for the tooth without referring to my record. The gutta-percha point, when worked into the canal, fills it in much the same way that a glass stopper fills the neck of a bottle. The glass stopper is ground to fit the neck by revolving in it, while the gutta-percha point is fitted to the canal by being moved in and out, friction on the constricted parts of the canal, aided by the solvent action of the oil of cajuput making an accurate fit.

The last chart (Fig. 12, page 32) illustrates the distances the different instruments extend into the canal. The 1 marks the distance to which the Gates-Glidden drill reached; 2 shows where the next sized instrument, a Beutelrock drill, stopped, and so on.

Dr. Lewis makes inquiry concerning the amount of time required and the difficulty experienced in opening root-canals. I have recently spent nearly three hours opening the canals of one tooth—a lower second molar—and the time was judiciously expended, for I felt that that tooth must be saved. When one undertakes to open the canals of a tooth his efforts should not cease until they are open, if it takes two hours or ten hours. Time should never be considered. If the tooth is to be saved it is not a question of time but one of saving.

One gentleman spoke about the drill striking the bend and making a little shoulder against which the next instrument would strike. These little instruments illustrated in the middle of that plate (indicating) should be used in a case of that kind, applying sulfuric acid before attempting to use a drill. You see these two, the long one and the short one with the stems; they are Beutelrock drills ground down to a fine point. The third one, that to the left, is a Donaldson cleanser with the barbs ground off. It can be used to good advantage, but the others have proved a little more satisfactory, as they can be more easily picked up, more easily handled.

The CHAIRMAN. We were to have a paper on the subject of "Pressure Anesthesia," but in the absence of the paper, and as Dr. R. B. TULLER, Chicago, Ill., has prepared a discussion on that subject, I will call on him to speak upon it.

Dr. Tuller then gave the following address:

A Talk on "Pressure Cataphoresis."

By R. B. TULLER, D.D.S., Chicago, Ill.

THE subject I was to discuss today is "perdentinal anesthesia," but as the paper bearing that title is not to be presented, I have been asked by Dr. Johnson to deal with the subject notwithstanding. As I interpret it, it is what has been called "pressure anesthesia," but it seems to me it would be more correctly termed "pressure cataphoresis." So far as concerns this discussion, at least, I will consider the three terms equivalent.

I presume there are few here who do not know that the terms refer to a mechanically induced penetration of a liquid anesthetic agent into the dentin and into the dentinal pulp. Its application has been directed more to exposed pulps, to enable their painless extirpation, than to dentin to obtund sensitivity.

The question of how it was discovered and came into use is somewhat obscure. Until recently my understanding was that it was first introduced some ten or twelve years ago by a Dr. Funk of Chicago, who went about selling the secret and privilege to use it. It could not long be a secret under such circumstances.

It came to my notice just about the time of the flood-tide of electric cataphoresis, or a little after. But not long ago I received a letter from Dr. Henry W. Gillett of New York, in which he says "The introduction of pressure anesthesia was much earlier than you place it. I used it in the late eighties, with syringe points exactly as shown by Dr. J. A. Johnson in the March *Items of Interest*. My use of it was due to a paper read before the Harvard Odontological Society by Dr. E. C. Briggs, and published in a now defunct journal that I do not remember the name of."

Now, however or whenever this pressure process was introduced, I want to emphatically indorse its virtues as nothing less than a blessing to humanity—including the dentist, who needs some consideration in the trials that afflict his patients. The full extent of its value seems not to have been known until more recently. I do not know that anyone has exploited it more than myself, though there may have been many; but what I have succeeded in doing I have published. I am quite free to admit, however, that I have not arrived at that stage where I can be positive and sure of producing perfect anesthesia in every case; on the other hand, I have encountered a number of cases so obstinate, or in which my manipulation or method of application was so faulty, that I had to give up. But I want to say this, that if one can succeed once in five times, that one time will win him over as an advocate and induce an affirmation of what I say as to its being a blessing to humanity—a veritable godsend in

many cases. And I believe we may yet understand it and have the application so under control that we can operate with positiveness and certainty in a large majority of cases, if not all.

I do not attempt pressure cataphoresis in every case, because it takes a little time and is of such a nature that I feel that I ought to be fairly compensated for such truly skilful service—when successful, at least; so I do not suggest it on all occasions. Often, however, it is to our own interest to employ it as far as time and facility of operating is considered and the strain on our own nerves is concerned. We all know that in a large part of our work we need nothing but to operate deftly with sharp burs and instruments, and I do not imagine you would apply pressure cataphoresis except in such cases as are excessively sensitive, or to extirpate pulps, though possibly in time, if we can be more certain of success, it may be demanded of us in a general way.

My early experience with pressure cataphoresis was in its application to exposed pulps, and my efforts were too frequently failures. But now and then one would succumb to the application so quickly and completely that I could not help feeling elated with the scheme. I determined to find out the reason for failures, if I could. I felt sure that in some instances it was due to not being able to confine the solution under pressure as it should be to be forced into the pulp.

I found really few cavities that had complete surrounding walls and were otherwise favorably shaped to confine a liquid under pressure. I sought out a means to confine my medicament to the exact exposure without regard to cavity shape other than being open and available to the method. I succeeded in this and found I could be positive and sure in a very much greater number of cases; so many, in fact, that I began to feel that I had a sure and certain way for every case. I have since found, however, some cases that do not respond readily and some not at all.

Now, from time to time I found instances where a considerable thickness of dentin still covered the pulp, and I applied my method, confining the solution positively in one spot directly over the pulp, and got as good results almost as quickly as when the exposure was complete. Of course, all understand that in cases of exposure or nearly so we begin pressure at *nil* and gradually increase it until we have used a considerable force. In my method this pressure is equal to several hundred pounds to the square inch.

My success in forcing the solution through a thin layer of dentin in the bottom of a cavity led me to the thought that the entire thickness of dentin from enamel to pulp might be penetrated by medicaments, and I began immediately to exploit that idea by making a special opening for my application of the pressure method and ignoring for the time the cavity of decay. I succeeded beyond all expectation. In a minute or two I found in most instances the entire crown of the tooth was so anesthetized that I could cut, bur, and grind at will without any pain. In cases where I wanted to extirpate the pulp I found I could do it directly from this special opening through the enamel, or utilize the cavity —and without pain in either case.

If, after getting into the pulp-chamber, sensitivity was found rootwise, it was only necessary to re-apply the cocain and pressure in the pulp-chamber. In some instances I have found canals

so obstructed or tortuous that I was slow in getting the pulp out, and sensitivity would return to some extent in other roots. In such cases it was only necessary to close the root I had cleared, charge the chamber with the solution and repeat the pressure for a few moments. I have in some cases left one root until another sitting and then cocainized it again by pressure. When we once reach the chamber we then have no trouble about confining the liquid by means of a piece of vulcanite rubber. I obtain the required degree of pressure and confine the solution in any way that seems best in each case, but one would find it a difficult thing to confine a liquid on a flat surface with a piece of vulcanite rubber. I can, however, do that with the means at my command and can anesthetize a tooth by grinding off a cusp until dentin is exposed and then proceed with my pressure cataphoric method.

When I desire to extirpate a pulp without bothersome post-operative hemorrhage, I use adrenalin. This, you know, is a preparation that injected with cocain into the soft tissues permits of what is termed a bloodless surgical operation. As adrenalin is a sterile solution I use it generally to dissolve the cocain whether the application is for sensitive dentin or pulp-extirpation. For the latter it is proper to apply the solution directly to the exposed pulp, or force in the adrenalin alone, since enough of it may not pass through the dentin to exercise its contractile effect upon the pulp, though the anesthesia may be complete.

The special opening or aperture is made usually near the cavity of decay in healthy tooth-substance, though I sometimes select a small defective spot that sooner or later must be filled any way.

When the opening is made in healthy tissue there is no danger of forcing septic matter into the pulp, as might possibly be the case in utilizing a cavity of decay. However, so far as my experience goes, I have had no serious trouble in utilizing the cavity of decay when that is convenient, first removing débris and soft decay and treating it antiseptically. There have, however, been some reports of tenderness or other evidence of disturbance for the first day or two after a tooth has been cocainized through the cavity of decay, and it has been attributed to the cocain. I am inclined to think it due to septic infection carried in with the cocain, and the special opening might obviate this; besides, I think healthy tubuli will conduct the anesthetic agent better than those clogged possibly with disintegrated dentin.

Producing, as I have done many times, both slight and profound anesthesia in the entire coronal part of a tooth through these special apertures, I have no hesitation in saying that it can be done in many cases; and to illustrate how these openings may be made where they will do the least damage if any at all, I published in the *American Dental Journal* last March an article with illustrations of all the teeth on one side of the maxilla, designating the places. In molars and bicuspids I would make the opening, when possible, where in extending the cavity it would be taken in, requiring no extra filling to repair it. If this is not practicable in a particular case, I endeavor to find in the occlusal surface some weak spot that might require filling at some future time if not then; this, of course, would have to be specially filled aside from the larger cavity. In the six anterior teeth, which would rarely be available through approximal

cavities, I operate through the lingual fossa, the special aperture requiring a separate filling. To force the cocain into any of these openings I sometimes use the old way of placing a pledget of cotton saturated with the solution in the opening and cover it up with soft rubber or gutta-percha to prevent regurgitation under pressure. I sometimes confine the solution *over* the opening so perfectly as to force it in under pressure. When using the soft rubber over the cotton I often use the automatic mallet instead of steady pressure.

The cases that will not respond to this pressure method I have pretty well determined are cases where secondary dentin has been deposited. There may be other abnormal conditions obstructing the canals, but I have found in a number that were of slow responsiveness that the pulp-chamber bore evidences of secondary deposit. Of course, there are many cases where it is not desirable to expose the pulp-chamber and we can only surmise the cause of failure to anesthetize the pulp.

Now, when I say "without pain," I mean without pain in most cases. The stubborn ones may yield after a time or may not yield at all, and of course, when not obtunded, or only partially so, may give rise to some pain and may require a second application. But when the anesthesia is complete there is absolutely no pain.

To cite a few instances, I have cut off a number of sound teeth one after the other, as high as eight in one mouth, that were to be utilized for bridge supports, and from the start to the finish have caused no pain beyond a mere suggestion of it as my bur passed through the enamel and entered into the dentin. I have removed a little enamel with a cutting wheel, exposing a little dentin, and confining my solution to that spot have produced anesthesia by pressure that permitted cutting and grinding of the tissues without pain.

In regard to the question of obtunding dentin, I labored for some time under the impression that the remedy must be applied directly to the cavity we desire to operate on, and that our medicament must saturate all the walls. In using my method comparatively few of the tubules are covered; but through these the cocain is carried to the pulp, and when a zone of that organ has become anesthetized all the fibrils or prolongations of the odontoblasts that penetrate the dentin from that zone are anesthetized. I have no faith in obtunding done in any other way than by making the agent act upon the pulp.

I believe this is to be one of the live and most interesting topics before the profession today, and worthy of our serious attention and investigation if we are to relieve the suffering of our patients in many, many instances. It is worthy, even though we fail four times and succeed once; one happy success will repay all our efforts and set us to thinking why we failed, and where many are searching for it someone may better find than I have the cause of such failures. I am looking for the dawning of an era of really painless dentistry, performed rationally and safely and without discouraging and unhappy sequences.

Discussion.

Dr. F. L. FOSSUME, New York, N. Y. I would like to have the essayist tell us in closing whether there is any pain under the tremendous pressure in injecting a solution of cocain after the small cavity is drilled in the central incisor?

Dr. TULLER. None in the least.

Dr. FOSSUME. Have there been any bad after-effects?

Dr. TULLER. Not to my knowledge. Pressure anesthesia, so called, has been used very extensively for more than ten years by way of the cavity of decay, but I have never heard of any unfortunate sequences.

Dr. FOSSUME. Are there any special instruments used?

Dr. TULLER. There are several on the market, I believe. The main point is the proper confinement of the liquid, used so that it cannot escape but can be absolutely forced into the tubules of the dentin, or into the exposed pulp. It has been thoroughly demonstrated that a liquid agent may pass under pressure through the entire thickness of the dentin and thoroughly anesthetize the pulp, but it should be borne in mind that the quantity is but the small fraction of a drop—not a flooding of the pulp-chamber.

Dr. J. I. HART, New York, N. Y. It is the proper confinement of the fluid in the cavity that makes the operation possible, and unless it is confined in the cavity the operation is *nil*. The essayist has not informed us how it is done, but it is done by the use of the instrument he has devised. There is another instrument in use, one devised by Dr. Meyer, and that instrument will also permit us to confine the medicament in the cavity, and it is only when that medicament is confined that we meet with any success. When cocain or adrenalin is pressed in with cotton and surrounded with soft rubber the liquid is almost bound to get out, but with the instrument it is forced into the tubules, and I can positively say that the result is admirable.

Dr. L. N. RUDY, Tooele, Utah. Instead of using a liquid solution of cocain I make a paste of cocain and glycerin, and place it in the cavity, after getting as nearly an exposure as possible. I use a piece of unvulcanized rubber that will more than fill the cavity, and finger pressure, gentle at first and increased as pain decreases.

The way to avoid failures is to make a very careful diagnosis of the conditions existing in the pulp when the case comes to you. I found in cases that came to me that the application of this agent was of no more avail than if I had used water, and in other cases in two or three minutes I could open the pulp cavity with a bur, run a broach to the end of the root and take the pulp out immediately.

Two months ago a young man came to my office with the pulp of a lower left first molar completely exposed. I applied this same treatment I have spoken of, and timing myself carefully, I found I had taken out the entire pulp in just four minutes from the time I made the application.

I find one source of failure is due to an inflammatory condition of the pulp. When the cocain is not readily absorbed, if you will investigate a little farther you will find a little pus pocket upon the surface of the pulp. When the pulp is in this condition the cocain will not be taken up because the circulation of the pulp is destroyed. In a condition of this kind the application may be left *in situ* for ten or fifteen minutes without getting any results; but in cases where the pulp has not been the seat of such disturbing phenomena, and its removal is necessary, it seldom takes more than three minutes for the cocain to act.

I have been more than pleased with pressure anesthesia for the extirpation of pulps, but it is likewise gratifying to have a method of painlessly preparing sensitive cavities.

Dr. H. G. ATWATER, Los Angeles, Cal. I desire information on one point made by Dr. Tuller which I did not understand; that is, why one point in dentin is sensitive and another is not.

Dr. A. M. LEWIS, Austin, Minn. A great many operators labor under the idea that a large opening will give better results, but I find the smaller opening gives the best success.

Dr. C. F. SHOOP, Central City, Colo. I would like to ask the doctor about his experience with carbolic acid in pressure anesthesia. I would like to know whether he would use it in sensitive dentin or to remove the pulp, and whether pericementitis follows such a procedure.

Dr. C. L. WHITE, Oklahoma City, Okla. I have never attained much success with pressure anesthesia in obtunding dentin for excavating where any considerable amount of tissue had to be penetrated to reach the pulp, but there is conclusive evidence that it is being accomplished in a most satisfactory way in skilful and patient hands.

I think the development of pressure anesthesia in the surgical removal of pulp is one of the greatest forward steps that has been made in operative dentistry in many years. It is my practice to follow the removal of pulp by filling the canals at the same sitting unless it is contra-indicated in the case at hand. There are many reasons urged against immediate canal-filling, but I consider it one of the chief advantages gained by pressure anesthesia. At first I used carbolic acid as an agent for producing anesthesia of the dentin and of the pulp, but about four years ago I commenced using a solution of cocain, and my success has been phenomenal. It seems that a very small percentage of dentists are using pressure anesthesia, but if given a thorough trial I think none would again be without it. In a great majority of cases where pulp is exposed, or nearly so, absolute anesthesia may be obtained even by crude methods, and used carefully and skilfully as Dr. Tuller describes, its field of usefulness is very broad.

In a certain class of cases my success has been only partial, but even in those cases where anesthesia is only partial or where it has apparently failed completely, I believe the pulp may be removed with as little pain as would follow the use of any other method and certainly with less danger of permanent injury to tooth and pericementum.

Dr. A. OWEN, Cisco, Tex. I would like to ask Dr. Tuller the percentage of cocain he uses and what is his favorite vehicle for carrying the cocain.

Dr. W. I. BRIGHAM, South Framingham, Mass. If we had always known of pressure anesthesia in removing the pulp and someone had discovered that arsenic properly applied would destroy the pulp without pain, I think we should hail it as a great discovery in dentistry. There are times when pressure anesthesia is valuable, but there are other times when something else is more valuable. There are times when pressure anesthesia can be applied for four or five minutes, but arsenic can also be applied to a sensitive or aching pulp immediately, the patient can be dismissed in two minutes, and in a week's time the pulp can be removed absolutely without pain. Each has its place. I would no more think of giving up arsenic for pressure anesthesia than I would think of giving up anything in the practice of dentistry.

Dr. W. KASSAB, Chester, Pa. I am glad someone broke the ground and spoke about arsenic. I do not have any trouble from the use of cocain in pressure anesthesia, but I only use it when I think I have time to complete the operation. I would like to ask the essayist whether he has any trouble with bleeding, and what his method is of stopping it.

Dr. J. A. TODD, St. Louis, Mo. I think it has been stated that in some cases troubles of infectious nature follow the use of cocain by the pressure method, and I would like to ask Dr. Tuller what his experience has been in that direction.

Dr. OTTO HOLLINGER, Chicago, Ill. I think we all know that the pulp is a part of the body the same as any other tissue, consisting of nerves, bloodvessels, and connective tissue, and therefore is subject to the same influences that other tissues are. A new element has been added to cocain, which is adrenalin. Adrenalin is a vaso-constrictor and is also slightly antiseptic and anesthetic, and therefore it has been adopted for use in combination with cocain. In inflammation of the pulp the bloodvessels are very much engorged, and adrenalin will produce anemia. Cocain will accomplish that as a rule, but not to the same extent as adrenalin, but where the pulp has been inflamed for any length of time and granulation or partial calcification or any other pathological process has taken place in it, the degree of degeneration which has taken place will of course determine the partial or entire failure of cocain. For instance, if the pulp is partly degenerated it will still be acted upon, but not so quickly or thoroughly. If totally degenerated, of course, it will not be affected by cocain at all. Surgeons in injecting cocain in secondary operations, as they frequently do when the patient is very much depressed, find cocain will not act because of the poor vascularity of scar tissue. In pulp nodules, or where the pulp has died completely and there is necrotic tissue present, cocain will not work, or if it does it will do so very poorly, but the addition of adrenalin will hasten the penetrating power of the cocain and the degenerated fibers will be affected more readily.

Dr. H. E. FRIESELL, Pittsburg, Pa. For about seven years I have been making use of cocain in pressure anesthesia, and have not found it necessary to have a special instrument, or to confine the liquid to the cavity absolutely. Old vulcanizable rubber, the largest instrument that can be inserted into the cavity, and a gradually increased pressure will give gratifying success in probably ninety-eight per cent. of the cases.

I have had cases of local sepsis in the pulp, but have never had a failure that could be attributed to such condition.

The greatest difficulty will be found with pulp-stones. Where a case does not respond quickly to pressure treatment, I now suspect pulp-stones and usually find them. Even in these cases considerable anesthesia will be produced, and one can drill as far as tolerated, make repeated applications of the cocain, and success will be attained.

Acute inflammation of the pulp has been given as a frequent cause of failure in this method; yet this is precisely the condition in which pressure anesthesia has been of the most benefit to me. Where the pulp is so highly inflamed that the application of arsenic is out of the question, the pressure method works like a charm is supposed to work.

Most of my failures I attribute to adulterated or deteriorated cocain.

I would like to have Dr. Tuller state whether he has ever observed any toxic effects from the use of cocain or formalin by this method.

Dr. L. D. MITCHELL, Arkansas City, Kans. I have used it for about four years, and the greater part of that time with perfect results. I do not mean by this that every case coming into my office is relieved in from three to five minutes and sent out smiling, but I do know that I can handle a case better with pressure anesthesia than with arsenic. If a tooth is aching and the pulp inflamed the application of arsenic will cause it to ache worse, with perhaps no results. In such cases it is better to apply a little oil of cloves to relieve the inflammation before attempting to anesthetize the pulp.

Dr. W. J. TAYLOR, Sacramento, Cal. We all know that as a general rule arsenic is contra-indicated for general use in the deciduous teeth. But cocain pressure anesthesia can be used there to splendid advantage, and carrying out the suggestion of Dr. Ottolengui, presented some time ago in the *Items of Interest*, I have used it in a number of cases to devitalize the pulp of deciduous teeth, and I must say, with the most satisfactory results. I think it is a splendid agent when it becomes necessary to extirpate the pulp at one sitting.

Dr. F. M. COCKRELL, Leavenworth, Kans. Pressure anesthesia, like all good things, is often overdone. I seldom use it to obtund sensitive dentin, but do use a perfectly sharp bur, touching the cavity lightly, so as to shave the tooth-structure. It seems no one here has had trouble with pressure anesthesia—only perfect success; but here is what I did once with pressure anesthesia: I removed the nerve in an incisor and at once filled the canal. Later I found I had passed the point through the apical foramen for quite a distance. I had anesthetized the tissues beyond the foramen and obtained no response from the patient when the point passed through the opening. Lately I have used formaldehyd and adrenalin, and once or twice the patient has had a very sore tooth, but I believe it was not permanent; I would like to know if anyone else has had trouble of that kind.

Dr. N. A. NEELEY, Christchurch, New Zealand. Success with pressure anesthesia is due to pressure, as I understand it, and success usually follows in proportion to the amount of pressure used. I have been using pressure anesthesia for some seven or eight years and within the last few months I had made a hypodermic syringe and a pair of forceps, the forceps to be used in connection with the syringe to obtain the greatest pressure. A special point was made for the syringe, on which was a little shoulder about 1/32 of an inch from the handle. On this was placed a little disk about ¼ of an inch, perhaps smaller, and on the disk a little rubber disk, which is made so it can be fitted over the cavity. I am speaking of approximal cavities in the front teeth. In this way the fluid can be confined to the cavity and the forceps used to put on extreme pressure by holding the disk with the left finger and using the pressure with the right. I have been very successful in producing practically painless operations on the front teeth.

Dr. TULLER (closing the discussion). I think Dr. Rudy is the first I have occasion to answer. In regard to the putrescent condition of the coronal portion of the pulp, it may be unwise to undertake pressure anesthesia (cataphoresis)

in such a cavity knowingly. There would be every chance of forcing septic matter into the pulp; but since we remove the pulp at once, I hardly think any damage can be done. In cases of that kind I think I would select preferably another point for application, say at the neck of the tooth with the probability of reaching a point where the pulp was vital. I have done that very successfully. I have perfectly anesthetized a pulp in an upper molar by application through a cavity well up on a denuded palatal root.

Dr. Shoop asked about the use of carbolic acid in pressure anesthesia. It may be a good agent; I do not know. All my applications have been in the line of cocain. I take a few drops of adrenalin on a slab and put in a few crystals of cocain and go to work. I do not aim to get any certain percentage.

Dr. Bowen spoke about stopping bleeding. That is done by the use of adrenalin. If not enough has been incorporated in the mixture it is easy to inject more into the pulp to be safe on that point, after it is anesthetized; or it may be pressed in with a rubber plug after the removal of the pulp.

In regard to the use of arsenic spoken of by Dr. Brigham. Arsenic certainly did its part well for many years because we had nothing better. I have not used arsenic for four or five years, except where the canals were obstructed, and in every one of these cases I failed, more or less, with arsenic, to the best of my recollection. When, after a good deal of effort, I was enabled to gain an entrance into the pulp, I almost invariably found a condition of secondary deposit or pulp-stones; so I felt that certain conditions of secondary deposit have an effect in rendering the action of arsenic to some extent valueless, the same as it seems to obstruct the action of cocain. The great point in favor of pressure anesthesia as against arsenic is the saving of time, as well as being painless. Frequently a pulp can be extirpated in three minutes; while with arsenic it will take from several days to two weeks before it can be removed painlessly. With the pressure method I have taken out a live pulp without the patient being aware of the fact until it was shown to him on the broach.

I think what I have said in reply to Dr. Bowen will answer Dr. Kassab's question about bleeding.

Answering Dr. Todd, who spoke about infection, I will say that I operated in cavities of all varieties before I discovered that the solution would go through the entire thickness of dentin. I thought I had to expose the pulp, and while I have done so again and again I have never had any serious infection in any cases. I have had a few cases where complaint was made by the patient of some sensitiveness in the tooth, but a little later it all disappeared. I think

that tenderness might follow the taking out a live pulp in almost any manner, or in forcing in an agent to simply obtund, but no serious sequences have been reported to my knowledge.

Speaking about toxic effect, I have never had any indication of it, nor have I heard anything that was in any way authentic. I presume in cases with a large apical foramen the cocain might be forced through in such a way as to get a toxic effect; but ordinarily I do not think we would experience any effect if we use any sort of discretion. Only a very minute quantity can be injected through the dentin at best, and only a minute quantity is used by any method I employ.

I have not said anything about immediate root-filling; I leave that to every operator's own judgment. I sometimes fill immediately and sometimes leave it until a day or two afterward, keeping the canal sealed with an aseptic dressing.

The subject was passed and the section adjourned until Wednesday, August 31st.

SECTION VII—Continued.

THIRD DAY—Wednesday, August 31st.

THE section was called to order at 4 o'clock P.M., by the chairman, Dr. C. N. Johnson.

The first order of business was the reading of a paper entitled "The Cement Problem in Inlay Work," by Dr. GEO. C. POUNDSTONE of Chicago, Ill., as follows:

The Cement Problem in Inlay Work.

By GEO. C. POUNDSTONE, D.D.S., Chicago, Ill.

No branch of modern dentistry occupies a more prominent position than that concerning the inlay. For esthetic reasons nothing can compare with an accurately shaped and shaded porcelain inlay. Great claims are made for it on account of its compatibility to tooth-structure, its resistance to thermal changes, and its tooth-saving qualities.

The dental profession has heard almost without number papers and discussions upon inlays. High-fusing and low-fusing bodies have been discussed with such fervor that lifelong friendships have been all but broken. The burnished matrix and the swaging process have been discussed again and again; but the one vital point has been almost overlooked, that is, the *cement*.

In almost every paper upon the subject of inlays we have heard the statement that the inlay has come to stay; but just therein lies the great drawback, —it will not stay, in many cavities.

Most dentists can with care and perseverance make a perfect inlay, exact in its shape and beautiful in its shading, but what does that signify if after a week, a month, or even a year, we find this work of art—if we can find it at all— hidden away within some vase among the other valuable family porcelains and jewels, or lying quietly in the corner of a pill-box in some upper bureau drawer.

To keep the inlay in position in the cavity without spoiling its original beauty is the problem before us. What cement to use is the question. Some cements will not stick, others wash out, others expand, so that what at first appeared to be a perfect joint is after a day or two a broad line of cement, while still others are permeated by the fluids of the mouth, micro-organisms, and débris, giving the inlay the appearance of being several shades darker than the tooth.

Until we can procure better cements, the inlay cannot reach the high degree of perfection hoped for it, and it is with that end in view that the work now presented to you has been undertaken.

What are the requisite qualities of an inlay cement?

(1) It must be capable of being com-

reputation of any of the cements tested, nor have I an object in recommending any particular brand.

I realize that this course may be open to criticism from the fact that many dentists are waiting for somebody to tell them just what to use, but since none of the cements that I have tested are perfect and many of them have defects that I believe can be remedied, I deem it advisable to give the manufacturer one chance at least to improve upon his product.

FIG. 1.

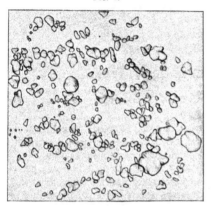

A, in glycerin.

FIG. 2.

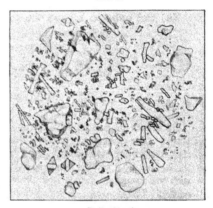

B, in glycerin.

pressed into a very thin film; at least as thin as the matrix used.

(2) It must have extra-adhesive qualities.

(3) It must neither expand nor contract.

(4) It must be impervious to moisture.

In giving the results of my observations and experiments the different cements will be designated by letters rather than by their commercial names, as it is not my purpose to in any way injure the

The first series of observations was made for the purpose of determining the general appearance of the various powders, the shapes and sizes of the granules, and their relative proportions in the mass. Microscopic slides were made from the different powders mixed with glycerin; the glycerin being used instead of the cement liquid to avoid chemical action. These slides were then studied with the binocular microscope, and drawings of carefully selected fields—that all the characteristics of the powder might be shown in one drawing—were made by the aid of the camera lucida. Lantern slides were then made from the drawings. Micrographs were made, but they were

Cement A, in glycerin. Large granules: few in number; from 25 to 35 microns in diameter; irregular in shape.

Medium granules make up the bulk of

FIG. 3.

FIG. 3.

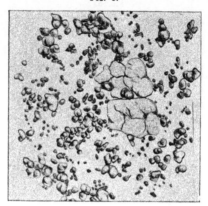

C, in glycerin.

FIG. 4.

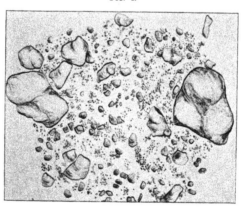

D, in glycerin.

not as satisfactory as the drawings, on account of the thickness of the films, in some cases exceeding 1/500 of an inch. Measurements were made with the micrometer.

the powder; from 8 to 15 microns in diameter.

Fine powder: small amount.

Cement B, in glycerin. Large granules: few in number; from 30 to 50 microns in diameter. Some of these appear to be zinc oxid, while others are flat, transparent crystals.

Medium granules: few in number;

to 5 microns in diameter and of small rod-like prisms, transparent, and square at the ends, from 2 to 5 microns in diameter and in length 3 to 50 microns.

FIG. 5.

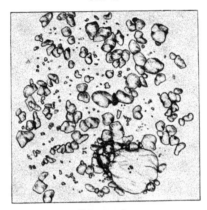

E, in glycerin.

FIG. 6.

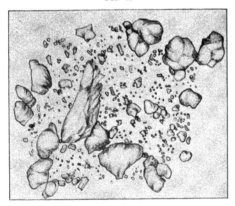

F, in glycerin.

from 10 to 15 microns in diameter. They resemble the large ones.

Fine powder: The bulk of the powder is made up of small granules from 2

There are in this powder a few bright red granules of medium size.

Cement C, in glycerin. There are two distinctly different kinds of granules in this powder, in all the different sizes. The somewhat regular shaped yellowish granules, apparently of zinc oxid, and a transparent, generally square crystal form.

Large granules: few in number; from 25 to 30 microns in diameter.

Large crystals: few in number; from 40 to 50 microns in diameter.

Medium granules: many; from 7 to 15 microns in diameter.

Fine powder: rather small in amount; made up of both granules and crystals.

microns in diameter, with an occasional scale-like, semi-transparent flake as high as 50 microns.

Medium granules make up the bulk of the powder; from 10 to 15 microns in diameter.

Fine powder: small amount.

Cement F, in glycerin. Large granules: few in number; from 30 to 40 microns in diameter, with an occasional flat one as high as 56 microns; very irregular in shape.

Medium granules make up the bulk

Fig. 7.

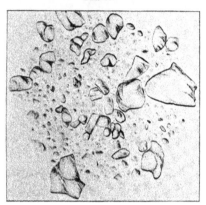

G, in glycerin.

Fig. 8.

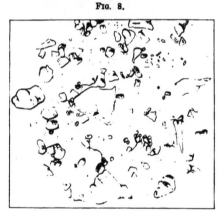

H, in glycerin.

Cement D, in glycerin. Large granules: very few in number; from 30 to 45 microns in diameter, with an occasional one as high as 56 microns. Very irregular in shape.

Medium granules: few in number; from 12 to 18 microns in diameter.

Fine powder: extremely fine and flourlike; of uniformly oval granules less than 2 microns in diameter; form the large proportion of the powder.

Cement E, in glycerin. Large granules: very few in number; from 20 to 25

of the powder; from 16 to 30 microns in diameter.

Fine powder: large amount; very fine; granules uniform in sizes and shape.

Cement G, in glycerin. Large granules: few in number; from 35 to 46 microns in diameter; irregular in shape.

Medium granules: many; from 18 to 22 microns in diameter; more regular in form.

Fine powder: a large amount, with particles irregular in form.

Cement H, in glycerin. Large granules—of three varieties. Granules of zinc oxid (apparently) very few; from 25 to 40 microns in diameter. A few semi-transparent crystals, irregular in form, from 50 to 60 microns in diameter; and many transparent broken crystals of all shapes and sizes up to 60 microns in diameter.

Medium granules: few in number; from 5 to 20 microns in diameter, and many broken crystals of medium size.

regular in form; from 8 to 15 microns in diameter.

Fine powder: a comparatively large amount of uniformly regular granules.

In this powder there is an occasional bright red granule.

For the second series slides were made from the various powders, each mixed with its corresponding cement liquid in the manner described by the manufacturer, to a consistence suitable for setting

FIG. 9.

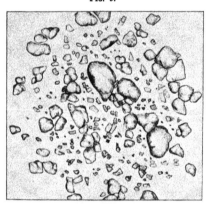

I, in glycerin.

FIG. 10.

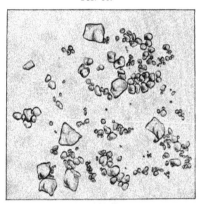

J, in glycerin.

Fine powder: small in amount, resembling the larger granules and crystals.

Cement I, in glycerin. Large granules: very few in number; from 20 to 27 microns in diameter; oval in shape with smooth rounded edges.

Medium granules make up the bulk of the powder; from 10 to 15 microns in diameter; oval in form.

Fine powder: small in amount; very fine.

Cement J, in glycerin. Large granules: very few; from 20 to 25 microns in diameter.

Medium granules: very many; quite

an inlay. Cover glasses were subjected to pressure in order to get a thin film of cement. These slides were then studied with the microscope. The process of setting was carefully watched for several hours, after which the slides were examined and studied and changes noted every few hours for a week or more, or until no further change was noted.

The important points of these observations are as follows:

Cement A.

Almost immediately the fine powder commences to unite with the liquid, the small granules begin to disappear and give off minute bubbles which increase in size and number until at the end of an the liquid. Very little if any change has taken place in the large granules except a slight diminution in size due to

Fig. 11.

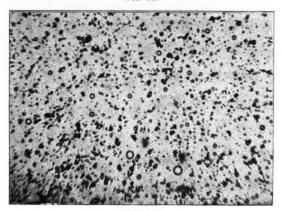

A—one hour.

Fig. 12.

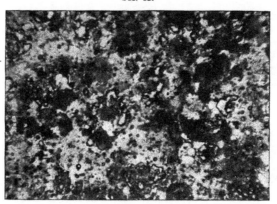

A—three days.

hour the field is pretty well covered with them.

By the end of 24 hours the fine powder seems to have about all united with the dissolving of the outer surfaces by the liquid. By this time many of the minute granules are surrounded by translucent areas which in three or four days develop into beautiful radiating crystals.

By the end of the week many of the

ules are still visible, the open spaces have become more irregular, and the mass is much more opaque in its appearance.

Fig. 13.

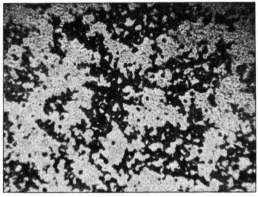

A—three months.

Fig. 14.

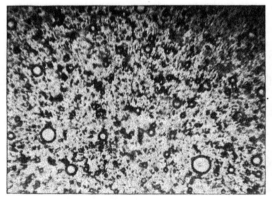

B—one hour.

bubbles have gone together, forming large irregular spaces, and the entire mass has taken on a grayish mottled appearance. In another week some of the largest gran-

Cement B.

Within twenty minutes after mixing the rod-like crystals in this powder have almost disappeared. The other granules show little change. The entire slide has a mottled grayish appearance.

hours a clear area forms around each bubble.

Around the edges of these clear spaces

FIG. 15.

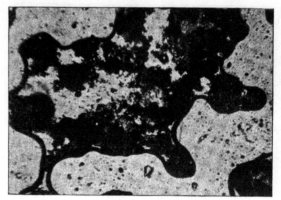

B—twenty-four hours.

FIG. 16.

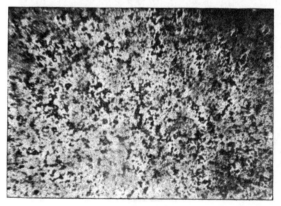

C—one hour.

Quite a number of bubbles appear soon after mixing; they expand considerably in size, and in from two to three

crystallization is quite apparent at this time and progresses rapidly. Within five hours there are large open spaces throughout the film. Circular areas of crystallization are numerous at or near the borders of the clear spaces. By the end of 24 hours the open spaces occupy

der dissolve readily in the cement liquid, but the action upon the other granules is slow. Very few bubbles appear.

By the end of an hour the film has a

FIG. 17.

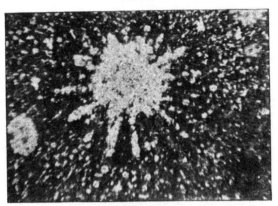

C—four weeks.

FIG. 18.

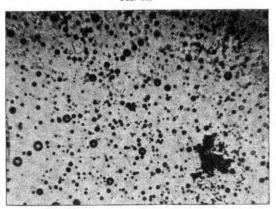

D—one hour.

at least one-half of the slide. Crystallization seems to be completed by this time.

Cement C.

The transparent crystals of this pow-

dark grayish granular appearance, with the zinc granules still plainly visible. Subsequent change takes place very slowly in this cement. In two or three days crystallization begins at intervals over the slide, building from a center, the crystals being formed successively in the form of rays, the area very much resembling the piece of jewelry known as a sunburst.

The outermost crystals are large with definite angles and pointed ends and are of a yellowish color. In viewing these crystallizing areas by transmitted light there is considerable iridescence.

Cement D.

Almost immediately after mixing and

no apparent change in the larger granules. In about four weeks the entire field becomes crystallized, the granules have almost entirely disappeared or have been covered by a mass of crystals projecting like the spines on a sea-urchin. The open spaces are also in many places fringed by crystals.

Cement E.

In this cement very little change is noticed in the first ten minutes except a gradual fading away of the smaller

FIG. 19.

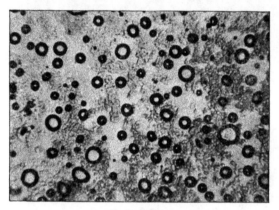

D—three days.

placing upon the slide a large number of small bubbles appear, arising from the finer particles of powder. The bubbles increase in size and number and, after a short time, unite with each other when coming into contact until they cover almost one-third of the entire field.

These remain as distinct circular bubbles for a week or ten days and then begin to assume irregular forms. By the end of the second week some crystallization is apparent around the edges of the bubbles. There is at this time little or

particles of the powder in its union with the liquid. This goes on until nearly all of the fine powder has disappeared. The medium sized and large granules have a decided tendency to group themselves into clusters or chains, leaving proportionally large areas of nothing but the liquid.

The granules show the effect of the action of the liquid by their diminished size and rounded edges. A few bubbles are present when this cement is first mixed, but no subsequent change takes

place. They are in all probability bubbles of air incorporated with the mass
in the mixing.

Crystallization is apparent after two

Cement F.

In this cement the fine powder unites
readily with the liquid, within a few minutes small bubbles begin to appear, aris-

FIG. 20.

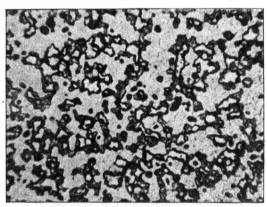

D—four weeks.

FIG. 21.

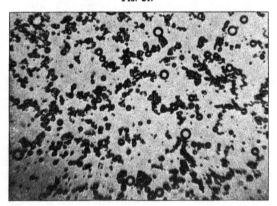

E—one hour.

or three days and continues in its formation for more than two months. The
crystals are all of the needle form, radiating from a center.

ing from the dissolving particles of the
fine powder.

These bubbles increase in size and
number for two or three days, after which

there is little or no change. The medium and large sized granules seem to undergo very little change other than

rather slow, the entire mass becoming crystallized in from four to six weeks.

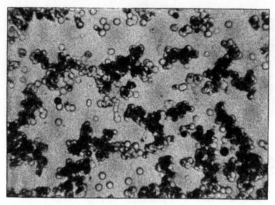

E—four weeks.

FIG. 23.

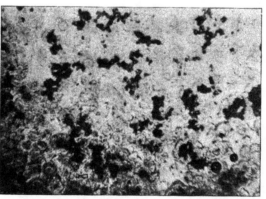

E—three months.

a slight diminution in size, the sharp jagged edges becoming smooth and rounded.

Crystallization is apparent in about three or four days, but its progress is

Cement G.

This is a rather slow-setting cement. Very little change is noticed within the first fifteen minutes except the appearance of a few bubbles arising from the particles of fine powder. At the end of an hour nearly all of the fine powder is still visible, and after 24 hours only the finest particles have disappeared. The

Cement H.

Quite a large number of bubbles appear in this cement soon after it is mixed. They increase somewhat in size.

Fig. 24.

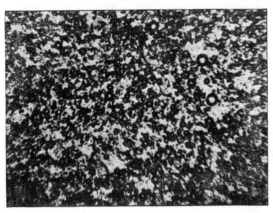

F—one hour.

Fig. 25.

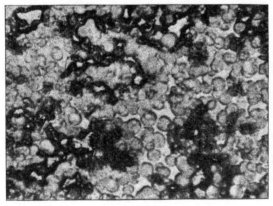

F—four weeks.

small bubbles that appear at first do not increase to any extent either in size or number, but remain as bubbles in the mass.

Very few of the granules or crystals of this powder seem to be readily dissolved by the liquid, for nearly all are still visible after 24 hours, though appreciably smaller. The slide at this time is of a grayish color and a few of the bubbles have commenced to assume irregular forms.

themselves into groups or chains with spaces of liquid between, as in Cement E.

Quite a number of bubbles appear in the clearer portions of the slide, appar-

FIG. 26.

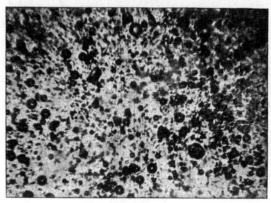

G—one hour.

FIG. 27.

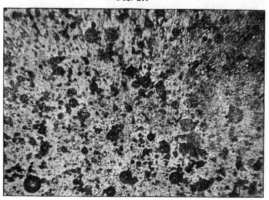

G—two days.

Cement I.

The fine powder of this cement unites very readily with the liquid. The larger granules have a tendency to arrange

ently coming from the particles of fine powder. By the end of a week there is a large amount of crystallization.

The bubbles have by this time changed

5

into large irregular spaces and the slide has a grayish mottled appearance much the same as that noted in Cement *A*.

disappeared and crystallization has advanced to a considerable degree. Two forms of crystals or of crystallizing areas

FIG. 28.

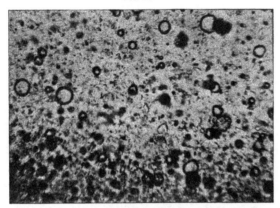

H—one hour.

FIG. 29.

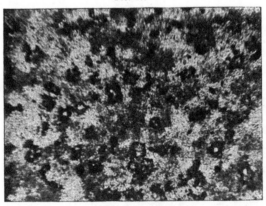

H—two days.

Cement J.

The fine powder quickly unites with the liquid and a few bubbles appear within the first half hour.

In two hours most of the granules have

are present: a rod or prism square at the ends, and the other in the form of a rhombus with the obtuse angles rounded.

There is no definite arrangement of

the crystals with respect to each other. In 24 hours there is little change except that the rounded angles of the large crystals are now straight lines, making six-sided prisms.

Slides of the different cements were made in the same way and kept in water at body temperature. They were studied from time to time with no appreciable difference in the results except a possible hastening of the process of crystallization. The bubbles and open spaces formed exactly the same as when dry, and in time became filled with the water, as will be shown in the slides for penetration.

FIG. 30.

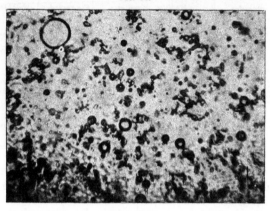

I—one hour.

FIG. 31.

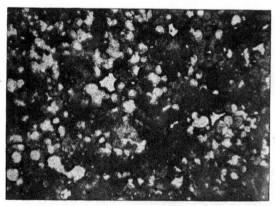

I—two days.

The foregoing observations may be summarized for a closer comparative study as follows:

ules of cement. As has been noted in the descriptions of the various powders many of the larger granules are very ir-

CEMENT	Large granules.		Medium granules.		Fine powder.	Bubbles in setting.
	Relative number.	Size of largest.	Relative number.	Average size.	Relative amount.	
A	Few.	35 microns	Many.	8-15 microns.	Small.	Many.
B	Few.	50 "	Few.	10-15 "	Large.	Many.
C	Few.	50 "	Many.	7-15 "	Small	Very few.
D	Very few.	56 "	Few.	12-18 "	Very large.	Very many.
E	Very few.	25 "	Very many.	10-15 "	Small.	Few.
F	Few.	56 "	Many.	16-30 "	Large.	Few.
G	Few.	46 "	Many.	18-22 "	Large.	Very few.
H	Few.	40 "	Many.	5-20 "	Small.	Many.
I	Very few.	27 "	Very many.	10-15 "	Small.	Few.
J	Very few.	25 "	Very many	8-15 "	Large.	Few.

As the cement granules do not dissolve when mixed with the liquid, and become a homogenous mass, it would seem from the foregoing measurements that some regular or flat in shape, and in microscopic examinations present the flat side to view. It is also quite evident that many if not all of these granules undergo

FIG. 32.

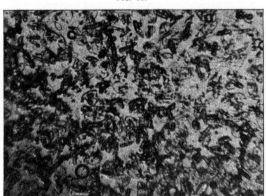

J—two hours.

of the cements tested would be unsuitable for the purpose of setting inlays, or if they were used a matrix of corresponding thickness would have to be used in order to get space enough between the inlay and the cavity wall for the gran- some change upon coming into contact with the cement liquid, whereby they are reduced in size; another series of experiments was therefore made to determine the exact thickness of these granules when set.

Two cover glasses were accurately measured in the micrometer and a mix of cement of proper consistence for setting an inlay was made and placed between them. that for not more than two or three minutes at a time.

At the end of fifteen minutes the cover glasses with the film of cement between

FIG. 33.

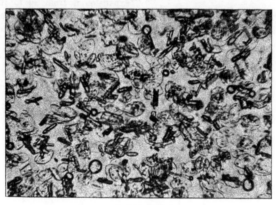

J—two days.

tween them. They were then subjected to a pressure of 25 pounds for fifteen minutes. This is the maximum pressure that would ever be brought by the fingers them were measured. They were again measured in 24 hours, and again in 72 hours, with the results shown in the accompanying table.

TESTS FOR EXPANSION OF COVER-GLASS FILMS. (DRY.)

CEMENT	Thickness of cement after setting fifteen min. under twenty-five lbs. pressure.	Thickness after setting twenty-four hours.	Expansion.	Subsequent change.
A	21 microns.	21 microns.	0 microns.	Slight expansion.
B	23 "	43 "	20 "	None
C	22 "	44 "	22 "	None.
D	24 "	25 "	1 "	Slight increase in expansion.
E	27 "	27 "	0 "	None.
F	30 "	34 "	4 "	None.
G	32 "	42 "	10 "	None.
H	26 "	27 "	1 "	Slight increase in expansion
I	31 "	35 "	4 "	Slight increase in expansion.
J	25 "	33 "	8 "	Slight increase in expansion.

upon an inlay and is far beyond that which most operators would use, careful tests proving that from 10 to 15 pounds is all that can be generally exerted—and Twenty-five microns is approximately 1/1000 of an inch. It would therefore seem that only five of the cements tested would permit the inlay to be placed into proper position if a 1/1000 matrix were used, and this would be under 25 pounds pressure. If this is true, then what will be the result in setting an inlay made to exactly fit the cavity by the swaging process?

This: The inlay if it be flat will remain just the thickness of the cement

liquid, will be more readily soluble in the fluids of the mouth.

The expansion of these thin films is also worthy of careful consideration. For example: In B, C, and G, in which the expansion is from 30 to 100 per cent., we have an explanation for the broad band of cement showing around the in-

FIG. 34.

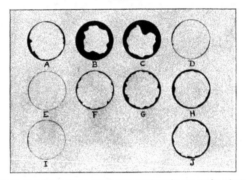

Cover-glass films after remaining in water-eosin twenty-four hours.

FIG. 35.

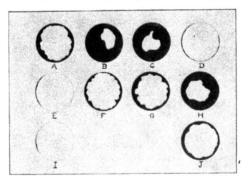

Cover-glass films after remaining in water-eosin two days.

film out of position, or if it be one with parallel or slightly converging sides the larger granules of the cement will be forced to the bottom of the cavity underneath the inlay and prevent it from being forced to position, while around the sides will be only the thinner portion of the cement which, owing to the excess of

lay after a few days when at the time of setting the joint appeared to be perfect. J also expands too much, while F and I could be better. A and E show no expansion, but A is filled with bubbles, and it will be shown later that E lacks in adhesiveness. D contains far too many bubbles, and H has troubles of its own.

FIG. 36.

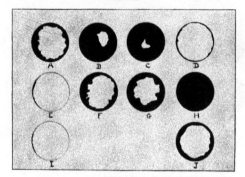

Cover-glass films after remaining in water-eosin three days.

FIG. 37.

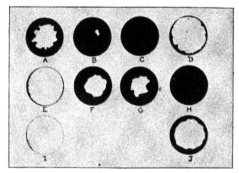

Cover-glass films after remaining in water-eosin four days.

FIG. 38.

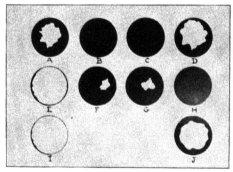

Cover-glass films after remaining in water-eosin five days.

FIG. 39.

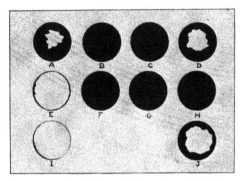

Cover-glass films after remaining in water-eosin six days.

FIG. 40.

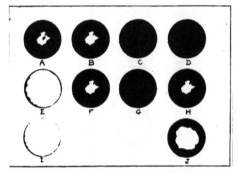

Cover-glass films after remaining in water-eosin seven days.

FIG. 41.

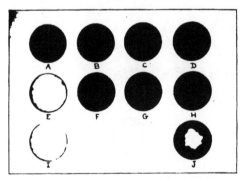

Cover-glass films after remaining in water-eosin ten days.

For the purpose of determining the adhesiveness of the different cements, tests were made as follows: Blocks of ivory were carefully prepared with the surfaces to be cemented together having an area of 60 square millimeters, approximately that of the surface of a large inlay. These surfaces were roughened with a vulcanite file and the blocks were then cemented together. They were kept dry for 24 hours, when they were pulled apart with the following results, the number of pounds given being the average of a number of trials in each case. The highest and the lowest tests are also given:

apart, considerable resistance was met with, the film of cement apparently interlocking into the uneven surfaces of the blocks on either side.

In these tests the capillary attraction between the cement and the ivory block is greater than the adhesiveness of the cement, and this has been the case with all of my tests except those in which the cement was covered with varnish, which would theoretically make it the same as if kept dry. But in the mouth we have all met with cases of old cement fillings in which it was necessary to chip away the last vestige of filling from the walls of the cavity, the adhesion being perfect,

TESTS FOR ADHESIVENESS. (Ivory blocks 60 sq. mm.)

CEMENT	Force necessary to separate after twenty-four hours.		
	Average force.	Highest.	Lowest.
A	46½ lb.	68 lb.	28 lb.
B	46 "	60 "	26 "
C	44¼ "	63 "	32 "
D	23½ "	30 "	18 "
E	81¼ "	87 "	20 "
F	45½ "	70 "	29 "
G	59¼ "	72 "	51 "
H	50¼ "	68 "	33 "
I	42¼ "	48 "	28 "
J	35¼ "	42 "	30 "

Repeated tests were made by cementing the blocks together and keeping them in saliva in the incubator at 37° C., but in every instance the force necessary to separate them was so slight that it was impossible to measure it with any degree of accuracy. These were flat surfaces, with the force applied perpendicular to the surface. When force was applied parallel with the surface, i.e. when an attempt was made to slide the blocks

thus proving that adhesion does, in some cases at least, take place.

It is my belief that most inlays are retained in position solely by the retention form of the cavity, the accurate fit of the inlay and the cement on the one hand, and the cavity wall and the cement on the other; and that after a few days there is a film of moisture between the cement and the cavity wall and between the cement and the inlay, the cement acting merely as a key in locking the inlay into the cavity by means of its projections extending into the irregularities of the cavity wall on the one hand, and the depressions in the inlay formed by etching or grinding on the other.

Cements that contain bubbles and open spaces will undoubtedly permit the penetration of moisture; but to more certainly demonstrate this another series of experiments was made. Cover glasses were carefully etched and cleansed, and

impervious-to-moisture cements; *i.e.* they will withstand the common test of rolling up a pellet of the cement and dropping it into red ink or anilin dye, and after immersion for days, weeks, or months show no signs of penetration of the coloring matter. But that test is of little or no value whatever, for the defect is not in the cement itself but in the joint between the cement and the tooth. The cement may be perfectly insoluble, but that will not prevent moisture pass-

FIG. 42.

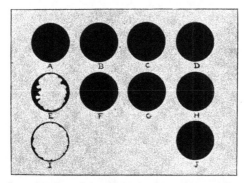

Cover-glass films after remaining in water-eosin two weeks.

a mix of cement placed between each pair. These were held firmly together until they had set, when they were placed in water-eosin and kept in the incubator at 37° C. They were examined from day to day and drawings were made showing the extent to which the eosin had penetrated. The results can best be shown by the illustrations. (Figs. 34-42.)

This penetration of the eosin is generally not within the body of the cement itself, but is between the cement and the glass, and a number of those cements which permit the eosin to pass between themselves and the glass are the so-called

ing between it and the tooth. If moisture can enter, micro-organisms will enter, and decay result. This is further proved by the fact that nearly all old cement fillings that are removed from cavities in the teeth are discolored completely over the surface that was in contact with the tooth, while in the center they are still as bright and clear as when first inserted.

The results of the foregoing observations and experiments may not offer much assistance to the dentist who is looking for the best cement; for it is difficult, if not impossible, to say which is the best, so much depending upon the particular purpose for which it is to be used. The individual case will in a large measure have to determine the kind of cement that will best fulfill its requirements. Again, so much depends upon proper mixing and care in keeping some cements that it is impossible to foretell the results of any one of them in the hands of different operators.

It is therefore advisable that every dentist shall do some experimenting, that he may know from experience what is actually taking place as a result of his own manipulation. In so doing he may be able to better his own work, or at least save himself from embarrassment through ignorance of that which he is using.

The hour being late, the chairman announced that the discussion of Dr. Poundstone's paper would be postponed until Thursday's session. Adjourned.

SECTION VII—Continued.

FOURTH DAY—Thursday, September 1st.

THE section was called to order at 2 o'clock P.M. by the chairman, Dr. C. N. Johnson.

The first order of business was the discussion of Dr. G. C. Poundstone's paper.

Discussion.

Dr. G. V. BLACK, Chicago, Ill. All I wish to say is simply to call your attention to the fact that this is another and a new method of studying cements; it is one that we have not had before us previously, and one that promises to give us very great and important information upon the subject. I have been over a number of these slides myself with the microscope and know there is more yet that can be said about these individual slides, as illustrating the character—the failures as well as the successful points—of these cements. The very important relation of cement to inlay work makes it one of the vital questions, and I am sure the manufacturers of cements will take up this plan and study and correct some of the elements of weakness of the cements as now presented.

Dr. J. N. CROUSE, Chicago, Ill. That cements are defective, that the weak point in inlay work is the cement, will not be denied by the most enthusiastic porcelain workers. It is the weak point of bridge work, it is the weak point in all lines where we have to use cement as a retaining material for fillings or crowns. Thus far nothing has been found that will take the place of phosphoric acid and zinc—a combination of them—to make cement. My belief has been, and I still have the faith, that the coming material will be a plastic material to correct the improper color, or to correspond with the color of the teeth.

The point I want to raise is, first, on the question of accuracy, by the use of twenty-five pounds pressure in cementing two slabs together with a view of ascertaining first the expansion or contraction, and second the solubility or penetration of the coloration around them. I can take the same cement, the same proportions, and mix them, and have an expansion in my test tube of from 2 to 10/1000 of an inch. I take the same proportions and pack in another way and have a shrinkage of 2/1000 of an inch. If I am accurate and have it stand pat, neither shrink or expand, by pressure put on the packing of a tube or by pressure put on the inlay in cementing it in, the expansion will be in proportion to the amount of pressure to a greater or less degree, the expansion being a great deal more with heavy pressure than where it is less. I have not set inlays enough to pronounce upon that, but I believe it is a mistake to put much pressure on an inlay when cementing it.

There is another question coming up, and I predict right here that the present method of making inlays will be absolutely revolutionized within a not very distant time. The change is going to be brought about by fusible cement. An exhibition was given in a clinic here this morning where the material was mixed into the form of a paste or cement, placed in the cavity, allowed to set and was baked without a matrix. In this material there is forty per cent. less shrinkage in the first bake than there is in porcelain. The cement will be absolutely fine, too, and the cement powder absolutely without crystal. In the illustration it was shown that those granules were so large as to make it impossible to fit an inlay perfectly and allow for the removal of the platinum and matrix. When I make this bold assertion that it is going to revolutionize the method of inlay and porcelain work I do so with the boldness that comes by experience. I have given it a great deal of thought and observation, I know what I am talking about, and when I say it will be one-third stronger than porcelain inlay I assert that with absolute assurance of being able to produce proof. I have watched a good many settings of other men's cements. I have seldom seen a dentist mix his cement right. I have been mixing barrels of it the last ten years and I know how it ought to be mixed. The spatulas are too small. I want a broad spatula, so that it will take up the whole mass, which should be thoroughly mixed. The question of adhesion of cement I consider one that is easily remedied. I have been using a good cement and it is sticky, it is so sticky that my girl said she could not mix it. There has been a great deal of complaint because it takes more elbow grease to mix it.

Dr. A. E. WEBSTER, Toronto, Canada. There is only one phase of this subject I desire to say anything about, and that is with reference to the permeability of cement by bacteria. I have done some work in connection with the subject, having found results corroborating what the essayist ascertained. I found that in nearly all cases cements are permeated by bacteria in from six hours to sixteen or twenty days, the extreme being about twenty days. The question that has always been asked me was, "Do the bacteria pass through the substance of the cement or around it?" I was not able to answer that question, but I think the essayist answered it thoroughly well yesterday. Where they contract at all the bacteria will pass around them, as was shown in the illustrations. Then there are other cements in which the bacteria will pass right through the substance of the cement. It seems to me very difficult to strike a medium where the organisms will not pass through or around the surface of the cements. That was the particularly interesting part of the paper to me and all I wish to discuss at the present time.

Dr. C. H. PARKER, Chicago, Ill. I would like to ask whether the bacteria that the doctor spoke of passing through the cement were of a harmful nature, were they of a destructive nature to the teeth proper?

Dr. WEBSTER. In respect to that, most of the bacteria I found that had passed through the cements were the ordinary pus organisms. I know they were the organisms that cause inflammatory processes.

The CHAIRMAN. I have much pleasure in introducing to this audience a man who has had as much experience in inlay work as any man in this country, and I take special pleasure in introducing Dr. N. S. Jenkins of Dresden, Germany, who will continue the discussion of this subject.

Dr. N. S. JENKINS, Dresden, Germany. This paper is a very important contribution towards the solution of one of the most important questions of our time. It does not deal with the chemistry of cement, but with its physical characteristics, and I know of no experiments in this direction which are so instructive and suggestive. The first step is to give us views of the various powders so enlarged that we can see that a family resemblance characterizes them, for they differ greatly in the size of the granules, but not so greatly in form. When, however, the powders become mixed with their fluids the difference becomes more marked. They behave very differently in mixing, and especially the difference in the number of bubbles is very suggestive. Of all the cements those marked E and I would seem to be most instructive, since they each possess very few large granules, very many medium granules, and few bubbles. E has no expansion. I has an expansion of four microns, and subsequently to the period of twenty-four hours has still a slight expansion. The adhesiveness of E is less than that of I, but both of them offer a far greater resistance to moisture than any of the others, with the odds in favor of

I. The experiments are of great interest, but they are still but a step toward the solution of the problem. We do not know of what the granules are composed, what the crystals are, or how pure the mixing fluid is. Phosphoric acid, which probably entered largely into the composition of the fluid, is notoriously unaddicted to purity. We cannot tell what proportion of dust and dirt had soiled the powders, nor how objectionable in bulk the coloring matter may have been.

From my experience of the extreme difficulty of keeping the material of which porcelain is composed free from foreign and deleterious substances, I feel great compassion for the manufacturers of cements who have been formerly influenced by the general delusion that some granular and resistant matter must be incorporated into cement and who have had special difficulties in obtaining and retaining pure materials. But in spite of all the imperfections of cement, it still remains an indispensable adjunct to inlay work. There are innumerable instances where cement practically fulfills the requirements of Dr. Poundstone's four propositions. Every experienced inlay worker knows that given the exactly made inlay he can in the vast majority of cases so set that inlay that no joint perceptible to the eye and visible disintegration of the cement supervenes. The color of the inlay and cement is preserved and secondary decay is far less frequent than with gold fillings. Moreover, the density and adhesiveness of the cement increase with time. The porcelain inlay which has been in place for ten years is removed with far greater difficulty than one which has been in for ten months. The mixing of any cement is an art. Powder and fluid should be inspected when placed upon the mixing slab, and if found in any way contaminated it should be discarded. Then a small portion of the powder should be thoroughly mixed with the fluid and gradually more powder added until the desired consistence is obtained. Then the inlay and cavity should receive a thin layer and the inlay pressed home. The edges should be freed from overflow, and then the final pressure, which should be firm but not excessive, continued until the cement has begun to crystallize, and the inlay still be kept dry for a time, according to the character of the cement. In the vast majority of cases there will then be a perfect operation, far more secure from accident than any other, and immensely more comfortable to the patient. But, however, we do not know why in the small minority of cases we have failure through weakness of cement. Whoever deliberately sets an ill-fitting inlay deserves to meet with failure, but the most skilful and conscientious man sometimes meets with a disaster which might be rightly attributed to imperfection of the cement. Therefore, these careful and intelligent observations of Dr. Poundstone have for us all a great significance.

Dr. G. T. EPLING, Keystone, W. Va. I have observed that cement when mixed on one slab and dropped on another will not adhere to the slab with as great tenacity as that with which it would adhere to the one on which it was mixed. Therefore, when I set an inlay now, after mixing my cement on a perfectly clean slab, adding just a small portion of the powder and thoroughly mixing before adding any more powder, I place some of the cement on the inlay and rub it thoroughly over the surface that will rest against the cavity.

Some of my patients who have been wearing inlays complain that the cement works out around the margins, and, in my opinion, there is no cement on the market at this time that is free from this fault. When perfection in the preparation of cement is attained, that is, when cement that will not be affected by the secretions of the oral cavity is produced, we then can abandon the inlay and use the cement. No matter how perfectly the inlay fits the cavity, one has to depend upon the cement to hold it in place. The cement problem in inlay work is, therefore, an important one and one that cannot receive too much consideration from porcelain workers.

Dr. J. N. CROUSE. I wish simply to speak of the destructibility, or the ease or liability of cement deteriorating before using. What brings this about I do not know, but it seems to be a change in the temperature. So a cement that will do well today, in two weeks from now will be very easily penetrated by moisture, so the anilin will show through in a few days. The same is true of the porcelains, and operators when mixing, if they want a little more powder dip the spatula in the powder, or if they want a little more liquid they dip the spatula in the liquid, and that utterly destroys the quality of the cement. We cannot be too careful about these things. I think the cement ought to be tested from time to time for its solubility.

Dr. W. V-B. AMES, Chicago, Ill. I have not heard the previous discussion, but there are some questions I would like to ask of Dr. Poundstone if I may, if he is here, in regard to the methods of procedure in making the mix in these tests. As I understand it he observed changes for days and weeks under some of those cover glasses, and I would like to know to what consistence this cement was mixed. I understood him to say it was mixed to about the consistence it would be used in setting the inlay, but I would like to ask the doctor to tell us about what he considers that should be, and whether all cements had about the same consistence. I do not realize how it is possible for some of the changes to take place which he described, unless those particular cements were of a very slow-setting variety and were used in more of a fluid form than was justified.

Dr. POUNDSTONE. I always mix each cement as nearly as I can according to the directions given by the manufacturer—to a consistence such that it will not drop from the spatula, but when placed in a heap upon the slab will retain its form. I use a non-corrosive German silver spatula.

Dr. AMES. You have noticed, of course, that there is sometimes a tendency to the formation of gases in cement during mixing, and as the essayist said there is danger of mechanical incorporation of air, but if it is carefully mixed I think there ought to be little danger of the latter sort. However, I can understand that with the use of a steel spatula we would almost necessarily have globules of gas forming from the presence of hydrogen from the action of the acid upon the steel or iron of the spatula. Then it has been noticed, that in some preparations of powder you get these bubbles from the fact that you have in the powder a little metal in a finely divided state, and this metal—zinc or iron—will necessarily give gas globules. You can see the formation of hydrogen during the mix as an effervescence. I have in a very crude way seen where there was gas in cement between two pieces of glass held between the eye and

a strong light, and this undoubtedly came from finely divided metal, and will probably account for some of the cases shown by Dr. Poundstone. I cannot reconcile myself to the fact that these changes should take place for weeks, as I got it from the doctor, after the mixing of the cement. It is hard to become reconciled to the fact that there is sufficient mobility of the mass to allow this air or gas to form and change them, as his experiments would show, and I would like to see it worked out further.

Dr. W. I. JONES, Nelsonville, O. I would like to ask Dr. Ames or Dr. Jenkins a question. I have seen the statement made that the fluid phosphoric acid would deteriorate with age. I believe the gentleman made the statement that it would deteriorate after three months' time. I would like to know whether that is true or not.

Dr. W. I. BRIGHAM, South Framingham, Mass. The essayist speaks of the value of a porcelain filling, he speaks of the durability of a porcelain filling and the little recurrence of decay. The durability of a porcelain filling does not depend on the porcelain. The porcelain forms only a part of the durability. It is upon the compatibility of the porcelain with the cement and the quality of the cement that depends the durability of the filling. The porcelain simply makes it a permanent filling. In cement we naturally have the best filling material if it were durable, and the porcelain simply makes it so. It has been said here that fusible cement may take the place of this and to a certain extent do away with the use of cement for filling, but if you have that fusible cement that filling in the end will have to be cemented in place, and the cement problem will be just as great then, if not greater.

The man who has had a great deal of experience in porcelain work will say it is a long time before we shall have a better product. I cannot help thinking what was said by Robert Ingersoll upon one occasion when introducing Henry Ward Beecher. He said, "We have waited a long time for Henry Ward Beecher and we shall wait a long time for another." We have waited a long time for the product of porcelain and we will wait a long time for something better. To my mind the cement is not the greatest problem; the cement problem is only secondary. The preparation of the cavity, to my mind, is of the greatest import. This discussion does not deal with the preparation of cavities, although this is the great factor in the problem. Cavities can be so prepared that fillings there inserted will last for years. As to the value of cement in preventing caries, we know that zinc oxyphosphate has antiseptic qualities, but is soon disintegrated by the fluids of the mouth. I believe that for a long time to come we will have to look for something better than porcelain as a filling material.

Dr. EDWIN T. DARBY, Philadelphia, Pa. It is undoubtedly true that the cement problem is one of the bugbears in connection with porcelain inlay work. It is generally regarded as the weak point in inlay work; I do not say it is, but it is so regarded by many men in the profession. It has been said, and truthfully said, that no chain is stronger than its weakest link, and they use that argument to say that no inlay is better than the cement with which it is set, but in my judgment almost any of the good cements are sufficient to hold a properly constructed inlay in place, barring accidents, for a number of years, anywhere

from five to ten years. I make that statement guardedly, and you will notice I premised it by saying properly constructed inlays. I think many failures are due not to the cement, but to the shape of the cavity or the shape of the inlay. Dr. Jenkins brought out one point, and my object in rising was to emphasize that point, and that is in regard to the mixing of the cement. Many men mix cement for porcelain inlays the same as they mix it for filling, and I contend that the cement used in porcelain work should be mixed with as much care as the most particular and painstaking artist uses in mixing his colors for painting the finest piece of porcelain. You cannot take a solution of phosphoric acid and zinc oxid, drop them on a slab recklessly and get good results. It should be, as Dr. Jenkins suggested, done by gradually incorporating the powder into the liquid, and furthermore it must be thoroughly spatulated. Most of the cements do not set quickly, and an expert can thoroughly incorporate his powder with the liquid and not have it set on his hands. If he has everything at hand in the way of instruments and assistance, the cavity dry, and everything all right and near at hand, he can mix it and mix for a considerable period of time, incorporating the powder with the liquid, and then when the inlay is set the chances are that the porcelain will stay in place as long as a gold filling or anything else.

We must not condemn the cements because of our failures, for I am within the truth when I say that very few inlays that are properly constructed and properly cemented in will be affected by the action of the secretions of the mouth upon the cement. I think we are on the verge of a period when there will be

6

great improvement in the character of
our cements as there have been improvements along all dental lines, and I think
within the next year we shall have cements as good as our porcelain, and that
will certainly be good enough.

Dr. POUNDSTONE (closing the discussion). I wish to thank the gentlemen
who have taken such an interest in the
discussion of this subject. There are a
few points I wish to speak of in order to
emphasize them.

As to the color of the cements tested,
in every case where it was possible I used
the light yellow powder. There is a difference in the different colored powders
from the same manufacturer. I have
found that the bubbling is greater in the
white, the bluish cast, or the pearl gray
than in the yellow powders, which appear to contain no foreign coloring matter. This point needs further investigation before definite conclusions can be
arrived at.

In the preparation of the cavity I repeat what I said in my paper, that it is
my opinion that most inlays are locked
into the cavity by the cement acting as
wedge or key. If the cavity is properly
prepared the cement will hold the inlay
in position for months and years, even
though it is not sticking either to the
cavity wall or to the inlay. There
must be retention enough in the cavity
to prevent the inlay from being moved
in any direction except that from which
it was inserted.

As Dr. Thompson has shown in his
contributions on cavity preparation, there
is but one way in which an inlay should
be set, that is in such a direction that the

stress of mastication will have no tendency to dislodge it. If this is done it
may not be absolutely necessary that the
cement should adhere perfectly to the
side of the cavity to retain the inlay in
position. If the cement does not perfectly adhere to the cavity wall bacteria
will pass between. Dr. Webster has just
shown us that these bacteria may not
always be harmful, but if harmless bacteria will pass through the way is open
for others that may produce pathological
conditions.

In regard to the matter of pressure
there may be a difference in the setting
of some cements under varying degrees
of pressure, but I do not believe with
Dr. Crouse that expansion is due to and
governed by the amount of pressure, for
in some cements there is no expansion
after being under high pressure, while in
others it amounts to as much as 100 per
cent.

In regard to grinding the cement powders finer; as has been noted in the
measurements there are but few of them
in which the largest granules are less
than 1/1000 of an inch in diameter. If
they can be ground finer I think it safe
to predict better results.

I wish to thank you once more for
your kind participation in the discussion
of this paper.

The subject was then passed.

The next paper on the program was
one entitled "The Enamel, and Its Consideration in Cavity Preparation; or Ten
Years' Progress in Cavity Preparation,"
by Dr. SYLVESTER MOYER, Galt, Ontario,
as follows:

The Enamel and Its Consideration in Cavity Preparation : or Ten Years' Progress in Cavity Preparation.

By SYLVESTER MOYER, L.D.S., Galt, Ont., Canada.

IF the attendants at this great fair—black, and red, and brown, and white, from "Afric's sunny strand," from the prairies of the north, from the islands of the sea, or from the centers of select civilization—could pass in open-mouthed array before us, one glance at their grinning teeth would enable us to write the history of those teeth—fresh and perfect from the Divine hand, then unclean areas, then vitiated oral fluids, then caries.

Teeth, like men, are "born free and equal," but to a greater extent than men are they subject to environmental conditions. With them it is almost altogether a question of environment. But this environment differs in respect to different teeth and in different dentures. Look at the subjects. Open a little wider, please. Now look at them. Inhale their breaths, notice what they had for dinner; test their saliva; see the tremulous tongue, the pale gums, the congested and hypertrophied gums, the turgid, languid, lazy circulation, the crowded and irregular arches, the congenital imperfections of the enamel; and, lastly, notice the infiltrated and impregnated caverns, and filthy cesspools of fermentation and decomposition. Note, too, evidences of care and attempts at cleanliness, and in how many cases also evidences of the dentist's skill.

How does all this compare with the teeth that were at the World's Columbian Exposition in 1893? They are worse, far worse. From twenty-five to fifty per cent. worse. The environment is less favorable. Civilization is moving faster, the telephone bell startles our nerves oftener, the "turmoil, and clamor, and din" of the mad rush of business on all sides; the greater social demands—green-eyed and ambitious. All of these conditions set our teeth on edge, and for some vague reason or other produce such conditions of the fluids of the mouth as result in increased tendency to caries of the teeth.

But the operative work looks better, far better. Bridge-work is better, porcelain work very much improved, and more extensively employed. Gum massage with its wonderfully curative and prophylactic powers is calling loudly to all of us.

But the greatest and most important improvement in operative dentistry in this decade has been in cavity preparation. For ten years the search-light of modern investigation has been thrown upon the enamel, and during the same time scientific genius has been chiseling, and cutting, and dovetailing, and squaring, and building until it would appear that we have now reached the ideal.

There were two great causes that ushered in the dawn of this new era. The first was a growing realization of the fact taught us by Dr. Black and corroborated by Dr. Williams, that certain areas of teeth are "immune to decay." Furthermore that this immunity is the result of perfect cleanliness, which condition of ideal cleanliness was produced by friction, resulting from the excursions of food in mastication, the movement of the tongue, lips, and cheeks, and from artificial means, such as brushing, etc.

The second great cause was the introduction to the profession of the nathodynamometer by Dr. J. H. Patrick at the World's Fair in Chicago. A pressure of hundreds of pounds to the square inch was a revelation to us. At once we became doubtful of the permanence of our cavity margins and filling supports. Prior to this time cavity preparation was almost wholly a mechanical operation; now it has reached the scientific. Then most of us cut back to secure easy access, and until we had produced good healthy cavity walls. Now there is "extension for prevention" as well as for retention. Then we prepared cavities which when filled were of the "ball and socket" order. Now we consider the enamel rods, their direction, histological structure, support, and nourishment.

No more noble ambition can inspire a dentist than the preservation of the natural teeth, and to this end cavity preparation is today the most important consideration that confronts us. This is equally true of inlays, of metal filling, or of plastic fillings. For until some method of prophylaxis, either of massage or medication, or of both, shall have been introduced, which will so influence the oral fluids as to prevent the gelatin-forming micro-organisms from building the little habitats on the surfaces of the teeth, and which will render inert any acid to be found in the mouth, up to that

time our only recourse will be to fill the cavities of such teeth as intelligently and conscientiously as we can. With the ever-increasing tendency of the teeth of each generation to be affected by caries, we will, if we live long enough, all prepare cavities with flat bases, with parallel walls, having steps and definite angles. We will carry the gingival margin under the gum line, level the peripheral enamel margin or cavo-surface angle, and gradually but surely more and more apply the principles of "extension for prevention."

All of these considerations may be observed, however, and the filling be very short-lived. The enamel rods must be considered, their histological structure, formation, direction, support, and nourishment. For if they are not, the filling, whether of gold or amalgam, will be liable to leak in a very short time. Unless we in addition leave the enamel prisms supported by healthy dentin and nourished at their basal extremities through its tubules, the prisms will either break away through the stress of mastication, or the intercolumnar cement will sooner or later lose its vital cohesive force, disintegrate, discolor, and the rods will crumble from their settings and drop out. Dr. Noyes is not far wrong when he says, "The enamel wall is no stronger after the filling is inserted than it was when the cavity was empty." This is true to a greater or less extent of all classes of cavities. All are surrounded by long, thin, irregularly formed five- or six-sided enamel rods cemented together, but not so firmly but that they may be easily separated. These rods have one end resting upon the dentin, the other extending to the surface of the tooth. With our chisels or cleavers we almost unconsciously learn to feel for their directions. Some are comparatively straight, and are easily cut or split apart; others are very irregular, interlaced, twisted about each other like gnarled wood, and therefore very hard to cut. You are all familiar with these different conditions. You meet with them every day. Ten years ago we referred to teeth as being hard or soft. We now speak of the histological structure of the enamel.

We will now consider the enamel surrounding pit and fissure cavities, commencing with those on the occlusal surfaces of bicuspids and molars. The peculiarity of the direction of the rods is their inclination toward the fissure. Elsewhere, with slight modifications, they stand at right angles to the surface of the tooth which they indicate, their inner ends pointing toward its center. The treatment of the enamel in this case would be as follows: First, with a chisel cleave away the enamel rods until there are no rods left that do not rest upon sound dentin. Next, the wall must be planed away until its margins lie in the axial plane. Then with a chisel—and a chisel only—slightly level the cavo-surface angle to prevent injury to it during the impact of the filling material. A glance at the enamel walls of the cavity thus prepared convinces me that they are left as strong as the hand of man can shape them. And it is necessary that this should be so, for the cavity margins here are subject to almost incomprehensible masticating stress; a pressure of a hundred pounds or more, sufficient to roll away or crush any unsupported enamel prism, may be suddenly pressed upon them. Cavities on the lingual surface of the upper incisors require special caution in preparation. Owing to the great danger of reaching the pulp, all cutting should be done with suitable chisels and hoes. Here the enamel rods incline more

and more as they near the incisal edge. So great is the inclination in large cavities that either the enamel margin will be weak or the fillings undesirably thin. If you remove all short rods by beveling the cavo-surface angle, you "hang on one horn of the dilemma." If you do not remove them, you hang on the other. How then, should they be prepared? This is the only case where the preparation of the enamel walls should be influenced by the material with which the cavity is to be filled. If for gold, leave no short rods. The thin margin of the gold will not chip. If for a plastic filling, it is advisable to cut the walls more nearly parallel, in order to have the margins of the filling as strong as the circumstances of the case will permit.

The only other class of pit cavities are those found in the occlusal half of the lingual and buccal surfaces of molars. The enamel in these presents little difficulty in preparing. Where the cavities are small, the enamel rods surrounding the cavities will always be very nearly perpendicular to the surface of the tooth, and parallel with the general direction of the cavity. In cases where the cavity extends so far toward the occlusal surface as to involve enamel rods whose inclination toward the occlusal surface is so great as to render the margin of the filling too thin to be considered permanently serviceable, it is advisable to open up the buccal groove, carrying it through the marginal ridge to the occlusal surface, leaving the base in the form of a step. Should the cavity thus formed extend to within the inner third of the occlusal surface, pass through the central fissure, and place the margin where it can be easily smoothed and finished, and where the friction of mastication will keep it clean, and thus free from the recurrence of caries. In considering smooth-surface cavities I shall take first those formed on the gingival region of the buccal and lingual surfaces of teeth, and then those formed upon the approximal surfaces.

Labial and buccal cavities begin very near the gum margin, where we find the enamel softened and broken in spots. We find also a growing area of uncleanliness, making greatest progress along the line of the gum margin.

Technique. Open with chisel, shape with inverted cone burs, and finish the enamel walls and cavity margin with a chisel. By extending the margin sufficiently far in all directions, the gingival border will be perfectly protected by the gums, while the open outline of the cavity will be kept clean by the friction of mastication, together with the friction of the lips, cheeks, and tongue.

Buccal cavities present similar conditions and environments, and require similar treatment.

The enamel margins of cavities in the approximal surfaces of incisors and canines require careful consideration. There must be judicious "extension for prevention." There must be extension for retention, a contact point for the filling, and sufficient thickness of the enamel for the proper preservation of its color. But here, as before, the consideration of the enamel rods is of first importance.

In the past it has been generally believed that the frequent recurrence of caries at the incisal margin of an approximal filling was due to insufficient care in the restoration of the contact point between the teeth. But after an examination of many such cases, and of the nature of the recurrent caries, my investigations lead me to conclude that

for every failure resulting from incorrect contact there are five failures the result of improper treatment of the enamel walls and peripheral enamel margins. The vulnerable points are at the gingival and incisal margins of the filling. If the former is extended back beneath the gum margin, it will be protected from decay. If the incisal margin is extended well past the contact point, we find that we shall involve rods that incline sharply toward the incisal edge of the tooth. If you square up this wall with a bur, you leave a corner of many rods unsupported by dentin, which will either become loosened by the impact of filling the cavity or later become dislodged by the stress of mastication. The result in either case is a deep, narrow cavity, as the first indication of failure.

In case an approximal cavity in an incisor approaches so near to the incisal edge as to leave no dentin to support the incisal angle except that which is detached from the main body of the tooth, or in case the cavity margin reaches the incisal edge, it is as a rule folly to depend upon the enamel for support. Drilling for anchorage between the labial and lingual enamel faces near the junction of their incisal edge is sometimes the only treatment of the angle that the circumstances of the case will permit, yet in the majority of cases the permanence of such preparation is very uncertain. When possible, therefore, recourse should be had to the dentin for additional retention and support, by building around them a band of gold of sufficient thickness to withstand any reasonable force that they may be subjected to. This is done by cutting back the enamel to the distal groove sufficiently to expose the dentin, known as the Johnston cavity, or by cutting away the incisal edge of the middle lobe of the tooth as recommended by Dr. Black. The former is more esthetic, the latter more likely to be permanent. In either case the gold is anchored in the groove composing the step in the dentin, and being built over the freshly exposed face of the enamel, forms a protection for it.

Let us consider the case of a typical approximal cavity on the surface of a bicuspid. In the past more fillings failed in this class of cavities than in any other. The future will, I am convinced, give better results. Ten years ago most of us would have separated these teeth, opened into the cavity, removed the decay, softened the dentin, and filled the cavity. Now we cut away more sound dentin and firm enamel than is required in any other class of cavities.

Preparation. Chip away as much enamel with a chisel and enamel hatchets as is possible. Then with a very small inverted cone bur cut through the marginal ridge and on through the central fissure, widening and perfecting the walls and margins as in previous cases.

When the approximal cavities in molars are large we frequently find the lingual cusp more or less undermined and very much weakened. In such cases it is better to cut back the enamel to the disto-lingual groove and toward the gingival margin until sufficient strength is found. Since the enamel of teeth from which the pulps have been removed loses much of its cohesive strength, the enamel plates cannot stand the stress of mastication. A filling inserted under such conditions, where the approximal cavities are large, will not long stand the stress of mastication. The more permanent treatment in such cases is to remove the whole of the enamel covering on the occlusal surface to a point beyond the marginal ridge, and then mastication force will thus all be upon the filling material.

In the treatment of the enamel surrounding all other variations and peculiarities of cavities, the rules laid down in the cases considered should be followed and applied.

In presenting this paper I have especially endeavored to emphasize the following points:

(1) That all enamel rods should be supported by sound dentin.

(2) That the enamel walls must be cut back, so that the stress of mastication will not bear too heavily upon them.

(3) That enamel which has lost its pulpal nourishment, either from the death of the pulp or from disconnection with it, will be weakened by the disintegration of the intercolumnar cement.

(4) That no enamel is proof against all forms of caries.

(5) That enamel that is kept clean will not decay; and finally

(6) That success in filling teeth, whether with inlays, or with gold, or plastic fillings, depends to a very great extent upon the careful consideration of the enamel in cavity preparation.

Discussion.

Dr. A. E. Webster, Toronto, Canada. As I take it, the important point in deciding what to do in dealing with decayed teeth is the general condition of the oral cavity. Second, the force to be applied in ordinary mastication to that tooth after the filling is in place. Third, the application of the filling to the cavity. These three things I think primarily decide the place of the enamel margin and the treatment of the enamel margin. They were beautifully illustrated at the clinics this morning. Every operator judged the condition of the mouth as to the location of his enamel margin, and judged also the force to be applied to the enamel margin. In one instance I heard the criticism offered that the enamel margin was not in the right location. Immediately the answer came, "There is no occluding tooth." That settled it. That had to be taken into consideration in the preparation of the cavity. There is always a difficulty in applying a metal filling, such as gold, to an enamel margin. Many have found that a perfect margin before the filling is in has been destroyed by the application of the gold to the margin. In such cases the margins are usually not as firmly supported by the dentin as they should be. There are cases wherein for esthetic reasons the enamel is not thoroughly cut away and to which it is difficult to apply gold. These are failures nearly always, sooner or later. There are perhaps more failures behind those walls in their preparation than in any other we attempt. Soon after the filling is made, after an interval of a month, or a year, a dark line will appear behind the enamel. In such cases, where the enamel is very thin, it is probably advisable to put something behind it or cut away more enamel.

Dr. EDWIN T. DARBY, Philadelphia, Pa. I will just say a word and I want to say it as a compliment to those gentlemen, not because they have not discussed the paper but perhaps because they do not need to discuss the paper. I take it those gentlemen are all reading men, they keep up with the literature of the profession, and I hope every one has read Dr. Johnson's paper on "Preparation of the Cavity for Filling." I think the dental profession is awake to the importance of the proper preparation of the cavity

before introducing gold; certainly the essayist has emphasized the importance of thorough preparation of cavities in connection with filling of teeth. I do not believe that intelligent men—and I take it that all men who come to this congress are intelligent men—fail to understand what is the more recent method in regard to the preparation of cavities. It is true there is a difference of opinion as to the extent of cutting that should be done— how much or how little the enamel margin should be cut away—and there may be an honest difference of opinion, but I think the men understand that they cannot prepare cavities as they did in former times and get as good results as they can get by preparing cavities as they are prepared by our best men of today. We had an object lesson this morning in the clinics that were given in the preparation of cavities, and no greater compliment could be paid to the men who gave clinics than to say that their operations were as fine as could be found anywhere in the civilized world. Operations were made there this morning that any dentist of America or Europe, or any place on the face of the earth, might justly be proud of.

Dr. W. R. CLACK, Clear Lake, Ia. We who live in agricultural communities know that the raising of bumper crops frequently so exhausts the soil that it becomes almost worthless; but I am glad to know that the soil that produced a Johnson and a Thornton is not too exhausted to produce other minds that are taking up the work along the same lines. I believe that men now beginning the study of dentistry will never be content to plod on in the old way. They will ever be reaching forward to that which is better and best in their chosen profession. Men who observe are already studying this matter of enamel margin. It was a stumbling block in my path for years. I hope I have gained some light and may be able to see the fillings I have made within the last few years stand on those margins. But I believe it is better to err on the side of safety. I think the cautious operator—understand, I do not say the timid operator—cares for those enamel margins and protects them from stress, so they will carry their load.

Dr. SYLVESTER MOYER (closing the discussion). I wish to thank you all for your kind discussion of my paper. I also wish to add my commendation to the clinics given this morning. It was the finest lot of work I have ever seen. All

of the cavity preparation was after my own heart. I wish to emphasize and repeat the great importance of carefully constructing the enamel margins. I find there is a great tendency to be a little careless, and if you were to ask me if I always prepare cavities with the care indicated I would have to tell you I do not, but the more nearly I approach to this ideal the more my conscience pats me on the back and the better pleased I am with my work when completed.

The next order of business was a paper entitled "Success and Failure in Operative Dentistry," by Dr. FRANK L. PLATT, San Francisco, Cal., as follows:

Success and Failure in Operative Dentistry.

By FRANK L. PLATT, D.D.S., San Francisco, Cal.

OPERATIVE dentistry may be defined as embracing all that part of dental science not concerned in the replacement of the loss of the natural teeth or the correction of their irregularities. For the purposes of this paper, however, the subject will be confined, so far as success and failure are concerned, to the ordinary and most frequently performed operations of dental surgery.

To properly define failure in any undertaking or application of science it first becomes necessary to decide what constitutes success, for when this has been determined failure is simply its antithesis.

The fundamental object of operative dentistry is the conservation of the natural teeth, either by prophylactic, hygienic and therapeutic measures, or the replacement of lost tissue with crowns or fillings.

The scope and purpose of operative dentistry being defined, we come at once to the consideration of what constitutes a successful operation.

The teeth under normal conditions, as evidenced in animals and savages leading a natural life, were no doubt primarily intended to perform their various functions throughout the life of their possessor, but as we are considering the teeth of civilized man allowance must be made for the degeneracies resulting from the habits, customs, and institutions of our civilization, for we have so far departed from natural modes of living that few individuals reach the age of maturity, and fewer still reach middle life or old age, without suffering the loss of one or more teeth as a result of dental disease, or without having had recourse to operative dentistry in one or more of its various branches. As it is impossible for the human race to revert again to savagery, or to recover at once its earlier vigor and freedom from disease, so it is equally impossible to remove by any operation the primary cause of degenerate and diseased conditions. We may successfully remove the local and exciting causes of dental disease, or replace with substitutes lost dental tissue, but as we cannot change or modify the diathesis which is the predisposing factor in each individual instance it is only logical to assume that the cause which first led to the disease may cause its recurrence. So, while it is quite possible that the predisposing cause of dental disease may be combated, and in a measure overcome by a continuous course of prophylactic treatment, it is not fair to say that dental operations should last indefinitely, nor is it just to assume that a given operation performed on different patients will give uniform results, for there must always be taken into consideration the predisposing personal diathesis, and also the habits, occupation, temperament, and age of each individual, and the circumstances and conditions governing its performance. As there are, however, certain objects to be attained in every dental operation, such as the relief of pain and the restoration of the usefulness and appearance of the teeth, a successful dental operation may be defined as one which under given conditions is productive of the most nearly ideal results in each individual case.

Under this definition there is at once presented to the mind of the careful, conscientious, thoughtful operator a vast field of study relating to the general and local conditions governing each case presented for treatment, and including the selection, preparation, and use of materials, the condition and adaptability of instruments, and the results it is hoped to achieve by operative procedure. All these considerations are essential to the successful practice of dentistry, and the operator who slights any of them, or adopts methods of empiricism, will sooner or later find he has been courting defeat and failure.

Much has been written on the bacterial origin of caries, on chemical action in the oral cavity, and the effects of habit and environment, but there is another point from which the failure of operations may be viewed, a point with which the dental profession has much to do and which reveals a state of affairs as deplorable as it is unnecessary. Every profession, trade, or general occupation is governed more or less by precedent, but there is no reason why the dental profession should adhere as tenaciously as it does to the unhappy precedents established in its earlier days or which have resulted from the unfortunate application of the rules of trade to a profession which should never have known their influence. The standard of value for dental services should not be fixed, as it too often is, by the cost of the materials employed, but should be in accordance with the actual results of the service rendered and the amount of time and skill required in its performance.

Experience, experiment, and scientific study have established rules for the preparation of cavities, the general principles of which are correct; filling materials have been the subject of countless experiments, and their virtues and failings carefully determined; instruments in almost endless variety have been devised for the preparation of cavities and the insertion of filling materials; calcareous deposits on the teeth have been the subject of much study, and their origin, chemical constituents, effect on tissue, and removal have been taught and illustrated extensively; artificial crowns in great variety and of varying value have been devised and their manufacture and application have been freely given to the profession; pulp-cavities have been treated and filled in countless millions, by numberless methods and with an endless variety of materials; and the history, development, and application of all these things is free and easily accessible to anyone who will read dental literature. When many men of many minds are interested in a common pursuit there will, of course, be a diversity of opinion regarding the best means of reaching a desired end, but as to the object to be attained and the general principles governing its accomplishment there is usually but little room for argument. Under such conditions it is reasonable to expect fairly uniform results from the operations of men specially trained and educated in all the principles and intricacies of dental surgery, yet our daily experience must lead us to believe that something is lacking in the system of operative dentistry as it is practiced to-day, for it is undoubtedly true that a large portion of the time of the average practitioner is spent in remedying the untimely failure of operations performed by himself or his contemporaries.

Leaving unconsidered the work of those who fasten their faith on a single method or material, for they are too hopelessly conservative to demand attention in a liberal age, we may study with interest the conditions presented in the mouth of an average patient who has suffered from a variety of dental ills and at the hands of a number of different operators. Here we may find a few fillings of gold or amalgam to which the patient points with pride as he says, "Old Dr. A did that work fifteen years ago, and I guess it's all right yet," a supposition which an examination proves to be correct; and we will further find that the cavities in which these fillings were placed were well prepared, perhaps not just up to the latest ideals of "extension for prevention," or the "prevention of extension," as the case may be, but with firm, smooth margins extending to the extremities of the fissures and compassing all that portion of the tooth involved by caries. We will find also that the fillings were well condensed, a feature which is essential to either gold or amalgam fillings, and they were also well finished.

Further conversation may develop the fact that "The old doctor charged an awful price for his work, but I guess it was worth it," all of which is food for thought as we continue our examination and find gold, amalgam, and oxyphosphate fillings undermined with decay, with rough surfaces and overhanging edges, in imperfectly prepared cavities whose margins have not been sufficiently extended, and from which the carious dentin has not been thoroughly removed.

We may also discover an ill-fitting crown, perhaps brazenly proclaiming its presence on an incisor or canine tooth, and we will undoubtedly find between the upper molars and on the lingual surfaces of the lower teeth rich deposits of calcareous matter and the usual débris of the oral cavity. Inquiry will reveal the fact that the teeth have not been cleaned for many months or even years, though several operators may have been consulted regarding other matters, and that most of the work has been hurriedly and cheaply performed and very obviously with no regard whatever for the established principles of cavity preparation and the proper selection and manipulation of tooth-conserving materials.

The patient will also be found to be almost totally ignorant of the methods and materials to be employed in the proper daily care of the teeth and of an intelligent appreciation of the true value of the various services which have been performed.

This is no idle picture, but one with which all of us are familiar, and it certainly does not bear out the frequent boast of the "wonderful progress" of dental science.

The conditions enumerated disclose the fact that the operations which succeeded were performed by a careful, conscientious operator, who demanded and received a fee commensurate with his skill and his integrity, and which permitted him to do the work as well as he knew how, while those which failed were executed by those who prostituted their art, their knowledge, and their skill to the god of mammon, and who signally failed in their duty to their patient, their profession and themselves.

It is not the lack of well-established theory or the fact that dental education is difficult to secure, nor is it always the lack of understanding which leads to failure, but it is a lack of moral courage and professional integrity, a lack of sufficient will power to overcome the evil precedents seemingly engendered by an unholy thirst on the part of the public for something cheap and of an equally unholy willingness on the part of the profession to give it to them.

Success cannot be universally attained, nor failure everywhere prevented, but the present condition of too prevalent failure may be modified by teaching our students and the members of our profession not

alone the correct principles of operative dentistry, but also the importance of educating the public to an intelligent appreciation of the actual value of skilled services and the part they must take in the care and preservation of their teeth; and above all our colleges, our societies, and our journals should teach that success, intelligence, and integrity walk hand in hand, while failure, falsehood, and deceit are spirits of evil bound together by inseparable ties.

Discussion.

Dr. C. S. STOCKTON, Newark, N. J. I didn't expect to discuss this paper at all, but there are some points which I should like to mention in this connection. First, Dr. Palmer, the gentleman who was a few minutes ago introduced to us by our chairman, recalls to my mind some fillings put in by that gentleman many years before, simply lining the cavity with gold and the rest of the filling with tin. Dr. Webster spoke a few minutes ago in regard to the preparation of enamel surfaces that in a few months sometimes would show dark lines. It was some thirty years after these fillings had been inserted when I saw them, and not a dark line in any of them. And if the patient had lived thirty years longer those fillings would have remained the same. It was soft foil that was put against the enamel; and, Mr. Chairman, I have sometimes thought, were I called upon today to decide whether soft foil should be abolished, or cohesive foil should be abolished, and we should have to depend entirely upon one or the other of these materials, soft foil would stay if you had my vote.

Excuse me if I mention something personal. Only a short time since a patient came into my office, and after doing some work I asked "How long has it been since I put these fillings in for you?" There were fourteen gold fillings in her upper front teeth. She thought a moment and said, "Doctor, that was thirty-one years ago." I say, I wish I could have that patient here today and have you gentlemen pass upon those fillings.

Referring again to the work of Dr. Palmer, we could not fix a price upon the fillings that he put in for that patient. No matter what he charged, they would be worth it. In speaking to the point in regard to the commercial value of our work, it is incomparable; we do not as a rule get enough for our services. There are few callings in life that are so trying, so exhausting. Comparatively few of us when we get to be as gray-haired perhaps as I am, have that accumulation of wealth which the work we render to our patients and to humanity would entitle us.

Another personal instance let me give you, showing, perhaps, that we must have a little discretion in regard to the kind of fillings that we put in. A lady for whom I had done work ever since she was a little girl, married and went to Cleveland. One of her front teeth decayed and gave way. The dentist there put in a very beautiful porcelain filling; it remained in only two weeks. Now if he had filled that tooth with gold, it would have been permanent. The stress was so great that it broke out. I am a great admirer of porcelain; I do some of it when I think it will stand. I am proud of my calling; glad that I have been a dentist and able to help humanity.

The CHAIRMAN. This is an international dental congress. We want to hear from some of the far-away countries. I am going to take the liberty of introducing to this section a gentleman who has come a long way; I think you have all heard of him; I want you now to become familiar with his face—Dr. J. M. Whitney of Honolulu. I shall ask Dr. Whitney to discuss this paper.

Dr. J. M. WHITNEY, Honolulu, Hawaii. For a year Dr. Stockton and I were in the same class together, and though we sat side by side here in this meeting I did not recognize him until his name was spoken by our chairman, and doubtless he did not recognize me.

Dr. STOCKTON. My hair got gray and yours didn't.

Dr. WHITNEY. Yes; it is over thirty-five years since we separated. I started out from my college fully impressed with the great value of gold. Soon after graduation I went to Honolulu. There I found a people who had, under the careful advice of a very conscientious man, been taught to greatly appreciate the value of their own teeth; and as he had retired from practice, I entered upon his labors. There was, fortunately, no question asked at that time about what material should be used, its value, or its cost; but I was asked to do everything I knew to preserve their natural teeth. For a young man starting out these were very favorable circumstances. I had been under the training of that eminent man, Dr. James Truman, and was fortunate enough to have been invited to his house, where he gave us out of his time and energy extra clinics on gold; and thus, though we were not taught the present methods, I started out with something of a system for gold operations. During the first fifteen years

I was the only dentist there, and probably knew every white person upon those islands. During the thirty-five years' practice there I have not averaged one plate of artificial denture in a year. Now why is that? Not because of my extra skill, but because I had a class of patients who valued their teeth, and I had only to do my best and use my best efforts to keep them in position. Scarcely a week, perhaps hardly a day, passes that I do not see the gold fillings that I put in thirty-five, thirty, or twenty-five years ago. I see them apparently as good as when they were put in. I can't say this of any other material. I have used, of course, amalgam in all its various manipulations, also cement and gutta-percha, and porcelain inlay. We were taught, in those early days, inlay by cutting out from a selected tooth the form of the cavity and inlaying it. But in all these different operations everything in my hands bears the stamp of gold; and so today my work and my thought is alone in gold operations.

Dr. H. G. ATWATER, Los Angeles, Cal. I realize that success—the paper being entitled "Success and Failure"—does not always depend, in fact seldom depends, upon the education of the man, but in the heart that he puts into his work; and I must say that every word uttered in this paper I know to be an expression of Dr. Platt's heart. I have seen his actions, and I have seen his work, and I know that every moment of success he has ever had is due to the fact that he puts his whole heart in his work.

Dr. T. M. WYATT, Bentonville, Ark. Dr. Palmer's remarks in regard to soft gold struck me very forcibly. I can show fillings that I made thirty years ago of soft gold by hand pressure, and the dark lines that have been referred to are not present. I am a strong advocate of soft gold yet. I use adhesive gold, but always start my fillings with soft, letting it lap over the margins. It would not be hard for me to decide which I would discard; I would drop the cohesive, as use can make soft gold cohesive.

Dr. A. F. MERRIMAN, JR., Oakland, Cal. I should regret very much indeed to allow this discussion to pass without saying a word about Dr. Platt, who is a personal friend of mine. He has been associated with us for many years in our society work in San Francisco, and certainly the paper speaks for itself—I want to compliment it; but one reason I rise is that, after such men as Dr. Stockton and Dr. Wyatt, who has just spoken, have paid such high tribute to non-cohesive gold, I feel very much in doubt of that myself after twenty-five years. This morning I gave a clinic demonstrating a combination of cohesive with non-cohesive gold, and after my experience I am perfectly satisfied that this is the best combination for a gold filling such as will last.

Dr. G. T. EPLING, Keystone, W. Va. I would like to ask the gentleman from Arkansas, who stated that he began the filling with non-cohesive and completed with cohesive foil, if he extends the soft gold completely to the margins of the cavity?

Dr. WYATT. It depends on the roots. I work from the enamel, starting it from the side of the cavity.

Dr. EPLING. Do you allow the non-cohesive gold to overlap the enamel margins?

Dr. WYATT. Yes, sir.

Dr. H. T. KING, Fremont, Neb. I see the discussion is getting into different materials, soft gold and cohesive gold, and is getting away from what I take to be the main point in the paper, and that is the care, the industry, the energy, and faithful work in the preparation that makes a perfect filling. The gentlemen have given a number of instances of fillings put in twenty-five years ago with soft gold, from which we may infer if they had been done with cohesive gold they would not stand. Now I have fillings in my own mouth put in thirty-one years ago last June, put in with cohesive gold, with a hand mallet, not one bit of hand pressure being used except to fix the first piece in the tooth. The fillings were made entirely of cohesive gold. I want to say one word in addition, in regard to the term that we use, known as extension for prevention. If it is true that is the proper way to fill teeth, then the gentlemen who filled teeth twenty-five years ago and saved those teeth must necessarily have practiced extension for prevention; but until the time Dr. Black gave us that description, it was known by other names. Marshall H. Webb describes in exact terms the thing that we mean by extension for prevention. If gold is skilfully and carefully packed, whether it be non-cohesive or cohesive gold, a good filling will be the result, one which will save the tooth.

Dr. J. W. O'KELLY, Fort Smith, Ark. I think, after all, the greatest success in preserving the teeth by filling depends largely upon the preparation of the cavity and the material used. Some thirty years ago I filled two teeth with non-cohesive gold foil, using hand pressure, and three or four years ago I saw them and they were in good condition, while a great many I have made since have not lasted that long. I have found from experience that the secret of success in fill- ing operations is in properly preparing the cavity and properly adapting the material to the cavity walls. I believe the greatest number of failures are caused by improper marginal preparation. The peripheral surface, for instance, and the marginal enamel edge should be burnished and polished before filling. Only a few years ago I observed this. In the case of an approximal cavity I remove the decayed tissue, and then with a burnisher I break down the fragile edge all around the marginal surface, then polish well with fine paper disks. This edge sometimes looks to be perfectly sound; but in burnishing it I find I have broken down quite a lot of soft, brittle enamel. Then I take a fine disk and run over the margin to make it smooth. I find when I do this and fill against the margins with non-cohesive gold and condense it thoroughly, that the result is a successful filling.

The secretary, Dr. Geo. E. Hunt, having been called to the chair, Dr. C. N. Johnson, chairman of the section, spoke as follows:

Dr. C. N. JOHNSON, Chicago, Ill. I had not expected to take part in the discussions of this section, but I am so impressed with the purport of this paper that I beg the privilege of saying a few words. We have heard from this gentleman and that gentleman about fillings— that one lasted so many years, and another lasted so many years. We have heard this method and that method described and commended or condemned as the case may be.

Now I think that success in operative dentistry, or in dentistry generally, depends upon many factors. It is not the material alone, it is not the method alone; it is, most of all, the man himself. Let us take a certain operation—one of these operations we have been speaking about—filling a cavity in a decayed tooth. Success depends not alone upon the preparation of the cavity; but, first of all, upon a thorough study of the conditions and of the causes of that decay in the first instance. It depends upon the recognition of the principles involved in the methods of decay. I was immensely pleased yesterday afternoon with the discussion of this subject on Dr. Miller's paper. All these things which seem to be abstruse and scientific are practical when they are applied properly. It depends upon a study of the environment of the case, the condition not only of that cavity but of that tooth; not only of that tooth but the other teeth in that immediate neighborhood; not only upon the teeth but the gum tissue surrounding the parts; not only that but the condition of the saliva; not only that but the constitutional diathesis.

All these things enter as factors in this question before we ever touch an instrument in the case at all. Then after all that, it depends upon the preparation of the cavity—the placing and proper condensation of the filling material; the integrity of the mass itself; the proper finishing of the filling; and then, more than anything else, as I see it, upon proper instruction to the patient to maintain that tooth in a hygienic condition afterwards. In other words, success in dentistry means taking the patient's case into our own hands so far as we can influence that patient and recognize the conditions present, and then so change the conditions that the mouth is rendered immune instead of being susceptible to disease. That, I take it, is success in dentistry.

It gives me the greatest satisfaction to hear these testimonies from these old gray-haired men who have borne the brunt of the development of this profession of ours and who have done service for humanity these many years. I would like to know what other profession gives to humanity the same definite and practical benefit for the same compensation as does the profession of dentistry. *I* do not know of any other.

I may be pardoned for mentioning one case in regard to the efficacy of dental operations properly performed. This has no personal application; I have mentioned it in public before, but I am so proud of it coming from the profession that I mention it every time I get an opportunity. I had in my chair some years ago an old lady more than eighty years of age. She pointed to a gold filling in an upper left lateral incisor, and said, "Doctor, there is a history to that filling. That filling was placed in there before I was twenty years of age." That filling had done service for that good old mother of Israel for more than sixty years. What an accomplishment that was! The dear old soul had even forgotten the name of the man who placed it there; she remembered the circumstance of the filling being inserted, but had forgotten his name. But that made no difference; I metaphorically took off my hat and bowed my brow to the memory of the man who could do that kind of work; and that work was accomplished upon the same principles that you and I try to do good work today. Those principles are involved in close application to the case in hand—concentration of energy in our work day by day, and above all, enthusiastic endeavor to practice dentistry to the highest possibilities of a very high art. I hope that the younger members of the profession will take a lesson from the older men. That is one reason I never fail to introduce an old practitioner, if I can, to the coming generation of dentists. I hope they will take a lesson and go into their work with the same enthusiasm and the same earnest application, and follow it out to the same success that these older men have; and with our increased numbers today, with the widening out of the profession, we can accomplish something for dentistry and for humanity—something that will leave its stamp upon the community to the effect that dentistry is something more than a mere trade.

Dr. Johnson then resumed the chair.

Dr. J. A. TODD, St. Louis, Mo. Dr. Johnson has told all I want to say. I want simply to confirm in his speech the keynote of the whole situation; that is, the care that the patient gives the work. One of my patients has in her mouth seven fillings put in thirty-one years ago, six made with cohesive gold and one with amalgam as black as your hat—all in perfect condition. She is fifty-one years of age, and every one of her teeth is perfect; not a single tooth in her mouth missing or in any wise defective, that is, outside of these gold and amalgam fillings. But she has religiously taken care of her teeth, and if she lives to be a hundred years old and keeps her present mental strength she will have need of no more fillings.

Dr. B. Q. STEVENS, Hannibal, Mo. I would not like to let this opportunity pass without saying a word, as I see Dr. Palmer and Dr. Stockton present, and when I think of Drs. Taft, Eames, and Patrick, who have passed away, I feel proud of them and call them my educators. It will be forty-five years the twenty-second of this month (September) since I became a student of dentistry, and I have been a pretty careful

watcher of my work. I believe I purchased one of the first diagram books ever published, that of Dr. Allport, issued in 1865, and I have a record of my practice.

We had no cohesive gold, so my practice up to this time was with soft gold. I could fill a cavity with soft gold that would stay in all right, but it did not look well, as I could not get it full enough. Then cohesive gold was introduced and I could make a beautiful filling, but I found it soon tumbled out. Then I put them both together and I could make a durable filling and one that looked respectable. In large cavities I always use soft gold, tin foil, or amalgam for the first half of my filling, then finish with cohesive gold.

I don't think gold is always the best material to use. We have many compositions now that will save the teeth if you will remove all decomposed material from the cavity and adapt the filling well to the walls. Amalgam should be rubbed in, and when the cavity is half full forced against the walls with a piece of cotton or bibulous paper. The cements should be given time to adhere while soft. The cavity should be dry for cements, but it is immaterial with amalgam.

And finally I want to impress upon the minds of our young men that it is not the filling material that saves the tooth, but the judgment one uses in selecting the material, and the man that inserts it.

Dr. W. J. TAYLOR, Sacramento, Cal. The title of the paper, "Success and Failure in Dentistry," I believe, can be summed up on the one side by certain remarks, and on the other by remarks diametrically opposed. I think the successes in operative dentistry can be summed up as follows: First, in proper preparation of the mouth and the oral tissues before operating upon any particular tooth. Second, the obtaining of proper separation before attempting to put in the filling. Third, the proper preparation of the cavity for the introduction of such filling as may be selected. Fourth, the proper introduction of the filling material selected. Fifth, the proper occlusion of the filling after its insertion. Sixth, the best finish that it is possible to give any particular material which is used for the filling. I don't believe one can finish or polish any filling too much; we all know that the débris of the mouth will glide more easily over a smooth surface than over a rough one. Seventh, keeping the mouth in a hygienic condition after the introduction of the filling. All of the foregoing to be successful must be backed up by the enthusiasm and the conscience of the individual operator, irrespective of the person for whom the operation is performed and irrespective of the fee which is charged. If we cannot do the work so that we have a self-consciousness that the work has been done to the best of our ability, I believe it is better for us not to do it and to send the patient to some other operator.

Dr. C. L. BOYD, Montgomery, Ala. There is one point in connection with this matter of success or failure in dental operations that I believe has not been touched on, that is the handling of the patient. Now I have seen defective fillings inserted by operators who as a rule do excellent work, and it was because in those cases they were unable to properly manipulate the filling materials, owing to the fact that they could not control the patients. That is one point; but there is another and a very important one that I likewise would call to your attention, namely, the adaptation of the material, half way, we will say, from the cervical to the grinding surface, at the margins, or just under the margins, a point along which we want to anchor the material which is being used. I have seen failures at these points, or leaks, whereas at other points, at the cervical margin and at the grinding surface, and at all other points, the fillings were entirely good, no discoloration at all. Now my idea is that we all at times fail to adapt the material closely to the margins at these points, whereas at the cervical margin and at the finishing up of the grinding surface we adapt it very much more perfectly, and therefore get better results. I think that many operators lose fillings more from leaks half way from the cervical margin to the grinding surface than from defects in their fillings at the cervical margins. Success, gentlemen, depends largely, too, on an intelligent and proper care of the teeth and gums by the recipient.

Dr. W. KASSAB, Chester, Pa. After listening to the essay and the discussion, and later to the discussion by Dr. Johnson where he asks the younger men to take lessons from the older ones, it brought to me the thought of my own work and the question whether it is going to stand the test of thirty years or not. I have to confess that I do not expect some of my fillings to last thirty years. I expect *some* of them to last that long—some amalgam and some gold—but some I do not expect to last that long; and the question comes to me now, Is it because I am doing inferior work, or is it because I do not work upon the same principles that these older men do, or is the percentage of their fillings which lasted that long greater than mine? That is one thing I would like to settle with my conscience. Some of these fillings put in thirty and thirty-five years ago have lasted all this time, but how many? Then again, we seem to consider every method that we use in every aspect except that of regard for the feelings of our patients. With some patients we can do work that will last thirty to sixty years; with others we cannot. Some patients will allow us to go on and do the work in that careful and thorough manner which is so necessary to insure success; while other patients will not, on account of their sensitiveness to pain or some other reason—simply will not permit us to do work that will last more than a few years at best.

Dr. H. L. AMBLER, Cleveland, Ohio. Upstairs in this building, in the educational department, in a case, may be seen a human tooth which has three fillings in it made of tin foil, and the tooth was worn in the mouth for thirty years and there is no decay around the tin filling. A gentleman who is sitting on the stage at this moment showed me a few years ago a tin filling which had done good service in the mouth for forty years. Dr. E. A. Bogue of New York, to whom the president so kindly and feelingly referred two days since, gave me a record of a well-authenticated case of a tooth that had been filled sixty years with tin foil and worn in the mouth and had no caries around the filling.

Dr. GEORGE E. DANIELS, San Francisco, Cal. We have all been discussing methods and materials, but it seems to me there is one important phase of the subject which we have failed to recognize. We oftentimes use our utmost skill and ability, use the very best material which in our judgment will save the teeth, but we do not have the full co-operation of the patient. We lose sight of the fact that we must have his co-operation. Many patients will hinder us; they are timid, they are afraid; they perhaps do not have enough confidence in our ability to perform that particular operation, or in some way they impede our progress and thereby render that operation a failure.

Dr. S. MOYER, Galt, Ont. Someone has said, "Success in life means to do one's best." I believe that applies especially to the practice of dentistry; and in order to do one's best in dentistry three things are necessary: First, education; by that I mean dental education and all the other education that we can get. That education will come in various ways —by reading, reflection, and discussion, and all those many ways that you know of. Second, manipulative skill; and third, conscience. Now with those three equipments, education, skill, and conscience, a man will be a success; that is, he will do his best. One cannot do his best without intelligence, education, and manipulative skill; and lastly, the operator must be a conscientious man. At some time or other I have failed in each one of these three; sometimes from a lack of conscience, or at any rate a want of sufficient care. I believe these old gentlemen we have heard from today have achieved their success because of a good education combined with manipulative skill, and a conscience back of it all which urged them on to do their very best.

Dr. WHITNEY. Excuse me for making one more remark. The gentlemen here from California may remember a paper read before the State Dental Association on the subject of "Gold vs. Amalgam," in which it was stated that having placed my ledger and record books into the hands of a bookkeeper, the personal equation might be eliminated. He was asked to take at random the names of twenty-one persons who had been under my care so far as I knew for twenty-one consecutive years, and follow each filling through the whole term of years and give me the result. After the conclusion of his labors he stated that not more than five per cent. of gold fillings had failed and been replaced within the twenty-one years.

Dr. STOCKTON. Dr. Whitney has hit the nail on the head; so did the gentleman who spoke a moment ago; it is the environment of the filling that very largely has to do with success. Just take an instance in the practice of old Dr. Waters of Boston. A young man asked him to examine his teeth; he did so, and made this remark, "Your teeth are not fit to be touched with a pair of tongs," and dismissed him. A few years after that, a gentleman presented himself to Dr. Waters to have his teeth examined. The doctor carefully examined them. Said he, "There is nothing the matter with your teeth; they are the finest set of teeth I ever saw, and in the most perfect condition. The care you have given to your teeth is simply marvelous; I never saw such a fine set." "You think you never saw my teeth before?" "No, sir; I never saw your teeth before." "Are you sure, doctor, that you never did?" "Yes, I am very sure I never saw your teeth before, nor have I ever seen so fine a set of teeth." Then the gentleman recalled the instance of a few years before "when you said to me that my teeth were not fit to be touched with a pair of tongs." That was a lesson for me, and I have never forgotten it. It is very largely the environment which affects the teeth one way or the other. Fillings will come out, and is it a wonder, considering

the lack of proper care on the part of patients? Is there anything more perfectly shaped than the teeth to avoid decay and destruction? Yet they do decay, and largely because of the lack of proper care. And I say to my patients sometimes when they come back—and I speak rather unkindly perhaps—"Why don't you complain of the Creator who made them? I did the best I could, but I only patched it, and if you had taken half the care that you should of the work that I did, or the work that your Creator did for you, your teeth would have been saved." Let us impress upon our patients that the great point in saving the teeth is to keep the teeth in proper condition after they are filled. Tell them they had better go out and throw their money into the river or into the street, unless they make up their minds to take care of their teeth, for otherwise the fillings will be a failure.

The CHAIRMAN. Now, ladies and gentlemen, Dr. Palmer has consented to say a few words to you—Dr. Corydon Palmer, one of the patriarchs of the profession. (Applause.)

Dr. CORYDON PALMER, Warren, Ohio. This subject is the one I feel most interest in, and always have; I consider it the vital principle in our profession. I want to say to you that I have been around and looked carefully over everything—looked carefully at the clinics and especially at the making of gold fillings; and according to my long experience and observation and what I have tried sometimes to teach, I found that there ought to be a reform in the manner of introducing gold into the teeth, especially the incisor teeth. I saw the clinicians introducing the gold with a single round point—a straight instrument—working in one direction only and without making any lateral condensation against the sides of the cavity, proceeding in that manner to build up a tooth and perhaps the broken-off corner of an incisor. I have been accused sometimes of being dogmatic, but I am going to try the other way this time and say in all kindness that I wish operators would get in the way of employing properly shaped instruments to introduce the gold, so as to make it possible to shift the instrument to one angle and to the other of the cavity, and carry the gold into the undercuts and against the labial thin wall where it is liable to show and be defective. Do the work carefully, and do not operate with an instrument that is seven inches long, nor stand off from the work and have somebody to mallet the gold who does not see or understand the technique of the work. I want to ask you to get into the habit of shifting the instruments across the cavity, carrying the gold into the angles and against the under side of the labial wall. Fine instruments with which to condense the gold laterally should be used. Do not fill beyond the cervical border before it has been properly finished, so that it will not require any further treatment after the packing is completed. Gold is not well condensed by just carrying it in one direction with the instrument; it must be condensed laterally as well as vertically. I do everything myself, with the mallet in my own hands—always have—and I use short instruments, so that I can see what I am doing, and endeavor to do a fine thing like an artist ought. Do not get into the way of putting all this mess of stuff in a cavity—cement or tin foil at the bottom, and then non-cohesive gold on top of that, and then cohesive gold. They do not make good operations. If non-cohesive gold is used to begin the filling without being careful to properly condense it, and then cohesive gold is adapted on top of it, it will not result in a good piece of work, as such a foundation is not a safe one.

Now, I would like you to make a good, clean foundation; begin with your cohesive gold—not necessarily the most cohesive kind, that will harden too quickly; get the filling started so it will not move, and then lay the gold across the cervical border, for there is where the failure occurs. Burnish the gold against the cervical wall, and instead of working in one direction only use instruments with which it will be possible to apply the condensing force in all directions. Lay the pieces on with a flat, serrated instrument, for that will make a smoother and handsomer finish than by trying to complete the filling with a straight point on the automatic mallet. I never put a machine on a tooth in my life; I never had such a thing by me— never did. The operations and fillings that I have seen made here look well; they finish up to look well. They spent a good deal of time with those little disks smoothing them up, but they could do better if they would work in the way that I speak of. (Applause.)

The CHAIRMAN. I want to find out how long Dr. Palmer has been in the practice of dentistry. How long have you practiced, doctor?

Dr. PALMER. Since 1839.

The CHAIRMAN. I beg the audience to rise to their feet before we adjourn, as a token of respect to this aged practitioner.

The entire audience then rose with applause, to which Dr. Palmer responded with a bow and "I thank you."

The session was then adjourned until Friday, September 2d, at 2.30 P.M.

SECTION VII—Continued.

FIFTH DAY—Friday, September 2d.

THE section was called to order at 2.30 P.M. by the chairman, Dr. Johnson. The first order of business was the reading of a paper entitled "Use of the Matrix for Tooth-Restoration," by GARRETT NEWKIRK, M.D., D.D.S., Los Angeles, California.

The paper was as follows:

Use of the Matrix for Tooth-Restoration.

By GARRETT NEWKIRK, D.D.S., Los Angeles, Cal.

WE talk too much and too indiscriminately to our patients and to students about *filling* teeth. Instead of filling, a part of the English-speaking race employ the term *stopping*.

The road-mender *fills* up holes with broken stone. The baker *fills* a crust with apples, pumpkin, or cherries, and after annealing calls the product *pie*. The apothecary *fills* a bottle with a liquid invention of Satan, and *stops* it with a cork. A railroad gang *fills* the approach to a bridge where the hold-up gang may later *stop* a train.

It might be well if we could fill our minds with correct ideas, and stop the abuse of terms in dentistry. We all know that many things we say are etymologically if not logically absurd, but we go on repeating them, and shall no doubt to the end of our chapter.

We say we fill a tooth. Do we? Certainly in a sense we fill simple cavities. In a sense we stop them from the ingress of air and fluids. But suppose that the cavity is not simple. There is not a hole merely, but an extensive breaking down. Suppose a cyclone strikes a house or a shell explodes therein, knocking out one end. Suppose that in Africa half a house is honeycombed by the insidious white ant. There is not merely a broken window or a hole in the wall. In either case, the house is in part a ruin. The hole could be *filled* or *stopped*, but the broken-down house would have to be rebuilt—restored.

That is what we are called upon to do continually—to build up and to restore, not of the same materials but a substitute. The comparison fails in this, however, that the house, new or old, is hollow, while our building is quite solid; it is more like the restoration of a broken monument of cement and stone, badly shaken by an earthquake.

The tooth is not a hollow thing like a glass jar which the mother fills with jam whereby to test the honesty and self-restraint of her small boy. No, indeed. It is a piece of masonry, broken down, whereto we add, if the foundation be sufficient, that which shall keep it in perpetuity, so we hope, during the lifetime of its owner.

The restoration of these broken monuments is no simple problem. The longer we are engaged in the work, the more we realize the fact. It involves a careful and continuous study of curved lines. None of the monumental forms are square or rectangular. They possess no straight lines and no plane surfaces. For every thirty-two there are sixteen forms. But the forms on separate sides are not always duplicated, and they are always reversed in position, making different studies for the workman. But more than this, you may observe and study ten thousand sets of those dental forms; they will be divisible into types and classes, but no two sets will be alike. To all general rules there are numerous exceptions.

Our problem, be it remembered, is not alone the restoration of a form. It is not limited to a study of the one broken building. Each body of ivory and bone stands in immediate relationship with two others; except that the monuments to wisdom have but one. Those stand at the end of each row, often inclined like the leaning tower of Pisa, but not so tall. This relationship of the monuments one to another is of great importance. They were not built originally for commemoration. They were not in-

scribed, but are often defaced. They are commemorative in a sense, and they may be ornamental, but their chief reason of being is for *use*. In this use and service they act not independently, but together.

In each restoration that we undertake we have to consider, first, a firm foundation, a good dovetailing of the part we add; second, a touching surface with the next building near the roof, so that the watershed is lateral, not between; third, a free ground space for gums, not vegetation.

Dropping metaphors, we will now speak of teeth as teeth. Each one has not only the double contact noted with its fellows of the same row, but a double relationship in normal articulation with those opposite, above or below. The point of approximal contact must be as a rule close and snug, only that a piece of silk floss will pass by the natural separation of the teeth under moderate pressure. This ideal condition is reached by slight over-building, careful experiment in finishing, and determined usually by an audible click when the thread passes the contact point. As a general rule, not always, the value of our building is conserved by a restoration of the original form of the tooth. But there are exceptions, where previous losses and abnormal spaces require variation, more or less. It is a question of conditions in the individual case and of forces present. There are mouths wherein irregularities —some by inheritance, some by accident, others by bad dental practice—have so disturbed relations that special and unusual forms of building are required to secure the best results.

I am now to consider briefly the use of the matrix for tooth-restoration, according to the principle above stated.

What is the dental matrix? Essentially, a temporary wall placed for the support of building material that is more or less soft or yielding. The builder of a concrete walk or wall uses boards to hold his material in form till it hardens.

The office of the matrix is threefold: ,

First, to serve as a wall of resistance, so that under pressure the building material may be thoroughly condensed and joined to the tooth.

Second, to give the general shape of restoration, with an excess of material—for the final form must be given in the later finishing. It is only in a general way, approximately, that the concavity of the matrix can represent the convexity of the completed part.

Third, for all plastic materials that require more or less time to grow hard, the matrix is kept in position till the new body can stand alone without danger of breakage.

MATERIALS AND FORMS OF THE MATRIX.

The ideal material is that combining the most strength with thinness and spring temper. It is now the consensus of opinion that no other material possesses so many excellences as rolled or hammered steel. Rolled or sheet steel, cut into ribbons, is best adapted to general use, being uniform in thickness and convenient. Tinned copper or German silver, rolled thin, are practicable materials for band matrices, being easily measured and soldered to fit special cases; for example, where the greater part of a molar or bicuspid crown is to be built up with amalgam, and wherever it is necessary to have the whole base encircled. In such cases it is not possible to get the best adaptation of the supporting wall without making a matrix for the one in hand.

For the restorations we are most commonly called upon to make, namely, the whole of an approximating wall with more or less of the occlusal, I do not consider the band matrix an ideal form. It is better than none, as "hand-me-downs" are better than no clothes at all, but not of the highest type. The ready-made band which passes all about the crown of a tooth is essentially the section of a cylinder. True, it may be sprung this way or that to change its diameters, but the circumference of its openings remains practically the same. A tooth-form has no relation to it, and we are trying to restore tooth *forms,* not those of washtubs or tin cans.

Nearly always a band matrix made to order for the case in hand will have its basal circumference smallest, and will have to be disjointed or cut for removal. The body it incloses should hold it fast. The smaller diameter cannot pass over the greater.

A solid band matrix to be used and removed entire must be of necessity too large in its rootwise circumference or too small at the crown. If large enough to provide for the approximal contact point, it must project far into the interproximal space. There is a gap left at the cervical base between the matrix and the tooth.

Theoretically, we are told that this condition is remedied by a wedge of wood, steel, or gutta-percha at the cervical margin. Practically, it cannot be done satisfactorily. It is a confession of unfitness. It is what our carpenters call a "Dutchman"—a wedge used to brace up an erroneous gap. Being of Dutch extraction myself, I may use the illustration.

How does it work? An attempt is made to force the steel forward at the crown and backward at the root. It resists at both places and the resistance reaches all around the band. Practically, in the majority of cases, the operator does *not* attempt the wedge. He fills to the matrix as it is; the material is projecting and ragged at the cervical base. He tries to smooth it down when it is half set after removing the matrix, or he leaves it till another time. Then he tries to cut it away with chisels, files, or corundum strips, lacerating the gums and feelings of the patient; or he forgets all about it and leaves the ragged ledge, like King Henry's brow, "o'erhanging its confounded base."

Perhaps the most serious objection has not been clearly stated. The edge of the matrix, when it is carried in at the first, should pass close to the tooth, between the tooth and the gum. It cannot be at first forced down midway upon the soft tissues and afterward wedged to position without injury. It should go at once where it is to stay.

The straight band matrix, jointed with screws and clamps, has an advantage, of course, over the fixed form. But every form of band matrix has this inevitable disadvantage. It comes short of the ideal in that it requires for itself the use of a second interproximal space. This involves often much difficulty of adjustment, with annoyance and loss of time; and it takes up just so much of space which is sometimes precious. It is where it is not needed and where it ought not to be. But it has continued to go there for many years on the plea of necessity that the matrix must have a rigid base of support. This apparent necessity no longer exists.

There is a man in Philadelphia who seems at times to be heaven-inspired, although he has a hard name. It is Ivory.

He knew that a matrix ought to go where it was needed, not where it was a detriment and in the way. In a dream, a vision of the night, he saw a marvelous instrument, and in his waking hours, with any amount of toil, he made his dream come true.

I know of no combination of mechanical principles in dental appliances that appeals more to my appreciation, not excepting the Perry separator. By the nicest adjustment of screw, lever, spring, and clutch, in a combination that it seems to me no other man could have imagined, the matrix finds its support along the opposing inclined planes of the tooth itself. When I discovered this instrument less than three years ago, I cried *Eureka!* And I have been crying it every day since. I have use for other forms of matrices, occasionally, but in the great majority of cases the Ivory matrix and its holder are a close approach to perfection.

A form of matrix which I cannot recommend is one widely advertised—a double matrix, consisting practically of two segments backed together and used for building up two walls at once in separate teeth. It seems to me that the principle is wrong—that one tooth should first be restored and finished, the other at a later sitting. With a quick-setting amalgam or cement, if haste were called for, the second filling could be inserted half an hour later. But one tooth at a time. Why? The teeth are not immobile, each moves slightly with any exercise of force upon it. The matrix should be fixed firmly to the tooth that is being operated upon. In the double form it is fixed to neither one nor the other. In the insertion of a single filling the material and the tooth move together as one body, and the former is in nowise disturbed. But with two teeth at once, each possessing independent motion, the material will surely be disturbed. The method is unscientific. Aside from these considerations, it is generally desirable to wedge the teeth apart slightly with gutta-percha, which is also the temporary filling during the interval between the first and second operations.

A valuable instrument for occasional use where the application of other forms would be difficult or quite impossible. is the "hand" matrix, so called I suppose because it is connected with a handle and controlled directly by the hand. Those made by myself I find the most satisfactory. Anybody can make one easily. Take any old instrument that has a sufficient body of steel for the blade—a spatula or thick chisel, for example; heat and hammer, heat and hammer, till you get it down thin. If you hammer enough you will make it tough; it will have a good spring and yet may be bent to any desired curve. No file should be used on it unless it be one that is fine and well worn.

For use, with everything in readiness for quick filling, the matrix blade is placed in position and held by the left hand of the operator. It is seldom that an assistant can manage it well. The handle is given a strong twist, so that the rootward edge is held firmly up to the cervical margin of the cavity. The opposite edge is held with equal firmness against the crown of the approximating tooth. If either or both of the teeth are at all movable a considerable separation may be obtained by this steady twist of the handle. A sense of firm resistance, too, will be experienced while pressing the material home. The separation obtained will be equal at least to the thickness of the blade, so that when it is with-drawn there will be the close contact desired.

For restoring the disto-occlusal walls of a second molar where it is sometimes impracticable to apply the dam, where the work were better done quickly, and for incisors in making large restorations with cement, the hand matrix is a very useful instrument.

A FEW DETAILS AS TO MANIPULATION.

Success with the matrix often depends very much on previous preparation. Deep-seated cavities are frequently bordered by swollen, sometimes overhanging gums. It is nearly always better, after a free opening and more or less of preparation, to let these carry a filling of gutta-percha for days or even weeks. It is not unusual with me to have in one mouth six or eight of these gutta-percha filled cavities waiting for the matrix and restoration.

Before placing the matrix for an operation, if there is any doubt of its fitness it should be tried in tentatively to ascertain whether it will pass, as it should, close to the tooth wall and not upon the gum. Sometimes an ill-fitting matrix may be fairly adapted by pinching in the cervical edge with pliers. The Ivory matrices, however, are so shaped and may be so inclined in their introduction that they go to the right place easily in most cases.

INTRODUCTION OF FILLING.

As a rule, I believe the matrix that is governed by any screw force should not be completely tightened at the beginning, whatever the material used, but should be after insertion of a third to one-half of the filling. And without doubt we may say that the great majority of operators do not take sufficient pains with that same first one-third. Of amalgam altogether too much is likely to be placed in the cavity at the start. Smaller pieces should be introduced at first and thoroughly condensed with smooth instruments all along the cervical wall and its junction with the matrix. This takes so much time with me that often a second mix of quick-setting amalgam is required to complete the operation. Often with extra dry alloy I have my assistant use the mallet.

In the second half or last third of the filling, whatever the material employed may be, enough force should be exerted against the matrix to induce separation of the teeth by a space not less but more than the thickness of the band. If the teeth have been prepared by guttapercha wedging, as above suggested, this necessary crowding apart is an easy matter. As before stated, there ought to be an excess of the new material to allow for final shaping, and there ought to be likewise a separation of the teeth at the completion of the filling beyond the normal. This to allow the final contact point to come slightly below and away from the border of the occlusal surface, as it ought, otherwise the contact point is a mere edge continuous with the occlusal surface, instead of being the rounded, finished knuckle of nature's plan.

There would be an improvement at this point, no doubt, if we were all to take the pains to make in each matrix a sufficient concavity, as we might with contour pliers, to bring the filling nearer to the ideal form. As it is, with any common form of matrix, the filling as the band leaves it shows only a straight profile from the cervical to the occlusal edge.

Every contoured matrix, however, would have to be left in position till the filling should be perfectly set. It could not be easily removed, like the straight band.

MATRIX REMOVAL.

With amalgam there are, as we know, advantages to be gained by leaving the matrix *in situ* till the material has become hard. In many cases it is necessary where the reconstruction has been extensive and the basal support relatively weak. The specially made band matrix of true form must be so left. But on the other hand, there is something to be gained by immediate removal. This is one of the advantages of an open matrix like the Ivory. When the clutch is loosened it lets go. It is readily straightened, being flexible, and touches the teeth only at the point of contact. With the lightly oiled surface a band should always have it is easily removed by gentle manipulation. Then, with a properly shaped blade, half knife, half burnisher, a trimming and close condensation of the material may be made all along the edges. I believe that perfect borders can be made in this manner with greater certainty than is possible otherwise.

The matrix is an indispensable instrument, but it has one inseparable disadvantage. We must acknowledge the truth that in relation to certain important margins we are working in the dark. There is no man living who can insert a matrix filling and leave it with the same mental certainty as to the integrity of all margins that he would have by visual or tactile exploration of those same margins.

And this brings me to the question that I wish to consider briefly in closing.

EMPLOYMENT OF THE MATRIX FOR GOLD
RESTORATIONS.

Undoubtedly there are a few operators
who can apply the matrix to a deep-
seated cavity and make good fillings from
start to finish. But I believe that in
general it involves a good deal of risk.
I am frequently called on to renew or
repair fillings that I have reason to think
were so inserted, that have failed at the
cervical or cervico-buccal or cervico-lin-
gual borders. I find others that are
spongy, or pitted, or grooved in those
places.

We know what the bevel of a margin
should be for gold; we know that for the
proper condensation of gold over such
a margin an adapted instrument must
have *free play*. We know that it is better
to have visual as well as mechanical access to the lines involved. If we have a
loose adjustment of the matrix along the
border, of what use is it? It is likely to
crowd unduly on the gum tissue, to draw
on the edge of the dam, and induce leakage. If it is *closely* adjusted, the matrix
with the margin forms a sharp, acute
angle into which the gold must be forced
accurately and condensed, or else there
is a weak line of union. I repeat that
it is risky. You do not know with the
same degree of certainty that you would
without the matrix. If science be knowledge the method is unscientific.

But after a body of gold has been
placed along the basal margin and angles,
then the matrix may be placed and of
service as a guide to the general form of
building, and of value especially for the
full extension and thorough condensation of the "knuckle" at the contact
point.

As a last word, I do not remember to
have seen a recommendation of the matrix in connection with gutta-percha fillings. Aside from those cases where it
is necessary to crowd away the gum for a
subsequent operation, the margin of a
gutta-percha filling should be carefully
made like any other. Patients suffer .
much discomfort and sometimes real injury from carelessly made gutta-percha
fillings. A matrix, especially the "hand"
form, is here valuable. It is better to
make the filling of form to begin with
than to crowd in an ill-defined mass to
be trimmed up afterward. If this be
done by warm instruments the heat is
likely to cause pain or discomfort, and it
is not easy to do the work well with sharp
and cold blades.

If you have not tried the matrix for
gutta-percha, you will thank me for the
suggestion when you do try it.

Discussion.

Dr. J. M. WHITNEY, Honolulu, Hawaii.
All must agree with the proposition that
for plastic fillings the matrix is almost
indispensable. Our only disagreement
lies in its use for gold. I think the cause
of this lies chiefly in the different ways
in which operators prepare the cavity,
and in the shape of the instruments employed in filling. We must ever bear in
mind that the cavity is to be filled by the
use of the matrix. Its cervical portion
should be at right angles to the tooth;
its lingual and buccal sides carved well beyond the zone of danger and made flat—
that is, not grooved or undercut, with the
borders cut to an obtuse angle. Cut from
thin rolled steel a strip of proper width,
curve it to form proper contour, and with
a matrix holder—such as Ivory's or one
regulated with screw and wrench, having
two double inclined sides with lower

points extending considerably beyond the upper—screw it firmly between the teeth until you obtain the proper width for the contour, if the teeth have not previously been separated. Lay the foundation of the filling with soft gold; mallet with a large flat-surfaced plugger, afterward with small flat surface. Begin with cohesive, using for borders small round-faced plugger (Royce's most nearly meet the requirements), being sure that the instrument carries the gold directly before it to the outer border where it strikes the curve of the matrix.

Our essayist says never use the matrix in but one tooth at a time. Now, with regard to this point, my invariable practice for the last fifteen years and more has been, where both approximal surfaces are defective, to prepare each tooth as before described, placing two curved matrices between them, and screwing the matrix holder firmly to place. This thoroughly protects the gingival space. Build gold or whatever material be used evenly in each tooth, giving each just the desired contour. These have been to me my most satisfactory operations. On removing the matrices be careful to see that the cervical borders are trimmed, which in my hands is best done by a thin, sharp instrument, that cuts off any projecting gold much more satisfactorily than carborundum tape. The remainder of the filling or fillings are easily and quickly finished with the usual tape. If any danger exists of flattening the contour, place a Perry separator and open a trifle. I have failed to see any serious objection to the use of the matrix when gold is to be employed as the filling material.

Dr. H. W. ARTHUR, Pittsburg, Pa. Having advocated the use of matrices of one form and another for years, I have been especially interested in knowing how the practice could be so summarily disposed of as the title of this paper would indicate. We are told "it is a dream." The form of matrix that will simplify the filling of cavities on the approximal surfaces of bicuspids and molars is most in demand. There is a difference of opinion as to whether a matrix should be rigid or flexible, or as to whether it should be closely wedged to the margins.

My practice has been to use a flexible piece of sheet steel, about 24 gage, shaping it so that it would not impinge on the gum tissue to the buccal or lingual surfaces, extending well beyond the margin at the cervical border and around the embrasure of the tooth to the buccal and lingual surfaces, with a lip bent over to rest on the marginal ridge, mesial or distal, as the case may be, of the approximating tooth. My practice is to wedge the matrix close to the margins at the cervical third, having it more or less free at the middle and occlusal thirds. The wedging may be accomplished with the "dream" of the author of this paper, or with simple orange-wood properly shaped and slightly moistened with sandarac varnish. I contend for this practice that the filling material can be adapted with such exactness at the cervical third that it will require but little more than a strip and trimmer to complete the operation at that point. The yielding of the matrix middle and occlusal thirds assures contour and approximal contact without special wedging. The buccal and lingual margins above the cervical third can be readily approached for finishing the contour and approximal contact. The holes punched in the buccal and lingual wings of the matrix afford a ready means for removing the tightly wedged matrix. The lip resting on the marginal ridge prevents rocking, also the driving of the matrix on to the gum.

Dr. A. F. MERRIMAN, Oakland, Cal. We see cases where it is necessary to wedge the matrix, and in other cases where we use cohesive gold it is better to allow a slight giving of the matrix, so that before the matrix is removed it will be possible to burnish the gold around the borders of the cavity.

In the condensation of the gold we should begin at the center and work toward the periphery. In many cases where we have not had the opportunity to watch our patients carefully we find, because of failure to use the proper instrument, after the matrix is removed and the burnishing accomplished that it becomes necessary to wedge again in order to get separation to complete the filling.

Dr. W. KASSAB, Chester, Pa. I would like to speak more with reference to amalgam than to gold. My experience with gold has not been so successful. About three years ago I had an amalgam filling placed in a lower molar in the approximal surface, and the matrix was used with a wedge. While I was having the filling inserted the thought came to my mind, Instead of having one wedge on one side why not have two wedges, one on each side? and I therefore used the Ivory separator, the one that has two fingers; the end of each is shaped like a wedge. I placed it between the matrix and the adjoining tooth and wedged it a little, and I have since come across nothing that has answered my purpose so well; I have become very enthusiastic over it and wish others would try it. It may cause the patient a little pain, but if you will whisper to him that it will make a much better filling, and with the steady pressure that is exerted, the patient will

forget the pain. Before taking the matrix out it should be pressed against the filling all around the edges, then with two fingers it can be removed without injuring the filling.

Dr. JOHN I. HART, New York, N. Y. The instrument described by Dr. Whitney has been also suggested by Dr. Dickinson. I have used that instrument, and I think it but right to call the attention of this body to it. The Dickinson instrument wedges the teeth to be filled to quite an extent, so that it produces practically a "knuckling" of the filling against the tooth immediately next to the one that is to be filled. There is little if any pain in the placing of the matrix, and it holds it in firm contact with the tooth that is being filled. The essayist suggested not screwing the matrix at the start as tight as he does later in the operation, and that is the only point I find to criticize in the paper. I think if there is any time when we should have the matrix in close proximity with the tooth to be filled, it is at the time we are filling around the cervical portion of the cavity. I think after that there may be no objection to slightly relaxing pressure, but at the start of the filling I believe the matrix should be placed as firmly as possible.

I think the discussion of this subject would not be complete without referring to the matrix suggested by J. F. H. Hodson of New York city, which permits of knuckling a filling as probably no other matrix will do. It consists of a strip of thin steel from which the temper is removed, and while in this soft state it is struck a few times with a round, smooth instrument which "oranges" the matrix, as the doctor describes it, and gives it a rounded surface similar to that we see on an orange. Two holes are then punched in the steel margins or smooth parts so that it may be readily engaged for removal and the matrix placed in position. If there is an adjoining tooth it is held firmly, but if it is not as tight as I desire at the cervical portion, that can be fastened or wedged. This form of matrix permits the shaping of the matrix for every operation.

Dr. N. A. NEELBY, Christchurch, New Zealand. I would like to explain a little wedge I use with the matrix. I take a piece of steel, about 30 gage, cut a strip about two lines in width, and bend it into a V shape; with this I wedge the matrix on one side where it strikes the adjoining tooth, and with the other I wedge the matrix in position. In this way I hold the matrix firmly in position. Of course, in different positions I would use a different thickness of steel, but usually it separates the teeth considerably.

Dr. Newkirk not being present to close the discussion, the subject was passed, and the chairman called for the next paper on the program, entitled "Tin-Cement and Sponge Tin: Two New Filling Materials and Their Use in Dentistry," by Dr. ARTHUR SCHEUER, Teplitz, Bohemia, Austria, as follows:

Tin-Cement and Sponge Tin: Two New Filling Materials and Their Use in Dentistry.

By Dr. ARTHUR SCHEUER, Teplitz, Bohemia.

A YEAR ago I published in the *Oster. Vierteljahrsschrift für Zahnheilkunde*—the Austrian dental quarterly —the method of preparation of a material which I called "sponge tin." This material is obtained from a solution of stannum bichloratum (bichlorate of tin by precipitation with zinc). The substances employed must naturally be chemically pure, and the precipitated sponge tin must be washed with running water until, when tested with blue litmuspaper, no trace of acidity is perceptible. This test alone is, however, insufficient; a small piece of sponge tin crushed in the mouth should not leave the slightest acid taste behind.

This result can be obtained after long and thorough washing and boiling. After every particle of moisture has been driven off by means of the drying oven, the sponge tin appears as a gray felt, consisting partly of light, dust-like tin particles, partly of metallic fibers and scales.

Sponge tin may be condensed between the finger-tips, and naturally much more readily when pressed into a cavity by means of a Solila or a Royce packer. It is of invaluable assistance in gold filling, since it may be mechanically united with, mechanically welded to any brand of unannealed sponge tin whatever.

Into the cavity, which need have no undercuts, I carelessly pack sponge tin nearly to the margin; it is quite the same whether with hand pressure or with the automatic mallet. Upon this I condense a layer of unannealed sponge gold— Watts' or Solila—then a layer of annealed sponge gold, and finish with annealed gold foil or cylinders.

My further experiments have yielded

the fact that a tin powder obtained from sponge tin when mixed with annealed zinc oxid produces a cement powder with certain qualities that render it of inestimable value in its application to dentistry. This powder is of a light grayish color, with here and there the shimmer of a fine particle of metallic tin, and may be mixed with any good cement liquid, producing a cement with far greater adhesive properties than that of the ordinary cement powder alone. This may readily be seen from the fact that the ordinary cement when it has hardened upon a metal spatula can be removed with comparative ease, whereas in the case of tin-cement it is accomplished only with the greatest difficulty.

Tin-cement is also quite remarkable for its hardness, as well as for its resistance to the wear due to attrition and to the attack of an acid saliva.

Furthermore, a ground and polished tin-cement filling, with its bright, silverlike surface, resembles a good gold amalgam filling, due to the rotation of one tin particle upon the other in polishing. Since the surface presented is practically of metal, its resistance to wear and to the attack of saliva is readily accounted for. Tin-cement fillings neither lose their own color nor do they discolor the tooth, consequently the usefulness of this material is considerably extended.

A still larger field for the employment of tin-cement is furnished by its quality of entering into intimate mechanical combination with any brand of unannealed sponge gold; and these combination gold fillings are in no particular inferior to the solid gold fillings.

The cavity should be filled nearly to the margin with tin-cement, and in the last stage of its hardening there should be condensed upon it a layer of sponge gold, unannealed, and of any brand whatever; upon this is packed a layer of annealed sponge gold, and the filling is finished with annealed gold cylinders or foil.

All this is done so rapidly that it can be completed in one-third the time required for a solid gold filling of equal size. And how precious is every minute to the busy gold operator, not to mention the saving in the amount of gold used!

If I call your attention further to my method of simplifying gold filling, it is because through its simplicity a faultless margin is rendered possible by the use of the materials here mentioned, especially of the tin-cement.

The cavity is prepared in the same manner as for a porcelain inlay, and the impression taken with No. 30 or 40 gold foil, this ·being well burnished to the walls of the cavity. Allow the edge to overlap $\frac{1}{4}$ to $\frac{1}{2}$ mm., and burnish carefully. If the foil at the bottom of the cavity is not torn, cut it with an excavator, fold the edges over and burnish to the walls. The bottom of the cavity should then be filled, either with sponge tin or, still better, with tin-cement, by means of which the impression is sufficiently retained in place, and that through a material which combines readily with sponge gold.

The balance of the cavity being completely covered with gold foil, the difficulty of further manipulation and completion of the gold filling is reduced to a minimum.

Discussion.

Dr. W. V-B. AMES, Chicago, Ill. In view of the fact that the essayist has furnished no data or experiments, I will pass around a bottle containing precipitate of tin, such as is described by Dr. Scheuer. He describes the tin as a precipitate. It is a powder of various grades, from a fine powder up to a crystal. In the mixture of such tin with the powder and oxyphosphate, the coarser tin, being in thin laminæ, would break into powder.

On being asked to discuss this paper I inferred from the title that the doctor had discovered some means of producing an oxyphosphate with tin oxid. This was the meaning conveyed, and it rather startled me, because I had gone through all the experiments possible with tin oxid without getting any result, so I found my task easy in discussing this paper when I found he simply meant a mixture of metallic tin and zinc oxid. I have gone through many attempts in the way of mixing such materials as this precipitated tin with oxyphosphate for this very purpose, and I must say with promising results. When I was practicing dentistry more than I am now, in my own work I made mixtures of precipitate of silver with oxyphosphate, the silver being in very much the same form, and I have seen excellent results from that, although I am inclined to believe there is something peculiar in the behavior of tin in connection with cement, especially when adopting the plan of making a filling and covering it with gold, owing to the peculiar gold-tin action. Dr. Shumway of Massachusetts told me at one time he had secured remarkable results when placing a thin veneer of cement over a tin filling, often filling the cavities of an incisor or canine nearly full of tin, and then placing a thin veneer of cement on it. He said the cement would last very much longer on a surface of tin than as a plain cement filling, and I have ex-

perimented at different times with some of this particular precipitated tin to further carry out his work in that line. I have found with an admixture of metals some very satisfactory results. The advantage comes from various sources, as I look at it. I often attempt to increase the strength and resisting power by the incorporation of various non-metallic materials, and at times it is an utter failure from the nature of the materials used, just as in the use of metals the filings or turnings will not give the result that the precipitated crystal will give. In the incorporation of foreign bodies a great deal depends upon the nature of the foreign substance.

The sponge tin I do not care to discuss; some others will be better able to speak of that than I.

In this connection, although it is foreign to the subject to an extent, I wish to speak of what can be accomplished by the admixture of materials other than the precipitated metals. Those metallic mixtures do not have a satisfactory color for the anterior teeth, so while we can use them in the posterior teeth, for the anterior we must look for something else. Here again the nature of the crystal or quality of material comes into play. I have secured a great deal of satisfaction for a few years past, especially quite recently, from the admixture of such materials as properly precipitated alumina or porcelain powders for inlay and other work. From the fact that we can obtain porcelain powders in various colors, we have in that the material which we can use to the greatest advantage for these processes, and I have found after over four years' observation of fillings in which a large amount of pulverized porcelain was incorporated with zinc oxyphosphate, that results have been brought about which were out of proportion to what might have been expected with plain oxyphosphate. I will say that it has been my experience with cement that on the occlusal surface of a molar or bicuspid it will last several times as long as upon an approximal surface of an incisor. In those cavities the destruction of the filling is brought about from the stagnation of fluids and the fermentation and putrefaction of food, but where such fillings of porcelain and oxyphosphate were put in more than four years ago, the results have been very satisfactory. I find I have made fillings which today are practically perfect, which, had they been made of plain oxyphosphate, would have needed renewal some time since. The theory, as near as I can advance it, is that the porcelain particles—after we have used about equal bulks of porcelain body and cement powder—are so near together as to make something like a very fine inlay joint, and the cement does not seem to waste to the depth of one layer of porcelain particles, so that in a short time we have a surface which is apparently all porcelain, and resembling an underbaked porcelain inlay. I myself have been deceived, having forgotten making certain fillings, and when some of these cases came back I would go to my book to see what I had done, finding that I had made one of these fillings I have mentioned. If it is as I say, that the porcelain particles are so close together as to form a very fine joint, we have a very valuable method in certain cases where we have thin walls which can be retained in that way. I have applied it in just such cases where gold had failed, and on the removal of fillings after secondary caries, I had such a condition that the walls were transparent, and operating in the way I have mentioned I have seen extremely satisfactory results in every way.

Dr. R. C. TURNER, Caldwell, Kans. I have been interested in the essay, and I have also been interested in the statement made by Dr. Ames. I would like to ask the doctor a question in regard to the incorporation of porcelain in the cement. I would like to know in what proportion he incorporates it to bring about the effect he has described.

Dr. AMES. I hope what I have said will not switch the discussion from the doctor's paper. There is a great deal of value in that, and one point is the therapeutic action that might come from the presence of the tin, so I hope this will not break into the discussion of the paper.

I do not claim that I have worked this out as to proportions. I put just as much porcelain in as I think is needed, so that it will be properly held together. I attempt to incorporate about an equal bulk of porcelain with cement powder. I do that by placing on the slab with the liquid, portions of the porcelain and cement powder. I mix the cement and porcelain, alternating in about equal proportions until I have made a stiff mix, as stiff as I can possibly make it. Make it just as stiff as you can with the spatula. Get in as much as you can of equal portions of cement and porcelain.

Dr. W. L. FICKES, Pittsburg, Pa. My experience is that any mixture of a foreign body with cement weakens it, and in mixing porcelain with cement I do not see why there should be any difference. Of course, they are closely allied chemically, and experiments have been carried on in the past to quite an extent and abandoned, but now it seems we are going back to the old experiments, and I would like to know why a mixture of cement with porcelain would be any different. I have made a mixture of cement with tin, and I find it weakens it, and I have come to the conclusion that cement is better without having anything mixed with it.

Dr. H. L. AMBLER, Cleveland, O. Strictly speaking it is not a tin-cement. That is misleading, but after the paper was read I knew what the gentleman meant. I will call your attention to a few historical facts.

In 1825 Ash of London made an extensive series of experiments in trying to produce crystals, or granules, or fibers of gold, and some of his product was put on the market to be sold as a filling material. But it was soon abandoned. In 1850, S. A. Main of Buffalo, N. Y., having probably read of these experiments, thought he could make something better and began to make experiments. The result did not meet with success, either commercially or in the hands of dentists. Two years after that A. J. Watts of Utica, N. Y., who was not a dentist, but a photographer, discovered the method of making Watts' crystal or sponge gold, which was put on the market, and with some changes is in use at the present time. As a commercial product it has been just moderately successful, and as a product for filling teeth it has been just reasonably successful. Since that time several other gentlemen up to the present year have tried to make precipitates, and crystals, and fibrous and sponge golds of different kinds, which have not been any great success commercially or in the hands of dentists.

Now if all these different products of gold that have been spoken of had been the best of anything that could possibly be made to fill teeth, why was it that from 1825 to 1904 the best operators in the world, both at home and abroad, did not abandon gold foil and use these

different products I have spoken of? Why did not Atkinson, or Webb, or Varney, and other men, throw away gold foil and take up these products? The method of producing the precipitate of tin, crystals of tin, has been known almost ever since tin was discovered. Pure tin may be precipitated in quadratic crystals by a slight galvanic current excited by immersing a plate of tin or clean strip of zinc in a strong solution of stannous chlorid; water is carefully poured in so as not to disturb the layer of tin solution; the pure metal will be deposited on the plate of tin at the point of junction of the water and metallic solution. Scrape off with a clean spatula, wash them clean, dry them, and you have crystals of tin. This is the old story over again, but I want to tell you that although this kind of product is put on the market as a filling material, it has very little integrity. These crystals I have just spoken of can be placed on the hand and with a spatula can be flattened down or rubbed nearly out of existence. Tin was put on the market in the shape of shreds by Dr. Slayton of Ohio. He made a machine for shredding tin, taking a solid bar of tin and shredding it up into a hairlike form, and then it was pressed into small mats and sold. Another form of tin is made by a similar machine which tears it up into shreds and fibers. I am bringing the history of these forms of tin right to the same date I brought the history of similar forms of gold. All these products of tin, such as crystals, shreds, precipitates, and fibers, stand in the same relation to tin foil as similar preparations of gold stand in relation to gold foil. If those preparations of tin were better than tin foil, why was not foil abandoned and those preparations taken up?

In 1859 Dr. Taft published in the *Dental Register* the methods of producing crystal tin for filling purposes, and dentists tried it for a short time, but discarded it as worthless. An electric current may be used to produce tin crystals, but they are no better than the above. There is no question that the mixing of some kind of metal filings with cement will add as a general rule to the life of fillings on an occlusal surface. Dr. Ames said he placed his mixture of the porcelain body with the oxyphosphate powder in the front teeth, and the mixture of cement with the precipitate of tin, equal parts, in the posterior teeth. I believe when you do make a mix in this way, that tin is the best metal to incorporate. I do not use powdered tin that you put on your hand and rub out of existence. I do not want the powder as fine as that, but ordinarily fine. I believe in the majority of cases the addition of the metal adds to the wearing service, and I believe as Dr. Ames does, that when a filling is worn down so that it almost presents a metallic surface, it wears longer than if made entirely of cement.

We know that cement is a poor conductor of thermal changes and electricity, and we know tin to be a poor conductor. Gold is four times as good a conductor of heat and six times as good a conductor of electricity as is tin, so with cement in a cavity where the pulp is almost exposed we still have a good non-conductor by combining it with tin. Now, if we can incorporate these two substances and make a filling for those difficult cases where the pulp is nearly exposed, I can see where it would be of great assistance to the dentist.

Dr. GEO. E. HUNT, Indianapolis, Ind. I want to say a word in regard to the admixture of amalgam and cement. If alloy is mixed with an insufficient quantity of mercury to make a homogeneous amalgam, and trituration is continued long enough, the whole mass will become a fine, dry powder. Equal quantities of this powder mixed with zinc oxid and made into a mass with the cement fluid in the usual manner make a hard and resistant material. The color is rather dark, but the filling will stand the wear of mastication, and does not seem to be affected by the fluids of the mouth nearly as much as when the amalgam powder is not incorporated.

The essayist not being present to close the discussion, the subject was on motion passed.

A paper written in French on the subject of "Preparation of Cavities," by Dr. J. D. LOSADA, Madrid, Spain, was read by title. The paper here follows:

Préparation des Cavités et Inconvénients de le "Extension for Prevention."

Par JAIME D. LOSADA, Madrid, Spain.

LA préparation des cavités est aussi importante que le placement de la matière obturatrice, et son succès dépend beaucoup de la forme de la cavité.

L'art de les préparer est difficile, car il s'y fonde sur des règles scientifiques et esthétiques qu'il faut en un instant harmoniser pour résoudre les problèmes de leur bonne préparation, que se divise en trois parties principales: ouverture, nettoyage, et forme propre de la cavité.

Dans la plupart des cas, les cavités sont visibles directement ou à l'aide du miroir. Quand il n'en est pas ainsi parcequ'elles sont approximales, il faut séparer les dents par les divers moyens connus. Quand la séparation que nous voulons obtenir n'est pas grande, nous donnons la préférence á la séparation immediate au moyen des instruments de Perry ou d'Ivory. Ce dernier qui a l'avantage d'être le moins encombrant, quoique quelquefois il gêne encore; on peut alors garder la séparation obtenue par celui-ci en ayant soin de mettre entre les dents séparées une cheville de bois d'oranger mouillée dans du vernis de sandaracque, qui empêche son glissement et nous permet alors d'enlever le gênant séparateur.

Quand l'espace dont nous avons besoin est un peu grand, nous employons presque exclusivement les procédés de lenteur, le coton serré et la gutta, proscrivant d'une façon absolue les coins en caoutchouc qui occasionnent toujours des pericementites traumatiques très douloureuses, et pendant l'acte opératoire nous conservons l'espace obtenu au moyen d'une cheville qu'a l'avantage d'immobiliser la dent, toujours plus ou moins ébranlée, et qui ainsi tenue est beaucoup moins douloureuse.

Si la gencive, comme il arrive souvent, rentre et ferme en partie certaines cavités on peut la pousser à l'aide de coton ou de gutta, mais si le mamelon est un peu grand il est préférable de l'enlever au galvano-cautère après l'avoir préalablement anesthesié à la cocaine.

Dès le début de la préparation, c'est-à-dire à l'ouverture de la cavité, nous nous trouvons déjà en face de trois règles très

importantes, fréquemment antagonistes qu'il faut concilier, donnant, d'après les cas, préférence à l'une ou à l'autre.

La première nous ordonne d'ouvrir la cavité de façon que son nettoyage et obturation soient faciles, ce qui nous oblige souvent à sacrifier une grande partie saine pour obtenir cet accès direct: la deuxième, par contre, nous oblige pour raisons d'esthétique à conserver la plus grande partie de la dent, tandis qu'une troisième nous conseille d'étendre les bords jusqu'à la zone qu'on appelle "self-cleansing," c'est à dire qui se nettoie d'elle même ou seule.

La prépondérance de ces règles au détriment des autres, dépend de la dent et de la place où se trouve la cavité. Comme règle générale dans les molaires et surtout à leurs faces distales et triturantes nous pouvons suivre avec liberté la première et troisième règles, tandis que dans les mesiales il ne faut pas oublier le deuxième pour éviter autant que possible que l'obturation ou une grande partie de celle-ce, se voie. Nous considerons ceci obligatoire pour les incisives et les canines, surtout pour les dames, et croyons qu'excepté dans quelques cas nous devons presque tout sacrifier à l'esthétique et conserver autant que possible la paroi labiale, faisant l'obturation par la face linguale. Il ne faut pas oublier que dans l'art dentaire l'acmé de l'art, c'est cacher l'art.

Je vous fais grâce de la classification des cavités d'après l'endroit qu'elles occupent et que vous tous devez trop connaître.

La facilité de l'ouverture de la cavité tient surtout de l'endroit où elle se trouve, et les instruments employés seront les fraises dentées, qui coupent rapidement l'émail et la dentine et sont beaucoup plus sûres que le ciseau qui casse plus souvent qu'on ne voudrait, quoique celui-ci et les meules soient utiles quand il faut détruire une partie relativement grande d'émail comme il arrive dans les cavités occlusales et distales.

Le ciseau doit s'employer avec précaution pour éviter son glissement dans les parties molles ou de faire sauter un morceau trop grand; l'emploi du maillet facilité l'opération. Dans les cavités occlusales des molaires, l'emploi des petites meules permet de couper d'une façon rapide les fissures et économise ainsi qu'avec le ciseau, fatigue et temps.

Une fois l'accès à la cavité obtenu, nous la laverons avec un fort jet d'eau tiède qui la nettoira de débris. Théoriquement nous devrions mettre aussitôt la digue dont les bonnes qualités sont incontestables, mais ce n'est pas toujours possible dès le début pour ne pas trop fatiguer le malade.

La digue permet de dessecher, à l'aide d'alcool et d'air chaud, la dentine que l'on rend de cette façon beaucoup moins sensible.

En général nous devons enlever toute la dentine cariée, mais dans quelques cas nous pouvons laisser une petite couche, qui recouvre la pulpe at la protège des agents extérieurs. Inutile de dire que ceci ne peut se faire que lorsque la pulpe est absolument normale et qu'il faut dessécher cette dentine et la stériliser complètement.

La méthode classique d'enlever la partie cariée, si fait au moyen d'excavateurs. Nous accordons notre préférence à ceux de Darby-Perry, avec lesquels on peut facilement soulever la dentine gâtée en couches minces en commençant du centre vers la péripherie jusqu'à arriver à la partie dure. L'excavateur permet une grande délicatesse de tact, et quand il est bien aiguisé comme il doit toujours l'être, cette opération est à peu prés indolore. L'emploi de la digue aide beaucoup car on peut mieux apprécier à sec certains détails et la sensibilité est moindre.

Aujourd'hui l'emploi des fraises est très étendu, car elles font la besogne plus rapidement mais elles n'ont pas la délicatesse de l'excavateur et font en général plus de mal.

Après avoir nettoyé la cavité, il faut la façonner de sorte qu'elle puisse retenir l'obturation pour ce qu'il faut avoir bien en compte les différentes forces auxquelles celle-ci sera assujettie et qui sont différentes dans les diverses cavités.

Comme nous avons déjà dit plus haut, il faudra souvent par raison d'esthétique nous efforcer pour rendre autant que possible, invisible l'obturation. Les parois doivent être resistantes en evitant avec soin de laisser l'émail sans une couche de dentine pour la supporter si ceci fut nécessaire et à fin de soutenir l'émail les bords devront être épais et lisses pouvant leur surface être plate ou biseautée d'après le cas.

Pendant toute la préparation de la cavité il faut avoir en compte le voisinage de la pulpe, si la dent est vivante, et il faut détruire aussi peu que possible la couche qui la préserve. Dans les dents mortes ce facteur n'existe pas et la forme rétentive de la cavité est plus facile à obtenir.

Les rainures et autres points de rétention doivent se faire aussi loin que possible de l'organe central de la dent, mais toujours dans de la dentine solide, jamais entre celle-ci et l'émail.

Pour façonner les cavités on emploie exclusivement les fraises, celles en forme de roue et cône renversé sont très utiles pour donner la forme rétentive.

Autant que possible le fond de la cavité doit être plat et les parois droites,

tandis que la ligne des bords d'émail
doivent être arrondis, evitant avec soin
les angles brusques, et il est préférable
une courbe bien grande à plusieurs
petites.

Comme nous avons dit plus haut, les
bords d'émail doivent être forts et leur
surface plane ou légèrement biseautée
aux dépens de la face interne de façon à
ce que la taille des prismes les laisse en
contact avec leurs voisins.

Pour obtenir la surface des bords, nous
croyons préférables aux fraises ordinaires
les fraises à finir les orifications, les
disques en papier émeri et certaines
formes d'excavateurs et ciseaux.

Avant de décrire la préparation de
quelques cavités typiques, nous ne pouvons passer sous silence un nouveau facteur dont l'importance est indéniable et
qui tient à diviser les grandes autorités
de l'opératoire dentaire.

Nous voulons parler de ce que nous
pourrons appeler en français "étendre
pour prévenir" et qui consiste comme ces
deux mots l'indiquent à étendre les bords
de la cavité pour éviter ainsi que ceux-ci
ou autres parties vulnérables des dents
obturées, se carient. Chose qui exige
quelquefois faire la cavité énormément
plus grande qu'elle ne l'etait.

Quoique le soutiennent les champions
de l'extension, ce procédé n'est pas tout
à fait nouveau, puisque le Dr. Webb en
parle déjà dans son livre sur la dentisterie opératoire dentaire, publiée en 1883.

Cette affaire sera probablement long-
temps encore soumise à un débat acharné,
des deux côtés il y a des sommités qui
offrent à leurs contraires des raisons ap-
paremment indiscutibles.

Nous croyons que la vertu est au juste
milieu: les deux ont raison, et tort, et
nous ne devons pas nous laisser entraîner
aux idées radicales qu'ils prêchent.

Il y en a beaucoup qui n'ayant entendu
qu'un côté de la question, ne veulent pas
se déranger à l'etudier et croyant, qu'ils
posent comme réformateurs éblouissent
leurs confrères et emploient sans discré-
tion et de la façon la plus radicale, le
nouveau procédé, sans comprendre ses
principes et peut être sans les connaître.

Nous n'admettons pas en général l'extension des cavités plus qu'il ne l'est absolument nécessaire, sur la face labiale
des incisives et canines, appliquant ce
principe quoiqu'avec moins de sévérité à
la face mesiale et labiale des bicuspides.

Les partisans d' "étendre pour prévenir,"
prétendent que toute cavité interstitielle
doit s'agrandir jusqu'à ce que ses bords
soient dans la zone qu'ils appellent "qui
se nettoie elle même."

Cette zone comprend les faces labiales,
linguales et occlusales, donc, d'après eux,
une cavité interstitielle, pour petite
qu'elle soit doit s'étendre jusqu'à pénétrer
bien en avant sur les dites surfaces. Quant
aux bord gingival de la même ils soutiennent qu'il doit être environ deux milli-
mètres sous la gencive brisant de cette
façon les dents, sous prétexte qu'elles
pouvent se carier, détruisant ainsi la
beauté et harmonie de bouches qui pourraient assurement se conserver en bon
état sans employer de si héroiques
moyens.

Le Dr. Black, prétend poser comme
dogme l'énoncé suivant, que nous tradui-
sons de la façon la plus fidéle "étendre
pour prévenir est étendre les bords
d'émail d'une ligne qui ne se nettoie pas
d'elle même à une autre qui se nettoie."

En parlant des cavités interstitielles
des molaires, il dit "dans ces cas tout le
bord gingival d'émail doit être recouvert
par la gencive," et pour les bicuspides
"que les angles buccaux et linguaux de
la ligne d'émail doivent s'unir directe-

ment par une petite courbe avec l'émail gingival et être couverts par un septum de gencive." On pourrait croire que les énoncés antérieurs ont rapport seulement aux molaires, mais la suivante aclaration de Black ne laisse pas de doute. C'est une érreur d'obturer des cavités petites aux surfaces approximales de n'importe quelle dent, incluses les incisives, car en général il faudra les obturer de nouveau dans quelques années, pour la simple raison que la gencive en se retirant laissera le bord d'émail exposé aux agents corrosifs. Pour cette raison les cavités petites ou moyennes à la surface interstitielle des incisives doit s'agrandir librement vers la ligne gingivale et élargir labialement et lingualement jusqu'à la zone qui se nettoie d'elle même. Tout le bord gingival d'émail doit être couvert par un septum de gencive assez profound pour que celle-ci en se retirant ne le laisse pas à découvert.

Il parait invraisemblable que certaines personalités puissent défendre ces doctrines, surtout en rapport avec les incisives. Il nous semble plus raisonable, les obturer par l'ancien système et attendre que la carie se reproduise pour les agrandir et les obturer de nouveau, mais il ne faut pas les défigurer dès le début par crainte d'un péril, qu'il est probable n'arrivera pas et que s'il arrive, est facilement réparable.

Même dans les cas les moins favorables, il vaut mieux être temporairement beau que toujours défiguré.

Nous ne devons pas non plus oublier que cette extension exagérée, affaiblir de beaucoup la résistance de la dent à cause de la grande perte de substance. Nous ne doutons pas que les obturations faites d'après Black, doivent protéger la dent et éviter la carie. Mais il est aussi impossible de nier que celles faites par les an-

ciens systèmes ont conservé et conservent les dents où elles se trouvent, et cònstituent un éloquent temoignage pour réfuter les idées de ces nouveaux "dentoclastes."

Des sommités comme Ottolengui et Darby, affirment qu'ils n'ont trouvé que de rares cas d'obturation cariée par le bord gingival et que dans la plupart de cas, il suffit que l'obturation touch à la partie en contact avec la dent voisine pour que la carie ne se reproduise pas.

Nous avons vu souvent des petites obturations faites par l'ancien système en or ou amalgame de vingt, treinte et même plus d'années et qui étaient parfaites.

Il est axiomatique en chirurgie générale qu'un tissu sain ne doit pas se sacrifier à moins de nécessité absolue: notre opinion est que l'on peut appliquer en grande partie cet axiome en chirurgie dentaire.

D'après les régles de Black il n'y aurait plus de cavités petites ni moyennes, car toutes, on les ferait grandes et les patients auraient à souffrir de longues séances pour les obturer en plus, de la douleur de la préparation par le nouveau système, celui de couper une grande partie de dentine absolument saine, chose presque impossible avec des personnes nerveuses ou très sensibles.

Ne pouvant pas d'une façon absolue, garantir l'immunité, nous sommes presque sûrs que, si l'on expliquait au client le pour et les contre des deux procédés, la plupart préféraient l'ancien.

Nous savons tous, les difficultés qu'il y a pour obturer sous la gencive et polir cette partie une chose presque impossible à faire, sans traumatiser le septum ce qui contribue a l'atrophier.

Que veulent dire "surface qui se nettoie seule" dont nous parlent tous les apôtres de l'extension? La dent ne peut pas se nettoyer seule, donc aucune de ses parties peut le faire. Sans doute, ils veulent se rapporter aux surfaces qui se nettoient sans besoin de brosse, par l'action de la langue, les levres ou les aliments : mais ces agents ne nettoient que les surfaces plates, et tout de même les faces labiales et linguales qui sont les mieux nettoyées et où en général l'émail est mieux formé, se carient assez souvent, ce qui nous semble une puissante réfutation de la théorie de Black.

Mieux qu'étendre les cavités à ces grandeurs exagérées que Black et ses partisans nous enseignent, il est préférable faire une bonne obturation et conseiller au client de la tenir propre avec la brosse et la soie.

Nous n'abominons pas absolument d'étendre pour prévenir et croyons qu'il faut inclure dans la cavité les parties voisinants dont l'émail est imparfait ou affecté de décalcification ainsi que les parois trop fragiles et qui ne peuvent pas être renforcées.

Quoique légèrement nous allons nous occuper de la préparation individuelle des cavités. Celles qui se trouvent à la surface occlusale des bicuspides et des molaires, sont les plus communes et les plus simples car elles sont accessibles et visibles généralement dans la fissure entre les cuspides des bicuspides et la partie atteinte. L'ouverture se fait généralement mieux avec un taraud ou une meule très petite ; les bords doivent s'étendre jusqu'à embrasser les deux dépressions qui se trouvent aux extrémités de la fissure, laissant la cavité de forme oblongue et un peu plus étroite vers le milieu : la forme rétentive s'obtient facilement en passant le long de ses bords une fraise en cône renversé, car cette cavité, comme toutes celles des surfaces occlusales en général, n'ont besoin que de très peu de rétention

car le grand effort qu'elles ont à subir, tend à repousser l'obturation dans la cavité. Dans les molaires, la préparation des cavités occlusales est similaire à celle dans les bicuspides. S'il y a plus d'un point carié au supérieures on pourrait les unir en faisant une seule cavité qui contiendra toutes les fissures et un peu des cuspides. Si les caries sont petites et l'émail qui les sépare est fort et sain, on peut les remplir séparément. On ne doit jamais laisser sans couper les fissures ou points soupconneux dans ces cavités et autres similaires. Dans les molaires inférieures, il faut aussi couper les fissures donnant à la cavité une forme de croix ou d'étoile et quant à la rétention nous appliquerons ce que nous avons dit pour les bicuspides.

Les incisives et canines rarement ont des cavités sur leurs bords coupants. Celles-ci se préparent en aplanissant premièrement avec une pierre ou des disques de papier émeri et creusant après une rainure avec un cône renversé entre les parties labiales et linguales, ce qui nous sert de rétention, couvrant les bords avec l'obturation.

Les cavités simples des surfaces labiales et linguales des incisives n'offrent pas de difficulté et n'exigent que très peu de forme rétentive, car elles n'ont qu'à souffrir pratiquement aucun effort qui tends à déloger l'obturation. Leurs bords doivent être arrondis et ne pas s'étendre plus qu'il n'est nécessaire. Les cavités approximales des bicuspides et des molaires ne sont généralement pas simples. Celles des bicuspides peuvent s'étendre quoique pas d'une façon si radicales dans la plupart des cas, comme conseille Black, et il faut toujours tenir en compte, en agrandissant les cavités, les conditions individuelles de chaque bouche, comme sont, la qualité des dents leur tendance plus ou moins grande à la carié, âge du client et soins qu'il apporte à la bouche.

Dans les incisives et les canines nous ne croyons pas necessaire étendre les cavités sur la face labiales que dans quelques rares cas, notre opinion étant qu'il est préférable attendre que la carie se reproduise, qu'abimer la dent dès le début. Il y a deux façons de préparer ces cavités : l'une quand elles sont très petites, consiste à séparer les dents suffisamment pour pouvoir les obturer en gardant la face labiale et linguale ; nous ne conseillons ceci que lorsque la cavité est très petite et la paroi linguale solide, dans les autres cas nous couperons cette paroi et introduirons par derrière l'obturation, en renforçant préalablement s'il est nécessaire avec du ciment ; quand cette cavité est très près du bord coupant il est préférable inclure la partie voisine du dit bord dans la cavité. Nous décrirons plus loin la préparation dans ce cas.

Les cavités mesio et disto labiales des incisives et canines se préparent de la façon que nous avons décrit pour ces cavités quand elles sont simples, les mesio et disto linguales exigent aussi un traitement similaire, la forme rétentive n'a pas besoin d'être grande. Les cavités interstitio-occlusales des incisives offrent quelques difficultés car l'obturation doit être fortement retenue pour pouvoir résister les efforts de la mastication, qui s'exercent principalement en deux sens, un suivant l'axe de la dent et vers la racine, et l'autre de dedans en dehors sur la couronne. Généralement la forme rétentive s'obtient en taillant une rainure assez profonde près de la paroi gingivale et une autre dans les parois labiales et linguales quand c'est possible : toujours naturellement dans de la dentine épaisse et un autre petit point près du bord cou-

pant. Dans beaucoup de cas, la forme antérieure est suffisante pour retenir l'obturation, tout de même, comme l'effort qu'elle doit subir est très grand, il vaut mieux la fixer plus solidement en taillant dans la paroi linguale une rainure de forme rétentive et qui remplit parfaitement l'objet voulu. On peut aussi comme conseil Johnson, au lieu d'une rainure, enlever tout le bord coupant lingual préservant autant que possible la paroi labiale.

Si la cavité est mesio-disto-occlusale on unit les deux côtés par la paroi linguale comme nous venons de l'indiquer, on peut aussi si la dent est morte fixer dans son canal une vis qui soutient l'obturation.

Les cavités dans les canines se préparent d'une façon analogue.

Les cavités proximo-occlusales des bicuspides et molaires sont fréquentes c'est à ces endroits que la carie recidive les plus souvent et sans aller aussi loin que Black, nous trouvons convenable les étendre suffisament pour que l'émail des bords soit parfait, poussant s'il est nécessaire jusqu'à en dessous de la gencive.

La rétention doit être forte pour supporter la mastication qui tend à déloger l'obturation dans un sens latéral. La taille des fissures facilite la rétention.

Dans les cavités mesiales des bicuspides on devra conserver la partie labiale pour éviter que l'obturation se voie trop.

Voilà à grands traits la préparation des cavités les plus usuelles et qui varie un peu si on emploie des matières plastiques au lieu de l'or, quoique l'amalgame exige le même soin pour sa rétention.

Nous avons omis à dessein la préparation des cavités pour l'obturation à la porcelaine, cette nouvelle matière exige une préparation spéciale et la décrire nous entrainerait trop loin.

Conclusions.

1. La préparation correcte de la cavité est de grànde importance pour le succés de l'obturation.

2. La dite préparation se fonde sur des régles scientifiques et esthétiques et se divise en trois parties: ouverture, nettoyage, et formation.

3. Les cavités se divisent en simples et composées, et reçoivent un nom différent, d'après la partie de la dent, où elles se trouvent.

4. Pour les ouvrir on emploira des fraises dentelées, des ciseaux et des petites meules: pour les nettoyer des excavateurs et des fraises, et pour les façonner les instruments, déjà nommés, des disques et des bandes d'émeri.

5. La cavité préparée doit remplir les conditions suivantes: forme rétentive suffisante pour que l'obturation puisse résister sans danger les différents efforts auxquels elle sera soumise, ses bords doivent être solides, et dans certains cas, plus étendus que la cavité primitive.

6. L'emploi de la digue est très utile et facilite l'opération.

7. Les théories "d'étendre pour prévenir" exposées par Black, présentent dans la pratique de grands inconvenients, et sont trop radicales dans la plupart des cas.

8. La dite méthode n'est pas admissible, pour les incisives, pour raison d'esthétique, étant préférable refaire l'obturation s'il y a recidive de carie.

9. Le nouveau procédé n'assure pas l'immunité absolue: et la méthode ancienne a conservé et conserve les dents, par des moyens moins héroiques.

10. Dans les molaires on peut suivre en partie les théories de Black.

11. La préparation des cavités est différente d'après la dent, et la place où elles se trouvent.

The CHAIRMAN. This concludes the work of this section. Before entertaining a motion to adjourn I want to express my thanks to the committee on Operative Dentistry for the splendid support they have given me in the preparation of the program.

I also wish to express my appreciation and my thanks to the secretary, Dr. Hunt, and also to Dr. Heckard, who acted as secretary *pro tempore* in Dr. Hunt's absence.

I wish to thank the stenographer, Mr. Long, for the assistance he has given us. He has been very faithful in his attendance on the sessions, and I appreciate it.

I also want to thank the members for their uniformly close attention and for their regular attendance at the sessions.

The chairman, Dr. Johnson, then declared the section adjourned *sine die*.

Fourth International Dental Congress.

SECTION VIII.

SECTION VIII:

Prosthesis.

Chairman—CHARLES R. TURNER, Philadelphia, Pa.
Secretary—H. W. CAMPBELL, Suffolk, Va.

FIRST DAY—Tuesday, August 30th.

THE section was called to order at 2.30 P.M. by the chairman, Dr. Charles R. Turner. Dr. J. Q. Byram acted as secretary *pro tem.*

Dr. J. P. Gray, Nashville, Tenn., was called to the chair, and Dr. CHAS. R. TURNER delivered the following address:

Chairman's Address.

We have assembled from the various parts of the world to participate in the work of the Fourth International Dental Congress, and the section whose duties we are called upon to begin this afternoon has for its especial consideration the subject of Dental Prosthesis.

As the wise men of the early civilizations of Egypt and Phœnicia visited far and wide to broaden and enlarge their knowledge by contact with men of other nations; as the Greek youth assembled in the market-place to learn the principles of argument and oratory from the lips of Demosthenes; as Paracelsus gathered from his travel the facts which he formulated into our first chemistry, so from time immemorial personal intercourse has been a fruitful means for the dissemination of learning. That they might counsel more closely together, by a process of easy evolution congregations of men have taken place in order that, in addition to the imparting of knowledge, theses might be debated and facts be established. Much wisdom has come from these deliberations. Modern scientific conventions have for their purpose the recording of observations, the deduction of principles from such records, the establishment of these conclusions by proof furnished again by the original facts. It is here that the earnest worker in pursuit of truth brings the findings of his careful search in contribution to his fellow-man; it is here that the painstaking toiler, following the single path of his own field of labor, is freed from the limitations of his scientific provincialism by the process of friendly criticism and discussion; it is here that the youth, by contact with such investigators, is inspired with enthusiasm to the undertaking of greater deeds, and it is here that he whom ability and experience have made a master of his craft comes to exhibit the fruits of his skill to his brethren whose activities have been directed along other lines.

To us in America it has seemed particularly fitting that the Louisiana Purchase Exposition should be the occasion of an international gathering in dentistry. In the words of our late lamented President McKinley, "Expositions are the timekeepers of progress," and no less is it true that a congress of its representatives from all portions of the world marks an epoch in the development of any science. It has been a hundred years since Thomas Jefferson secured from Napoleon, the First Consul of the Republic of France, the tract of land whose acquisition the city of St. Louis is now celebrating. It has been more than a century since Lafayette's army came from that same country to battle in behalf of American liberty, and is it not an event of equal importance in the history of dentistry that at that time there arrived upon American soil practically the first dentists to come to this country? And have not the developments of these two contributions of France to the New World been parallel marvels of unusual wonder?

The portion of dentistry with which we shall have to do in this section is dental prosthesis in its broadest sense, and includes the replacement of any or all the tissues pertaining to the masticating apparatus. If we may believe that the date assigned is correct, the findings in Etrus-

can and Phœnician necropoles seem to show that prosthesis is as old as dentistry itself. Whether it be as crude as the use of a vegetable fiber blanched by mastication by the courtezans of the port of Athens in a vain attempt to lure the unwary by the borrowed integrity and whiteness of their dentures, or whether it be as unsatisfactory as the teeth with which the divine Cleopatra may have charmed Mark Antony (although she might only have been able to endure them when he was present), prosthesis, since its beginning, has endeavored to supply to frail humanity portions of tissues lost through the curse of disease or the ill fortunes of accident, in order that form might be preserved and function prolonged. One may hardly be so sanguine of the possibility of dental prophylaxis, of dental hygiene, or of dental surgery as to fear that the need for dental prosthesis may cease to exist. In spite of conservative dentistry, and in addition to its careful ministration, the field of prosthetic dentistry will continue to enlarge and develop. And along what line will its further evolution take place?

Thomas Huxley said that scientific knowledge differs from common knowledge only in its greater accuracy, and in our own particular field of human inquiry it is evident that the tendency of investigators will be along the line of exactness in their search for ultimate truths. There must be an improvement in our knowledge of physics and mechanics which shall permit the construction of artificial substitutes in such a manner that the present difficulties attending their use may be overcome. We must enlarge our acquaintance with form and color—the fundamentals which are necessary to an analysis of the requirements of our creations—so that the lost parts may be supplied by substitutes in such perfect harmony with their environment that they shall escape detection after careful inspection. We have room for improvement in the technique of present processes, and a fertile field for labor in the search for materials of greater cosmetic and mechanical possibilities. We may still strive to deserve that encomium which Dr. Oliver Wendell Holmes thirty years ago pronounced: "The dental profession has established and prolonged the reign of beauty; it has added to the charms of social intercourse, and lent perfection to the accents of eloquence; it has taken from old age its most unwelcome feature and lengthened enjoyable human life far beyond the limit of the years when the toothless and purblind patriarch might exclaim, 'I have no pleasure in them.'"

In thus formally opening Section VIII, I wish to make public my grateful thanks to the Committee of Organization which has seen fit to select me to preside at its meetings. I trust its sessions may result in substantially furthering the cause of its special sphere of labor, and I hope that any failure on my part to serve it wisely may be laid at the door of my inexperience rather than to the score of unwillingness.

Dr. GRAY. The first item on our program for this afternoon is a paper by Dr. CALVIN S. CASE of Chicago, Ill., entitled "The Mechanical Treatment of Congenital Cleft Palate." I will ask Mons. B. Platschick of Paris, France, to occupy the chair during the reading of Dr. Case's paper.

Dr. CASE. I had thought to present after the reading of my paper a number of models illustrative of the points discussed therein, but I think that it would be better to present the models at once, so that all may have an opportunity to examine the various kinds of artificial palates which I propose to describe.

He then read his paper, as follows:

The Mechanical Treatment of Congenital Cleft Palate.

By CALVIN S. CASE, M.D., D.D.S., Chicago, Ill.

AT the meeting of the National Dental Association in 1902, and at the Illinois State Dental Society of 1903, I presented descriptions of a new form of artificial palate. And now after a more extended opportunity, with a greater number and variety of cases to study the development of this principle and its possibilities, I am more convinced than ever that it represents a system that is both practical and scientific for the mechanical correction of every form of congenital cleft palate, and one, moreover, that is absolutely sure of affording means for the perfect correction of speech in these cases.

Some authors have made quite a distinction between an obturator and a velum, so that the profession has come to regard an obturator as any cleft-palate instrument which is composed of hard material, gold or vulcanite, and a velum as one composed of flexible rubber after the form of the Kingsley palates. Both

9

are essentially for the correction of speech by restoring a lost or undeveloped portion of the natural palate by artificial means; correctly speaking, therefore, they are both artificial palates.

When Dr. Wm. Suersen proposed the insertion of a cleft-palate instrument which could be worn with comfort and, in conjunction with the muscles, enable the patient at will to close the connection between the oral and nasal cavities, he presented a scientific principle that is as true today as then, and one, moreover, that must be successfully attained to be of value to the wearer, whatever the form of the instrument or the method of its construction.

He called the instrument which he devised for this purpose an "obturator," because it was intended to close and prevent the passage of air, which is the vehicle of voice, from escaping into the nares.

Later, Dr. Norman W. Kingsley, who will always be regarded as one of the greatest geniuses of his day, realizing the difficulties of constructing and successfully applying the Suersen device, invented a flexible-rubber palate, with which you are all familiar. He named it an artificial velum, because its posterior extension was intended to imitate the action of the natural velum, by bridging the cleft and restoring the palate to the possibilities of a normal organ of speech.

It doubtless has done more than any other device that has ever been invented to relieve the ills of this most unfortunate deformity, principally because it could be inserted and worn with comfort, even though quite imperfect in its adaptability to the parts, and though more or less inadequate in possibilities for the acquirement of perfect enunciation and tone. But Dr. Kingsley and others who adopted this method of practice, I believe,

have always been convinced of its inefficiency when considered as a permanent appliance, if for no other reason than the early deterioration of flexible rubber when worn in the mouth, requiring that the palates be renewed about as often as once a year to keep them in the necessary form. This is not difficult for those who construct individual molds for each case, in which the palates can be easily vulcanized and mailed to any part of the country. But in a long experience of its use I have found that three-fourths of the patients soon tire of this régime, and either discard their palates altogether or get along in some way with what must be very poor apologies.

So that at best the most ardent admirers of the Kingsley velum regard it as only superior to a perfectly constructed obturator for the early stages of a completed operation.

Dr. R. Ottolengui, in discussing my paper at the National meeting, said: "The only advantage of a soft velum over an obturator seems to be that it enables a more rapid progress in the acquirement of speech, but later in life, perhaps at the time when the patient needs a new instrument—in any event speech having been perfected—it is usually preferable to make a hard-rubber appliance, which will be more permanent and more cleanly than one of soft rubber. Thus the obturator apparently comes into use after the patient has been educated to speak by means of the soft-rubber appliance, which should, in every sense of the word, be a velum."

Though Drs. Kingsley, Ottolengui, myself, and others have always advised the changing of vela for metal or hard-rubber instruments, the instances are rare when this has been done, principally because it involved another complete operation considerably differing from the first, with added fee, etc.

In some instances there has been an attempt to change the Kingsley vela for hard-rubber obturators made after the very ingenious method and form devised by Dr. Grant Molyneux; but, largely because the shape and conditions were so entirely different, with the consequent irritation to the sensitive tissues, the patients could not be induced to wear them, and insisted upon continuing with the original palates which gave them no discomfort and when new and perfectly fitted enabled them to speak with the most satisfying results.

Then the question arises: If the hard rubber or other so-called obturators are ultimately superior, why not make them in that way at first?

To say nothing of the extra irritation to exceedingly sensitive tissues which a hard rubber or metal appliance would at first produce, even if absolutely correct in form, those who have had considerable experience in the fitting of artificial palates know very well how difficult, and in most instances impossible, it is to make a *first* palate that does not require considerable change in form before it perfectly subserves the purpose of vocal articulation. Nor can this always be accomplished skilfully until the palate has been worn for some time, and the tissues allowed to become accustomed and adjusted to this foreign body in the mouth and throat.

Through a desire to take advantage of the benefits afforded by a soft-rubber appliance on the one hand, and a hard-rubber obturator on the other, and at the same time avoid the possibilities of the final inefficiency of the one and the difficulties in construction and adjustment presented by the other, has arisen the present artificial palate, which it is the object of this paper to present.

It essentially consists of a form of palate which can first be made of soft rubber and possess all the advantages of the Kingsley velum, and then, when the patient has become accustomed to it in its flexible state and its present form is assured, by packing the same casts in which the soft rubber palates were vulcanized with another quality of rubber, a hard-rubber palate is produced which possesses all the advantages of a perfect obturator.

If made of soft rubber and vulcanized within specially constructed metal molds, as this system demands, the operation is a perfectly painless one, and the first palate can be worn without irritation or special inconvenience; after which, desired changes in its form, such as are nearly always required in order to perfect the palate, can then be easily made by slightly enlarging or contracting the mold.

In my first paper I presented it as composed of soft rubber alone, not having had an opportunity to judge of its merits when made of hard rubber. Dr. Ottolengui, in opening the discussion, said: "I had always thought until to-night that it would be necessary for those who treat these cases mechanically to decide between a hard-rubber obturator and a soft-rubber velum, but Dr. Case has brought us a new appliance. He states that it differs essentially from the Kingsley velum, and it certainly does, not only in form but in action and every feature. Of course, it is not a hard-rubber obturator, but I consider it an obturator rather than a velum."

Those who are familiar with the Kingsley palates, which I am pleased to say I have used with great satisfaction in my practice for over twenty years, will remember that the veil or posterior portion of the palate is sustained by extending the central thickened portion into it, and from this point it is gradually flattened to a comparatively thin edge, where it is more or less curved in conformity to the pharyngeal wall, against which it is intended to rest during the contraction of the pharyngeal and palatal muscles.

In this particular it is quite different in form from the palate I am about to describe, in that with the latter all the central portion of the palate is thin,

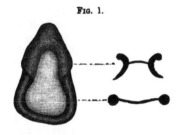

while the edge of the veil is thick, in the form of a solid roll about one-fifth of an inch in diameter, or preferably triangular, with rounded corners, so that its outer flattened surfaces exactly and firmly fit the pharyngeal walls *when the muscles are in a contracted state.*

Fig. 1 represents the lingual view of the artificial palate, with transverse sections. Figs. 2 and 3 show the palate in position.

In extensive clefts the borders of the veil extend forward along the lateral walls of the pharynx and posterior nares, and becoming thinner, form the borders of the nasal extensions which rest upon the floor of the nares.

When the cleft does not extend into the hard palate, the veil is shaped in a similar manner, but with the nasal portion abridged to meet the requirements of the case.

Where the cleft extends into the hard parts, the body of the palate which covers the borders of the cleft and forms the lateral wings on the roof of the mouth should not extend back of the attachments of the bifurcated velum palati, nor in any way interfere with the free action of the muscles; neither should it extend upon the roof of the mouth any farther than is necessary to give a firm seating for the palate. This portion should be about as thick as an ordinary rubber plate, being thinned along its oral borders and thickened to form the nasal borders.

There are a number of important advantages in this form of palate, even when made of flexible rubber and used for the purposes of a velum:

First. The early deterioration of the rubber, causing the curling up of thin edges of the veil, is entirely prevented. When this occurs, as it frequently does with ordinary vela, the vocal usefulness of the palate is impaired—if not destroyed—in proportion as it permits the escape of air at the curled-up portion of the border.

Second. The heavy border of the veil is sufficiently yielding and flexible to be worn with comfort if properly fitted, and it also presents sufficient stability and breadth of surface to permit firm contact of the pharyngeal muscles in closing the naso-pharyngeal opening.

Third. In more or less extensive clefts the thin central portion extending forward into the body of the palate permits a resilient yielding of the lateral portions of the body, which frequently allows one to spring it into place with sufficient grasp of the irregular borders, along which it should accurately fit, to hold it in position without other aid. Whenever this can be accomplished with the soft

In taking an impression for the construction of this palate where the cleft

Fig. 2.

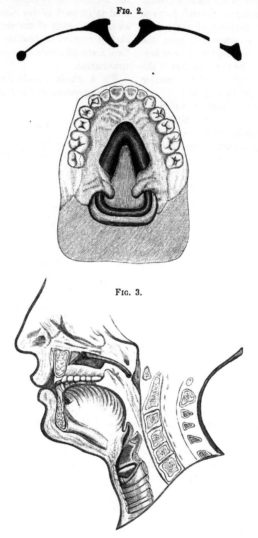

Fig. 3.

palate, it will readily be continued when it becomes hard.

is extensive or even extending somewhat into the hard palate, it is my object to obtain a perfect model of that portion of the roof of the mouth over which I wish the palatal portion of the plate to extend, and along the borders of the cleft forward of the pendent portions of the velum palati, extending somewhat upon the floor of the nares and representing as perfectly as possible the nasal borders of the cleft and lateral surfaces of the posterior nares. (See Figs. 11 and 12.)

These surfaces, a part of which lie above the pendent and unstable tissues of the velum palati, are frequently susceptible of being perfectly reproduced in the model of a plaster impression. It will usually be found in a typical case that the posterior nasal openings are laterally constricted, from which point the nasal fossæ widen to form the floor of the nares. By obtaining a perfect impression of these somewhat unyielding surfaces, which otherwise, on account of their position, would be very difficult to reproduce, the anterior borders of the artificial veil can be perfectly fitted to them as they merge into the nasal borders of the body.

I lay particular stress upon this portion of the operation because I have found it important, not only as a great aid to the proper action of the pharyngeal muscles, but in clefts of considerable extent the overhanging nasal borders of the artificial palate can be easily sprung into place, and when fitted perfectly patients soon learn to place and sustain the palate without the aid of a supporting plate.

I would advise, however, that the supporting plate be always made, to enable patients to more readily adjust and sustain the palates until they have learned to wholly do without it.

When no artificial teeth are required, or when, if required, a bridge denture is practicable, the supporting plate should be made to cover as small an area of the roof of the mouth as is consistent with the demand for strength. I rarely extend it forward of the second bicuspid, leaving as much of the anterior palatal surface exposed as possible, which I believe materially aids in acquiring perfect enunciation.

Fig. 4, which is made from the model of an impression of the mouth with the

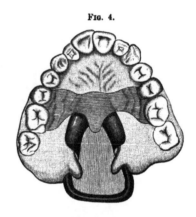

FIG. 4.

apparatus in place, shows the form of the supporting plate I usually make.

Preparatory to taking the impression for an artificial palate, I study well the cleft and surrounding tissues to determine the character and extent of the impression. For all clefts that involve the hard palate, an accurate plaster impression of the parts outlined is not more difficult than most impressions for partial dentures.

There are two ways of taking these impressions: One by forming a base of modeling compound upon which to lay the plaster, and the other by using plaster alone.

For the first the compound is wrapped

around the forefinger (Fig. 5), and pressed gently to place. Removing, softening, and perhaps slightly reshaping and cutting away surplus, this is repeated several times, with the view of finally obtaining a modeling-compound

plaster in position, need cause no fear of its easy removal, even though an excess of plaster be used—providing it does not come forward of the alveolar ridge in extensive double clefts—as all that portion which extends above the border of the

FIG. 5.

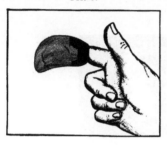

FIG. 7.

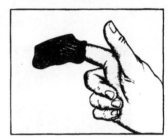

impression that will not displace the soft posterior borders, and that will perfectly support the plaster for the final impression. (See Fig. 6.)

cleft forming the impression of the nasal fossæ will readily break from the smooth, oiled surface of the compound when the impression is removed, it being otherwise

FIG. 6.

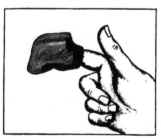

FIG. 8.

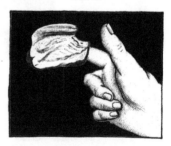

The palatal surface is then roughened so the plaster will cling to it, and all that portion of the compound which extends above the nearest approaching borders of the cleft is cut away and the cut surface smoothed and oiled. (See Fig. 7.)

This, when carried to place with the

unattached to the lower parts, as the compound completely bridges the cleft from its nearest approaching borders. The nasal section can then be teased back toward the more open portion of the cleft, and allowed to fall on a mouth-mirror, from which it is replaced upon the impression. (See Fig. 8.) Fig. 9 shows different views of a plaster impression taken in this way.

As a rule, I prefer plaster alone, dividing it as above in sections at the borders of the cleft. Fig. 10 shows different views of an impression of an extensive cleft taken entirely with plaster. The first

plaster introduced in a flat impression tray. The impression does not need to extend even to the gingival borders of the teeth.

In filling and trimming the models from these impressions, nearly all that portion back of the attachments of the soft palate is cut away, and the nasal

FIG. 9.

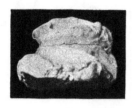 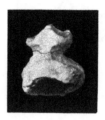

a   b

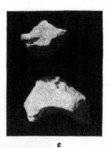

c

section is passed freely into the nasal cavity with a spatula, stopping it abruptly at the nearest approaching borders of the cleft. The under surface is then lubricated with a solution of white vaselin, and the first part of the second section is delicately laid on with the spatula, so as not to lift or dislodge the upper section. The plaster is spread out over the roof of the mouth with a spatula, and when partially hard is strengthened for removal with fresh

portion open and freely exposed to the extreme nasal borders, produced by the impression.

This is done to facilitate shaping the modeling-compound model of the palate, and its ready removal and replacing during the process of repeated trials in the mouth.

Fig. 11 shows lingual aspect of the finished model. The nasal aspect would look very similar.

The model of the body of the palate,

as shown in Fig. 12, is formed first and then inserted in the mouth for trial, etc. At this time the lateral nasal extensions of the palate model should be abridged to facilitate introduction. They can be added at the time of investment, and, upper surface of the palate model. (See Fig. 13.)

The loop is drawn out to about the proper size and shape, and the palate model inserted into the mouth for correction, etc., until the wire is seen to rest

FIG. 10.

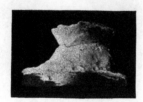
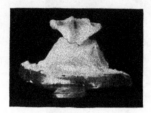

L.

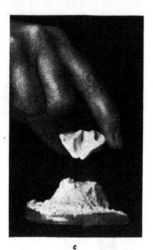

c

if desired, still further extended by scraping the metal molds.

The position for the border surface of the veil is determined with a loop of small soft copper wire No. 20, the ends of which pass into thin tubes about half an inch long, embedded in the along a zone of the pharyngeal walls that is best adapted to unite in their muscular action with the artificial veil for the ultimate closure of the naso-pharyngeal opening.

The path of this pharyngeal zone, which practically should extend from the lateral extension of the nasal borders on each side back to a line immediately in front of or slightly above the greatest contracted ex-

illation of the surface, and, what is of the greatest advantage, the pharyngeal walls above and below the wire can be

FIG. 11.

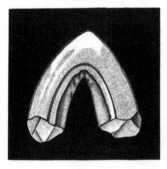

FIG. 12.

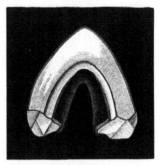

tension of the superior pharyngeal muscle, is carefully chosen to avoid imping-

readily seen through the open loop, and the action of the muscles studied.

FIG. 13.

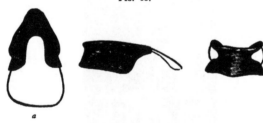

FIG. 14.

ing upon the Eustachian opening, and to obtain the most active possibilities of the muscles. The surrounding muscles can be made to contract by a slight tit-

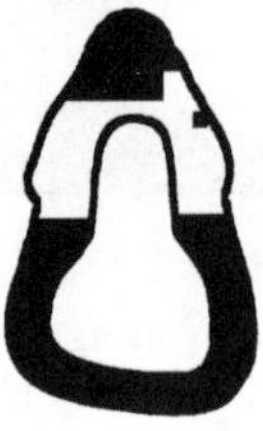

As the loop turns forward to pass beneath the Eustachian opening, the pharyngeal surfaces will often be found corrugated and thrown into irregular folds, so that in finding the smoother path across these ridges, to prevent the escape of air at the border of the veil through these sulci, it may be found desirable to raise or lower the wire upon one side more than the other. Forward of this it soon comes in contact with the upper surfaces of the palatal muscles, as it enters the posterior nares.

After fitting the wire to mark the desired outlines of the veil, the roll of compound which is to form the model of the border, as shown in Fig. 14, may be attached to the loop, following the outlines of its peripheral surface. This is placed in the mouth warm, and the patient told to swallow, which being repeated several times will produce a perfect impression on its outer border of the desired zone when the muscles are contracted.*

The object of the veil or pharyngeal portion, as Suersen pointed out at the birth of scientifically constructed artificial palates, is to give the greatest possible aid to the muscles, principally the superior constrictor of the pharynx, to form a complete closure of the nasal passage in producing the enunciatory parts of the consonants, and then to be immediately followed or preceded by the largest possible opening when the muscles drop back to take a position to form resonating or open tones.

It will be seen by this that the relative position of the border, or contact surface of the veil, should be only that which is consistent with the possibilities of the muscles to completely reach and close the space, in order that resonance or the power of freely throwing the tone into the sounding-chamber of our vocal organs—which is quite as important to perfect

* Dr. Grant Molyneux was the first to use a wire loop to obtain plaster impressions of pharyngeal walls.

speech as distinct enunciation—may not be obstructed.

I can see no reason, furthermore, why the pharyngeal contact surface of the palate should be any wider than necessary to enable stability of muscular contact, as seems to be presented by the Molyneux pattern, nor do I see that the central portion of the palate needs to be thicker than is sufficient to stop the air, which is the vehicle of voice.

If the diaphragm be a thin plate of rubber or gold, valuable resonating and nasal breathing space will not be obstructed.

I at first named this palate the "velum obturator," because it stands for both, but as Dr. Ottolengui has said, it is more of an obturator than a velum, and yet it is one which, if made of soft rubber vulcanized within metal molds and properly constructed according to the method and principles I have outlined, presents to the patient and the operator all the advantages of a soft-rubber velum.

The principal advantage in this system of preceding the operation with a soft palate is not that it can be worn with greater comfort from the start, nor that it enables the patient to more readily acquire perfect speech—though these are important—but that it admits of more readily determining the slight variations in its form that may be necessary and possible to alter by changing the molds in which it is vulcanized, until you have reached a form that is exactly suited to the demands of the surrounding tissues for the acquirement of perfect enunciation, resonance, and tone. When this has been accomplished, the palate is easily changed from a soft to a hard-rubber obturator by simply packing the same molds with hard vulcanite instead of soft.

The fact that this change can be made

without subjecting the patient or operator to another complete operation, and also that the hard-rubber palate is the same shape as the soft one, which the patient has become accustomed to, are features of incalculable importance.

Again, this change can be made gradually by packing a portion of the mold with hard and the balance with soft rubber.

When I am ready to change it to an obturator, it is my custom to make the first ones with the body, or naso-palatal portion, of hard rubber and the veil of soft. This will not subject the sensitive tissues to a too sudden change.

A favorite method will be to make the thin central portion of gold plate rolled hard and as thin as No. 38. The gold plate is cut the proper size to permit its edges extending partly into the thick border of the veil. This is then laid in place in the mold, and the rubber packed as before.

If the border of the veil is made of soft rubber and the central portion of gold, I have no doubt the palate will last for years without harmful deterioration. This would permit a slight elastic movement of the veil that is always desirable.

I here present a variety of palates of practical cases [exhibiting], made in the different ways I have described, which will give you a far better idea of its form than has been possible with the illustrations.

———

Dr. CASE. We have with us today Mr. Seaton of New York, who has kindly consented to be present to show the practicability of this new "velum-obturator." I made an artificial plate after the Kingsley form, for him a number of years ago, and a week ago last Saturday

I took the impression for the present instrument. On the following Wednesday he had the soft rubber palate inserted; on Thursday the plate partially hard and partially soft, and on Friday night the hard rubber obturator. The change has been very radical, as you can see by the shape of the plate which he has, and of course his speech may not be as perfect as it will be when he becomes used to it, being unused to the bridge denture which takes the place of the incisors that were originally attached to the sustaining plate. I will give him a number of words to pronounce.

Mr. Seaton stood beside Dr. Case and repeated the following words as rapidly as they were pronounced by Dr. Case: "Certainly," "success," "He thrusts his fists," "Call Charles," "go," "give," "James," "George," "church," "choose," "shame," "they," "thou," "these," "positively," "difficulty," "preacher."

Dr. CASE. I am going to ask you, Mr. Seaton, to say just a word or two in your own way, if you do not object.

Dr. Ottolengui requested Dr. Case to have Mr. Seaton pronounce the name of Norman W. Kingsley.

Mr. Seaton clearly repeated the name.

Mr. SEATON. Well, doubtless Dr. Case wants me to speak further in order that you may judge of my ability, but really I am glad of the opportunity, for I want to express to you my thanks as well as those of Dr. Case for your kind attention to this paper, and I would like also to express my gratification at the advance which has been made by your profession which has done so much for me. I would like to add that I have been wearing a soft rubber velum for about ten years, and while I found it very satisfactory indeed, I think, in fact I know, that in the hard rubber obturator which

I now have I have an artificial palate which is far superior in every way.

I am of course not yet quite accustomed to it; it is with some difficulty that I handle it, but I believe that within the next thirty days I will be able to speak in a way that will deceive almost anyone.

Dr. H. J. GOSLEE, Chicago, Ill., who had been called to the chair, announced that the discussion of the paper would be opened by Dr. Ottolengui of New York.

Discussion.

Dr. R. OTTOLENGUI, New York, N. Y. Before opening, I wish to say that I have been requested by the chairman to make the following motion: That the discussion of papers read in this section be limited to ten minutes by those opening the discussion and five minutes by those who follow in discussion.

The motion being duly seconded, a vote was taken and the motion prevailed.

Dr. OTTOLENGUI. This paper, and one or two others on the same line, mark a distinctive era in our work on this subject. I must also admit that at the present time I am speaking theoretically; I have not had an opportunity to try Dr. Case's method, and I reserve the liberty to take back anything that I say now.

Since visiting Dr. Case's office I think I have made an important discovery there. I think that a part of his lack of faith in soft rubber is due to his method of vulcanizing, also to the fact that he has not had so good a rubber to work with as Dr. Kingsley has had. At the present time, I myself do not have that high-class rubber. In the first place, Dr. Kingsley has used an exceptionally fine quality of rubber. I have asked him

many times for his formula but he has lost it. He had a large quantity made up and at the present time he is using rubber that has been in those boxes twenty years and that material is superior to any that has been produced within the past twenty years.

One point will help; I understand through Dr. Case's son that he vulcanizes at high heat for a short time. In Dr. Kingsley's practice and in mine the rubber is started at the low heat of 240° F., where it remains about an hour, 250° about an hour, 260° about five hours— nearly a day's work to cook this rubber. At a higher temperature it is nearly always spoiled. The moment it is removed from the flask if you detect an odor like a parched peanut, it is burned, and you may be sure that the rubber will not last nor be as durable as that prepared by long vulcanization at a low heat.

To pass from that to the remarks the essayist made about the difficulty of making an obturator at the first attempt; that is true in a sense, but in many cases, in fact in all cases that I have had anything to do with, the model for the final obturator has been formed successfully.

I want to say this in regard to the wire loop: In all my own writings I abstain from giving anyone credit for being the first to have used any device. In this instance it may be that Dr. Molyneux was the first to use this device with plaster. Nevertheless, it is also true that Dr. Kingsley always used the wire loop in getting his pharyngeal wall. He used a combination of gutta-percha and wax. So that, while Molyneux may have been the first to use that method exclusively with plaster, Kingsley was doing that long ago. It is a little dangerous to record who first used a method, or who first published it.

Now I want to make a remark about this Kingsley palate presented by Dr. Case. At the last discussion of one of Dr. Case's papers, I advanced the opinion that his new device was rather an obturator than a velum. Now I would certainly say this so-called Kingsley velum, made by him for Mr. Seaton, is not a true Kingsley velum, but is likewise an obturator in effect. There is in this instrument too much of the soft rubber to allow of the play that it should have; it is a great deal too rigid. Now, I hesitate, because Dr. Case's patient is present —am I at liberty, and will the patient understand the nature of this discussion?

Dr. CASE. You may go on.

Dr. OTTOLENGUI. I believe Dr. Case's new instrument is satisfactory in this case with one very important exception. I believe that gentleman would be better off with a regular obturator—I believe that it would do away with a certain nasal resonance. I believe that the anterior part is not sufficiently closely adapted to his mouth. I have found that very often the addition of even a little, a very little thickness, will make all the difference in the world in the escape of sounds. For that reason, instead of taking my impression of the nares at the outset, I leave that for the very last; I get the impression of the palate, then that part that goes back in the throat; and the last thing I do is to take the plaster of Paris and press it up in the roof of the mouth—and that must be very carefully done, so there will be a close adaptation—and in many cases, not all cases, for there is no rule that will control all these cases, the nasal resonance which this gentleman has at present will disappear, because of the close fit thus obtained.

Dr. M. S. MERCHANT, Giddings, Tex. I would like to ask Dr. Ottolengui a question or two. I did not think that the defect he referred to was a nasal resonance, and I would like to hear Mr. Seaton speak again.

Mr. SEATON. Well, as you are the ones to judge as to that, I feel that I am working a little bit under a difficulty; I have been wearing a soft rubber velum for probably ten or eleven years—of course the velum being changed every eighteen months or so—and this obturator Dr. Case has made is quite a change, which I feel is beneficial, at the same time, making that change has caused me to lose control to a great extent of my power of articulation, and I hope to regain that before many days.

Dr. MERCHANT. Do you whistle?

Mr. SEATON. I have done so. (Mr. Seaton whistled a few notes and then whistled a tune.)

Dr. OTTOLENGUI. You notice that when the gentleman whistles, the sound is not of sufficient volume to come out loud. I believe that a closer adaptation will enable him to do that.

Mons. B. PLATSCHICK, Paris, France. I wish to say that I am familiar with the very splendid results obtained by my confrères in France, among whom are Drs. Martin and Delair, and I recognize the fact that Dr. Case has obtained a very splendid result in this patient; for although Dr. Case speaks well, I think that his patient speaks better than Dr. Case, because I can understand him better.

The CHAIRMAN. If there is nothing further to be said, Dr. Case will now close the discussion of his paper.

Dr. CASE. I want to say you can hardly judge from the speech of any one person, as has been fully exemplified by the remarks of my distinguished friend from Paris, as to the resonant tone and articulation of a voice in its relation to an artificial palate. The speech of anyone who has a natural palate may be imperfect, as I am perhaps in my vocal tones. So that it is not admissible to establish a standard of perfection for patients.

Again, when you bring a patient with an artificial palate before an audience he is more or less embarrassed, and sometimes you are disappointed and surprised yourself at what seems to be a nasal or a catarrhal tone which you have not before discovered in his speech. Now, in ordinary conversation, Mr. Seaton does not have that tone. You must remember this obturator was a complete and radical change and the first one was only inserted a day or two ago.

The sound to which Dr. Ottolengui refers is due perhaps to the fact that the back of the bridge is open, presenting a very uneven surface. I at first closed that with a piece of gutta-percha, but knowing that he could not wear anything of that kind, and that he would soon accustom himself to the conditions, I discontinued it. I know that within a short time Mr. Seaton will be entirely free from the slight imperfect tone he has at present. You can see that his enunciation of the most difficult words is absolutely perfect.

The subject was then passed.

The next order of business was a paper by Dr. B. J. CIGRAND, Chicago, Ill., entitled "Facial Guide Lines as Taught by Artists and Sculptors."

The paper was illustrated with fifty-six stereopticon views.

Dr. Turner here resumed the chair.

The next paper on the program was one by Dr. G. H. WILSON, Cleveland, Ohio, on the subject "Some Properties of Plaster of Paris and Its Compounds," as follows:

Some Properties of Plaster of Paris and Its Compounds.

By GEORGE H. WILSON, D.D.S., Cleveland, Ohio.

IN some form, plaster is the material upon which all dental substitutes are constructed; hence it is pertinent that the material and its peculiar properties should be well understood. I opine that most of our failures in prosthetic dentistry are due to a lack of knowledge of the materials we use and a comprehension of the underlying principles of manipulation; that is, they are not due to an insufficiency of material, but to lack of knowledge and dexterity.

Prof. C. J. Essig, in the "American Text-Book of Prosthetic Dentistry," states: "Plaster of Paris (calcium sulfate, $CaSO_4$) is prepared from a native calcium sulfate, containing two molecules water of crystallization ($CaSO_4 + 2H_2O$), called gypsum when found in opaque masses, alabaster when it presents a semi-opaque appearance, and selenite when it occurs in transparent prisms. The first is the common source of plaster of Paris. It is prepared by heating the mineral in an oven where the heat does not exceed 127° C. (261° F.), by which the water of crystallization is expelled. It is afterward reduced to a fine powder, and when mixed with water it solidifies after a short time from the re-formation of the same hydrate; but this effect does not happen if the gypsum has been overheated and its affinity for water destroyed. In setting there is always a slight evolution of heat and more or less expansion."

Gypsum is a more or less impure hydrated calcium sulfate, and the plaster produced from the rock of different sections of country will have different working qualities, and each be suitable for some special purpose; also the method of manufacture will produce certain properties; therefore it becomes necessary to know the nature of any brand of plaster before we can know whether it is or is not adapted to a specific use.

There are two properties of plaster of Paris to be considered in this paper—*expansion* and *compressibility*.

EXPANSION.

The expansion of plaster of Paris has been studied more or less thoroughly at different times for the past sixty years. Probably the most accurate investigation from a scientific standpoint has recently been made by Dr. Prothero of the Northwestern University Dental School, with a specially constructed micrometer. During the past two years various articles have appeared in the journals by Dr. Stewart J. Spence, detailing various experiments. The writer of this paper believes that some of the experiments were misleading and some of the doctor's deductions were incorrect.

I desire to state this proposition as a truism: That a material (such as plaster of Paris) must be judged by the results obtained when it is manipulated by the best known methods.

I assume that all accept the statement quoted from Professor Essig, that "Plaster expands more or less." Upon experiment it is found that there is much difference in the expansion of the various brands upon the market; also that the method of manipulation makes a marked difference. For scientific accuracy it is necessary to have an instrument that will measure one ten-thousandth of inch, but for practical purposes a very simple and inexpensive method will demonstrate what kind of plaster will give practical results. I have adopted for this purpose a beaker of thirty-five to forty grams, or nearly one and one-half ounces capacity. It is slightly tapering and nearly one and one-half inches in diameter at the top. This beaker is thin, is of well-annealed glass, and sufficiently strong to stand the slight expansion of some brands of plaster, when properly mixed. A plaster that expands somewhat more may make a single crack in the beaker in twenty to thirty minutes' time; while another may shiver the glass into many pieces in from five to ten minutes. I have used several dozens of these beakers in this manner and have not had one break after thirty minutes from the time of placing the plaster in the receptacle, yet at the time of writing this paper some of these beakers have been standing eight months.

A plaster when properly mixed may not fracture the glass, but will, if improperly handled, show marked expansion. There are two essential factors in mixing plaster: First, a definite ratio of plaster to water so as to produce the maximum strength without perceptible expansion. Second, excessive agitation in mixing the plaster causes expansion and reduces the strength; due to a disturbance of crystallization. I have found that while one plaster may require two measures of plaster to one of water to make a proper mix, another may require as much as three and one-fourth measures of plaster to one of water; also that plaster when freshly ground will require more water than when it has been standing exposed to the atmosphere.

Lineal expansion. The first test was made by filling a seven by three-fourths inch test tube, which gave a negative result; there being perceptible to the eye no cracks in the glass or bulging of the plaster at the open end of the tube. For the second experiment, I had made a frame for molding bars of plaster eighteen inches long; upon either end was securely fastened an end-piece one and one-half inches thick; a piece of one-fourth inch thick plate glass was placed upon the base between the end-pieces, and two sliding bars one-half inch thick were placed over the glass between the end-pieces, so that a bar of plaster one-half inch thick, and any width up to two and a half inches wide, could be molded. All the parts were kept thoroughly oiled to prevent adhesion of the plaster. It is reasonable to suppose that if there were any perceptible expansion of this eighteen-inch bar that it would show itself in the direction of least resistance and consequently would be bowed upward. The results were practically *nil,* so far as the eye could detect. I believe we are justified in concluding that if a plaster when properly manipulated will stand the test of the beaker and the eighteen-inch bar, its expansion does not necessarily account for a misfit denture, but that the imperfect adaptation is due to an unsuitable plaster or faulty manipulation.

French's regular dental plaster was used for these experiments. This plaster is probably obtainable at all dental supply houses.

COMPRESSIBILITY.

The writer is not aware that special stress has ever been laid upon this property of plaster; but if so, this contribution is offered as corroborative testimony. The writer believes that this property of plaster accounts for more failures in prosthesis than all other causes, barring a lack of knowledge and manipulation.

The testing of this property of plaster has been done with a lever upon a freely sliding plunger one-half inch in diameter. The plaster was placed in the lower half of a vulcanite flask, as the unconfined plaster would crush and give no satisfactory test of compression. The first series of tests was with French's regular dental plaster, to determine the time at which it reached its greatest degree of hardness. The conclusions were, that with two measures of plaster to one of water, and with minimum stirring, the greatest resistance to pressure was reached in from twenty to twenty-five minutes. The tests were carried through a period of twenty-two hours. Other brands of plaster varied very materially, some requiring between one and two hours.

The next series of tests was to determine the length of time during which compression took place. As near as the eye could determine the compression was complete in about five or ten seconds; fifteen minutes' application of a given pressure made no perceptible increase.

It was observed in another series of experiments that the compression increased much more rapidly than the force applied; thus seven hundred and fifty pounds made fully twice the compression produced by five hundred pounds; and the same was also true of a thousand pounds compared with the seven hundred and fifty pounds.

10

I find that French's regular dental plaster is practically non-expanding, is fine-grained, mixes smoothly, sets quickly, reaches its greatest hardness in about twenty-five minutes, shows but slight compression at two hundred and fifty pounds, but excessive at one thousand pounds pressure—between five and six one-hundredths of an inch. Thus far the plasters I have examined show much more marked expansion and generally considerable less compressibility than French's.

The Spence plaster compound is a remarkable preparation. It requires a small quantity of water and much kneading. A suitable mix can be made with three to three and one-fourth measures of plaster to one of water, which will not break the glass beaker; but upon working in more compound some expansion will be developed. In thirty minutes the material will resist a greater force than French's regular dental plaster, but its maximum strength is not developed for about two hours, when one thousand pounds pressure will not make the impression that two hundred and fifty pounds will upon ordinary plaster. The material is hard to mix and is very coarse grained. I use it for making casts by lining the impression with a thin layer of regular dental plaster, and the Spence compound is packed into the soft plaster lining. By this means I obtain a cast that is smooth and dense upon its surface and has great strength. The compound is also most valuable for articulating casts, being very hard, strong, and sharp in outline.

Appreciation of the fact of compressibility of plaster is of great importance in vulcanite and celluloid work. When the prosthetist has obtained an accurately fitting base-plate, and having proved the ar-

ticulation by trying in the mouth, finds that in the finished denture the teeth are too long upon one side, or the plate warped out of shape, it does not imply expansion of plaster or shrinkage of plate material, but rather an excess of rubber or celluloid improperly placed, and undue pressure. If there was an expansion of plaster in the flask there would be a thinning of the plate, because the investment plaster would compress the wax form, while the trouble is a thickening of a portion or the whole of the plate. These statements are proved by the fact that a perfectly fitting denture can be produced of these materials. While it is true that all plaster expands and rubber contracts in the process of vulcanization, it is equally true that these inherent properties are so minute when the best materials and processes of manipulation are employed that they make no practical difference in the finished denture.

Unvulcanized rubber is an exceedingly tenacious material; it will flow under slight pressure if given time, but will resist a tremendous pressure momentarily. The flask is closed under screw pressure; probably one to three tons pressure is often applied.

In considering the power of the screw in the flask press, we must consult physics, which informs us that the screw is a wedge and lever, and the work is equal to the power multiplied by the circumference described by the power, multiplied by the pitch of the screw, less the friction of the screw. The very convenient press, No. 2 of the Buffalo Dental Mfg. Co., will serve us for illustration. The circumference is twenty-five (plus) inches, the pitch one-tenth of an inch; allowing one-fifth for friction we have each pound of power producing two hundred pounds of work; and when we consider the tremendous force so easily applied upon compressible plaster, we have a sufficient explanation for all misfit vulcanite and celluloid dentures, provided a perfect plaster impression and cast were used.

CONCLUSION.

A perfect fitting vulcanite denture can be made from a properly prepared plaster cast, or, what is safer in the hands of most men, a Spence-compound cast with a plaster facing, attention being given to packing and vulcanizing.

The rubber should be placed according to the space to be filled. It is better not to use sufficient rubber to entirely fill the mold at first; but use the wet cloth to separate the case, and add the necessary amount of rubber for the second or even the third closing of the flask. The cloth separator can be used over a vulcanite base plate as well as over a plaster cast. The flask and contents must be well warmed and the pressure applied lightly and increased at intervals of a few seconds.

The vulcanization should be accomplished at a low temperature and given a long time.

We should study our failures, for by them much is to be learned.

Discussion.

Dr. J. H. PROTHERO, Chicago, Ill. It is with much pleasure that I have listened to Dr. Wilson's most excellent paper and noted the many excellent points of interest touched upon. Only those who have taken up original lines of research and carried them through until a greater or less degree of success has been attained can appreciate the efforts of the essayist. I heartily welcome this paper as a valuable contribution to prosthetic literature.

The principal subject of this paper and the one on which the essayist lays the most stress, namely, the compressibility of plaster, has been almost totally disregarded by many in practice. Its importance is unquestioned, as the evil results pointed out by him in denture construction are sure to occur if proper precautionary measures are not observed.

While aware of the fact that a large surplus of rubber under heavy, rapid pressure will distort the face of almost any ordinary plaster model or of the entire matrix in some cases, my own ability to lessen such occurrences by proper measures has led me to neglect investigations along this line for what appeared of more importance, namely, the expansion of plaster. In my capacity of teacher, however, I have laid considerable stress on the error resulting from compressibility, as all beginners unless forewarned are liable to meet with more or less difficulty. I have been pleased as well as benefited greatly to hear Dr. Wilson's ideas on this subject, as I am sure all those who have heard them have been, and I will therefore offer no criticism on this phase of the subject, except to state that his means of measuring the compressibility of plaster seem somewhat too crude to secure accurate comparative results.

Nothing impresses upon the mind more clearly the expansive, contractile, and compressible qualities of a material under like or unlike conditions than a record of such movements in fractions of an inch or in millimeters.

In regard to the use of Dr. Spence's or some other hard plaster for the body of models, the idea appears to be a good one and will largely overcome the evil results caused by the careless packing of rubber, or faulty manipulation in closing flasks, which, as Dr. Wilson states, are common sources of error.

I will state here that I have been conducting a number of experiments lately with a combination of Portland cement and plaster of Paris. I am getting fairly good results and think will soon arrive at a point where I can tell what is the correct formula for a dental plaster, so that you can manufacture it yourself.

I must, however, take exception to Dr. Wilson's experiments on the expansion of plaster and to the deductions he draws from those experiments. In the first place, the use of the beaker—which is cracked when expansion passes beyond a certain limit and which maintains its integrity when under that limit—is too crude for practical purposes. Could the present accurate knowledge of the behavior of dental amalgam alloys have been determined, or could these alloys have been brought to their present almost perfect state without the use of the amalgam micrometer? I am sure it would not have been possible. For years before Dr. Black took up the study of alloys, various men were engaged in filling cavities in ivory blocks, test tubes, and steel matrices with alloy, and testing microscopically whether shrinkage or expansion occurred. No accurate results, however, were arrived at until an accurate instrument was devised for recording any and all changes that might occur under varying conditions. In the amalgam tests the object was to find a material which, in addition to other necessary qualities, would neither expand nor contract. So in the study of the physical properties of plaster, we wish to discover some mode of treatment of the material or method of manipulation that will con-

trol expansion and contraction, and this can only be done by careful and accurate experiments with suitable instruments. Therefore, I feel justified in stating that the tests on expansion, as recorded by Dr. Wilson, are inaccurate and not to be compared with his tests on the compressibility of plaster. The essayist states that he finds French's regular dental plaster non-expanding, fine-grained, mixes smoothly, sets quickly, and reaches its greatest hardness in twenty-five minutes. From my own experience as well as experiments with this brand of plaster I can say that it expands fully as much as ordinary plaster unless precautions are taken to obviate this movement. All plasters expand to a greater or less extent. The degree of expansion depends largely upon the manner of manipulation as well as upon the proportions in which the plaster and water are mixed.

A mixture of French's dental plaster manipulated in the ordinary way and in bulk the width of an ordinary impression, expands about sixty ten-thousandths of an inch in twenty minutes. The amount of expansion noted is sufficient to bulge an ordinary impression upward in the palatal portion to a very noticeable extent, thereby producing an incorrect copy of the mouth. A model poured into such an impression under similar circumstances will also be distorted in like manner. A denture constructed over such a model regardless of its density and resistance to compression, even though the manipulative steps were accurately carried out, would result in a misfit, therefore it appears to me very important that the expansive property of plaster should be overcome if possible, or at least reduced to the minimum to obviate error in the initial steps of dental construction.

Dr. Wilson says, "A plaster, when

properly mixed, may not fracture the glass, but will, if improperly handled, show marked expansion." He further says, "There are two essential factors in mixing plaster. First, a definite ratio of plaster to water, so as to produce the maximum strength without perceptible expansion. Second, excessive agitation in mixing the plaster causes expansion and reduces the strength due to a disturbance of crystallization.

"I have found that while one plaster may require two measures of plaster to one of water to make a proper mix, another may require as much as three and one-fourth measures of plaster to one of water."

These statements are contradictory from the fact that in the first instance a definite ratio of plaster and water are recommended, and in the second instance the statement is made that various plasters require different quantities of water.

I agree with the essayist that the plaster and water should be mixed in definite proportions to secure the best results, and following out this idea I conducted many experiments to determine the proper quantity of each.

The following proportions were found to give the most uniform results:

Plaster,	gr. lv;
Water,	40 cc.;
Sulfate of potash,	gr. v.

Very slight agitation.

The sulfate of potash is used to control expansion and should be dissolved in the water previous to sifting in the plaster.

Dr. WILSON. In the experiments conducted by me, I placed in a triangular receptacle 6 inches long a mix of French's dental plaster mixed in the ordinary way. Placed in that, it would expand ten one-thousandths in twenty-five minutes and in the second expansion not less than ten one-hundredths. Now, as compared with conditions in which it has not been used, I am unable to state. I know this, we have secured excellent results with sulfid potassium when incorporated with water in the fitting of dentures, but when the rubber is placed in the flask there is a certain deterioration of the face of the model and perhaps of the entire matrix. I have models showing expansion of at least one-tenth of a millimeter.

Dr. B. J. CIGRAND, Chicago, Ill. I would like to say a word in regard to this very excellent paper of Dr. Wilson's. It seems to be the old story—the subject we at times think we know the most about is the thing we really know least about. Within the past two years men like Dr. Wilson and Dr. Prothero have shown us that we did not know much about the manipulation of plaster of Paris. I rather agree with Dr. Prothero that the beaker is not as accurate a measurement as would be the micrometer, for the reason that the glass is largely affected by the temperature of the plaster poured into it.

Dr. WILSON. It is the same mix.

Dr. CIGRAND. But you cannot tell how absolutely alike were the beakers—you cannot tell that. The thin one would be the first one to fracture. I believe the micrometer would be the better way of measuring it.

Another point Dr. Prothero brought out, which I appreciate very much, that of the change in the mouth and in the tray, and third in the model, and possibly there is a fourth.

This is a matter we ought to be very much interested in, because many a plate which has been carefully constructed has not been entirely satisfactory for this very reason.

Dr. WILSON (closing the discussion). As far as my experience with the beakers was concerned, they were not designed to be of scientific accuracy. Dr. Prothero has gone into that in detail. My object in undertaking this work was to make a simple test of the plaster we are using, because I know many men have the habit of purchasing builder's plaster; yet that expands far more than the French regular dental plaster, although much harder.

How many students or practitioners can detect a ten-thousandth part of an inch. What difference does a ten thousandth or two ten-thousandths of an inch make in an artificial denture?

Dr. Prothero compares the amalgam with the plaster experiments. In the case of amalgam we must fill cavities properly to keep out microbes: we are not trying to keep out microbes. With plaster the case is different. We do not need so close an adaptation, but we do not want differences of one-quarter, one-eighth, or one-sixteenth of an inch.

I say that the ordinary plaster can be worked in such a way that it will give good results; but if we do not work it properly we do not get good results.

Dr. Prothero criticizes the paper upon the point of the ratio of plaster to that of water. He states that there is a given ratio. The given ratio in the case of French regular dental plaster is two measures of plaster to one of water. I will state that it will be found that it requires one and three-quarters of plaster to one of water.

Another point brought up is that there might be a difference in the thickness of the glass. In this instance I performed this test with the idea that the one would break and the other would not; I used no care in the selection of the glasses.

The object of my work was to make a practical test. We cannot all have a micrometer—could not all afford it, but we will be glad to have Dr. Prothero do this work.

Dr. PROTHERO. I am now just as much in the dark as I was before in regard to the correct method of manipulation so that the plaster will not expand, and I would be very much pleased to have Dr. Wilson enlighten me.

Dr. WILSON. I consider the essential point is to ascertain the proper measure of plaster, and to stir sufficiently with the proper amount of water. I would be pleased to have Dr. Prothero test this and see if it is not correct. I will say, in making these tests I mix a mass with very little stirring, and then stir in the rest until it begins to crystallize, because I consider the degree of stirring causes the difference in the expansion of the plaster, for the reason that it was the same mix of plaster, only the one portion was stirred longer than the other.

Dr. PROTHERO. Yes, I recognize the fact that much stirring will greatly increase the rapidity with which it expands.

Adjourned till Wednesday afternoon.

SECTION VIII—Continued.

SECOND DAY—Wednesday, August 31st.

THE session was called to order at 2.30 P.M. by the chairman, Dr. Chas. R. Turner.

The CHAIRMAN. I take pleasure in calling upon Dr. REUBEN C. BROPHY of Chicago, Ill., who will read the first paper upon the program for this afternoon's session.

Dr. Brophy then read his paper, entitled "The Rationale of Materials Used in the Construction of Dental Base-Plates," as follows:

The Rationale of Materials Used in the Construction of Dental Base-Plates.

By REUBEN C. BROPHY, M.D., D.D.S., Chicago, Ill.

IT is demanded that the profession of dentistry be credited with having made great progress in development, and that acknowledgment be made that it is upon a sound and substantially scientific basis; yet, in my opinion there are some infractions of this generally existent rule, one of which I have the honor of considering upon this occasion under the title "The Rationale of Materials Used in the Construction of Dental Base-Plates."

The profession of dentistry as a learned, scientific body, should not regard lightly any phase of its practice, but all subjects should command equally earnest thought and study. The branch of dental practice comprehended in the substitution of artificial for natural teeth through the use of plates, is of sufficient importance to merit the earnest and most thorough consideration of the profession.

While it is true that the prime motive actuating the truly professional dentist in his labors is to prevent the loss of the natural teeth, and thereby to prevent the necessity of plate work, yet the acknowledgment is forced from us that with all our skill, with all our earnest effort, that demand for this particular work will endure perpetually.

So long then as we must recognize plate work as a fixed, permanent department of practice, it is demanded that we attach as much importance to its development to a general standard of excellence as we attach to any other department of practice.

In the comments which I shall make upon this subject in this essay, I hope to cover somewhat broadly the general adaptability of the various materials in use in the construction of dentures dependent upon contact with the soft contiguous tissues for their retention, from a standpoint of physiology, hygiene, and influences reflecting upon the standards of mechanical skill of our profession.

I place physiology first, you notice. If my conception of this matter is correct the requirement of paramount importance for the dentist is conservation of humanity's physiological interests.

The teeth serve an important purpose in the animal economy; we strive to preserve them, and when lost we reproduce them, with the well-grounded conviction that the physical interests of the patient demand it.

Thus far, however, we have no direct connection with our title argument, for any kind of material may be employed in carrying teeth which will restore the dental function.

I have laid stress upon the physiological importance of restoration of the teeth, as generally and rightfully regarded, merely to more forcibly call attention to the peculiarly inconsistent practice employed by our profession of using materials or substances in making artificial dentures which in themselves to a great extent are physiologically incompatible. It is proper that we should first consider the properties which a material should possess in order to be physiologically compatible.

I believe that a material to be compatible to animal tissue, when fixed in contact with those tissues as a base-plate is fixed, first of all must be a ready conductor of heat, and must be of low specific heat. This, to my mind, is the characteristic of first importance from a standpoint of physiology.

There can be no restriction of the radiation of the body heat without a physiological effect, and I think that it will be admitted by physiologists that beyond a certain limit restriction of such radiation cannot be maintained without pathological effects.

The upper base-plate particularly, when perfectly adapted to the superior maxilla is held in contact with the tissues upon which it rests through complete exclusion of the air from beneath it. We are told that plates are held in position by capillary attraction, but inasmuch as there can be no such thing as capillary attraction in the presence of the atmosphere it has always been a question with me whether it would not be fully as proper at least to term the force which retains plates in position atmospheric pressure. Atmospheric pressure certainly exists whatever other forces are exerted.

In a paper read by me before the Chicago Dental Society November 15, 1899, and published in the *Dental Review,* vol. xiii, No. 11, I reported experiments I had made to determine heat transmission, or conductivity, and specific heat of vulcanite and of metal. These experiments showed that vulcanite conducted heat very much slower than did the metal used, which was aluminum. I made use of that metal because of the fact that it approaches vulcanite more nearly in the matter of cost than any other metals in use for the purpose of making plates, and because of the fact that it makes invalid the argument that the cost of metal plates debars them from general use.

Knowing then that vulcanite—and what is said of vulcanite may also be said of the other vegetable compound, celluloid—is a very much slower conductor of heat than the metals, and the further concomitant fact that it absorbs and retains heat to a greater extent, or is of much higher specific heat, and knowing that as a result of these physical characteristics the tissues which are held in contact with them are constantly maintained in a superheated condition through excessive prevention of normal radiation of the animal heat through them, we may well conclude that the unquestionable fact that in the great majority of mouths in which these plates are worn the underlying tissues are found to be in a pathological condition is most plausible evidence that this lack of conductivity is very largely if not wholly the cause of such pathological condition.

Placing conductivity, then, first as an essential to physiological compatibility of dental base-plates, I would name as a second essential quality, freedom from constituent substances which might in any way exert toxic influences upon animal tissues when in contact with them, or indirectly by chemical action upon the animal physical economy. It is known that the metals are free from constituents, and that those we may or would use for base-plates are free in themselves of such chemical action; while it is also known that in the vegetable compounds used the qualities do exist which yield such influences.

In the characteristic of dental base-plate materials which come next for our consideration, as stipulated by me at the outset of my essay, i.e. hygiene, a very important connection exists between it and the quality of physiological compatibility just considered.

An unhygienic base-plate cannot be physiologically compatible. Nature rebels against uncleanliness. Give us absolute cleanliness, a perfect hygienic condition, and bacteria are repelled. Uncleanliness in some form or another is the precursor of practically all disease.

What qualities in the base-plate are essential to hygiene?

First, the material of which the base-plate is made should be solid and dense and its surface should be capable of receiving and should receive a smooth finish and polish in order that there may be no mechanical retention of substances coming in contact with it, and it should be made of material for which the oral secretions have a minimum affinity.

The metals only possess these qualities to an extent desired. Not only do the vegetable bases not possess them, but, through the application of the heat to which they are subjected when in the mouth, latent odors are brought out, and, through association with odors thrown off by the fermentative processes of the secretions within the mouth, they are intensified to an extent approaching very nearly the limit of obnoxiousness.

I have considered the qualities pertaining to the interests of the laity we serve which base-plates should possess—physiological compatibility, and hygiene. I now come to the consideration of my theme from the last standpoint from which I am to consider it—that of the influences of materials used for base-plates, or more properly in this instance for dental plates, upon the standard of mechanical skill in our profession. This is an important consideration.

At the outset of my paper I said that while our profession had made great progress in the past, there were some infractions of that generally existent rule. To my mind the present standard of skill made use of in our profession in the line of plate work is a most striking infraction of that rule. Men of our profession who express themselves honestly will freely acknowledge that not only has the standard of skill exercised in dental plate work not advanced, but for the past fifty years, or since the introduction of the vegetable compounds, it has been constantly degenerating.

Whence are we to look for the cause of this condition? Wholly to the fact of the metals having been so generally superseded by vulcanite. In the first place the dentists of half a century ago or more regarded this branch of the practice with much more interest than it is regarded now; they regarded it as of sufficient importance then to do it themselves, and, as a result of their individual efforts, they became artisans in metal working; they felt that they had to be; to construct a plate demanded skill, they considered.

What is the condition existing today? You all know, gentlemen; it is unnecessary for me to dwell upon this. With the introduction of the vegetable plates progress in skill ceased, and interest in this particular department began to wane. Now the greater percentage of dentists take the impression and turn it over to someone else to construct the plate. Skill in plate work and the application of science in the work have largely become dead letters.

The question of the greatest importance before the dental profession today is, Will it continue to tolerate this its greatest and practically only barrier to the title of a skilled and scientific profession, and is it to indefinitely suffer without dissent and unopposed the continued use of vegetable compounds in prosthesis?

Discussion.

Dr. GEORGE H. WILSON, Cleveland, Ohio. I want to say that I feel the paper is in the right direction. The opposition that I will offer is not with the purpose of opposing Dr. Brophy, but with the idea of possibly having him work harder to bring about the desired results.

Unquestionably the first part of the paper is correct in stating there is not the appreciation for prosthetic dentistry there should be. Only a few of us who are especially interested in this branch give our direct attention to it, and it devolves upon these few to bring about the perfection that we desire. So, that while this paper is in the right direction, in trying to improve and correct the faults of the practitioners, I feel that the essayist has made some progress, and that he can still improve in some directions.

There is no question as he states, that first of all the material must be a ready conductor of heat. He speaks of certain undesirable materials being of a low specific heat. I cannot comprehend why this should make any special difference. The specific heat is the property of absorbing heat in carrying it from one certain temperature to another. This heat is so little, I cannot see how that would of itself do harm. I can comprehend how the radiation of heat can be of importance, but how the specific heat can be so, I do not fully comprehend. I would like to have Dr Brophy make that more plain.

Then he speaks of the plates being held in place by capillary attraction and adds that there is no such thing as capillary attraction in the presence of atmospheric pressure. As I understand, capillary attraction occurs when two plates are held in quite close contact, when moisture and some air will of course be drawn up between the two plates. I do not see why we cannot have capillary attraction between the soft tissues. He says that we should call that atmospheric pressure. We cannot have atmospheric pressure as long as there is to any great extent absolute contact so as to have a vacuum. If we have a space so the pressure can be reduced, then of course we have atmospheric pressure. If that space be filled in with moisture, then I cannot understand how we can have atmospheric pressure.

Regarding the expensiveness of the material, Dr. Brophy considers that aluminum is equally inexpensive as vulcanite. This, I think, is a mistake; the expense of labor in construction is the great and important factor. The labor in the construction of aluminum is as great if not greater than in vulcanite, and if it is greater then it is more expensive.

I think I heard Dr. Brophy say at one time that he could make nine successful cases out of every ten attempts with vulcanite. We ought not to have any such percentage—it ought to be correct every time. If one plate in ten is a failure, it adds very materially to the expense of construction.

Another thing, I have my doubts as to whether anyone has yet perfected aluminum to the extent that the secretions of the mouth will not act in a detrimental way, as is the case now in many instances. I have two cases in mind that do not prove its durability; in the summer of 1878 or 1879 I constructed a plate, and in ten years it was completely perforated. Another plate had to be replaced in five or six years. I have seen other cases in other mouths that were perforated in five or six years. It is usually necessary to replace the plate in five or ten years, which adds materially to the cost of the material. Aluminum is no more expensive than vulcanite so far as the material *per se* is concerned.

Dr. Brophy makes two charges against vulcanite: one is its retention of heat, which is well taken. This is one of the greatest objections to the material. The next one he speaks of is the injurious ingredients in the coloring matter. We can obviate this by using black rubber, but pure vermilion, which is mercuric sulfid, is perfectly insoluble in the fluids of the mouth and cannot therefore act injuriously upon the tissues of the mouth or systemically.

Dr. R. M. SANGER, East Orange, N. J. I listened to Dr. Brophy's paper with a great deal of interest because it is a timely protest on the part of Dr. Brophy against the all too careless construction of artificial dentures, not from a mechanical standpoint but from a physiological and hygienic one. I believe the purpose of his paper is to call the attention of the profession to this neglect and try in a measure to correct it.

Dr. Brophy has only suggested a remedy, and I would like to supplement his suggestion by the statement that in my opinion the rising generation of dentists allow the fee to stand ahead of their better judgment. They permit the patient to dictate to them what that fee shall be, rather than dictating it to the patient, and because of their fear they do a class of work which in their heart of hearts they know is not the best that can be done for the patient if the question of cost is eliminated. Do you question the cost of the doctor when your life is in danger, and should you question the cost of a dentist when your health is in danger thereby?

It is time for us to array ourselves with Dr. Brophy on the side of a higher standard—of more scientific dental prosthesis—to have gold, and platinum, and porcelain reinstated in their rightful places in dentistry. We do not need to compromise by substituting aluminum.

Dr. H. J. GOSLEE, Chicago, Ill. Possibly you can now appreciate why I wished Dr. Sanger to speak first, as he has so correctly and beautifully expressed my sentiments. I am heartily in accord with the paper and with the somewhat idealistic views of the author, and as Dr. Sanger has said, I believe that we have been working away from the ideal toward the cheaper or more commercial aspect of this phase of dentistry for too long a time, and that we should now endeavor to reinstate a class of work which has given so much satisfaction in years past, and which is not used now as much as it should be.

Dr. BROPHY (closing the discussion). I want in the first place to express my appreciation of the frankness with which everyone has spoken who has taken part in the discussion of my paper. That is one thing I like under all circumstances—frank, honest expression of views. While Dr. Wilson does not agree with me, I feel nevertheless that he is entitled to congratulations equally with those who have more nearly agreed with me, because I do not doubt the honesty of his convictions.

First, in regard to specific heat. There is a connection between conductivity and specific heat; any material which is a slow conductor of heat will be found of high specific heat. The two taken in combination, in the matter of a base-plate, are the things which tend to maintain the underlying tissues in a superheated condition.

Upon the question of capillary attraction, I said in my paper that such a thing was impossible in the presence of the atmosphere. I may be wrong, but if so I shall have to ask that it be demonstrated to me.

I feel that it is unfortunate that I spoke of aluminum in my paper. I infer from the remarks of Dr. Sanger and also of Dr. Wilson that they took it that I was especially championing this metal as a material for base-plates. As a matter of fact I did not do so. In my paper I advocated the use of the metals in preference to vulcanite. As clearly stated by me, I referred to aluminum because it fairly represented in desirable characteristics all metals used for the purpose of making base-plates, and principally because it most nearly approaches vulcanite in the matter of cost. Dr. Wilson was wrong in his inference that I made the claim that aluminum plates could be made cheaper than vulcanite plates, for I did not.

The argument of Dr. Wilson that vulcanite is durable is a very poor argument in favor of this material for use as base-plates, for, because of its non-conductivity and high specific heat qualities, absorption is so furthered by it that in order to insure constancy of adaptation or fit, changes or new plates are demanded in this material much more frequently than in the metals. In my opinion the fact that a vulcanite plate that has been worn fifteen to twenty-five years, as Dr. Wilson stated, is not much of a recommendation. I believe that in every case these plates should be discarded for the best interests of the wearer long before the lapse of that much time.

The CHAIRMAN. Before announcing the next paper, I notice that Dr. Charles Godon of Paris, France, president of the International Dental Federation, is in the room, and I wish to invite him to occupy the chair as honorary president.

Dr. Godon took the chair.

Dr. CHARLES GODON. Mr. President, I thank you for the honor.

The CHAIRMAN. I have pleasure in stating that the next paper is a contribution from Germany, and will be presented by the author in person. I am pleased to introduce Zahnarzt Dr. HERRMANN RAUHE of Düsseldorf, Germany, who will read his paper entitled "A New Suction Chamber."

The paper was as follows:

A New Suction Chamber.

By Zahnarzt Dr. HERMANN RAUHE, Düsseldorf, Germany.

IN the course of years, many kinds of suction chambers have been recommended with the common object of securing artificial teeth to the palate without the use of clasps.

First there were the chambers formed in a rubber plate by the use of an oval or heart-shaped tin plate; then we had pearl and star plates which covered the surface of the rubber with a number of suction chambers.

These were soon given up for the reason that on one side they soon lost their effectiveness because the pearls sank into the membrane, irritated it, and shortly rendered it spongy. Then the manufacture of double suction chambers came in. But they lasted only a short time because violent irritations took place even with them, and they were also unclean. In the year 1872 a suction chamber was placed on the market which consisted in the attachment of a little rubber plate in the vault of the denture by means of a rivet and small metal plate, which was forced to the center of the rubber surface, giving it the form of a shallow cone. This possessed great power of adhesion, but two distinct disadvantages: the rubber plate soon became spongy and could only be renewed by the dentist and not by the patient, and the border of the rubber plate pressed so strongly against the membrane of the palate that irritation and frequently necrosis occurred. In the beginning of 1890 this plate was improved by a Frenchman, who vulcanized a little nut on the plate instead of the rivet. This facilitated the change of plates, but the rubber was still pressed hard against the palate and the same irritation resulted.

The new suction chamber that I wish to show you is similar to Hall's, but the defects of the old are avoided, and the replacement of the rubber disk is made very simple. On the center of the plate (Fig. 1), in the circular depression, we have placed a button-like addition, over which is placed a disk of rubber. The button is so constructed that the rubber disk assumes a slightly concave shape whereby it may be readily pressed up tight against the mucous membrane, but without any injurious effect. It works as a leather sucker instead of as a sucking bowl. As it almost fills the circular depression, the membrane is prevented from being drawn into this cavity, and thus irritation is avoided.

The replacing of the button is accomplished by means of a plate that we have designed. This plate—Figs. 2 and 3, the latter much enlarged—consists of three parts which in Fig. 2 are marked with the letters A, B, and C. The parts B and C are zinc, and by a slight pressure are joined together. Part A, between them, is made of gold.

This plate is placed as the former heart-shaped tin plate upon the center

now under the button plate, is partly divided to permit its easy removal.

With an excavator bend the ring, and then slowly withdraw it from beneath the button. Part A, the gold plate, is now bound fast to the rubber, as the hole in the center of the plate (D) is filled with hard rubber. This hard rubber and the little gold plate formed the button over

FIG. 1.

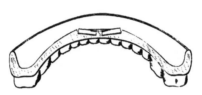

FIG. 2.

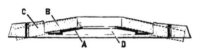

FIG. 3.

of the plaster cast with the opening upward, and is held by three little pins. In order not to injure the plate it is recommended that a piece of tin foil be laid over the cast, which, of course, must be removed subsequently. Now the case is packed with rubber as usual, paying particular attention, however, that the center of the vault has an abundance of rubber. After vulcanizing, remove the zinc plate and then the part C. which has the pins in it. The zinc ring B. which is

which is stretched the rubber ring. The position of the rubber ring after buttoning is shown by the dotted line in Fig. 2. After removing the zinc parts B and C. the button is flattened and polished, and after a rubber ring is put on the chamber is completed. So far as the shape of the chamber is concerned, for different jaws, it is important to look first of all for the flat portions of the palate—looking for the best location. When the palate is high and vault-like, or has a hard center, two chambers may be used. In plates for mouths in which the canines remain the chamber should be placed far back in the mouth to avoid a tilting of the plate during incision.

The advantages of this appliance are as follows: The plate is easily adapted to the model and the button plate stands away from the palatal surface of the plate to the extent of about one-fifth of a millimeter, that is the thickness of the base of part C. By this means irritation of the tissues by the button is prevented.

It is possible to button and unbutton the rubber ring without the use of tools.

The rubber disk will not irritate the palate because of its vaulted shape.

After a few days the rubber ring fills the concavity so perfectly that the mucous membrane cannot be drawn into it. Finally, the easy method of adapting the disk is an advantage which must not be undervalued, and the use of clasps is rendered entirely unnecessary.

This appliance does not possess its full adhesive property at first, but after a little use it becomes very strong. This should be explained to the wearer, and also that the rubber ring must be frequently changed and always as soon as it becomes larger than its corresponding chamber. As a suggestion, it is best to have two, keeping the one not in use quite dry and alternating daily.

Discussion.

Dr. R. M. Sanger, East Orange, N. J. The device which the essayist has shown us is a clever one, but in this country it is not new. It may be new in Germany, but here it is not. We knew of the same principle under the heading of the Scott suction disk. Whether you have all become familiar with it or not, I do not know, but Dr. Scott introduced the same principle in the seventies. Dr. Rauhe has made a slight improvement on Dr. Scott's idea, in that he makes the disk smaller and in that he protects his disk pretty nearly to the rim, so that the objection to the Scott disk is in a measure overcome— that is, that it will not become ball-shaped until the plate no longer comes in contact with the mucous membrane.

Now the fact that this is interchangeable, is not new, for Dr. Scott's disk was equally interchangeable and it had the same objection which Dr. Rauhe's invention will have in a modified form. In the first place, partially vulcanized rubber is affected by the mucous secretions, and in a little while it becomes soft and foul. He provides for this by putting in a new disk. In the second place, when this rubber begins to deteriorate there is a gathering of the secretions of the mouth, which makes it offensive.

Now there are mouths to which this device would be a godsend; fortunately for us, they are few, and consequently I should say that while this device from my standpoint would be applicable in those exceptional cases, I would hesitate to recommend it in general practice.

The secretary, Dr. H. W. Campbell. here took the chair.

Dr. C. R. Turner, Philadelphia, Pa. I differ in general with Dr. Rauhe upon the principle on which the use of the appliance is based. But, granting as Dr. Sanger has said, that there are a few cases which arise in practice in which a device of this type is about the last resort, I feel that the method which Dr. Rauhe has presented will be of considerable assistance to us.

I wish to particularly call attention to the careful detail with which the technique of the placing of the device in the denture has been worked out. The tin plate for holding the gold head of the pin, which has been passed around just now, makes a depression of fixed size in the palatal surface of the vulcanite denture, and the soft rubber disks are cut carefully to fit this, so that when the tin plate has been removed, and the rubber disk inserted, there is no space left into which the mucous membrane may be drawn.

The ease with which the soft rubber disk is taken off and replaced seems to me to be also a valuable phase of the use of this device, inasmuch as it is possible for the patient to be supplied with a box of the disks and to remove and replace them at will without the necessity of consulting the dentist.

I wish to express my personal thanks to Dr. Rauhe for being present and for reading the communication in person, and I trust the device he has presented to us will find its proper field of usefulness in this country.

Dr. H. J. Goslee, Chicago, Ill. I do not like to lose the opportunity of expressing to the gentleman who has come so far to give us this little idea, my personal appreciation of it in the very limited number of cases in which it might be applicable.

As Dr. Sanger has said, however, in America there is no longer much use for this or other similar methods, and it is only in extreme cases that we can utilize it.

With Dr. Turner, I appreciate the cleverness of the technique and construction of Dr. Rauhe's device—it is better than the Scott method and will be more permanent.

Along this line, however, I am in favor of the retention of dentures by other means, and am of the firm opinion that the sooner we get away from all such devices and work toward securing a close and uniform adaptation of the denture to the tissue upon which it rests, the sooner we will be contributing to the successful wearing of artificial dentures.

Dr. Rauhe (closing the discussion). I have little more to say in closing the discussion of my paper. I have used the little invention in many cases within the past two years with the greatest satisfaction.

Dr. Turner then resumed the chair.

The Chairman. We have another paper on the program for this afternoon, the author of which is not here; as we shall be much pressed for time I should be disposed to read this paper by title.

Dr. Goslee. I move that the next paper be read by title.

This motion being duly seconded was unanimously carried, and the secretary read the paper by title—"Which is the Ideal Crown—the Banded or the Bandless Crown?" by Edward G. Christiansen, Drammen, Norway. The paper here follows:

Which is the Ideal Crown—the Banded or the Bandless Crown?

By EDWARD G. CHRISTIANSEN, Drammen, Norway.

WHEN I received the kind invitation to read a paper before this section of the Fourth International Dental Congress I gladly availed myself of the opportunity in order to bring about a discussion upon a theme that I have been occupied with for a long time—and which all present, I am sure, have puzzled their brains about—well knowing that here in the native country of fine prosthetic work this theme would create a prolific discussion among the first masters in this domain.

The crowns mostly used have been the barrel and the collar crowns, as well as single crowns used as abutments for bridge work, and I am sure that it will create a great sensation to try to reduce the applicability of these appliances to a minimum of what they are now. In fact, this is what I intend to do. I am surprised that nobody has hitherto urged this, especially in view of the literature yearly published on the subject of crown and bridge work.

Most people have surely taken it for granted that a crown always ought to have a band about the root in order to strengthen it and to support the crown. Only in cases where the root has so deteriorated that it is impossible to place a band around it, have other methods of making a crown without a band been mentioned. From the time when ready-made crowns such as Bonwill's, Logan's, etc., have been used, we have seen excel-lent work—crowns that have remained in the mouth for years, and are still doing good service. It is therefore natural to ask why we have abandoned these crowns when their record is so commendable. The question is easily answered—the work of inserting them was too troublesome and the assortment from which to select them too limited.

The Logan crown is mostly used, but everyone who desires precise work must admit that it is an exceedingly laborious, not to say impossible, task to grind it so that it will adapt itself accurately to the surface and circumference of the root. The work was, therefore, as a rule, badly accomplished and dissatisfaction the result.

As to the collar crown the root is plainly covered by the cap and therefore not so exposed to be injured by caries. This therefore looks ideal in the beginning, but after some experience we will find that the collar crown also has its defects and that its applicability is highly overestimated. In the first place, how difficult it is to prepare the root in such a way that it is fit for the reception of the band. The root ought to have a slightly conical form in order to prevent the band from standing out from it anywhere and thus irritating the gum; but how often is not this impossible, when we at the same time are to have the band well under the margin of the gum! How many teeth do not slope down against the apex

11

of the tooth directly under the margin of the gum—and in such cases the fashioning is at any rate very difficult besides being inconvenient for both operator and patient. The adjustment of the band requires in many cases, I may say in most cases, an ability, a preciseness, and a patience greater than most dentists possess. For this reason alone the collar and barrel crowns are in many cases contra-indicated. In the second place, though the work be done as well as possible we nevertheless see in many patients that the gum does not bear the contact with the metal, but that the gum recedes from the metal, the consequence being that the band appears and the root is laid bare. As a rule we see this unacceptable consequence of the collar and barrel crown where the gum as a thin film only covers the neck of the tooth, *i.e.* on the labial or buccal sides.

Thus I think that apart from the inconvenience to the patient and the waste of time, there are sufficient reasons to limit the use of these crowns to very few cases, such as where the force of mastication will be exerted in one direction only, or where the root is very weak or short, precluding the placing of a sufficiently long post within the canal.

Everybody will no doubt admit that from an absolutely ideal point of view a crown forming a direct continuation of the root is the most correct, *i.e.* a crown filling only the place that was occupied by the lost substance. From the foregoing it follows, that in the case of the molars the barrel crown as a rule is contra-indicated, as the pressure here comes vertically on the occlusal plane, for which reason it is unnecessary to have a band around the root, which strengthens the crown against lateral pressure. Most of you will no doubt admit that it is very

seldom that we find the interproximal space absolutely normal between two barrel crowns. On the bicuspids, especially in the upper jaw, the band will often be necessary, namely, where the root is exceedingly weak and where the opposing teeth have grown up so that the crown has to be prepared more like a canine, and thus the pressure is directed particularly lingually and buccally. But here, as with canines and incisors, a half-band is sufficient, and the inconvenient consequence of the gum receding on the labial part is prevented.

May I here add that the term "half-band" is not precisely correct, as it is three-quarters of a ring that is used, the band extending from the mesio-buccal angle round the lingual side and to the disto-buccal angle of the tooth. As the term half-band has, however, become firmly established in literature, I do not want to alter it. The band is to be there either in order to strengthen the root or the post, and at all events three-quarters of a band will be sufficient for that purpose. When we have carried the band round the entire circumference of the root I think it has been with a conservative view, although the result is in most cases a failure.

A half-band is also much easier to adjust than a full band, as the half-band can be polished down to the root when soldered to the root-plate. I hold therefore that a usual band is contra-indicated in any and every case, and that only the half-band should be used—*i.e.* half-bands always ought to be used where the crown is to become an abutment for a bridge, also where molars are wanting, so that the mastication is performed by the front teeth, and briefly, wherever the root has to bear more than usual heavy pressure. It will be seen that we have innumerable examples in support of my theory; everything depends upon the accuracy with which the details of the work are carried out, and this only requires patience on the part of the practitioner. No greater difficulty is connected with the work. This alone gives it a great advantage over the usual banded crown. In most cases where a crown without a band would be too weak, the error is that the post has been too weak or that the root-plate is not regularly adjusted to the root, or that proper attention has not been paid to the articulation.

The post must be quadrangular and flattened, absolutely not round or square, as is usually the case. Further, the post must be placed in the root in such a way that the pressure when clinching the teeth influences the short side, as the post has its greatest strength in that direction.

How to prepare root-plates that exactly fit the root is nothing new. I shall, however, with your permission explain the method I have used for years, and by means of particular instruments. Some of my colleagues have perhaps heard of Messrs. Ash & Sons' Christiansen's crown-swaging outfit, or the American imitation of the same, the Ajax swager. I still use this outfit, but of course with an altered working method, as it is constructed with the barrel crown in view. In the first place the root is polished down to at least one-half mm. below the margin of the gum and care is taken that the gum is well pressed away in order to get an exact impression of the surface of the root. This is the next stage, and is made by means of Stent's composition. The best method of making it is to roll the mass to a point between the fingers and to bring it up to the root in a semistiff condition. The impression is well cooled and trimmed, and is afterward placed in one of the rings or cups which forms part of the outfit. The ring is filled with sand mixed with oil; the sand is laid round the impression in such a way that the surface rises about one-half mm. A second ring is placed on the top of the first and Spence metal is poured into it. Thus we obtain a model of the surface of the root, and then we quickly swage a gold plate by means of the compress. The whole work requires only a few minutes. For myself, I always leave it to my assistants to accomplish everything when the impression is taken, while I myself drill out the root-canal in the desired fashion. For incisors, canines, or single-rooted bicuspids the canal is made to fit a flattened square post. When ready the root-plate is placed on the root surface and fastened to place by means of a strong, sharp instrument (a tin or gold plugger answers the purpose) while a hole for a square post is made by means of another instrument of such a shape that the hole can be made to fit the post accurately, being conically pointed and in accordance to the shape of any of the four sizes of posts that I use. When the hole is ready a post is put through and the whole thing is taken out and soldered, after which it is replaced and a new hole is made either in front of or behind the first hole; then a post is carried into it and soldered to the plate and first post. In this manner I obtain a flattened, strong post. Of course the last post may be smaller than the first in the proportion that we desire the first post more or less strengthened. Now the exact adjustment of the root-plate is to be made. The plate is polished and finished so that it completely adapts itself to the surface and circumference of the root. The root-plate is made of 0.21 mm. pure gold, or of 0.18 mm. platinum, if a crown with porcelain backing is to be used. The posts are made of iridio-platinum. If a half-band is to be used a strip of 22-k. gold 0.2 mm. thick and as wide as the band is soldered to the outside of the plate, but with care that no surplus of solder runs down to the underside of the plate. The soldering finished, the plate is replaced in the mouth, where the half-band is polished exactly to the root, whereupon the whole thing is taken out and the half-band strengthened by means of solder.

The same method applies to incisors and canines, but for bicuspids and for molars it is essentially different. I here use an entirely new and, as I think, excellent method. Formerly I employed porcelain teeth as found in the market for this purpose, filling the space between the root-plate and the tooth with porcelain, but after having practiced this method for several years I have now abandoned it. I had found out that the porcelain bodies that we can now purchase are not strong enough for the building up of crowns except in very few cases, where the bite is exceptionally high. However, this method did not satisfy my desires because I could not always trust the durability, and further because these teeth are far from having an ideal shape and size. I therefore employ this method more seldom now. When constructing bicuspid or molar crowns after the new method I do it in this manner: The root-plate with the post being in position, with Stent's composition the bite is taken and the crown is completely modeled in the composition. This done, the crown is

tried in the mouth in order to examine if the articulation be correct, the patient being asked to masticate, to ascertain whether the contact-points are correctly adjusted, as it is impossible by means of an articulator only to carry out all these movements of mastication. Finally, the crown is placed in sand, as mentioned before, with the impression of the root and front side up, so that this part may be later on substituted by porcelain for the sake of appearance. Over this a ring is placed and Spence metal is poured into it. In the mold obtained by this means a gold plate of 24-k. gold 0.21 mm. thick is swaged. A drawing plate as used in the making of seamless crowns renders in this connection valuable assistance. The gold cap thus obtained is soldered to the root-plate, a correct articulator having been previously obtained. The porcelain body is now applied, thus adding strength and beauty to the finished piece. For the soldering 22-k. gold is used, as this does not melt at the fusing-point of Jenkins' enamel, which is the one I prefer for this work. In this way, in an easy manner I arrange to make a crown forming a direct continuation of the root and exceptionally strong, with a good exterior, and last but not least, with a correct articulation.

Dr. F. EWING ROACH, Chicago, Ill., read a paper entitled "A New System of Anchorage for Partial Dentures," after discussion of which,

The section adjourned until Thursday, September 1st, at 2.30 P.M.

SECTION VIII—Continued.

THIRD DAY—Thursday, September 1st.

THE section was called to order at 2.30 P.M., Dr. Chas. R. Turner, chairman, presiding.

The CHAIRMAN. I have great pleasure in announcing that the usual program for this afternoon has been slightly changed so that a paper may be presented by Dr. Ch. Godon of Paris, France, in behalf of his *confrère* Dr. LEON DELAIR, on "An Artificial Larynx and Glottis." The paper will not be read, as it has not been translated into English. Dr. Godon will give a brief description of the appliance with which Dr. Delair's paper deals.

Dr. CH. GODON, Paris, France. I am sorry this paper has not been put into English, because it is very interesting; I bring it to you from Professor Delair, of L'École Dentaire de Paris. He has made many appliances for the restoration of the tissues of the face. He is well known in Europe on this sort of work. One of the latest things he has made is an artificial larynx and glottis for a man who had to have those organs removed.

(Dr. Godon then gave a *résumé* of the paper illustrated with lantern slides.)

The paper was as follows:

Larynx et Glotte Artificiels.

Par LEON DELAIR, Paris, France,

PROFESSEUR SUPPLÉANT À L'ÉCOLE DENTAIRE DE PARIS.

AVANT de passer à la description de l'appareil phonateur qui fait l'objet de cette communication, je vais brièvement mentionner les travaux antérieurs entrepris dans un but analogue pour le remplacement post-opératoire d'un organe aussi essentiel que le larynx.

Billroth, le premier, pratique l'ablation totale du larynx et ce fut Gussembauer qui eut l'idée de remplacer l'organe supprimé par un appareil résonnant, en forme de fuseau. La partie supérieure de ce larynx artificiel était constituée par une anche formée de deux lames de métal extrêmement minces que faisait vibrer le passage de la colonne d'air sortie des poumons. La partie inférieure de l'appareil consistait en un tube où venait s'aboucher la canule trachéale. Pendant les repas, pour éviter la pénétration des aliments dans les voies respiratoires on obturait à l'aide d'un bouchon l'orifice inférieur de l'appareil.

A ce larynx rudimentaire Bruns apporta deux modifications primordiales : tout d'abord, il remplaça le tube inférieur rigide par une genouillère articulée permettant à la base de l'appareil de suivre les mouvements du pharynx et du cou, puis il supprima l'anche métallique pour mettre à sa place une pièce similaire en caoutchouc mou plus douce à actionner.

Julius Wolff vint ensuite qui modifie à son tour l'appareil, en enfermant l'anche dans une sorte de gaine qu'obturait un grillage de toile métallique s'opposant à l'introduction des particules alimentaires et des mucosités : Cependant ce larynx nécessitait toujours l'emploi d'un bouchon inférieur pendant les repas.

C'est au Docteur Cl. Martin de Lyon que revient l'honneur d'avoir apporté à l'appareil combiné de Gussembauer, de Bruns et de Wolff un dernier perfectionnement. Il y ajouta un tube œsophagien qui permet aux liquides et mucosités ayant pénétré dans la boîte de phonation de passer dans le tube digestif, et cela sans nuire au bon fonctionnement de l'instrument, ainsi sont assurées la phonation et la déglutition simultanées que les inventeurs précédents n'avaient pu réaliser.

Le larynx perfectionné par le Docteur Cl. Martin nécessité une pièce de prothèse immédiate insonore en caoutchouc mou. Elle est introduite dans la plaie aussitôt après la laryngectomie jusqu'à la cicatrisation complète des tissus et maintient la communication entre la bouche et la trachée, enfin elle réserve la place du larynx artificiel en caoutchouc durci qu'on posera quelques semaines après. Ce dernier, affecté à peu près la forme de l'organe naturel, il en a les mêmes dimensions. C'est une sorte de boîte conique dont la base supérieure est bouchée obliquement par un grillage métallique qui s'oppose à l'introduction des aliments.

L'appareil est terminé à la partie inférieure par un tube articulé, percé d'un trou transversal, pour l'introduction de la canule trachéale. A l'intérieur est placée l'anche vibrante qu'avait imaginé Bruns. Cette anche en tube de caoutchouc mou mince, est maintenue par une cage métallique conique et rectangulaire ; l'air expiré s'y engoufre en quelque sorte et son passage fait vibrer l'anche, le son produit est alors transformé en mots articulés par les organes accessoires de la phonation.

Enfin un tube ovale long de 30 mm. environ, se branche à la partie inférieure et postérieure de la boîte, et selon l'expression du Docteur Cl. Martin : "ce conduit à cheval sur l'éperon trachéo-œsophagien descend dans l'œsophage."

Aussi le porteur de cet appareil peut à la fois respirer parler et déglutir. Les aliments solides glissent facilement sur la grille oblique et pénétrant dans l'œsophage, les liquides la traversent mais s'écoulent sur l'anche conique, ils viennent retomber dans l'œsophage par le tube inférieur, ingénieux perfectionnement qui fait le plus grand honneur au si distingué prothésiste le Docteur Cl. Martin. La seule critique qui puisse être faite de cet appareil c'est qu'il faut le retirer souvent, manœuvre qui ne laisse pas que d'être très délicate. Il est nécessaire en effet de nettoyer l'intérieur de la boîte où fermentent les débris alimentaires qui y pénètrent à chaque repas, d'autre part l'appareil étant en caoutchouc durci, ne peut être, par crainte de détérioration, stérilisé à l'eau bouillante.

Un autre appareil phonateur est celui inventé par le Docteur Gluck. Il est très simple mais plutôt destiné aux trachéotomisés pendant la période de guérison. Il consiste en un tube de caoutchouc long de 25 cm. et de 8 mm. de diamètre s'adaptant à la canule trachéale et dont l'autre extrémité pénétre jusque dans le pharynx nasal.

L'appareil producteur du son est placé immédiatement à l'ouverture de la canule. C'est un tube métallique à la partie inférieure duquel est ménagée une ouverture ronde fermée par un mince clapet de métal. A l'instant seulement, ou l'opéré veut parler il fixe l'appareil sur sa canule, alors, à chaque inspiration le clapet s'élève et laisse pénétrer dans la trachée une certaine quantité d'air, l'expiration le referme et refoule l'air dans le tube. En outre, en travers du tube, se trouve, tendue transversalement une mince et étroite bandelette de caoutchouc flexible qui entre en vibration au moment de l'expiration et le son produit est conduit dans le pharynx nasal. Cet appareil extérieur peut rendre de grands services aux trachéotomisés mais la phonation obtenue est forcément très faible. De plus certains sons articulés qui exigent pour être émis dans la cavité de résonnance buccale l'occlusion normale complète du naso-pharynx sont produits, en sortant du tube, par la seule résonnance des sons dans l'arrière cavité des fosses nasales et dans les sinus, car le bord postérieur du voile du palais appliqué contre la paroi du pharynx s'oppose à leur passage. Ils ont donc une tonalité sourde et sont peu compréhensibles. Il faut cependant reconnaître que les sons articulés gutturaux sont plus en usage dans la langue allemande que

chez nous. Aussi l'appareil de Gluck peut-il rendre de plus grands services à ceux qui s'expriment en allemand qu'aux individus parlant des langues latines.

En terminant ce court historique je mentionnerai une ingénieuse tentative de Hochenegg qui imagina une machine à parler externe, sorte de boîte contenant une anche bruyante entrant en action grâce à une soufflerie que mettent en mouvement soit les mains, soit le bras. Cet appareil perfectionné depuis par d'autres a été peu employé, car l'immobilisation continuelle d'au moins une main ne le rend guère pratique.

Maintenant que nous connaissons les différents moyens employés pour faire parler de malheureux laryngectomisés nous passerons à la description de mon appareil dont le principe original diffère absolument de ceux décrits ci-dessus.

Le 17 Mars 1904 M. le Professeur Pierre Sebileau faisait dans son service d'oto-rhino-laryngologie à l'hôpital Lariboisière, une laryngectomie totale sur un homme de 44 ans, ouvrier plombier, atteint d'épithélioma du larynx. Puis quelques semaines, après, il présentait à la Société de Chirurgie son malade parfaitement guéri, et décrivait son procédé opératoire. A la suite de cette communication il me faisait l'honneur de me poser ce problème:

1°. Faire parler son laryngectomisé dont la bouche ne communiquait plus avec la trachée, sans qu'il soit nécessaire de lui faire même la plus petite opération.

2°. De ne pas employer le larynx artificiel issu des combinaisons de Gussembauer, Bruns, Wolff, et Cl. Martin, la pose de celui-ci nécessitant dans le cas présent une opération.

3°. Ne pas utiliser l'appareil de Gluck, ce dernier ne pouvant guère être utilisé comme un appareil définitif.

4°. Imaginer un système permettant simultanément la déglutition et la phonation.

tivement et qui m'a semblé répondre aux conditions qui m'avaient été posées. Je dois dire tout d'abord que je n'ai voulu

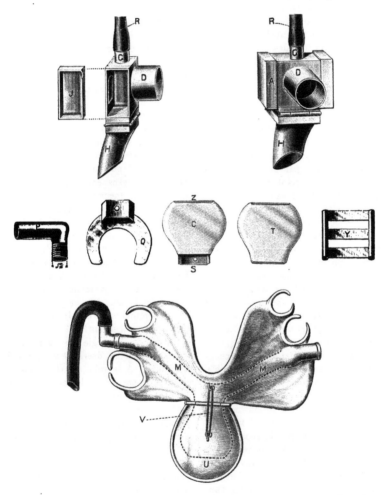

5°. Faire un mécanisme pouvant fonctionner sans l'aide des mains ni soufflerie.

Je passerai sous silence mes recherches et mes nombreux essais pour décrire l'appareil, auquel, je me suis arrêté défini-

faire ni un larynx, ni une machine à parler ; je me suis arrêté en dernière analyse, à la combinaison d'une glotte artificielle dont le principe m'a été inspiré par le simple appeal qu'emploient les oiseleurs pour attirer leurs victimes. L'appareil se compose de **trois** éléments: Un externe (A), la boîte à clapet trachéal; deux intra buccaux (B), la pièce palatine (c) la glotte artificielle.

derrière laquelle se trouve tendu, en rideau, le clapet de caoutchouc (G); par cette issue l'air pénétré dans la boîte et de là, dans la trachée. La partie supérieure est terminée par un tube cylindrique

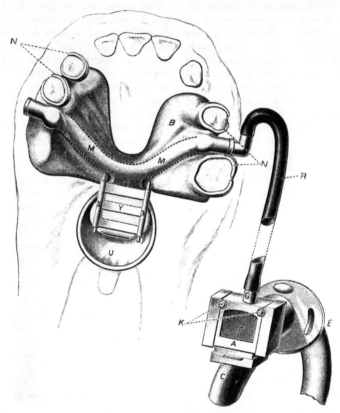

La boîte à clapet est en argent fin; elle est rectangulaire et renferme hermétiquement un clapet de caoutchouc extramince; à sa paroi postérieure est soudé un tube (D) de 13 mm. s'emboitant exactement dans la canule trachéale (E) pour l'introduction de l'air dans les poumons; en face, c'est-à-dire à la paroi antérieure, est ménagée une ouverture rectangulaire (F)

(H) de 7 mm. de diamètre, pour la sortie et le refoulement de l'air dans la pièce palatine; au fond inférieur de la boîte, un petit bouchon rectangulaire à charnières (I) facilite le nettoyage: enfin deux autres bouchons latéraux (J) permettent l'introduction du clapet et de son support (K) ainsi que le vissage des deux boulons d'arrêt (L). On conçoit facilement le fonctionnement de cet appareil; à chaque inspiration l'air soulève le clapet tendu verticalement en avant de la boîte et envahit la trachée et les poumons. A l'expiration, le clapet repoussé par l'air obture hermétiquement l'ouverture antérieure et ce dernier vient ressortir par le tube supérieur. De celui-ci part un tube de caoutchouc de 5 mm. de grosseur qui contourne le menton, passe dans la barbe, et pénétre a gauche par la commissure de la lèvre dans la bouche où son extrémité s'adapte à la pièce palatine. L'appareil est en or. Il est formé de deux plaques de 15 mm. de largeur et soudées ensemble sur le rebord (M). Entre ces deux plaques est ménagé un vide de 8 mm. de largeur sur le milieu de cet espace, les plaques sont écartées de 2 mm. pour être réunies à zéro, en M sur les bords. C'est en somme une sorte de tube fusiforme très aplati pour ne donner à la langue que le minimum de gêne. Cette tubulure est appliquée transversalement contre la voûte palatine immédiatement au dessous de la portion aponévrotique du voile. La pièce est maintenue en place par quatre anneaux d'or soudés à la plaque. A droite sur deux prémolaires restantes (N) à gauche sur la seconde prémolaire et la seconde grosse molaire. De chaque côté, manque la molaire de six ans. Ces deux vides sont utilisés pour le passage des deux extrémités de l'appareil creux qui se termine cylindriquement au niveau de la face jugale des dents voisines, et qui ont subi un filetage de 6 mm. de longueur sur 5 mm. de diamètre (o). Sur un de ces filetages vient se visser un coude de métal (P) de 1 cm. de longueur. C'est sur ce coude articulé, grâce au taraudage, que vient obliquement s'adapter l'extrémité du tube d'arrivée de l'air. A la partie postérieure de l'appareil une ouverture ovale de 10 mm.

de long sur 2 mm. de large est ménagée pour la sortie du souffle. On conçoit maintenant que l'air expiré et refoulé par le tube dans la plaque creuse vient ressortir avec pression par cette petite issue.

C'est à cette ouverture que se fixe l'appeau de caoutchouc. Cet appeau est constitué d'un tuteur en forme de croissant mince en or (Q); il est enveloppé d'un tronçon de tube de cacutchouc extrêmement mince (R). A la partie postérieure est soudée un tube ovale de 3 mm. de longueur et de 9 mm. de diamètre pour l'emboitage de la pièce dans l'ouverture correspondante ménagée à l'arrière de la plaque palatine (S). L'appeau (T) a 22 mm. de large et 20 mm. de long. Les deux branches du tuteur écartent l'appeau de caoutchouc dont les deux lèvres restent intimement accolées ainsi d'ailleurs que le tube de caoutchouc tout entier.

Que le souffle soit projeté par l'opéré dans l'appareil avec plus ou moins de puissance, selon la tonalité, qu'il veut donner à sa parole, les deux lamelles de caoutchouc s'écartent plus ou moins de leur base à leur extrémité dont les bords, agissant comme une véritable glotte se mettent à vibrer vivement au passage de l'air qui entre en vibration à son tour.

Ce phénomène se produit à l'extrémité centrale du voile du palais immédiatement en avant de la luette. L'ouverture de l'appeau est donc placée obliquement en arrière du voile du palais. Ainsi le son produit est projeté du côté du pharynx, et, selon les sons articulés à produire il est dirigé soit du côté de la cavité de résonnance nasale soit du côté de la bouche où les organes secondaires de la phonation le transforment en parole. De plus, les lèvres de la glotte étant intimement accolées s'opposent à la pénétration des aliments dans l'appeau pendant la déglutition, ce qui permet au sujet de parler et de manger sans quitter l'instrument.

Cependant cet appareil très simple en principe, ne fonctionnerait que très imparfaitement s'il ne lui était appliqué un petit perfectionnement. Nous savons que pendant l'émission des quatre cinquièmes environ des sons articulés le voile du palais s'élève en se contractant et vient s'appliquer contre la paroi postérieure du pharynx, formant ainsi cloison entre la bouche et les fosses nasales.

Pendant ce phénomène physiologique, l'appeau se trouve isolé entre la langue le pharynx et le voile. La glotte artificielle dans ce cas, peut donc vibrer sans obstacle. Il n'en est plus de même au contraire lorsque des sons simples et des sons articulés nasaux sont produits ; car pour cela le voile du palais s'abaisse afin de laisser la colonne d'air expiré vibrer librement à la fois dans les deux cavités de résonnance nasale et buccale.

L'appeau pendant l'émission de ces derniers sons se trouve en même temps comprimé par le voile du palais et par la langue. Un dispositif spécial imité de mon appareil pour voile du palais artificiel et articulé sur la pièce palatine évite le contact du voile contre lequel il s'applique.

C'est une plaquette mince autour de laquelle est soudée un fil rond pour en rendre le contact plus doux à la muqueuse (u). Un petit ressort de caoutchouc lui imprime des mouvements d'élévation et d'abaissement suivant ceux du voile (v). Cet isolateur est de 2 mm. plus large que l'appeau. Au dessous de celui-ci deux tiges parallèles (x) vissées sur l'appareil palatin soutiennent une petite grille de métal (y) qui empêche à la langue d'entrer en contact avec l'extrémité de l'appeau c'est-à-dire la glotte artificielle (z).

Comme on l'a compris par la description ci-dessus, j'ai surtout cherché à combiner un appareil pouvant être exécuté par le chirurgien dentiste.

En effet rappelons nous les travaux de prothèse exécutés par les Kingsley, les Delalain, les Michaëls, les Cl. Martin, nous nous rendrons compte qu'ils n'ont guère fait école ; et précisément à cause des extrêmes difficultés de toutes sortes qu'il ont vaincu dans l'exécution de leurs ingénieux appareils ils n'ont réussi souvent qu'à éloigner de la prothèse restauratrice ceux-là même qui auraient eu des aptitudes pour l'exécuter. Simplifions donc le plus possible la conception et la production de ces pièces délicates et le chirurgien dentiste pourra s'y adonner davantage pour le plus grand soulagement de nombreux mutilés et conséquemment pour l'honneur de l'art dentaire.

Lorsque M. Sebileau et moi nous avons présenté notre malade à la Société de Chirurgie, puis à l'Académie de Médecine une seule objection sérieuse a été faite : la glotte se trouverait trop profondément placée. Eh bien ! Cette situation nous ne nous l'étions pas imposée. C'est la seule qui corresponde aux desiderata physiologiques et physiques de mon appareil, nos études dans ce sens et nos patientes recherches nous l'ont amplement prouvé.

En effet, ne l'oublions pas, le mécanisme de la parole exige que, pour la production de celle-ci, plusieurs organes accessoires entrent simultanément en action (langue, voile du palais, joues, lèvres, dents, pharynx). Rappelons nous aussi que physiologiquement le son phonique est produit par la pression de la colonne d'air expiré des poumons venant frôler la glotte et la faisant entrer en vibrations de même que l'archet fait vibrer la corde d'un violoncelle. Mais pour la transformation des différents sons simples a,

e, i, o, u, et leurs composés qui, eux, peuvent être produits par le plus ou moins
grande écartement des cordes vocales supérieures sans aide d'autres organes, le
son est arrêté en trois points définis de la
cavité buccale : les lèvres, le bord palatin,
le voile du palais. Je ne m'étendrai pas
davantage sur les lois de la phonétique
qui ont fait, de ma part, l'objet d'une
communication en 1902 à Montauban au
Congrès de l'Association Française pour
l'avancement des sciences. J'insisterai
cependant sur ce fait qu'après avoir es-
sayé de placer ma glotte artificielle à la
voûte palatine j'ai du me résoudre à la
fixer plus en arrière pour l'obtention des
sons que, ke, gue, xe, et de leurs dérivés ;
Ceux-ci ne peuvent être émis que si le
son produit par la glotte éclate, après
avoir été arrêté dans l'arrière bouche,
dans une cavité de résonnance formée
par : en avant, la base de la langue en
contact avec le voile du palais relevé, en
arrière par le pharynx. Il était donc indispensable de placer la glotte artificielle
le plus loin possible pour obtenir les
mêmes résultats phonétiques qu'avec le
larynx humain dont le son arrive dans le
pharynx de bas en haut alors que celui
de ma glotte y est projeté en haut et
d'avant en arrière. Le son obtenu ainsi
peut varier selon les dimensions données
au tuteur de l'appeau, plus en effet, les
lèvres de la glotte sont longues plus le
son est grave, c'est au prothésiste à régler
la tension de l'appeau pour donner à son
sujet un timbre de voix en rapport avec
son âge, son sexe, sa force, ses occupations. Il peut sembler à l'examen de
l'appareil qu'il soit difficile d'habituer un
sujet à une pièce en apparence étendue
et gênante. Il n'en a rien été dans le
cas présent et je pense que ce la ne doit
pas être si la plaque palatine creuse est
parfaitement appliquée au palais et si

ses moyens de fixation ont été minuti-
eusement réglés d'avance. Obtenir semblable résultat n'est pas difficile pour le
chirurgien dentiste et tous ceux qui se
sont occupé de prothèse vélo-palatine
savent combien les sujets porteurs d'appareils voient vite disparaître l'effet des
réflexes, c'est ce qui se passe notamment
pour l'accoutumance de mon voile physiologique à clapet. J'ai posé d'abord à
mon sujet une large plaque palatine en
caoutchouc durci s'arrêtant à la portion
aponévrotique du voile. C'est porteur
de ce premier appareil d'accoutumance
que j'eus l'honneur de présenter mon
sujet à la clinique spéciale de prothèse
restauratrice bucco-faciale, lors de la ré-
cente visite officielle à l'Ecole Dentaire
de Paris du Directeur et des principaux
membres du Conseil d'Administration de
l'Assistance publique. Je leur exprimai
alors la conviction que j'avais de par-
venir à faire parler le laryngectomisé et
j'ai reçu d'eux à cette occasion de pré-
cieux encouragements. Quinze jours après
j'ai remplacé cette plaque par une semblable pièce s'étendant, cette fois, jusqu'à
la luette et terminée transversalement
par un bourrelet de la grosseur d'un
crayon. Sitôt le sujet habitué à déglutir
sans quitter cette pièce très gênante je
lui posai, le 25 Juin, un appareil définitif
en caoutchouc creux auquel était fixé l'appeau. Il le supporta immédiatement
bien et ne fut gêné au début que par les
vibrations de la glotte contre son voile,
par moments même le contact de celui-ci
empêchait l'appeau de fonctionner pendant la production de certaines articula-
tions. C'est alors que j'imaginai d'isoler
l'appeau du coile par une plaque articulée
intermédiaire. Puis je fus amené à protéger aussi l'appeau contre la pression de
la langue ce qui nuisait à la sonorité des
sons.

Afin l'accoutumance obtenue, la phonation rétablie, la déglutition permise avec l'appareil je pensai que le sujet devrait se trouver plus à l'aise avec une pièce plus mince et plus légère que le caoutchouc. J'exécutai donc celui-ci en or pour la présentation du malade par M. le Professeur Sebileau et moi à la Société de Chirurgie le 19 Juillet et à l'Académie de Médecine le 26.

Au point de vue esthétique, le passage du petit tube sur le côté du menton, laisse certes, à désirer, mais comparativement au résultat phonétique obtenu, c'est, on en conviendra, un bien petit inconvénient. D'ailleurs mon sujet, quelque peu coquet, sait très bien, à la promenade, dissimuler avec sa main gauche maintenant un fume cigare à la commissure de sa lèvre, le tube que sa barbe cache un peu déja.

En résumé nous pensons avoir créé un appareil appelé à rendre d'importants services; il permet de faire parler un laryngectomisé sans lui imposer une opération si petite soit elle. Nous avons satisfait à toutes les conditions du problème qui nous avait été posé par M. Sebileau. Nous sommes surtout heureux d'avoir exécuté cet appareil dans des conditions telles que tout chirurgien dentiste est capable d'établir le semblable, faisant en quelque sorte du travail du prothésiste le complément nécessaire à l'œuvre du chirurgien pour le plus grand bien des malheureux.

Discussion.

A MEMBER. I think, as Dr. Godon states, that this appliance will have a wider application than ever before. There are many instances where the posterior walls become diseased and ulcerated, and the back of the throat may become attenuated. I had a gentleman in my office a year or so ago whose soft palate had become adherent to the back part of his throat so that the only aperture was about the size of a lead pencil. I found within my own province I could do nothing for him, because the throat was defective and the slightest occlusion prevented him from breathing. This box appliance would have served as an occlusion for him and afforded a passage of air. There is going to be a tremendous use for this most ingenious appliance.

Dr. Hart J. Goslee, Chicago, took the chair.

Dr. TURNER. One feature of the appliance which Dr. Godon did not enlarge upon should not be overlooked. He has stated that by the use of this appliance it is possible for one to have a tenor voice at one time and at another a basso profundo.

I think the attachment of a vocal apparatus to an artificial denture is an entirely original idea. I am not acquainted with the use of this means of attachment in any previous case. I wish to express my own appreciation of the presentation which Dr. Godon has made of the valuable work of his *confrère*.

Dr. Turner then resumed the chair.

The CHAIRMAN. Is there anything further to be said in the discussion of this paper? If not, I will call upon Dr. Godon to close the discussion.

Dr. GODON (closing the discussion). I have only to thank you for your attention to this paper; I will be pleased to tell my friend Dr. Delair of your kind reception of his paper; he has devoted many years to this work. He has retired from the active practice of dentistry and for the past few years has been devoting his time exclusively to this line of work. He does a great deal for the working people of his country and does not charge anything for his services. This is a new and interesting work. He has made many devices that I could not present to you. I will be pleased to talk to any of you on this subject. I thank you very much for the words of appreciation you have spoken in regard to the paper of my friend Dr. Delair.

Dr. R. OTTOLENGUI, New York. I am sure we all appreciate very much Dr. Godon's presentation of the paper by Dr. Delair, and I move that a special vote of thanks and congratulations be sent to our confrère Dr. Delair through Dr. Godon. (This motion being duly seconded was unanimously carried.)

Dr. GODON. I thank you, gentlemen, for your kindly expression in this matter.

The CHAIRMAN. The next paper on the program for today is by Dr. Hart J. Goslee. Dr. Goslee needs no introduction. I have great pleasure in calling upon him to read his paper on "The Mechanical Requirements and Cosmetic Possibilities of Modern Artificial Crown Work."

Dr. HART J. GOSLEE, Chicago, Ill., then read the following paper:

The Mechanical Requirements and Cosmetic Possibilities of Modern Artificial Crown Work.

By HART J. GOSLEE, D.D.S., Chicago, Ill.

IN view of the more or less exhaustive contributions to our periodical literature which have been published during the past ten or fifteen years relating especially to the methods of restoring the crowns of natural teeth, it would perhaps seem to the casual observer that the subject in general must have been so well covered as to almost preclude the further presentation of views possessing any features of intrinsic value.

And yet, notwithstanding the conspicuous evidence of the progress made in this particular field which is so forcibly manifested by the splendid character of much in our current literature, and by the class of operations now being performed as compared with similar efforts of even a decade ago, the field is in a measure so broad and so diversified as to doubtless always offer possibilities of still greater advancement.

Indeed, when opportunity for improvement in any line of human effort ceases, then progress ceases, and therefore, in consonance with common philosophy, since we cannot rest permanently at anchor on the turbulent waters of the sea of human activity, retrogression must otherwise be inevitable.

The practice of truly modern dentistry in its composite specialties, however, offers an opportunity for combining *art and mechanics* which, while limited in scope, is yet of so high an order and of such a diversified range as to warrant the assertion that the millennium has by no means yet been reached.

Of the specialties which go to make up our young, vigorous, and useful profession, no individual one—unless perhaps it be that of orthodontia—affords greater or even equal opportunities for the closer blending of these two important phases of human endeavor—art and mechanics—or contributes so largely to the development of a higher conception of the possibilities incident to their combined application, than is afforded in the methods which pertain, from a mechanical aspect, to the preservation of the roots of teeth and to their more or less permanent restoration to a normal degree of usefulness; and, from a cosmetic aspect, to the close simulation of or improvement upon the natural organ to a degree such as to defy detection in the substitute.

While "dental" mechanics has perhaps not contributed much to the fundamental principles of this particular science upon which all of our efforts are so largely based, yet a review of the advent and development of artificial crown work in itself will afford convincing evidence that in the natural progress of the profession it has contributed liberally to the arts and to many of the other sciences of modern times, and that it has at least in no way retarded nor proved a barrier to the natural advancement of all mechanical pursuits.

Since it is the very highest achievement of true art to copy nature, we have contributed liberally thereto by the development of procedures which enable us in our particular field to so closely simulate nature in her perfections and imperfections as to be able to substitute the natural with the artificial in such manner as to preclude detection.

While I make the statement that we are now able to accomplish this in a large degree, yet I must also acknowledge with profound reluctance that many of us do not do so, and that still more do not even try. Hence, I find a logical excuse for this effort in the attempt to stimulate others to aid in the elevation of the profession in general, and of dental art and dental mechanics in particular, to a sphere beyond that of the mere artisan, and more in accord with the higher degree of art which modern possibilities offer.

Such possibilities, however, are not the product of the day, but are the outgrowth of a gradual process of development, and a knowledge of the various stages of this development should constitute a portion of the education of everyone whose ambition is to achieve results beyond the ordinary.

In reviewing the development of this particular class of work, it will be observed that the cosmetic requirements were early recognized by our progenitors, and that their primitive efforts were largely concentrated upon the production of a substitute for the natural crown which would, first of all, closely resemble it; and, secondly, be capable of more or less universal application.

To this quite laudable ambition may be attributed the advent of porcelain, and subsequently of porcelain crowns; but as the art side encompasses only one phase of the requirements, and as the efforts were for some little time directed mainly toward this phase, the more or less temporary nature of the results quite naturally caused an awakening to the fact that the very highest artistic achievement was practically but wasted energy, unless constructed with due observation of those aseptic requirements which afford comfort and immunity from subsequent disturbances, and with a further observation of the mechanical requirements which insure a high degree of permanence in the operation.

This demanded the adoption of procedures based more largely upon the fundamental principles of mechanics, and hence was recognized the inadequacy of the former crude methods of root-preparation and of crown-attachment.

The cosmetic possibilities were then for a time subordinated to the mechanical requirements, and soon the era of the glaring gold crown was upon us. While this practice has reigned to a more or less flagrant extent ever since, yet, as the profession advanced, the desire for higher artistic attainment increased, and in proportion as this tendency advanced among the more conscientious members of the profession, so also did it develop among their patrons, until now the employment of the gold crown on any tooth within the range of immediate vision is generally considered an offense against the refinement and culture of the patient, and an acknowledgment that the professional and ethical standing of the dentist is not of the very highest order.

Since the application of gold crowns offers a useful and highly indestructible method of preserving the teeth, however, and since there are some teeth, of course, which are not within the range of immediate vision, the employment of such methods will doubtless always be often indicated. Indeed, when properly adapted to roots which have previously been placed in a condition favorable to permanent comfort and usefulness, and when the application is confined to such posterior teeth as are beyond the range of vision, there is no other method of procedure which offers so great a degree of general adaptability, and of opportunity for obtaining reasonably permanent results, as the gold crown.

In view of the combined requirements, however, the field of adaptability embraces but a small area of the normal denture, and hence we may ask how and by what method may the remaining teeth in the denture be restored and preserved in a manner which will conserve to the maximum degree of perfection in all of the requirements?

That the cosmetic requirements demand the employment of porcelain is acknowledged, and that the mechanical requirements also demand a pronounced degree of strength in the crown and of stability in the attachment is also conceded, and yet again how may the composite of these requirements be best obtained?

An effort in this direction was marked by the advent of the porcelain facing, and its use in combination with gold, and the so-called "Richmond" crown with its various modifications was suggested and is still much employed. While this general style of construction embraces advantageous features in line with both of the general classes of requirements, still it involves detail which is necessarily somewhat circuitous, and possesses disadvantageous features so pronounced as to preclude its universal employment.

While the mechanical requirements are perhaps adequately conserved in so far as attachment to and protection of the root is concerned, the particularly objectionable features are that a thin veneer of porcelain can never possess that degree of translucency necessary to closely resemble the natural teeth when it is placed in contact with a surface of metal; and that a maximum degree of strength in its attachment to the metal can scarcely be expected from the simple attachment afforded by the pins.

These very objectionable features, when combined with the necessarily circuitous detail incident to the construction of this style of crown, and when further supplemented by the apparently innate desire of an unfortunately large proportion of practitioners to avoid the expenditure of as much effort and energy as possible, soon led to the suggestion and manufacture of ready-made porcelain crowns.

The stupendous sales of some forms of this particular style of crown which the manufacturers have recorded each year since their introduction, silently attest to the willingness of a large proportion of the profession to use and of the manufacturers to supply and to create and increase the demands for those methods which offer only the advantage of simplicity in application.

In this particular connection, is the employment of any ready-made style of crown for immediate adjustment conceded to afford the same opportunity for obtaining a maximum degree of permanence incident to the preservation of the roots of teeth, as is offered by the crown which is skilfully constructed for the special case? Is it possible to secure as close an adaptation between the base and periphery of the crown and root by grinding the one to fit the other, as is obtainable by the burnishing or swaging of a metal base? Is the joint secured by the former procedure as impervious to the penetration of the secretions of the mouth as is the joint which may be obtained by the latter? Do we not depend largely upon the closeness of this joint for permanence in the operation? and are the opportunities for the protection and preservation of the root as favorable by the former method as by the latter?

My answer to all of these manifestly logical queries is emphatically negative, and I can scarcely believe, in view of the present methods for obtaining a maxi-

mum of all of the combined requirements incident to the application of artificial crowns, that the continued more or less extensive employment of ready-made products is indicative of the progress which the profession is making.

Indeed, it occurs to me that the general use of ready-made crowns by the ambitious and conscientious practitioner of today is as deplorable a practice as the employment of the so-called "shotgun" prescription by the modern physician; and I believe that the sooner the progressive practitioner arrives at this conclusion, and abandons the use of all forms of ready-made crowns—except perhaps in rare instances—the sooner will he be adopting more conservative and reliable methods, putting forth better efforts, and conducing to more permanent results.

In order that we may more fully appreciate the possible logic of these conclusions, that such efforts may be made, and that such results may obtain from our efforts, it is necessary that we should first carefully consider and analyze the requirements of modern artificial crown work.

As applied particularly to the ten—or possibly twelve—anterior teeth, where the use of gold is contra-indicated, these constitute in the composite, first, a degree of adaptability which will make the application more or less universal, and which will offer opportunity for the reasonably permanent protection and preservation of the root; and, second, the substitute must possess that degree of translucency which will impart a harmonious and life-like appearance, and thus enable it to closely simulate the natural teeth. Thus it will be observed that while each of these two classes is of equal importance with the other, one pertains only to the mechanical phase of the question, while the other ap-

12

plies more exclusively to the cosmetic side.

While it is true that one or two styles of ready-made porcelain crowns are so constructed as to make it possible to achieve cosmetic results in their use, it is also equally true that their employment in the usual manner of adjustment for which they are designed, does not in a similar manner conform to the mechanical requirements. Hence the principal advantage claimed for them, that of "simplicity of adaptation and attachment," can only be regarded as an affront to the ambition and skill of that class of practitioners who are diligently striving for the best rather than for the easiest methods. And, indeed, these are the practitioners who are doing the most to elevate the profession, and to make it possible for themselves as well as others to do better operations and in turn to procure better fees.

Because of their inherent cosmetic qualities, however, such crowns may be employed, but not in the simple and expeditious manner for which they were originally designed, because this adjustment does not insure the maximum degree of permanence which is demanded.

As pertains to the class of requirements which have been and are thus designated in the composite as being mechanical, and upon which depend the protection and preservation of the root, and consequently the permanence of the operation, I have already emphasized the importance of securing the very highest degree of accuracy in the adaptation of the crown, and asserted that this essential feature may be accomplished only by conforming a metal cap or base to the exposed end of the root.

Early recognition of this fact led to the construction of crowns with a metal base adapted directly to the end of the root, and subsequently to the employment of a cap entirely encompassing a short projecting end. This procedure was advocated as a means of carrying the immediate joint between crown and root to a point where it would be less accessible to the secretions, and thus more immune to their deleterious action, as well as for the purpose of adding increased stability to the attachment between the two, and of insuring greater protection to the root.

The advisability of such a procedure has precipitated much vigorous discussion, and has always been more or less a debatable question, and the fact that it continues to be so regarded by many, probably accounts for the extensive use of ready-made crowns.

This question seems logically debatable on the ground that the presence of a band often detracts from the cosmetic appearance of the crown by being more or less conspicuous; and further, and more important, that it almost invariably becomes a source of irritation, inducing gingivitis and subsequent recession of the soft contiguous tissues, not infrequently to an injurious extent.

While some have contended that this condition when present is caused by an electro-chemical action induced by contact between the metal and the soft tissues, through the medium of the secretions, it is the belief of the large majority, and of myself, that such a theory is only hypothetical, and that the true cause of such manifestations may invariably be traced to mechanical irritation. It is my further belief, however, that when such conditions do present, the fault is not with the principle, but in its application.

Hence I maintain that if the periphery of the projecting end of the root is properly and skilfully prepared—a procedure, however, which is usually performed in the most flagrantly perfunctory manner —and then if a *narrow* band made of a gage of metal sufficiently heavy to retain its given shape under the stress of fitting is well and closely adapted to the sides of the root, and allowed to pass only a short but uniform distance within the free cervical margin upon all surfaces, so as to closely follow the cervical curvature of the gum and offer no impingement upon the peridental membrane, the presence of a band will offer *no* mechanical irritation, and the objections to this style of construction will thus be largely, if not entirely, removed.

In proportion, then, as these statements seem to be logical, the employment of a band in the manner indicated is practicable and warrantable, and in a large percentage of cases will afford a type of construction which will without question offer the most permanent results. Where it may not be so adapted, however, its employment is contra-indicated, and the adaptation of a simple plate to the end of the root will doubtless offer the next best means of conserving this phase of the requirements.

In recapitulation, the requirements classed as mechanical, demand, first, the construction of a well-adapted base, and second, the possession of sufficient inherent strength to sustain the stress of mastication; and those classed as cosmetic demand the employment of porcelain in accordance with the indications mentioned.

With this conservative analysis of the respective requirements, let us now consider how they may be so combined as to be productive of the highest and most modern type of construction. These requirements may be obtained by the employment of such crowns as the Davis,

Logan, and Justi designs, when the employment is made in conjunction with a base of either gold or platinum, or otherwise perfectly adapted, and such method of procedure is the only means by which reasonable permanence may be obtained in their use.

This may seem a somewhat radical statement, in view of the fact that such crowns, mounted without such an observation of the combined requirements, have been known to restore the function and usefulness of roots for almost a score of years.

It must be conceded, however, that such instances are the rare and extraordinary occurrences, not the average experience and observation of the general practitioner. Also, that the longest service has probably been with bicuspids, where the occlusion favors their retention, whereas with the six anterior teeth mastication provides a stress constantly tending toward their labial displacement. Furthermore, irrespective of how long such crowns, so mounted, may do service when they are finally lost through failure from whatever source, it will be observed that the root itself is usually beyond redemption. This is not true, however, of the root which has supported a crown having a well-adapted base, and when the removal of such crowns is for any reason demanded, the fact that the supporting root is usually found to be in a good state of preservation should serve to prove the logic of my contention.

Incident to the use of these crowns in the proper manner, however, and for other than temporary purposes, it may be said that the variety of molds and colors in which they are now manufactured offer favorable opportunities for a close simulation of the natural teeth. And yet, in justice to the varied requirements in this connection, their employment does not offer the same opportunity for selection, nor for a close adaptation of the peripheral outline of the crown to the base, which is afforded by the use of simple facings, for the reason that such crowns are made in a far more limited number of molds than are the ordinary facings. Neither can we as accurately secure the necessary circumferential approximation when compelled to use a ready-made porcelain substitute having the proportions of a complete crown.

For these reasons, then, it would seem that the combined mechanical and cosmetic requirements may be best obtained in the large proportion of cases by the employment of facings and the construction of modern porcelain crowns.

The advent and development of porcelain work; the recognition of its possibilities and limitations; the large range of adaptability of the compounds now prepared, and the improved facilities for their employment now at our command, make it possible for every progressive practitioner to achieve results which combine both of these general classes of requirements to the highest possible degree, and to an extent not to be attained by any other modes of procedure.

The special advantages to be obtained from the application of porcelain crowns lie in the artistic manner and facility with which the natural conditions and varying characteristics may be closely simulated, together with the increased possibilities for securing a degree of strength exceeding any other style of construction. For these highly important reasons I beg to submit that the construction and application of porcelain crowns is destined to become the universal, if not the exclusive, practice of the

future, as applied to restoring the ten anterior teeth.

In conclusion, I desire to call your attention to the various principles underlying the construction of this particular class of work, with the aid of models, and to assure you that the possibilities of porcelain work, as pertains to this application, are only limited by the ability of the operator to acquire skill, and by his desire to adopt modern progressive methods.

As the time of this session is so well taken up, I shall not go into a detailed description of these models. They simply illustrate the variations of principles underlying the construction of porcelain crown work, and I will be glad to pass them around and have you observe the principles and possibilities which I have mentioned.

Discussion.

Dr. W. A. CAPON, Philadelphia, Pa. In this paper I have nothing to oppose, nor is there anything of much importance that I can add, for the essayist has stated all that can be said as to what is the best practice derived from an experience gained from constant and the best attention to these important points. There cannot be a difference of opinion as to the relative value of a crown with band or without, nor can there be a comparison between the metal and porcelain crown when used individually.

There are those who use ready-made crowns from choice, and there are others who use ready-made crowns from force of circumstances. To those using them from choice, I have nothing to say in their defense. There are others who use ready-made crowns because their patients will not allow them for financial reasons to perform the higher grade work. I allude to the hosts of dentists who cater to that class of patients who demand a lower grade of work. This applies to dentists who operate on people who work in mills or where time is not paid for according to its real value.

In making bands for crowns, of course that work has my undivided support because I do not think there are many here who have worked any longer than I have in that line. I am speaking of band crowns with porcelain attachment. It may not be just the same as the essayist has described, but there are other methods of great value, and I am only too glad to be able to support what he has said. The band crown is one that can never be done away with, in spite of the many beautiful operations which have been done in the clinics today, where platinum has been done away with entirely. Much can be said in favor of platinum as a band. I advise it in my different visits to cities all over the country, because the irritation of the platinum band is very small, in fact almost *nil*, although there is tissue that will be disturbed by anything that may come in contact with it; but the platinum band, or iridio-platinum, which is the same or almost the same thing, has the advantage of stability and cannot be praised too highly.

I have a crown in my own mouth which has been there eleven years. There is not the slightest irritation of gum tissue, and there is no drawing back from the edges. If a band crown must be used in connection with solder work, I think the advice of all of us would be to use platinum as the first base, which will amply repay us in after years, for there is very seldom recession. I have a thousand crowns in use today with platinum bands, and it is decidedly pleasant, and it makes me feel better to see the majority of these crowns free from any irritation in the use of platinum. I say, All hail! to platinum wherever it can be used. All colleges should teach such work in preference to the gold work. I believe in teaching students the work advocated by this essayist. The work should be compulsory, otherwise the student is not properly equipped for his work, nor is he able to compete with those who have this knowledge.

The future of porcelain and its many branches has never been outlined to such an extent as in these clinics within the past few days—all proving that the evolution of this branch of our art is most active.

Dr. E. PARMLY BROWN, New York. It seems almost superfluous to say anything on this paper which is so up-to-date, or on this exhibit which is up to the very minute. Nothing that has ever been presented in a paper or exhibit has compared in its completeness and its perfection and in its artistic detail with this of Dr. Goslee's. But it is no more than I expected from him when I knew that he was coming here from Chicago.

Twenty years ago I introduced this porcelain work before the First District Dental Society, and the report was published in the *Cosmos*. I showed two or three models, all porcelain bridged and all porcelain crowned, and after reading my paper the wise men looked at each other and laughed a little; but they are not laughing now. They are coming round to find me. I got a little hysterical then, but upon second thought I said to myself, "You can't drive things into men's heads; it will not be twenty-five years before this system of mine will be right on deck."

Taking up Dr. Capon's remarks, there is only one thing I want to say in explanation in regard to platinum: They will be using platinum on the teeth of the angels of heaven—and no other metal.

I never put in one Richmond crown, nor a single gold band around any, except where I insert gold crowns on posterior teeth.

Dr. N. S. JENKINS, Dresden, Germany. I can only congratulate the essayist on his most instructive paper and with all my heart agree with all of his propositions. I rejoice to see that he has emancipated himself from the indiscriminate use of bands. My friend Dr. Capon is an advocate for the use of bands, but only in certain cases. Dr. Capon always avoids a band when he can consistently do so; is it not so, Dr. Capon?

Dr. CAPON. When I speak of a band, I mean the same as the essayist has in his model. I use the same pattern; it does not hurt the tissue in any way.

Dr. JENKINS. It has come to be my experience that in the great majority of cases it is wholly unnecessary to have any band whatever, for the reason that after long-continued experiment I have reached what I believe to be an absolutely irresistible strength in the iridio-platinum pin, when of appropriate size and exactly fitted to the root. That strength is reached by a 20 per cent. alloy of iridium with platinum. Ten per cent. with platinum affords the most desirable alloy for caps and in the infrequent cases where bands or half-bands are indicated. But with a pin of 20 per cent. alloy—a pin which accurately fits a countersunk root to which a thin 10 per cent. iridio-platinum cap has been exactly fitted—a band is very seldom desirable.

Lastly, I would say that the making of

an all-porcelain crown or an all-porcelain bridge is an operation which every dentist ought to make as his regular daily work, not as an exception but as the only thing which a civilized dentist should put in the mouth of a civilized patient.

Dr. R. OTTOLENGUI, New York, N. Y. We get the idea in entering in a discussion that one is a disputant. It is as difficult to get up a discussion on this paper as it would be to discuss a sermon on the proposition that "Honesty is the best policy."

This paper is simply an appeal for ethical endeavor, and I cannot argue against that. It is an appeal for the standard that a man must do the best that is in him in every operation in crown and bridge work.

I will only make one additional remark, and that is the only point which the essayist has left out. I had the pleasure of reading this paper in my camp this summer at the Adirondacks. I could have told the doctor then about this point, but I was afraid I would have nothing left to say for myself in this discussion.

When we make a gold plate with porcelain attachments, we find the gold itself is not cleanly. The worst place is the crevice between the porcelain and the gold to which it is attached—and it is doing away with the space between the backing and the porcelain which is the most important feature of the all-porcelain crown, making it absolutely instead of only moderately hygienic.

Dr. R. L. SIMPSON, Richmond, Va. It was not my intention to try to add anything to Dr. Goslee's most excellent paper. I came here to sit at the feet of these skilful and learned gentlemen, and become a humble learner. But while sitting here the thought came to me that those whose patients have summer homes in the Adirondacks can well afford to use platinum and porcelain; but it is another matter to the practitioner who is giving his services to the mass of the American people—the great middle class who are only moderately able to pay for dental restorations of any kind. Can he in duty to himself and them take up this more artistic and more expensive work, and is it best for the patient from the standpoint of durability?

I had the pleasure of seeing Dr. Parmly Brown's beautiful specimens several years ago, and from that time have held them up as ideals. And today when I look at the work of Dr. Goslee I can only wish I were as skilful.

Porcelain and gold are used in an entirely different manner. With porcelain we have to do an immense amount of artistic guessing, for we do not know how much it is going to shrink in the baking, and we must add just exactly as much as is needed and no more; but those who use gold have a great deal more liberty and latitude to overcome defects. With gold we can copy nature's cusps perfectly, knowing the gold duplicate will neither shrink nor change its shape; whereas with the other material we must do all the carving, and have to guess at the size.

My efforts have been to perfect the prosthesis of gold and flatbacks and saddlebacks, making the gold stiff enough to stand the strain. You will find that porcelain workers use saddle bridges to add strength to their porcelain by bulk. So much bulk to gold is not needed, and self-cleansing bridges seem to be the best in my experience.

A great deal of discussion has taken place about the use of bands, or half-bands, or none at all, but the difficulty to my mind is that they are improperly made.

The only point I would leave with you in making gold-porcelain bridges is to so grind your facings that they will be supported both at the cutting edge and the cervix by a kind of cup, and not to depend on pins alone. Then add enough solder to make the bridge inflexible.

Dr. E. A. BRYANT, Washington, D. C. I took great pleasure in listening to this paper. It pleases me equally as much if not more to see before us almost the entire foreign delegation to this congress listening to the subject and interested in the papers on prosthesis.

Some of the discussion in regard to the use of porcelain has gone a little bit farther than I think is entirely safe for the average man to attempt. My friend Dr. Brown who taught me in my school days, and who first reached out the hand of fellowship to me when I came to New York from the Rocky Mountains, when bringing out my system pertaining to gold bridge and crown work, has for twenty years at least confined his practice to porcelain work, and has attained that proficiency which gives him the ability to construct porcelain dentures strong enough to stand perhaps the greatest strain of mastication; but the point I wish to bring out, and which I have followed in my own practice entirely, is to attain a structure which under any condition can be repaired in every part, generally without removal from the mouth.

If a facing is broken from a porcelain bridge, it has to be removed in order to be repaired. In a great many instances, perhaps in a majority of the cases, the breakage of any portion of that bridge requires a removal and the making of a new bridge. That is not so in the use of gold bridges and replaceable facings or removable bridges.

I think, gentlemen, we should always put into a patient's mouth a denture as strong as can be made and as artistic as we can make it, and one according to a method which the man himself is able to handle intelligently in all the phases of his work.

Dr. M. KRAUS, Vienna, Austria. It afforded me great pleasure to listen to the reading of the paper and also to the discussion that followed. I am from Vienna, a city where a civilized public resides. (Laughter.) I perfectly agree with Dr. Parmly Brown that a civilized people feel disinclined to carry jeweler's work in their mouths for show.

During my education in dentistry at Chicago I had the good fortune to see and to admire the exquisite work of my present friends Drs. Parmly Brown of New York, George Schwartz, Haskell, and Goslee of Chicago, and Dr. Capon of Philadelphia, as also that of many other men whom I have since learned to admire. My utmost endeavor was to acquire the knowledge of that art I appreciated so well, inasmuch as I am convinced that porcelain work is the only art by which the deficient natural tooth, or parts of it, can be best artificially supplied.

I only wish to warn my fellow-practitioners against the use of low-fusing bodies in the making of porcelain crowns. I thank my friend Dr. Goslee for his instructive exhibition and paper, which indeed is an excellent and charming piece of art.

Dr. G. D. SITHERWOOD, Bloomington, Ill. I want to say that Dr. Goslee has not only written a paper that is up to the very minute, but he has also written an up-to-date book, and every man who has not read that book is not up to date. Dr.

Goslee did not know I was going to say this.

I am an eclectic in practice, but rarely ever put on any sort of crown except a porcelain crown. It takes no longer to make a porcelain crown than a gold one. It is merely a matter of practice. The smallest amount of metal consistent with strength—the narrower the band the better. There are cases in which I make a porcelain crown without a band, but I advocate the band; it makes a better adaptation.

Attention has been well called to the singular facility with which the gum tissues take to the burnished metal platinum in place of gold.

Bear this fact in mind, as stated in the paper: A porcelain crown is as readily, as easily, and as quickly made as any other crown. It is artistic and permanent, and it is the up-to-date crown.

Dr. BROWN. I understand the statement has been made that porcelain work cannot be ground, cannot be added to, and cannot be taken from. This is an error. You can cut and polish the surfaces of porcelain work and add to it to an unlimited extent.

Dr. GOSLEE (closing the discussion). Permit me to assure you of my gratitude for the manner in which you have received and discussed my paper. I should like to feel that I would be justified in taking this opportunity to close the discussion in a fitting manner, particularly after listening to the closing remarks of some of my confrères, but such is quite out of the question.

I want to agree with what Dr. Parmly Brown has just said in reference to the grinding or the adding to or subtracting from the previously glazed surfaces of porcelain. If the body is properly packed and manipulated it can be ground and polished and the result will be a smooth and well-vitrified surface.

With reference to the advantage of placing platinum next to the soft contiguous tissues of the mouth, I believe that these tissues take more kindly to platinum, or the alloy of iridio-platinum, than to any other metal, even pure gold.

Dr. Jenkins has referred to the employment of a band, but I believe he slightly misunderstood my paper. I said that I employed a band in a large proportion of my cases, and I do, even on the anterior teeth wherever there is to be any lateral strain. Where the strain is to be more direct, however, all that is necessary is a close and accurate adaptation between the base and periphery of the crown and the root. Especially on the upper anterior teeth, however, I regard a very narrow, well-finished band as a decided advantage. But its success depends upon its accurate adaptation to the root on which it rests.

Dr. Simpson has said something regarding the use of porcelain by the country practitioner, or by those who may not have every facility for doing this work.

In this connection permit me to say that from an economical viewpoint you can construct a porcelain crown at an expense not very much greater than the cost of ready-made crowns, and it does not take much longer to make a suitable cap, properly adapted to the root, than it would take to prepare your root, select a ready-made crown and then properly adjust it.

Dr. Brown referred to the statement that porcelain could not be ground or altered like gold after finishing. I do not think it should be necessary to grind gold any more than it would be to grind porcelain. I think that we can and should do our work in either instance so that it will not need grinding.

The CHAIRMAN. The next paper on the program is a contribution by Mons. B. PLATSCHICK of Paris, France, entitled "Tube Teeth, and Their Modern Applications." This paper will be illustrated by stereopticon views. I take pleasure in introducing my *confrère*, Mons. B. Platschick of Paris.

Dr Ottolengui was invited to occupy the chair.

The paper here follows:

Tube Teeth, and Their Modern Applications.

By Mons. B. PLATSCHICK, Paris, France.

EVERY time that I have undertaken the study of the history of dental prosthesis I have been surprised to see that one of the most fertile inventions of our specialty, tube teeth, have not found a greater field for application in practice either in Europe or in America. America was in ignorance of this method for more than fifty years. Harris' "Prin-ciples and Practice of Dentistry" contains but two pages and Litch's text-book hardly ten lines on this subject. It was only at the time of the World's Columbian Dental Congress, held in Chicago in 1893, that Dr. Girdwood of Scotland gave some valuable suggestions. Yet notwithstanding this remarkable communication, the literature on tube teeth is very limited. The articles published occasionally in reviews and such standard treatises as Essig's, Richardson's, etc., merely quote Dr. Girdwood's suggestions, and the work of the last mentioned is only fundamental. It is due to this lack of knowledge relative to the use of tube teeth in the practice and theory of prosthesis that I thought it would be interesting to address you these few notes and to call your attention to this old-fashioned method which is worthy of resuming its place in the laboratory. In fact, is the abandonment of this procedure since 1837,* as if it were worthless and incompatible with the modern progress of prosthesis, justifiable? Cannot new and artistic results be obtained by the use of tube teeth in combination with the latest scientific invention? These are the questions I shall endeavor to answer.

The abandonment of tube teeth is not justifiable, but is explained by a study of the evolution of prosthesis in the last fifty years. Rubber—a new invention—opposed the development of this method almost at its beginning. Everyone may have had an opportunity of observing in some historic collection the first "terrometallic" teeth of Fonzi. Compared with those manufactured today they are simply horrible, being badly carved, dull, and black. They possess features which destroy their purpose of imitating the natural organs. Successive improvements finally placed at our disposal teeth that were certainly superior to Fonzi's from

* According to the details furnished by the firm of Ash & Sons, Claudius Ash, founder of that house, manufactured for the first time tube teeth with a gold sheath. We have analyzed the metal of these sheaths with the following result: Gold, 9.32 per cent.; silver, 8 per cent.; platina, 52 per cent.; other metals, 8 per cent.

the standpoint of the quality of the porcelain and from an esthetic point of view; but all have continued, as is the case with those of today, to present the defects due to the pins inserted in the body of the teeth, whereby the resistance to shock has been diminished. The bicuspids and molars for metal plates have the same crude form, with a narrow masticating surface. The invention of tube teeth in 1837 remedied in an admirable manner all the defects of pin teeth. At last we had front teeth and, above all, molars that from the point of view of form and resistance possessed a real superiority over all those hitherto produced. There were to be no more horrible teeth—nonanatomical, fragile, breaking under the slightest force of mastication—in short, we now have perfect teeth approximating in form the natural teeth and strong enough for all uses.

It is interesting to know that at the time of the appearance of tube teeth they presented another timely advantage, namely, that of replacing those made of hippopotamus ivory. Even in the case of considerable absorption the shape of the neck portion of the tube tooth could be made to replace the absent tissues. Later on, before the use of vulcanite had become general, the upper portions of these teeth were notched and a little gutta-percha was inserted to represent the gum; but often the row of teeth was left untouched, as the exaggerated length could be hidden by the beard or lips. In view of these advantages tube teeth found at once extraordinary favor with prosthetic dentists.

I am sure that many of you have had occasion to see full sets made with tube teeth mounted upon a metallic base, without any other substance to take the place of the absorbed tissue. These full sets, with springs and tube teeth, were then in frequent use. The pin tooth was dethroned and the tube tooth earned its place throughout Europe.

Some time after their invention, tube teeth were in general use in France, Germany, Spain, and Italy, and particularly in England—the land of their birth. It is surprising that America did not adopt the method so universal in Europe, and it is astonishing that the Atlantic should limit its spread to the confines of Europe precisely at a time when relations rich in results between the old and the new world were becoming closer.

We are justified in believing, although literature gives no evidence, that this novelty of all others ought to have been placed within the reach of the American dentist; and although some voices, not impartial perhaps, attribute this to their English origin, the reason has appeared insufficient to me, and I am desirous that American dentists clear up this historic point. Although the date of first manufacture is remote, I was inclined to think that Americans, preferring teeth of their own manufacture, for reasons which I shall not go into in this paper, did not wish to use the English teeth, and were therefore forced to renounce the tube teeth, being restrained from manufacturing them in America on account of patents. Particulars obtained from Ash lead me to believe that such was not the case, as this firm say that patents were never taken out on the tube teeth.

The introduction of vulcanite in dental prosthesis dealt tube teeth their deathblow. Winderling's invention stopped the development of the method introduced by the Ash firm. The novelty of the new substance forced all other less useful inventions into oblivion, mainly by reason of its ease of manufacture and cheapness of production. Vulcanite once

discovered, everybody used it in every possible case. Metal plates became rare and were substituted entirely by vulcanite plates. Let us add that the improvements in porcelain teeth introduced at about that time contributed largely to this. Tube teeth, even in cases of extensive absorption, were considered useless inasmuch as rubber would substitute the missing parts to better advantage.

For these reasons many metal plates were substituted by rubber plates, and tube teeth continued to be less used and were even abandoned in cases in which their use might have been preferable. It was a pity. No one could reasonably question this class of work from the esthetic and hygienic point of view, as well as its strength and ease of replacement. I do not insist upon their value; the experience of this honorable assembly obviates the necessity of entering into a more detailed exposition of the subject. I shall confine myself to reminding you that the opinion of writers is unanimous upon the advantages of tube teeth, and that the few faults attributed to them may be easily overcome. Let us now determine whether the reasons which prevented the propagation of the use of tube teeth still exist, or whether they have been modified, and if there is still room for the method in the present condition of dental prosthesis.

We shall see that if rubber was detrimental to its development on the one hand, on the other the continuous progress in dental prosthesis facilitates the renaissance of that method by entirely modern applications. Conditions have changed vastly in the last fifty years; prosthesis has become of more general use. If the progress of operative dentistry permits us to save a great many teeth which formerly were sacrificed, that of dental prosthesis permits us to replace better than formerly the masticating organs of persons who have lost them through age or in spite of the services of the dentist. These conditions, united with the general culture of a more enlightened public, can tend only to increase the number of prosthetic appliances. The tube tooth finds itself, on account of very favorable conditions, suited to a large field of usefulness in prosthesis. The difficulties in its use should not be taken into consideration inasmuch as they have been exaggerated, and besides may be overcome by that knowledge which is the result of familiarity with their use. Habit eventually renders the most difficult manipulation quite easy. Although matters of commercialism should not be alluded to in an assembly where scientific questions are discussed, I think it necessary in order to study the subject in all its phases, to say one word regarding its economy. While the tube tooth now costs double the price of the pin tooth, I am convinced that were manufacturers to lower the price to that of other teeth they would be working to their own interest, to ours, and to that of the public. In my opinion, this is a very important point. The profit on a piece of work should not be considered, and only the experience of several years of labor should influence the price. Still more, the unwillingness of dental depots and of dentists themselves to carry a considerable stock of materials, the purchase value of which is far superior to the intrinsic value, should be taken into consideration. I trust that the manufacturers will agree with my views, and thus earn the gratitude of the dentists.

In regard to this, I beg to mention an idea which I believe the manufacturers could utilize. It consists in the use of a nickel alloy similar to that used for some time in a certain kind of pin tooth. It does not enter into the theme of my paper to discuss the advantages or conveniences of this new invention, but I believe that it would be of service to us when applied to tube teeth. Laboratory experiments have confirmed the fact that a nickel or gold post attached with sulfur in a nickel sheath would hold just as well if not better than in a platinum sheath. Theoretically, there is no objection on the ground of any chemical change that tube teeth with nickel sheath might undergo in the mouth, the sulfur playing the rôle, as it did with the former teeth, of a filling, and the oral fluid could not thus penetrate between the two metallic parts.

I shall not further insist upon the different methods of employment of tube teeth, nor repeat their manifold advantages. Neither shall I linger to refute the unusual disadvantages which are found only by those who have erred in trying to apply them in all cases without distinction. But the resolution I formulated, and which was adopted in the Congress of 1900, encourages me to urge the return to the use of tube teeth in continuous gum dentures, their employment for this purpose being the object of my communication to the congress. I am forced to treat the matter in a complete way and will try and make it as short as possible.

But few of our colleagues here present had opportunity to admire the first application of continuous gum for tube teeth made by M. Feuvrier at the Exposition of l'Ecole dentaire de Paris in 1889, and probably few of you know of his communication presented by our lamented Dubois to the Société d'Odontologie de Paris May 7, 1889. It is therefore indispensable to a thorough understanding of my work to recall in a few words that first and brilliant essay. M. Feuvrier prepared his plate with the usual rim employed in continuous gum work. The teeth were adjusted and the pin soldered as for an ordinary piece. After having determined the position of the teeth and finished their adjustment they were withdrawn from the pins, and soft platinum rings were placed around their necks, and when they had been replaced the rings were duly soldered. The teeth were then replaced in order to be absolutely sure that none was out of alignment and that the setting was still perfect. Nothing further is necessary except the placing of the body and enamel, and subsequent baking. After the teeth have been removed, when the baking is finished, they have only to be cemented in place. I need only mention that what started Feuvrier on the right road in his technique was his desire to make a continuous gum plate superior to all others obtained by the use of the old-style teeth; and also the impossibility of leaving the teeth on the plate during the baking of the Allen body, as they would have fused during this procedure. At this time this was the only way that could be employed by the practitioner who was in love with his art and was desirous of making a continuous gum denture with tube teeth. Today Feuvrier's method is the only one available when using Allen's body or others similar to it. But for some years past the manufacturers have furnished us with a tooth body which enables us to employ tube teeth in a simpler way than that of Feuvrier. It is precisely this method that I desire to describe in a few lines, taking as an example a full upper plate. It is well no note that this same method may be employed with partial upper and lower plates. Still, before describing the technique of the making of the plate, a little digression is necessary to throw some light upon one important point. For this kind of work, the platinum tube in the tooth is entirely unnecessary.

Recognizing the value of a tube tooth without the tube, my colleagues at the congress of 1900, passed the following resolution that I had the honor to present: "That the manufacturers should make teeth of the form of natural teeth with a canal extending longitudinally through them as in the tube tooth, but omitting the platinum tube. These teeth should have in addition to the neck, a large portion representing the root. These permit the construction of continuous gum plate—very pretty, practical, economic, and not so heavy as those made with any other teeth."[*]

It is my duty to state that Mr. Cunningham had already theoretically devised this tube in 1890 at the annual meeting of the British Dental Association. That suggestion has not as yet had its merited success; but I do not despair, and I believe that the American manufacturers will not delay entering this field which is so full of promise, and will give us teeth which outside of their other qualities will permit us to employ the high-fusing bodies, of which I am an ardent advocate.

To resume the description of the plate: A platinum plate of the desired size is swaged up as usual. Then swage a narrow plate covering the first only where the pins are to be soldered. The plate is then tried in, which is done with a view of ascertaining in the mouth itself where the plate should be cut to give free play to the muscles of the cheek and the fre-

---

[*] Proceedings of the Third International Dental Congress (Paris). vol. i. page 424.

num of the lip. Solder all along the buccal and labial margins of the plate a wire of special form, that obtained from

FIG. 1.

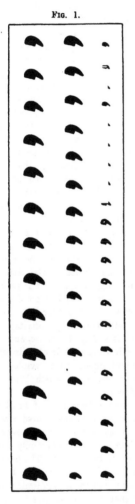

a draw-plate (Fig. 1) made for the purpose. As you see, the wire (Fig. 2) presents, first, a convex part, A, on the external side in contact with the cheek or lip; second, on the internal side the half, B, slightly flattened and destined to be soldered to the extremity of the plate; third, a groove part, C, that has the same function as a turned rim; that is to say, to receive and maintain the margins of the porcelain (Fig. 3). The next figure (Fig. 4) shows the cut of the plate, the wire being soldered. It is unnecessary to insist upon the advantages of this wire, which can be of any given diameter by reason of the use of the special draw-plate. Besides forming the border this wire serves to reinforce the plate, and it likewise permits

FIG. 2.

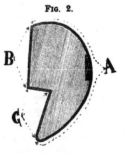

any adjustment that might be necessary notwithstanding the careful trial of the plate. This adjustment is impossible with a plate with a turned rim, which in addition could not have been tested in the mouth.

The teeth are then adjusted roughly on the plate. I say roughly advisedly, as a careful adjustment would mean a loss of time. As the small interstices between the teeth and the plate would be easily filled with body and baked at the same time with the body, that will serve to fill the holes in the tube teeth on the masticating side. The teeth having been adjusted to the plate with wax to maintain them in alignment, a plaster wall is made over the external surface, and after the wax is removed the teeth are replaced, which, thanks to the plaster wall, are held in correct position, and you may with a

FIG. 3.

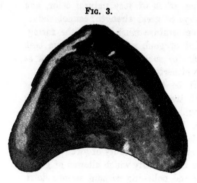

FIG. 4.

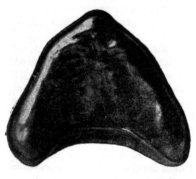

sharp point mark the place to which the pins are to be soldered. After soldering the pins (Fig. 5) and after all due precaution to free the plate of plaster and to clean it and the teeth, begin to apply the body. (Fig. 6.) The pins should be slightly painted with the porcelain body and a small quantity placed at the base. This will serve to fill the gaps left by the rough adjustment. The teeth are then

slipped on the pins, which have been left a little short so that they cannot be seen on the masticating surface, which will be

FIG. 5.

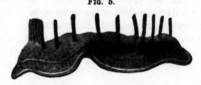

filled anyhow with a small amount of porcelain as said above. One or two bakings will definitely fix the teeth to their places, establish perfect contact with the

FIG. 6.

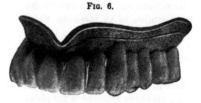

plate and, finally, fill the hole in the surface. We have nothing further to do except to apply body and enamel as for other continuous gum plates. (Fig. 7.)

FIG. 7.

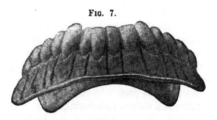

The lingual side of the plate may be covered or not, as you choose, although it is useless in most cases. In this way you obtain a plate which answers all esthetic requirements and which besides having all the good qualities of continuous gum work is much lighter, of much simpler execution, and lends itself to greater ease of repair.

If this new application of tube teeth is capable of interesting the eminent colleagues forming part of this congress, I am sure it will succeed in convincing the manufacturers of teeth that they should work for the progress of our profession.

Discussion.

Dr. N. S. JENKINS, Dresden, Germany. Our thanks are due to the essayist for calling attention to an invention which has had and may still continue to have great usefulness. Tube teeth were designed to be attached to metal plates through pins soldered to the plate. These pins were to pass through the tubes and the teeth were to be attached to the plates by melting sulfur to fill up the interstices. Very beautiful and very cleanly work could be done by this method, but it possessed certain disadvantages. These disadvantages were, First, instability. It was not possible to solder a pin suitable to the caliber of a tube tooth which, through the slight attachment of sulfur, should always permanently endure the force of mastication. In many cases either the tooth broke away from the pin, or, which was a worse disaster, the pin broke from the plate. In the latter case repair was a serious undertaking.

Second, the adjustment of the teeth was hampered by the unavoidable perpendicularity of the pin. Bound by this unchangeable condition it was not always possible to place the tooth in the desired position.

Third, the spaces between the necks of the teeth could not be filled up to advantage, for the teeth would not endure the heat then necessary to add and fuse porcelain for increased strength, beauty, and cleanliness. Tube teeth, although very dense, often of very natural color, and always of great strength, cannot endure a temperature much beyond the fusing-point of gold, and therefore have been unfit for such continuous-gum work as has hitherto been advocated.

It is, therefore, not surprising that with the advent of vulcanite these teeth should so generally have passed out of use. "The day of their destiny was over, and the star of their fate had declined." In spite of their beauty of form and color and that density which allowed of grinding and polishing without serious detriment to the surface, they were easily displaced by teeth of coarser texture which could be advantageously set upon a vulcanite base.

It is difficult to speak justly of the introduction of vulcanized rubber into dental practice. It greatly simplified and cheapened prosthesis, but at the expense of destroying, for a time, worthier and more artistic work. It supplied the masses with practical substitutes for the natural organs, but it led in many instances to the reckless extraction of teeth which could have been preserved in health and comfort for a lifetime, and to the general degradation of the standard of prosthesis.

But at the present day there is an almost universal revolt against this unhygienic and inartistic prosthesis; a revolt to which the concluding paragraphs of this interesting paper gives welcome evidence. The essayist gives us a graphic description of his method of employing tube teeth to make what is practically a piece of continuous-gum work, and this ingenious process excites only admiration.

But here I would venture to mention what I have at last achieved in this same direction. For years I have been working to produce a porcelain which should do for prosthesis what porcelain enamel has done for inlays, viz, to bring continuous-gum and porcelain crown and bridge work within the scope of the practice of every skilful dentist. This has been accomplished by the recent completion of a body which I have called "prosthetic porcelain," as it has been designed only for prosthetic purposes. Through its use tube teeth can be attached to iridio-platinum plates after the manner of M. Platschick, with the greatest ease and certainty; and also the teeth of all other manufacturers can if desired be united and combined in the same denture. This universally applicable porcelain fuses sufficiently below the melting-point of gold to permit the use of pure gold solder, a matter of great importance. I earnestly hope that this or some similar body may so far fulfil the wishes of M. Platschick as to still further advance the use of tube teeth which he justly commends so highly.

Dr. E. PARMLY BROWN, New York. The gentleman from the other side has presented a most excellent paper; as I understand, it relates to continuous-gum work.

I wish to describe a method of making porcelain plates which in my opinion is extremely valuable. I take a No. 34 gage or thinner iridio-platinum plate, whether making full upper bridge, partial bridge, or continuous-gum work; I make two dies, a zinc die and a lead die. I swage up that, anneal it, make a duplicate, and then cover the upper side of the first one with pure gold, and the inner side of the duplicate—using blowpipe. I place between these two four or five thicknesses of No. 4 pure gold foil, use wet flux between those two, solder and swage, repeating that three or four times, and then have a third plate, soldering as before, getting a stiffer plate than ever has been made. The third plate is punched full of holes, about 500, like a sieve, to receive the porcelain, and when that is under white heat you have something like cast steel—you can't budge it—the gold and platinum have mingled.

M. PLATSCHICK. I must thank Dr. Jenkins and the other speakers for their kind remarks, but it astonished me to hear Dr. Jenkins' suggestions against the use of the tube teeth. He consequently does not agree with all the authors and writers mentioned in my paper, who have successfully employed the variety of teeth under discussion.

Dr. Turner resumed the chair.

The CHAIRMAN. The next paper on our program is one by Dr. FRANCISQUE MARTIN, Lyons, France, entitled "Immediate Prosthesis in Cases of Resections of the Jaws, According to the Method of Dr. Claude Martin." The paper will be read by Dr. Masson.

The paper was then read, as follows:

Immediate Prosthesis in Maxillary Resections: Method of Claude Martin of Lyons.

By Dr. FRANCISQUE MARTIN, Lyons, France.

GENTLEMEN: I wish to revert to the question of immediate prosthesis after maxillary resections, and to lay before you the present state of my father's practice and my own.

The question, as you are of course aware, is not a new one. Dr. Claude Martin's work on "Immediate Prosthesis," giving a summary of twelve years' practice, dates from 1889; the work also gives technical details on the construction and application of the apparatus, and makes numerous observations. Five years later, Claude Martin published a new work, giving the later results of his method.

It is not my intention to reproduce here the numerous and conclusive observations presented by Claude Martin at different congresses and learned societies. I wish simply to recall to your minds the essential points of the method and lay before you the state of my father's practice which has varied but little since 1893, the date of his last work on "Resultats éloignés de la Prothèse immediate," and also to refute certain objections that are continually being made, several of which appear to us to be unfounded.

I will not dwell at length on the construction of apparatus of the immediate prosthesis class; all the details referring to this question are fully explained in the treatise on "Immediate Prosthesis." I shall refer, therefore, in a cursory way to the molding of a natural maxilla of average size. This operation gives us a hollow mold, which we fill with melted wax, and as this mold is composed of several parts it is easy, as soon as the wax is cold, to remove it without injury. We thus obtain a wax maxilla absolutely identical with the natural one, and which may be modified by molding it according to requirements. We now hollow out canals in the middle of the thick part of this maxilla, two for the ascending branches and one for the horseshoe. In these canals are placed zinc tubes filled with flake-white, the ends of which are stopped with wax. We afterward put it into a muffle as an ordinary set of teeth.

To render the filling easier, we only make a three-quarter maxilla, that is, the horseshoe and one ascending branch. When we have to place a complete maxilla we take two halves, which we join together with plates and screws. These apparatus being very thick and of black india-rubber, we bake at a low temperature, 145° C. for three hours. We afterward soak in diluted hydrochloric acid for one or two days in order to dissolve the zinc tubes, and we now have an apparatus for immediate prosthesis. We have only to pierce the surface with several holes communicating with the canals made by the zinc tubes; through one of these holes in the front and upper part of the horseshoe and which has been made a little larger, we drive a metal tube that joins a second india-rubber tube by which we make our irrigation at high pressure.

We now prepare our plates and screws for fixing the apparatus ready for use at the moment of operation.

Such, gentlemen, is a rough outline of the way we make the apparatus, and for many years we have only modified some of the minor details.

As regards the first application of the prosthetic apparatus during the operation, I shall not go into minute details, but simply insist on certain points of the operative manual

(1) As to the choice of an apparatus: Before making an immediate prosthesis apparatus, it is indispensable to take the impression of the patient's upper maxilla, especially if it be a question of replacing the mandible, so as to establish an apparatus of such a size, that what will be the alveolar border in the prosthetic piece corresponds as exactly as possible with the normal articulation of the patient. It is therefore most important to make an apparatus of a proper size, so that when it is replaced by the definitive piece there is no risk of establishing a defective articulation of the artificial teeth with the upper teeth; this is a matter to be well considered from the outset and which has a definite value.

(2) The manner of fixation: As soon as the apparatus is completely finished we screw on to it the plates, which must also be fixed by screws to the remaining fragments. Here I beg to call your attention to a new arrangement that Claude Martin presented and explained at the Munich congress in 1892. He used to fix his apparatus to the bones behind with a large metal plate bearing on the lingual face of the maxilla, and before by two horizontal lamellæ. These two latter he has modified by placing longer ones and

crossing them like an X, so that the lamella which is fixed to the lower part of the apparatus is screwed to the upper part of the remaining fragment and inversely.

This arrangement prevents all movement of the apparatus, which consequently no longer rubs against the remaining fragment in the movements of the jaw, and it insures an absolute fixity even if there be but one fragment. We shall see farther on the importance of this fixity of the apparatus, when we consider the question of a relapse after prosthesis.

(3) Another point on which we have insisted for many years, although practitioners do not appear to attach the importance to it that it deserves, is the absolute necessity of making during the days following the operation, frequent irrigations under high pressure. When we have been able to attend very closely to our patients we have not allowed a single day to pass without calling several times to see that these washings have been carried out by reliable persons according to our instructions; we have thus been able to form an opinion of what may be expected from our method.

An objection has been made that these washings, begun immediately after the operation, cause hemorrhage in displacing the clots of blood. We do not consider this objection well founded; frequent washings do not appear to us to injure the hemostasis, especially if they are made with a very warm antiseptic solution; and besides, by preventing infection, they also prevent secondary hemorrhage. In fact, we have only observed hemorrhage in two cases, in which instances the surgeons had forgotten a plug in the wound. Hemorrhage may also take place through the laceration of one of the temporal arteries, which are not always sufficiently obliterated by torsion in the disarticulation of the ascending branch of the maxilla. Prosthesis, however, cannot be held responsible for this accident.

(4) Another objection made to immediate prosthesis is the difficulty experienced in replacing the primitive apparatus and the length of time required before it may be substituted by the permanent one. I do not think this objection is justified, even in the case of an operator of even average skill. In fact, if the screws are near the ascending branch and consequently somewhat distant from the commissure of the lips, it is sufficient to use a chisel as a lever on the head of the screw in order to easily remove it.

In other cases we have resorted to the following plan: As frequently the two halves of the apparatus are fixed to the median line by a screwed plate, all that is required is to unscrew the four screws that fasten it in order to set the two halves of the maxilla free, and then by grasping with the left hand one of these halves it is possible, without causing much pain to the patient, to pull forward the branch of the corresponding bone, bringing it sufficiently in front to enable one to easily remove the screws that fix it to the apparatus.

The provisional apparatus once removed, the permanent one has to be placed. The following is the technique usually followed by Claude Martin: Before changing the apparatus we take an impression of the mouth of the patient, of the remaining fragment or fragments, and the upper edge of the temporary apparatus. We cast this impression, and then construct an apparatus in such a

way that it will have, by means of clasps and laminæ, a solid hold on the teeth of the remaining fragment; and at the point where the dental arch of this piece corresponds to the temporary apparatus there is a groove into which the ridge of the apparatus fits. As soon as the temporary apparatus is removed we place it in that groove and fix it there with two or three screws. Add the time required for adjusting all these apparatus on the model of the remaining fragment that we obtained by the first impression, to place the model and apparatus into plaster, and the time the latter takes to set, and all is finished. The few minutes this operation takes up will certainly not give time for the cicatricial filaments to draw the fragments nearer to one another, for as soon as the plaster is dry the groove screwed to the primitive apparatus, the canals of which have been stopped with hard wax, is replaced into the mouth of the patient just as a simple set of teeth, and there is ample time to construct a definitive apparatus that will thus be made exactly like an intermediary arrangement, since the immediate apparatus adjusted to the piece fitting to the teeth of the remaining fragment has given us, by placing it in this last mass of plaster, the complete casting of its lower edge.

All this is much more quickly executed than described, for it requires just the time to screw home two screws and to wait the few moments necessary for a small quantity of plaster, mixed with salt or alum, to become sufficiently hard.

Such are the principal and different points of the operative manual to which I wish to call your attention.

Before concluding I wish to discuss, and to refute before you, the principal objections that have been raised against immediate prosthesis. These are principally two, viz—first, that it favors the infection of the wound; second, that later on it becomes the cause of a relapse.

The first of these objections was made twelve years ago by Boennecker.* "The piece of rubber," says the German author, "that covers the soft and bony sectioned parts does not allow a free discharge of the secretions, and one cannot be sure of the asepsis of the apparatus. In the prosthesis of Dr. Martin a backward step is made as regards the treatment of the wound. . . . He places a foreign body which promotes retention, and hence, the disinfection of the mouth being impossible, it is a serious fault against antisepsis."

As Claude Martin replied long ago, these objections are entirely theoretical, and appear to be puerile to those who see us daily practicing our method. Let us, however, discuss them in order to enlighten the members of the congress upon the important question.

The disinfection of the buccal cavity is quite possible, and even quite easy to effect, if the rules we have laid down be carried out. The question of the antisepsis of the mouth after operations followed by prosthesis has always been Claude Martin's desideratum. "It is for this reason," he writes, "that we have in our prosthetic pieces hollowed out canals of irrigation opening on to all points of the cruentous surface and through which it is easy to make antiseptic washings." We were so convinced of the efficiency of the means we have adopted that we did not hesitate to make the washings

ourselves in the hospital wards when the temperature of the patients rose, to prove that with a little care a complete disinfection could be effected and a stop put at once to the accidents of retention.

Boennecker, continuing his remarks, calls attention to the fact that we mention in our observations a case of erysipelas and another case in which there was a particular fetidity of the mouth.

It suffices to reply that the complications referred to by Boennecker took place in 1878, a period when antisepsis was in quite a rudimentary stage and when we had not yet made use of our apparatus fitted with irrigation canals. We think, indeed we are certain, that in taking as a basis our practice of the last twenty years, and with our apparatus facilitating the washing out of the parts, every infectious accident should disappear, especially if care be taken to make, as we recommend, irrigations of the buccal cavity under high pressure. From this point of view, and we cannot insist upon it too strongly, Esmarch washings must be absolutely given up. This manner of irrigation, which we too often see employed by ill-trained hospital attendants, does not give sufficient pressure. Eguisier's irrigator must infallibly be used, which gives a pressure of $7\frac{1}{2}$ meters. *In frequent washings under high pressure lies the whole secret of success.*

We now come to the question of a relapse after immediate prosthesis.

Immediate prosthesis has often been incriminated, and even is today by some surgeons, as inducing a relapse. This opinion is based, we think, much less on an examination of facts than on a generally admitted idea that the causes of mechanical irritation are also the causes of tumors. This idea of general pathology is correct, but in the particular case re-

---

* "Ueber Unterkieferprothese," *Verhandlungen der Deutschen Odontologischen Gesellschaft*, Berlin, 1892.

ferred to an ill-judged application of it was made. In fact, the prosthesis apparatus, solidly fastened, cannot be compared to a mobile foreign body, which by its frequent change of place is necessarily a cause of irritation. Although the fixing arrangement, described above, has only been presented a short time, relatively, my father nevertheless had already made use of it for a considerable time before, and I hasten to describe it to you, being convinced that henceforth such a reproach can no longer be laid to the charge of immediate prosthesis.

A strict examination of facts, in the numerous observations that my father possesses, some of which date as far back as twenty-five years (see the publication mentioned above), refute entirely such an objection. Moreover, we do not hesitate to say that immediate prosthesis offers, on the contrary, a guarantee against a relapse. In fact, the prosthesis apparatus, whatever its size may be, is just as easy to fix; consequently the surgeon, when he has recourse to immediate prosthesis, is more at ease in making a large ablation of the tumor, which indeed is the principal guarantee against a recurrence.

Such, gentlemen, are the conclusions my father has arrived at after nearly thirty years' experience with immediate prosthesis. This method has always given both to him and to me excellent results. It has the great advantage of replacing at once the resected bony fragment by an apparatus of the same size and form and capable of fulfilling the functional rôle of the resected part. Lastly, it does not expose the patient to the least danger, either immediately or later, to infection or relapse, assuming that the rules we have laid down be carried out and that even the slightest details be carefully observed.

Discussion.

The CHAIRMAN. The discussion on Dr. Martin's most instructive and interesting paper will be opened by M. Platschick.

M. PLATSCHICK. We are happy to see that Dr. Francisque Martin has advanced along the line of his father's work on immediate prosthesis of the maxillæ and restorative prosthesis.

Dr. Claude Martin was the first to make use of an apparatus of the "immediate prosthesis" type. Dr. Francisque Martin in his paper today says particularly that, contrary to the affirmation of surgeons, the late results of this prosthetic procedure are most brilliant and successful.

We are convinced that if the American dentist could ally himself with the surgeon, as does Dr. Martin of Lyons, he would obtain equally as good results. For this reason we hope that Dr. Martin's text-books may be translated into English, as they have been into German and Italian.

The CHAIRMAN. Though the hour is late, I cannot let a paper of such proportions as this go by without saying a word. I am familiar with the work of Dr. Claude Martin, and have carefully read the exposition of that work as presented in his book. I have not had personal experience with the apparatus which he has designed, but upon theoretical grounds I feel satisfied of its effectiveness, and wish to compliment him most sincerely upon its ingenuity. If we may judge from the photographs of cases in which portions of the maxillæ have been removed, and this appliance inserted, there has been a marvelous preservation of form.

This method seems to me to be the logical means of preventing the deformity which follows such resections—the deformity resulting from the falling in of the soft tissues and due first of all to the fact that they are not supported by a bony skeleton, and, secondly, to cicatricial contraction.

It seems a rather heroic procedure to put into a freshly made wound a foreign body of any sort, and, as he has said, it is absolutely necessary that it be so constructed that a state of asepsis be maintained as nearly as possible. The canals which traverse the entire appliance permit an effective lavage of the wound, and an antiseptic wash is used frequently, I believe as often as every two hours. The

utilization in some cases of the periosteum which is left, as the basis for a socket into which the prosthetic appliance fits, is an extremely valuable addition to the use of such an appliance. I feel that in this contribution of Dr. Claude Martin, and in this exposition of it by his son, we are given a very valuable means for the preservation of the form of the face after resection of the jaw.

A paper by Dr. RUDOLPH WEISER, Vienna, Austria, entitled "Some Cases Illustrating the Present Development of Conservative Dentistry and Dental Prosthesis," was read by title. It here follows:

Some Cases Illustrating the Present Development of Conservative Dentistry and Dental Prosthesis.

By RUDOLPH WEISER, M.D., Vienna, Austria.

I SHOULD like to describe a few cases out of my practice, intended to show the great success that modern dentistry has attained in replacing lost parts of teeth, rows of teeth, and even the alveolar processes, and in utilizing curable teeth or parts of teeth to serve as abutments for dental and oral prosthetic appliances.

First, I will describe a bridge replacing fourteen teeth of the upper jaw. I have chosen this particular case out of my rich collection of bridge specimens not because of the size of the bridge, for—like very many other practitioners—I possess a large number of examples of such prosthetic pieces. Remarkable circumstances about this case were the conditions which led me to construct a bridge for a patient of about sixty-five years of age.

The patient (Dr. C. K.) had worn for years an upper and a lower plate replacing the premolars and molars, but in spite of this his front teeth become more and more worn, and the original normal position of the lower jaw changed into a progenetic one (Fig. 1). On account of this deformity which interfered with mastication the replacement of the teeth became more difficult with every new plate.

Perhaps a bridge is not exactly the appliance indicated in the case of a patient in the sixties accustomed to the use of plate, and although in this case the patient seemed quite satisfied with the plate I nevertheless decided to make one. The upper right and left third molars were treated for pulpitis gangrænosa; the upper right and left centrals and canines eroded to a great degree, but were free from pyorrhea alveolaris and the pulps of them were largely calcified. These were devitalized and the bridge made to rest on these six supports*; the

FIG. 1.

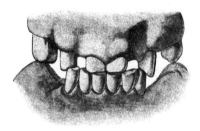

front teeth projected sufficiently beyond the lower incisors to enable me to counteract effectively the malocclusion mentioned above. (Figs. 2, 3, and 4.)

Secondly, I should like to describe a

FIG. 2.

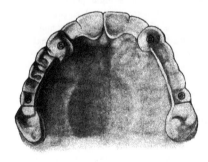

case in which both the antra had been opened many years ago according to Cooper's method, through the alveolus of

---

* The bridge is detachable for the dentist.

a molar or premolar extracted for the purpose. The patient had already lost before my treatment all the molars and the second premolars. As the axes of the cylindrical operative wounds were not parallel, but formed an angle to each other of about 30° (Fig. 5) it was not

FIG. 3.

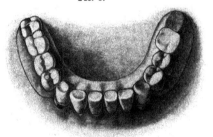

possible to fasten both pins to the palate piece of a single plate, because the plate could not have been introduced. I therefore divided the plate into two un-

FIG. 4.

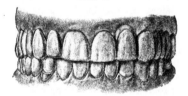

equal parts, each with a pin. (Figs. 6 and 7.) The plates partly covered each other (Figs. 8 and 9) and when placed in their right position they fit upon each other and rest immovably. This is brought about first by the non-parallel pins acting as a suspending apparatus, secondly through a four-cornered projecting guide on the palate plate (Fig. 8, *g*) which fits into a corresponding sheath on the palatal side of the plate (Fig. 9, *s*) and thirdly by two clamps attached to the premolars (Fig. 5); one of these proceeds from the plate on the palate side, the other from the plate on the tongue side.

(Fig. 9) with large gold fillings had been split deep into the root during mastication; of the left lateral incisor only a root overgrown with granulating gum was left. The left central had extensive metallic fillings. As both the last mentioned teeth also gave the patient much trouble from chronic alveolar abscesses, with fre-

FIG. 5.   FIG. 6.   FIG. 7.

FIG. 8.   FIG. 9

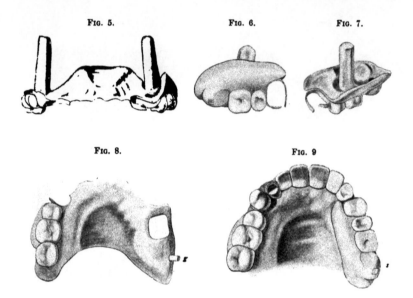

The same case, a very hale old lady of sixty, offers further details which show what progress dentistry has made in making use of teeth apparently fit for the forceps. Of the six incisors it was only possible to preserve the crowns of the canines by means of gold and porcelain fillings; the other four were very much affected, partly by caries and partly by erosion and abrasion. The very defective root of the right lateral incisor showed (Fig. 9) penetrating caries with consequent pulpitis; the right central incisor

quent acute recurrences, the apices of the roots were resected.

As it was a case of the front teeth of a lady, and as pyorrhea alveolaris was not present, and the line of the gums therefore a normal one, visible on speaking and laughing, I concluded that crowning was indicated and not extraction. The uncertainty of a permanent success, however, in view of the split right central and the great destruction of the left lateral incisor root decided me to construct a bridge. This embraced with root-caps the roots of the right lateral incisor and the left central, of which I had removed the crowns for the purpose, as well as the roots of the split right central, and sent a projection without a cap into the root of the left lateral.

In the mandible the right premolar was replaced by a crown, which was em-

In order to carry this out successfully, crowns and bridges are very often necessary in view of the wretched condition of the teeth of most persons affected with cleft palates. The same is true of the non-operable cases, in which the obturator is much more extensive and is intended to be worn for life.

FIG. 10.

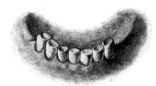

FIG. 11.

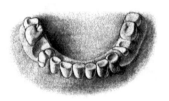

FIG. 12.

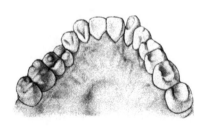

FIG. 13.

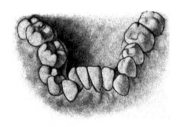

braced by the clamp of a plate replacing the lost teeth (Figs. 10 and 11).

Cases like the last described form a transition from specifically dental to surgical prosthesis, or rather a combination of both.

To this group the treatment of cleft palates quite commonly belongs. With the exception of those cases operated in early childhood, they are as a rule sent to the dentist to have an obturator fastened to the teeth to assist in speech.

My case (D. F.) forms a classical example of this kind. It is a case of cleft palate (uranocoloboma posticum mediale) extending to the middle of the hard palate. The lower dental arch which runs into an irregular W-shaped line is, when the mouth is shut, forced into the wide and almost semicircular dental arch of the maxilla like a wedge, so the latter has in the course of years been enormously enlarged. (Figs. 12 and 13.)

As regards the occlusion I found the

following conditions present before treatment. The premolar and molar teeth of the maxilla had ground with their lingual surface the buccal side of the opposed teeth to such a degree, that not only the muco-periosteum of the alveolar process had disappeared, but in consequence of the resorption of the alveolus the roots of almost all the molars of the mandible were exposed (Figs. 14 and 15). The only lower teeth which occluded normally were the right first and second premolars. Only the gum and the alveolus of the lower canine (Fig. 16) failed to show symptoms of resorption (Fig. 13). The four lower incisors, on the other hand, appeared to be pressed upward in the shape of a fan, and the

gum had receded almost to the end of the roots (Fig. 13).

The unfortunate patient was in other respects a completely healthy, good-looking, strong, and intelligent girl; and in order to save her from the imminent danger of all her lower teeth falling out so

FIG. 14.

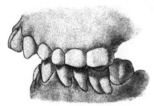

With half-opened mouth

FIG. 15.

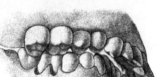

With half-opened mouth.

FIG. 16

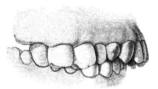

that a plate could not then be fitted in consequence of the abnormal character of the occlusion, no course remained but to extract all the exposed teeth and then to construct a bridge which would articulate normally with the expanded maxilla. For this bridge the roots of the lower canines and the third molars, which had been freed from the gums by an operation and were still impacted, had to serve as supports. Their pulps were removed and their crowns cut down, to raise the bite, so that only their filled roots could be used as supports (Figs. 17, 18, 19).

The second stage of the treatment consisted in the construction of an obturator

fitted with suitably shaped gold crowns. The patient can now masticate without trouble, and has learned to speak quite intelligibly after several months' instruction.

FIG. 17.

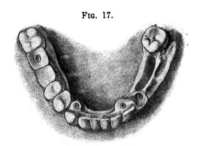

FIG. 18.

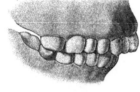

FIG. 19.

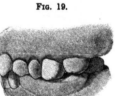

FIG. 20.

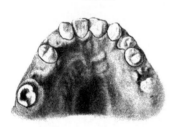

FIG. 21.

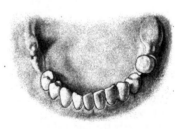

of gold, which was fastened by a gold plate to the right and left upper first molars. But in order to prepare these teeth for this purpose and to protect them for the future against wear and caries, they were ground to a cylindrical shape and

In a second case of uranocoloboma posticum mediale, in which the teeth of the maxilla had already been partly lost and partly much damaged by caries (Figs. 20 and 21), a bridge was made for the right side and an artificial crown for the left (Fig. 22), in order to give a firm hold to the palate-plate which carried the obturator (Fig. 23). The vulcanite plate was on the right side allowed to project into the so-called self-cleaning space of

mediately after the operation. In a great number of cases, models for the construction of splints, immediate and temporary appliances could be prepared from impressions taken before the opera-

FIG. 22.

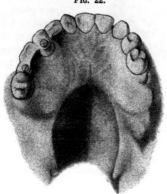

FIG. 24.

FIG. 23.

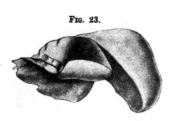
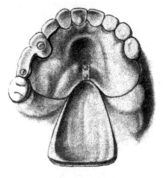

the bridge, and on the left was fastened by a clamp to the artificial crown on the second premolar-root (Fig. 24).

Finally, I would like to point out how important it would be for the success of prosthesis if the dentist were consulted by the surgeon before, during, and im-

tion. Whereas after the sewing up of the wound and bandaging, and especially after the scar has begun to shrink, the preparation of models from which any good work can be done is made more difficult if not quite impossible.

A dentist present at the operation

could decide whether certain teeth should be saved in.order to use them as supports

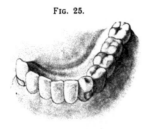

FIG. 25.

for future appliances or whether they should be extracted. I will only mention one out of various examples, which forms a striking proof in support of this plea.

In the case of a high naval officer a partial resection of the lower right alveolar process and an extensive plastic operation of the mucous membrane was performed by Professor Eiselsberg on account of a malignant tumor which, originating from the mucous membrane of the right cheek, had attacked the mandible. The taking of an impression and the construction of a plate was only begun many weeks after the opening of the mouth had been already much contracted owing to the shrinking of the scar, and so it was only possible with great difficulty to obtain models that could be used.

The maxilla was toothless and the mucous membrane tightly stretched extended to the cheek in the neighborhood of the right alveolar process, and from this to the floor of the mouth, bridging over the upper surface of the mandible which had here lost its alveolar process. The vestibulum oris and the alveolar process were thus completely on the same level on the right side.

The construction of a plate to replace the lower left premolars and molars pre-

sented no serious difficulties, since it could be fastened on to the six lower incisors which were available (Fig. 25).

But since all the teeth of the maxilla were wanting any dentist can estimate how difficult it would have been under the circumstances described to insert an upper plate. In the course of a close examination I discovered under a granulating spot of the mucous membrane a root corresponding to the upper right canine. I was on the point of removing this root in accordance with the rule to extract all roots before constructing a plate, when it suddenly occurred to me to lay this root bare from the covering mucous membrane and to examine it more closely. I then found to my surprise and joy that the root was well developed, strong, and firm, and curiously enough was filled with a bleeding and very sensitive tissue

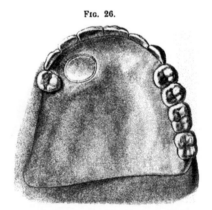

FIG. 26.

(living pulp?). The conservative treatment was successful and this root has now served for years as the point of attachment of a plate replacing the left premolar and molar teeth (Fig. 26).

The patient, who looked very much

run down before and immediately after the operation, today enjoys excellent health and has gained weight in a surprising manner, a thing which would certainly not have come to pass if he had not possessed a good masticatory apparatus. Thus the preservation of a single root may under some circumstances be the cause of a considerable prolongation of life.

Dentistry is the daughter of surgery; it has developed and is built upon the doctrines of the mother science, and gratefully devotes its services to the latter, and in the moment of its highest consecration, when it performs its most difficult exploits, becomes again a part of the widely ramifying composite subject general surgery.

A paper in the German language, presented by Dr. LUDWIG WARNEKROS, Berlin, Germany, on the subject of "Obturators," was read by title.

The paper here follows:

Obturatoren.

Von Prof. Dr. Med. LUDWIG WARNEKROS, Berlin, Germany.

BEI den Spaltbildungen, mögen sich dieselben nur auf den harten oder weichen Gaumen erstrecken oder auf beide, indem sie den harten Gaumen bis zum for. incisinum vollständig-entweder einseitig oder doppelseitig-spalten, so sind mit den verschiedensten Hilfsmitteln gute Erfolge erzielt worden.

Einerseits sind genügend Fälle beobachtet wo nur durch operation, durch Staphyloraphie und Uranoplastik sowohl ein Kosmetischer, sowie auch ein vollständiger Spracherfolg, selbst bei ausgedehntester Spaltbildung erreicht wurde, so dass nur noch Stellungsanomalien einzelner Zähne oder die häufig stark ausgebildete Progenie noch einer Nachbehandlung durch Prothese bedurfte.

Andererseits sind viele Operationen, vervollständigt durch nachträglicher anfertigung eines Schiltskyschen Obturators, und endlich sind nach gänzlich misslungener Operation oder bei Operationsscheuen Patienten die besten Erfolge nur durch einen Obturator allein erzielt worden.

Auch was die Obturatoren selbst betrifft, kann der Nachweiss geführt werden, dass nicht etwa nur nach einem bestimmten System angefertigte Obturatoren einen Erfolg sicher stellen, sondern die gebräuchlichsten arten derselben sind alle erfolgreich zur Anwendung gekommen.

Anders gestaltet sich die Sache, wenn wir zu entscheiden haben, welcher Obturator die meisten Vorzüge besitzt und gegebenen Falles zur Anfertigung zu empfehlen ist. Als Nachteil der Suersenschen Obturator ist stets mit Recht die Grösse und der Umfang desselben angeführt worden.

Ich habe schon früher angegeben, dass es nicht nötig ist, die Verschlussplatte so gross zu formen, wie Snersen es gethan hat, dass viehlmehr-wie an den Modellen ersichtlich-ein kleiner Obturator in den Fällen, wo der gespaltene weiche Gaumen noch vorhanden ist und jederseits bei dem Verschluss des Nasenrachenraums als Verschluss zwischen *cavum nasale* und *c. orale* mitwirken kann, dieselben Erfolge erzielt, und dass in den Fällen, wo nach der Operation das Material zum völligen Verschluss nicht ausreicht, nur ein kleiner Pflock nötig ist, um die Stärkung des Musculus Constrictor pharyngeus superior genügend zu bewirken dass derselbe die Funktion des weichen Gaumens mit dem Zöpfchen tadellos übernimt.

Zur Anfertigung eines Gaumen-Rachen Obturator ist nicht ein Abdruck des ganzen Defekts nötig, sondern es genügt ein Abdruck, der es gestattet die Gaumenplatte anzufertigen. Ich verschliesse gewöhnlich beim Abdrucknehmen den Defekt mit einem Watepflock.

Über die Herstellung will ich mich kurz äussern. Ich verfahre in folgender weise: nach Anfertigung der Gaumenplatt, die mit einem in die Spalt hineinragenden durch Metalleinlage verstärckten Fortsatz versehen ist, wird dieser angeramt und an denselben bis zur Flüssigkeit erwarmte schwarze Guttaperchemasse angeschmolzen.

Wenn die ersten Lagen der Guttaperchemasse am nächsten Tage oder sofort durch Einlargerung in Kochsalz mit Eispackung erkaltet sind, werden neue Guttaperchemassen aufgetragen, und der Patient gebeten Sprachübungen zu machen. In dieser Weise wird der Verschluss des Spaltes etappenweise in 8-14 Tagen zu erreichen versucht.

Die Guttaperchemasse darf aber nur in so geringer Menge an dem Fortsatze angetragen werden, dass die seitlichen Helften des gespaltenen Gaumens nicht gespert werden, sondern dass nur, wenn der *tensor* und *levator veli palatii* beim Schlucken und Sprechen den gespaltenen

Gaumen heben, ein Kontakt mit der Guttaperche erreicht wird.

Für die Formung der hinteren Rachenwand ist es allerdings notwendig dass wir uns die Abdrücke der Tubenwülsten verschaffen. Diese geben dem Guttaperchekloss den Halt welche notwendig ist, um durch sorgfältige auftragen der Guttaperche die Eindrücke des *m. constrictor pharyngeus superior* zu erlangen. Diese letztere stellt sich bei Patienten, die noch nie einen Obturator getragen haben, meist nicht in der Form eines Querwulstes wie es gewöhnlich beschrieben wird, sondern als zwei hinter den Tubenwülsten beginnende schräg nach unten convergirende Muskelzüge dar, die sich an der Raphe im spitzen Winkel treffen und bei deren Contraktion nicht selten die bindegwebige Raphe knopfartig hervorspringt.

Sind alle beschriebenen Partieen an dem Guttaperchekloss deutlich abgedrückt so lasse ich den Patienten denselben noch mehrere Tage bei täglicher Revision tragen, wo bei ich mich durch muldenförmiges Aushöhlen an der oberen und unteren Seite bemühe der Prosthese eine möglichst kleine Form zu geben und dadurch dieselbe den Patienten möglichst angenehm zu machen.

Durch die obere Mulde wird dem Rachenschleim ein bequemer Abfluss geschaffen. Die Schluckbewegungen dürfen in keiner Weisse behindert sein, und die Respiration bei geschlossenem Munde durch die Nase muss ohne Anstrengung vor sich gehen können.

Zum Schluss entferne ich mit einem heissen messer die Eindrücke der Tubenwülste die jetzt keinen Zweck mehr haben und ersetze die Guttaperche durch Kautschuck, wo bei es bei der Kleinheit des Obturator, nicht nötig ist den Kloss hohe zu stopfen.

Es bieten auch diese Obturatoren die

meisten fortzüge hinsichtlich der Sauberkeit und Haltbarkeit, was ich gegenüber
dem Obturator aus weich bleibendem
Kautschuck besonders hervorheben will.

Mit recht ist der Schiltskysche Obturator nach ausgeführter Uranoplastik
und Staphyloraphie als eine bedeutende
Errungenschaft der Zahnheilkunde hin-
gestellt worden; und doch machte sich
ein Mangel bemerkbar.

Da nämlich der elastiche Ballon welcher mit einem Spiralfeder verbunden
ist und den Nasen-Rachen-Raum ausfüllt,
sich leicht zersetzt, und der Patient bei
der Reinigung auch eine Beschädigung
fürchtet, so wird derselbe einerseits selten genügend gereinigt und andererseits
auch noch getragen, wenn in dem Ballon
durch die Risse die bald in demselben
entstehen, sich Zersetzungprodukte an-
gesammelt haben. Diese Unsauberkeit
welche mit dem material verbunden
ist, habe ich dadurch zu verhüten
gewusst, dass ich statt des elastichen
Ballons eine Platte aus hartem Kaouts-
chouck an der Spiralfeder befestigte.
Dieselbe wurde in der Weise geformt,
dass an der Spiralfeder schwarze Guttaperche solange aufgetragen wurd, bis die
Eindrücke des *m. const. phar. sup.* deutlich erkennbar waren. Es wurde durch
den so hergestellten obturator eine
gleiche Stärkung der Musculatur wie
durch den Schiltskyschen erreicht, so
dass er in manchen Fällen nach ein-
iger Zeit überhaupt entbehrt werden
konnte. In anderen Fällen, wo er
dauernd getragen wurde, bot er den
Vorteil der Sauberkeit und leichteren
Reinigung.

Derselbe Nachteil, nur in grösserem
Masse, macht sich geltend wenn ein
Schiltskyscher Obturator getragen wird,
ohne dass die Staphyloraphie und Uran-

oplastik ausgeführt worden sind. Der
grosse elastische Ballon bedarf häufig eine
Erneuerung die der Patient, zumal wenn
er keinen Zahnarzt am Orte hat, nicht
immer selbst auszuführen im Stande ist.
Auch hier lässt er es bei kleinen Beschädi-
gungen des Obturators, aus Furcht, den
Schaden zu vergrösseren an der nötigen
Reinigung fehlen, ohne zu bedenken dass
derselbe in diesem Zustand grosse Gefah-
ren für die Gesundheit in sich birgt!
Auch bei erworbenen Defekten wurden
deshalb die Obturatoren stets aus hartem
Kautschuck angefertigt.

Die Überbrückung des weichen Gaumens wurde von mir nicht durch die
Schiltskysche Feder, sondern durch einen
unbeweglichen halbrunden Goldstreifen
bewerckstelligt. Hierbei ist aber darauf
zu achten dass dieselbe in solcher Entfer-
nung vom weichen Gaumen angebracht
wird, dass Letzterer, wenn er sich beim
Sprechen und Schlucken bewegt, keine
Verletzugen erleidet.

Die meisten erworbenen Defekte sind
auf Syphilis des Nasenrachenraums zu-
rück zu führen und zeigen die grösste
Mannigfaltigkeit. Besteht die Perforation nur im harten Gaumen, so genügt
eine einfache Gaumenplatte wie sie beim
Zahnersatz verwendet wird; ist aber ein
Defekt des weichen oder des weichen und
harten Gaumens eingetreten, so muss in
der vorher geschilderten Weise ein Obturator aus hartem Kautschuk angefertigt
werden.

Ganz unerquiklich werden die Zu-
stände wenn bei Syphilis des Nasen rach-
enraums nicht nur eine Perforation sondern auch eine Verwachsung des weichen
Gaumens mit der hinteren Rachenwand
eingetreten ist; aber gerade hier hoffe ich
dass die Erfolge, die ich mit den kleinen
Obturatoren erzielt habe, ein Zusammen-

14

arbeiten der Laryngologen mit den Zahn-
ärzten herbeizuführen im Stande sind;
denn der Operateur braucht sich nun
nicht mehr zu fürchten die Sprache des
Patienten zu verschlechtern, wenn er den
Defekt durch Lösen des angewachssenen
Teiles vergrössert und uns den Patienten

zur Anfertigung eines Obturators über-
weist.

———

There being no other business before
the session, Dr. Turner, the chairman,
declared Section VIII adjourned *sine
die*.

Some Interesting Exhibits: Gold Medal Awards.

Archæological Exhibit.

ANCIENT AND MODERN DENTAL INSTRU-
MENTS AND APPLIANCES.

AN interesting archæological collection, prepared under the auspices of the
École Dentaire de Paris, was exhibited
in Sections XIX and XX in the Palace
of Liberal Arts.

The first prize of a gold medal offered
by the Committee of Organization for
the best and most instructive array
of ancient and modern dental instruments and appliances was awarded to
the custodian of the exhibit, Dr. EMILE
SAUVEZ, delegate of the French Government.

Prosthetic Pieces.

Dr. VINCENZO GUERINI, Naples, Italy,
presented a great many prosthetic pieces
in different systems and materials (vulcanite, celluloid, gold, platinum, aluminum—the last with and without soldering). Among the many bridges (removable and immovable) in gold, platinum,
and porcelain, was especially noticeable
a full bridge, upper and lower, in which
all of the twenty-eight teeth were made
in gold, with quite perfect anatomical
forms. He presented also specimens of
his system of palatal prosthesis.

Dr. Guerini was also awarded a gold
medal for his exhibit.

Fourth International Dental Congress.

SECTION IX.

SECTION IX:

Education, Nomenclature, Literature, and History.

Chairman—TRUMAN W. BROPHY, Chicago, Ill.
Secretary—WINTHROP GIRLING, Chicago, Ill.

FIRST DAY—Monday, August 29th.

THE section was called to order at 3 P.M., by the chairman, Dr. Truman W. Brophy of Chicago, Ill.

On motion, the paper by Dr. GEORGE VIAU of Paris, France, entitled *"A propos* of a Portrait of Pierre Fauchard,"* was directed to be presented for reading at a general session of the congress. [For this paper, with the discussion thereon, see report of the second general session, in Vol. I of Transactions, pp. 31-38.]

On motion, the session adjourned to meet on the following afternoon.

SECOND DAY—Tuesday, August 30th.

THE section was called to order at 3 P.M., by the chairman, Dr. TRUMAN W. BROPHY, who then read his address, as follows:

Chairman's Address.

Setting aside the fact that I may be charged with a misconception of the duties of chairman of a section in an international congress when I treat of the subject that I am about to discuss—a subject of interest to Americans chiefly —yet, in view of the fact that I have already presented addresses on dental education from the international point of view in foreign lands during the past five years, may I not here and now talk on a topic which occupies our thought in America? Therefore, inasmuch as the subject (in which I have concerned myself not a little) is of vital importance to our profession, our colleges, and our student body, I venture to present this topic that is engrossing us now.

The problem before us is the elevation of the standard of preparation of a dental student.

Briefly stated, I am going to consider informally (1) The prerequisites of the student's education; (2) the *time* element in his professional work; (3) how to assist the student to accomplish his aims.

No matter what subject you may name, whether you refer to character, architecture, road construction, national or international laws, educational standards, educational institutions, all must be built, if we would have them endure, on deep, broad, and well-laid foundations.

Our section stands out conspicuously as the most important section of this great congress. Education and educational methods are now and ever will be the themes which claim the thoughts of our distinguished men, and elicit their best efforts from pen and rostrum.

A thorough education is the foundation upon which a professional man must rely if he would attain a high degree of success as a practitioner.

Men who have not thought deeply on the subject of dental education, particularly on the preparation most essential to equip students for matriculation in dental colleges, insist on certain standards of high-school and college work, in the belief, no doubt, that such standards are ideal ones; but while such preparatory training is quite sufficient for entrance upon the study of law, theology, or medicine, such instruction, followed by the conferring of the degree of A.B. and all that the degree implies, cannot, as taught in most of the schools and colleges, properly prepare a student for entrance upon the study of dentistry; nor can such preparation in the highest degree prepare a student for the study and practice of surgery in any of its branches.

We are all of us agreed that a thorough education is essential as a foundation for entrance into a professional school, but when we ask ourselves the question, To what use are we to put this education? then we are brought to realize what kind of a preparatory equipment a student needs to enable him to make the best and most satisfactory progress as a dental student.

In the advanced high-school and college courses, too little attention is paid to the subjects of physics and manual training. No matter how far a student may be advanced in his college course, his classical education and linguistic proficiency will not alone qualify him for the practical duties of the dental student.

Before entering the dental college a student should have taken, some time before or in connection with his higher educational work, a thorough course in manual training, and have acquired a knowledge of digital manipulations, and have become skilled in the use of instruments. Such a course of manual training is of inestimable value alike to the dental student and the medical student who expects to practice surgery.

Digital training, to make it of the greatest value, must be a youthful training, for manipulative skill is seldom acquired after the age of twenty-five.

The late Dr. W. C. Barrett, in discussing the value of digital training, related his experience in matriculating a freshman student, thirty-one years of age, who was a college graduate, and whose education in English, French, and German was very thorough. He told how the members of the faculty were pleased with the scholarly accomplishments of the candidate, and to one another remarked that, "If all our students were as well educated as this one, what superior practitioners they would make!"

In Dr. Barrett's words: "That man had the best-trained mind and most ignorant hand of any student we ever had in our college." With all his knowledge of the classics and his delightful personality he was ignorant of technology and lacked the manipulative skill so essential and indispensable to the dentist. Moreover, he was not able to acquire digital skill.

I am firmly of the belief that the preparatory education for matriculates in our dental colleges will soon be exactly what our faculties require. If we should publish in our annual announcements that three years hence all matriculates must have completed 48 counts, or the four years' high-school course, including a technical course in manual training, students would prepare themselves and come to us thus qualified. In justice to prospective students it would only be fair to notify them long enough in advance, so that they might be able to comply with the higher requirements.

Holding a professorship in the Rush Medical College during the past twenty-four years, I have seen the admission requirements advance in that institution from a very low standard to the present high one. The requirement at the present time is fulfilled by the completion of the second year's course in the university.

While Rush Medical College exacts that its matriculates take a longer preparatory course than our National Association of Dental Faculties requires— necessarily barring many young men from admission—nevertheless its classes are large, and have greatly improved in scholarly attainment.

The faculties in our professional schools seem to overlook what I feel to be a duty to students who seek advanced standing. No matter how much knowledge a young man may possess, how thoroughly he may know branches of the curriculum, he cannot be examined, be given credits for his knowledge, receive advanced standing, and so shorten his college course.

It seems to me that the International Commission on Education, in co-operation with this section, in justice to young men who possess certain qualifications for advanced standing, should devise a plan by which the knowledge they possess can be determined, and by which the students may be graded according to their merits. I am confident that each nation participating in this congress could create for their respective countries a representative board, made up of men whose scholarly attainments, professional ability, and unswerving integrity eminently qualify them to examine applicants for advanced standing. Such boards of examiners would, I am satisfied, have the confidence and respect of the public and the profession everywhere; a board which would give each one examined such a certificate of credits as would enable any dental college to which the student might apply to give him the standing and classification among the students, and in the schools, to which his knowledge would entitle him.

STATUS OF AMERICAN DENTAL COLLEGES.

Recently the discussion of American dental colleges and the legislation of the National Association of Dental Faculties has brought out the fact that many gentlemen who write on the subject of dental education and who are administering the dental laws are not fully acquainted with the status of our dental colleges.

It seems, then, as if it were only just to our American colleges to place before the representative men of the dental profession of the world, as well as other professions and the public, facts regarding our dental institutions of learning. Moreover, the Committee on Foreign Relations of the National Association of Dental Faculties, through the strenuous efforts of its late chairman, Dr. W. C. Barrett, whose labors we all appreciate, has made us acquainted with the standing and courses of study of all foreign dental colleges, and is it not fair that the schools abroad should be informed in regard to the standing of our colleges, that our foreign co-laborers may have the same knowledge of our dental institutions of learning which we have acquired of theirs?

Let me first call your attention to statements frequently heard at home and abroad, to the effect that university schools are on a higher plane, and are entitled to higher consideration than other schools, whether connected with local universities or built up on their own individual merits.

It has been said that state university schools are endowed, or that they receive liberal appropriations from the state, and consequently are not dependent on the students' fees to defray the expenses of conducting educational work.

There is not a dental college in the United States, in the universities or out, that has an endowment of a single dollar. There is not a state university dental school which receives a state appropriation, if they receive any at all, equal to the fees which the treasurer of a university collects from the dental students. All the dental colleges in the United States, therefore, are dependent upon the fees of the students to defray their expenses. The assumption of men who are not correctly informed, and whose voluminous writings on commercialism in dental schools state that colleges are conducted for commercial purposes, is unworthy of them, unjust, and misleading. Little do the men who make these statements realize the struggle of the founders of the Baltimore College of Dental Surgery, the first dental college in the world, and of the Ohio College of Dental Surgery, the second dental college; how hard Harris and Hayden, and Taylor and Taft worked as builders of dental educational institutions.

The Baltimore College of Dental Surgery was our first institution of dental learning, and every American dentist, every foreign dentist, should stand uncovered and bow his head in reverence when the name of its founder is pronounced, the name of Chapin A. Harris. Our hearts beat with pride as we recall the work of those distinguished men to whom the world owes a great debt of gratitude for the labor and sacrifices made in establishing dental colleges, and developing systematic courses of instruction.

While Harris was the founder of the first dental college, one of his immediate successors, Dr. R. B. Winder, was the founder of the National Association of Dental Faculties, an organization whose influence has been and will continue to be active in dental educational work, and it ranks among the foremost educational organizations of our country.

The achievements of Harris, Hayden, Taylor, and Taft were not easy; there were no endowments, no government appropriations for them; the colleges stood then as the American dental colleges do today—dependent upon the students' fees to carry on their work, and when the fees were inadequate these founders paid the bills out of their own pockets, as college faculties of dentistry do now, and in many instances received no compensation for their services, except the satisfaction of doing their duty in conscientiously teaching their students. Commercialism? Is it not necessary for an educational institution to pay its debts? Is there a man in this or any other country who has any practical experience in dental college management, who has not ofttimes been nearly at his wits' end to know how to get funds to enable him to add to the equipment of the college, in apparatus, furniture, etc.? It is owing to the statements previously mentioned, that our dental colleges are conducted for the purpose of making money, that I have referred to the subject, and in justice to my co-laborers, the dental teachers of our country, I declare that the strictest economy is necessary to meet the expenses of the colleges; and the compensation of the teachers, if they receive any at all, is in most cases insufficient for the time, ability, and energy expended.

The action in Washington in changing the course from seven months to six months was approved by some prominent men, who, apparently without analyzing the advantages or disadvantages of the situation, adversely criticized the action at St. Louis, by which action it was decided that a student might complete his studies within a period of three years, of which thirty teaching weeks in each year—of six days a week, exclusive of holidays—would constitute a full curriculum, and admit the student to the final examinations for the degree of Doctor of Dental Surgery.

The figures before you show that the St. Louis decision provided a course only forty-four days shorter than the four years' course of seven months, and fifty-two days longer than the four years' course of six months, adopted in Washington.

It is too apparent to require argument that the action of the association at the St. Louis meeting placed the educational work of our colleges on a much higher plane, and marked a decided improvement over the four years' course of six months. The four years' course of seven months would make it necessary for a student to spend either nearly half of his time outside of college, or, intervening the courses, remain in the infirmary (provided his college had a summer practice course), and receive only practice instruction, with no didactic work whatever. Furthermore, he would be required at the close of his third year of the four years' seven months' course to wait twelve months longer, and get only forty-four days' instruction more than he would in the course arranged at St. Louis.

The National Association of Dental Faculties has a membership of fifty-four colleges. Of these, four are organic parts of the state universities — Michigan, Iowa, Minnesota, and California. These colleges are owned by the states and controlled by boards of trustees elected by the people of the respective states. I do not hesitate to say that the good work to the credit of the dental faculties of these schools has been handicapped by frequent and unjustifiable interference on the part of politicians, who have in many instances caused friction in the dental faculties, and through political influence have forced superior teachers and excellent men, who have ornamented our profession by reason of their greatness, to resign their professorships.

There are other dental schools which have a form of affiliation or a business contract which will enable them—if the conditions of the contract are carried out —to eventually become departments of universities. The universities, however, which have such contracts with professional schools, do not supervise the educational work, nor do they assume any responsibility—financial or otherwise— in conducting the school.

There are other dental colleges which are organic parts of local universities. Among these latter universities are Harvard, University of Pennsylvania, Northwestern University, Washington University of St. Louis, etc., none of which are in any way under state or government supervision.

The impression which has prevailed abroad to some extent, that certain of our university dental schools are under government supervision and that the educational work is conducted by teachers working under direction of the government bureau of education, and that the diplomas of such universities bear government indorsement, is incorrect. There are no dental schools under the direction of the United States government, consequently no diplomas bear its seal. If the state universities would appropriate sufficient funds to meet ever-increasing expenses to properly carry on the college work, or if endowment were provided to aid such schools, there would be some advantages derived from university connection. But as it is, the name "Department of the University" is of little or no practical value in assisting educational work.

By reason of the efforts of the National Association of Dental Faculties, which was organized in 1884, the educational standards of our dental colleges have been from year to year advanced (prior to which an applicant for admission to certain colleges, whose private instruction and practice extended over a period of five years, might matriculate in the senior class, and become a candidate for the degree of D.D.S. at the close of one course of instruction of five months). This standard was raised by the association, first, to two courses of six months each, with one year's high-school work as an educational requirement for admission; next, to three courses of six months each, with two years' high-school work as a prerequisite; and, finally, at Milwaukee, in 1901, the association adopted a resolution to the effect that the course of instruction beginning with the session of 1903-04 would be four years of seven months.

The dissatisfaction which arose among some of the colleges, in regard to the length of the sessions, led the association, at its annual meeting in Washington, to change the length of the term from four years of seven months to four years of six months. This decision was a compromise measure, but soon after the meeting adjourned many of the colleges tendered their resignations and announced to the secretary that they had decided to make the length of sessions eight or nine months, and complete the course in three years.

I received letters from the deans of four of our oldest and strongest dental colleges informing me that they had resigned. At once I wrote them, urging them to reconsider their action, and at the same time I called a meeting of the deans of the Chicago colleges, and finally persuaded them to join me and get the officers of the National Association of Dental Faculties to assemble a meeting and adopt a course which would save the association from dissolution. This was done, and the association convened in St. Louis, where the following resolutions were adopted:

RESOLVED, That the minimum time for dental teaching required by this association to qualify students for examination for graduation shall be thirty weeks of six days each, in each of three separate academic years, exclusive of holidays; this resolution to take effect at once; and be it further

RESOLVED, That all rules or parts of rules in conflict with this resolution be and are hereby repealed.

All the catalogs of the colleges have been issued in accordance with the resolutions quoted, and it is now of interest to know exactly what the change in the course has been, as to actual teaching days, and in other respects.

I have made a careful tabulation of the actual time in days of college work, so that you may note the changes, in days, in the length of courses of the past and present. Let us compare the seven months' course of four years with the six months' course of four years, and with the course last arranged, of three years of thirty teaching weeks in each year, exclusive of holidays. [See table, page 220.]

The courses in American colleges begin about October 1st and the seven months' course would end May 1st. We have, in these seven months, 212 days. There are 20 holidays, 31 Sundays, and the 30 Saturday afternoons, which would make 15 days more. A total of 66 days must be subtracted from 212 days, leaving 146 days of actual college work done in each scholastic year. This, multiplied by 4, the number of years, gives us 584 teaching days in the four years' course of seven months.

In the four years' course of six months, we get 181 days. From this number we must subtract holidays and Sundays, 59, which subtraction leaves us 122 days. This result, multiplied by 4, gives us 488 teaching days in the four years' course of six months.

The course adopted in St. Louis in July last is of three years, each year to consist of thirty weeks of six days in each week, exclusive of holidays. In thirty weeks of six days each we have 180 days. This number, multiplied by 3, gives 540 teaching days. The advantage in time which the seven months' course of four years has over the six months' course of four years is 96 teaching days.

The advantage of the four years' course of seven months over the three years' course of 30 teaching weeks of six days in each week is only 44 teaching days.

The advantage of the three years' course of thirty teaching weeks of six days per week over the four years' course of six months each is 52 teaching days.

If we take out the Easter holidays and every Saturday, in accord with the custom of some of the colleges, we must subtract twenty more holidays from each course of seven months. We have then in the four years' course of seven months each 504 teaching days, and as the present course is 540 teaching days we have, consequently, 34 days more college work in the present course than in the four years' course of seven months each adopted in Milwaukee.

And if the four years' course of six months had prevailed, the student would have been 48 months getting 24 months' instruction, and would have had 52 days' instruction less than he would get in such a course as has been arranged at St. Louis.

I believe the student and his parents are entitled to some consideration. To

TABLE SHOWING THE ACTUAL VALUE, IN DAYS, OF COLLEGE COURSES OF FOUR
YEARS OF SEVEN MONTHS, FOUR YEARS OF SIX MONTHS, AND THREE YEARS
OF THIRTY TEACHING WEEKS IN EACH YEAR OF SIX DAYS A WEEK, EX-
CLUSIVE OF HOLIDAYS.

The 66 holidays and Sundays are made up of the following:

	Days.		Days.
Alumni	1	Lincoln's Birthday	1
Election	1	Washington's Birthday	1
Thanksgiving holidays	3	Saturday half-holidays	15
Christmas holidays	13	Sundays	31

Total 66 days. (31 full days; 6 days Easter vacation.)

	Days.
Course of four years of seven months each year (per year)	212
Less holidays and Sundays (per year)	66
Total teaching days in one college year of seven months	146
Course of four years of seven months each year	4
Number of actual teaching days	584

	Days.
Course of four years of six months each year (per year)	181
Holidays and Sundays	59
Total teaching days in one college year of six months	122
Course of four years of six months each year	4
Number of actual teaching days	488

	Days.
Present course of instruction, three years of thirty teaching weeks, exclusive of holidays	180
Course of three years of thirty teaching weeks	3
Number of actual teaching days	540

Summary.

	Teaching Days.
Four years' course of seven months	584
Four years' course of six months	488
Three years' course of thirty teaching weeks (each year)	540

	Teaching Days.
Four years' course of seven months	584
Four years' course of six months	488
Excess of four years seven months' course	96

	Teaching Days.
Four years' course of seven months	584
Three years' course of thirty teaching weeks (each year)	540
Excess of four years seven months' course	44

	Teaching Days.
Three years thirty teaching weeks' course	540
Course of four years, six months each year	488
Excess of three years thirty teaching weeks' course	52

exact twelve months' time, one year's college course fees, and living expenses, equal at least to six hundred dollars, and to give only 44 days' instruction within the twelve months, seems unjust, but to require the same expenditure of time and money, to compel him to wait six months without instruction, and then to attend college six months longer, and thus to spend a whole year, giving him 52 days' less instruction than the present course provides, would be unworthy of the National Association of Dental Faculties.

It is of little consequence to the profession and the people *where* a dentist gets his knowledge, or whether he spends fractions of three years, fractions of four years, or fractions of ten years in a dental college, before entering in practice. This is not the question. The question that demands an answer is: How can our colleges best produce educated men, proficient dentists, and safe, reliable practitioners?

The action of the Faculties Association at St. Louis was *not* a step backward. It was a provision for a better course and a more exact course than had ever before been inaugurated. It fixes the days and hours that the student must attend college. Had I been able to control the action, the course would have been made 32 teaching weeks, exclusive of holidays, with an advance in educational requirements for admission, but the action of the association is most commendable in adopting a course which is a great improvement over the four years' course of six months. Such a course is equal to three years of nine months, including holidays.

Every teacher realizes that the vacations which occur in the short courses of six and seven months keep the college work in a state of constant confusion.

The present course will in a great measure remove this embarrassment.

The experience of the dental school of the University of Michigan, which established a four years' course of nine months, five years ago, demonstrates in a practical way that no dental college can make a standard far in advance of other institutions and maintain an existence.

In 1900, the number of students enrolled in the Michigan University dental department was 247; graduates, 76.

In 1904: students, 94; graduates, 6.

The board of regents of the University of Michigan found it necessary to either conform to the rules of the National Association of Dental Faculties or discontinue the dental department.

As I have said in the beginning, our questions under discussion may perhaps claim an international interest.

Let no man assume that dental education in America is likely to become a retrograde movement. To do so would be un-American and contrary to the traditions of our institutions. We are proud of the history of the dental colleges of our country, and while the National Association of Dental Faculties has in some matters taken steps which I wish had never been taken, and which I heartily wish it could retrace, on the subject of the course of instruction and how to instruct this great body stands for the highest and the best. The dental profession everywhere, and our sister institutions in foreign lands, may rely upon the work started by Harris and Hayden to be carried on by the distinguished men who are assembled here today, and who, when the next International Dental Congress convenes, will have advanced our educational institutions to a higher position; and the American dental graduates of the future, as in the past, will take high rank with the members of our profession throughout the world.

[For the discussion of Dr. Brophy's paper, jointly with the following paper by Dr. Hunt, see page 227.]

The next order of business was the reading of a paper by Dr. A. O. HUNT of Omaha, Neb., on "The Count System of Students' Credits."

The paper was as follows:

The Count System of Students' Credits.

By A. O. HUNT, D.D.S., Omaha, Neb.

AT the request of the chairman of the Section on Education, Nomenclature, Literature, and History, I have consented to present a paper on this subject, with some misgivings as to whether the proper time has yet arrived. The system is entirely new in its application to the dental curriculum and is unfamiliar to teachers and managers of dental schools. It is adapted to all other conditions, however, and there is little doubt of its final success; but its practicability is yet to be tested in this relation.

The public-school system is the foundation of true Americanism and the bulwark of our strength. It is the standard of excellence and the standard by which all things are finally tested. It produces the best morals, the best politics, the largest amount of intelligence (per capita) and that superabundance of energy observed in every avenue where human effort is displayed.

The system begins with the primary school and extends through the secondary or high school to the state universities. It is under the control of the government, national, state, and local.

While the purpose of having good schools in each grade is general, yet methods would necessarily vary, as well as the subjects taught. There are high schools of one year, of two years, of three

years, and of four years, in which the teaching is not the same even in those with the same length of time.

It has been necessary in some cases to have preparatory departments as part of the universities in order to equip the student for entrance into the university proper. As a considerable number of the high schools of a state advanced to four-year courses, or to an equivalent to what has been taught in the preparatory departments of the universities, these latter departments were dropped by the university, and students of such high schools were admitted to the universities without examination and became what is called accredited schools. There are also other schools in existence that are private, or special in their character, over which the state or government exercises no control. They also have their own methods of teaching and arrange their own curricula.

This lack of uniformity produces the condition that the credentials or diplomas for the same degree issued by the various schools do not always represent the quality or quantity of work the student may have had.

In 1784, by the act of the New York legislature, there was established the University of New York, composed of nineteen regents. Each appointment was made for life. It was reorganized in 1787. The Governor, Lieutenant-Governor, Secretary of State, and Superintendent of Public Instruction are members *ex officio*.

As the count or credit system originated with this body, and has been used by it for nearly half a century, it may not be out of place to quote from the *Bulletin* what their function is:

UNIVERSITY OF THE STATE OF NEW YORK.

Object.—The object of the University as defined by law is to encourage and promote education in advance of the common elementary branches. Its field includes not only the work of secondary schools, colleges, universities, professional and technical schools, but also educational work connected with libraries, museums, study clubs, extension courses, and similar agencies.

The University is a supervisory and administrative, not a teaching institution. It is a state department and at the same time a federation of more than one thousand institutions of higher and secondary education.

Government.—The University is governed and all its corporate powers exercised by nineteen elective regents and by the Governor, Lieutenant-Governor, Secretary of State, and Superintendent of Public Instruction, who are *ex officio* regents. Regents are elected in the same manner as United States senators; they are unsalaried and are the only public officers in New York chosen for life.

The elective officers are a chancellor and a vice-chancellor, who serve without salary, and a secretary. The secretary is the executive and financial officer, is under official bonds for $10,000, is responsible for the safekeeping and proper use of the University seal and of the books, records, and other property in charge of the regents, and for the proper administration and discipline of its various officers and departments.

Powers and Duties.—Besides many other important powers and duties, the regents have power to incorporate, and to alter or revoke the charters of universities, colleges, academies, libraries, museums, or other educational institutions; to distribute to them funds granted by the state for their use; to inspect their workings and require annual reports under oath of their presiding officers; to establish examinations as to the attainments in learning and confer on successful candidates suitable certificates, diplomas, and degrees, and to confer honorary degrees. They apportion annually an academic fund of $350,000, part for buying books and apparatus for academies and high schools raising an equal amount for the same purpose, $100 to each non-sectarian secondary school in good standing, and the remainder on the basis of attendance. The regents were also granted in 1901 $20,000 for the benefit of free public libraries.

Regents' Meetings.—The annual meeting is held the first Thursday in December, and other meetings are held as often as business requires. An executive committee of nine regents is elected at the annual meeting to act for the board in the intervals between its meetings, except that it cannot grant, alter, suspend, or revoke charters or confer honorary degrees.

Convocation.—The University convocation of the regents and the officers of the institutions in the University, for consideration of subjects of mutual interest, has been held annually since 1863 at the capitol in Albany. It meets Monday, Tuesday, and Wednesday after the fourth Friday in June.

At this convocation, though it is primarily a New York meeting, nearly all questions discussed are of equal interest outside of the state. Its reputation as the most important higher educational meeting of the country has in the past few years drawn to it many eminent educators not residents of New York, who are most cordially welcomed and share fully in all discussions. A council of five is appointed to represent it in intervals between meetings. Its proceedings, issued annually, are of great value in all educational libraries.

For a better consideration it may not be amiss to refer to a subject now under discussion before the regents, relating to the combined baccalaureate and medical courses, which shows the care and consideration exercised in reaching conclusions involving important changes. Again quoting from the *Bulletin:*

SHOULD THE REGENTS REGISTER COLLEGE COURSES AS THE EQUIVALENT OF THE FIRST YEAR IN A MEDICAL SCHOOL?

In 1902 an amendment to the medical laws of the state of New York provided that the regents might accept as the equivalent of the first year of the full four years of at least nine months each, including four satisfactory courses of at least six months each in four different calendar years of a medical school, evidence of graduation from a registered college, provided that such college course should include not less than the minimum requirements prescribed by the regents for such admission to advanced standing.

At convocation in 1902 a thorough discussion of the requirements for admission to medical schools, including the combined baccalaureate and medical course, was participated in by representatives of both the medical and liberal arts faculties of representative New York institutions.

In continuation of the study a suggested outline was prepared and sent to many leading educators, both of New York and other states of the Union, to learn their opinion regarding the outline of subjects and their treatment during the first medical year as follows:

Suggestions: Anatomy 150 hours, laboratory 50 hours at least. Biologic sciences 150 hours, laboratory 50 hours at least.

The course is then definitely outlined as to the teaching of histology and microscopy, botany, zoölogy, and bacteriology.

Chemistry 150 hours, laboratory at least 50 hours. Physics 100 hours, laboratory 40 hours. Physiology 100 hours, laboratory 50 hours.

Correspondence was had with the representatives of the following interested institutions:

Independent colleges: Hamilton, Colgate University, Princeton, Oberlin, and others.

Independent medical schools: Long Island College Hospital, Albany Medical College, and others.

Universities: Cornell Medical College, Syracuse University Medical Department, Harvard University, Yale University Medical Department, University of Pennsylvania, University of Michigan, American Academy of Medicine, etc.

To supplement the information gained by this correspondence there was also presented the action of the Association of Medical Colleges, as follows:

At the meeting of the Association of American Medical Colleges, held at Atlantic City, June 1904, Dr. Henry L. Taylor of the New York State Department of Education, presented a paper on the subject which elicited much discussion. At this meeting the following resolutions were adopted:

"RESOLVED, That the Association of American Colleges approves of the so-called combined system of college and medical education, and of giving time credits not exceeding one year, to the holder of A.B., B.S., or other equivalent from a reputable college or university, provided such a student has had at least 900 hours in physics, chemistry, osteology, histology, embryology, anatomy and physiology, and provided the applicant for such time credits satisfies the professors attached to the medical college as to his proficiency in the first year medical studies."

"RESOLVED, That a committee on national uniformity of curricula be appointed to co-operate with a similar committee appointed by the National Federation of State Medical Examining and Licensing Boards for the purpose of presenting a minimum standard of medical education, together with such recommendations as the committee may deem proper to make as to the division of the subjects in a four years' graded course. Said report to be presented at the next annual meeting and to be printed and distributed at least one month before the annual meeting."

"RESOLVED, That no student shall be admitted to advanced standing without a direct communication from the dean certifying as to the applicant's credits and moral qualifications."

All these matters are introduced to show the importance of the careful consideration of the system of counts in establishing a safe, inflexible, systematic standard upon which to base the work of advancement so much desired.

There might be profitably selected quotations from speeches made before the annual convocation of the regents, where men representing all sides of any movement both within and without the state of New York take part.

The *Bulletin* issued by the regents is replete with the opinions of all of the best men interested in the advancement of education on every topic that may come before the body for consideration.

It will be well for us, then, in the interest of the advancement of dental education, to become familiar with the methods of a body of men who are entirely free from the entanglements of politics, sectarianism, and personal aggrandizement, who for more than a century have fulfilled their trust faithfully and well, and for more than half a century have tested the virtues of the count system and applied it to all the phases of education of whatever character, holding always to the one idea that when the regents' certificate has been issued to any individual it represents a definite amount and quality of instruction as scheduled by them in various publications.

Independent of the sources from which it may be obtained, their system is so hedged about with precautions that are just and equitable, that it cannot but be accepted as final by any body of men called upon to act upon their credentials, whether in America or elsewhere, if they

are familiar with their methods, which are published to the world.

The count system in itself is a very simple affair. Its application to the varying conditions is not so simple but is not in any way incomprehensible or impossible.

It consists in the establishment of a "unit" that stands for something definite. Their unit for the academic courses stands for one day of a week of five days of not less than forty minutes each day for ten weeks' instruction in each branch of study included in any course as counting one.

The year's course is expected to include forty weeks of work, so that any branch of study pursued for one school year through four terms will have credited to it at the end of the year four counts, or forty-eight counts for the full four years' high-school course, three studies for each term or period.

In other states of the Union the principle of the system has been adopted but the basis of the unit may be different. In our section, in Nebraska, for instance, the year is divided into two semesters of twenty weeks as the basis of the unit instead of ten. Each student in a four years' course of high-school work understands clearly that he must carry four studies for the year, or when he comes up for graduation at the end of his four-year course he must have to his credit thirty-two counts, or eight for each year, before he will receive his diploma. There are additional branches that may secure thirty-six counts. Nothing can be more simple and capable of understanding by both pupil and teacher.

There are two well-organized bodies of men, the National Board of Dental Examiners and the National Association of Dental Faculties, in this country, com-

15

posed of representative men who are all without exception interested in the advancement of dental education. While their motives are identical, many things intervene to make their actions not always harmonious.

Let us first consider the National Board of Dental Examiners—a body without any legal status itself, yet made up of representatives of bodies that have the highest legal standing by state enactments. This comes from the conditions that exist in the organic laws of the country. The national government has certain rights that are not delegated to the states, and beyond which it cannot go. Each state is competent to make laws that may suit itself and are legal so long as they do not encroach upon the position occupied by the national government.

It is evident, then, that each state may pass laws for its own guidance that are entirely independent of laws that any other may pass. This has produced variation in the laws regulating the practice of dentistry in the various states. Some are in advance of other states on this account, and there is not opportunity in this paper to discuss them further, only to state the fact. However, the point that affects all alike is the difficulty presented in each case for the state examining boards to fix a standard that shall be uniform and have a definite basis.

Many of the laws contain this clause, which is a stumbling-block: "To accept the diplomas of all *reputable dental colleges.*" Now the boards have never been able to come to a decision as to what a *reputable* dental college is. Some of the laws attempt to define it by enumerating the various branches taught in all well-organized dental colleges. It happens

that a college of low standard may teach the same subjects, so that under this definition all schools are reputable that teach those subjects.

The boards as yet have not been able to perfect an arrangement acceptable to all, whereby a person fully licensed in one state may remove to another and be allowed to practice there. In a few words, there is no standard as yet established that is acceptable in all parts of our country. Many of these conditions will be changed eventually by state enactments or by an arrangement between the various boards. The count system of credits is undoubtedly the only means when fully understood and inaugurated that will secure a standard that will form a basis for reputability by which this can be accomplished.

The National Association of Dental Faculties, another body that is vitally interested in the consummation of the universal standard, has been working along its lines and according to its lights, in the furtherance of this object.

In 1884, when the body was organized, there could not be conceived a more unsatisfactory condition existing than then existed as to the standard of dental education. No preliminary requirements. No uniformity in the course of instruction, and all things in a chaotic condition.

This organization has steadily advanced along its course, bettering things continually from the beginning. It is not necessary to go over the many episodes that have happened in twenty years. It has, however, raised the preliminary requirement in twenty years from nothing to the entrance into a third year of a four years' high school or to an equivalent of twenty-four counts by the New York regents' standard. In 1895 this association adopted a minimum entrance requirement, at that time but little above the finish of a grammar grade, with progressive advancement for each year. This was rescinded in 1896. Had the action of 1895 been continued we would have had an entrance requirement at this time (1904) of the completion of the high-school course, or forty-eight counts by the New York regents' standard. This would have come about without any hardship to either students or schools.

The National Association of Dental Faculties has adopted the count system again this year, with the preliminary requirements of entrance into the third year of a high school, or twenty-four counts. It has also adopted the count system to be applied to the regular curricula of the schools. The following is the schedule: Unit—1 hour per week of lectures for a semester of 15 weeks, equal one count. Unit—2 hours of laboratory work to be equivalent to one hour's lecture. Special subjects, two of which constitute one count—Embryology, electricity, diseases of the antrum, jurisprudence, facial art, hygiene, regional anatomy, dental ethics.

This is the keynote to the situation. If all of the bodies interested in the advancement of dental education in this country and elsewhere will apply the same earnestness and conservatism freed from personality, politics, prejudices, etc., and study this question, and discuss it freely (after obtaining the necessary information relating to the count system) with all interested, in the opinion of the writer nothing but the perfect advancement of the cause is possible, and it will secure a standard that can be accepted by all as just, equitable, and fair.

Perhaps it will not be possible to get the best results without a new organization or committees with supervisory and administrative powers selected from the National Association of Dental Examiners, the National Association of Dental Faculties, and from the International Dental Federation, to whom all matters would be willingly relegated and with whom all schools which desire a full recognition of its standard may register.

Certificates issued by such a board will constitute a standard based upon something definite, and will carry with it the positive assurance of value, correctness, and authority of an organization that will be recognized throughout the dental world as having supreme authority in such matters.

This can only be accomplished by the use of the count system, which will regulate the quality and quantity in every branch of instruction established; it will carry with it a dignity and respectability that does not now exist. Students upon entering the study of dentistry will have a higher estimate of the profession, and will themselves, both as students and graduates, be interested in forcing the standard up to the highest point consistent with good results.

Discussion.

Dr. H. L. BANZHAF, Milwaukee, Wis. I can only express my hearty approval of what Dr. Brophy said concerning the entrance requirements to our dental colleges. I think that the high-school diploma is the most rational requirement, and believe that the high school comes nearest to solving the perplexing problem of preliminary education. It seems to me there can be no doubt that it can safely be considered the best instrument for preparation within the reach of the general public. The adoption therefore of the high-school diploma as a preliminary requirement to our colleges will unquestionably be found to be an efficient means of uniformity.

Another point which Dr. Brophy has brought out appeals to me very strongly: It is just as necessary to deal in definite quantities as to the teaching months, days, or hours required in our curriculum as it is to adopt the count system in the grading of credentials presented by the student.

Dr. Hunt's paper has been particularly instructive to me, and I want to express my hearty approval of the suggestions which the essayist has made in regard to establishing a board to be composed of representatives of the National Association of Dental Faculties, the National Association of Dental Examiners, and the International Dental Federation. If this were done I believe it would insure the selection of men eminently fitted for such a position, and this board, with supreme power, could settle many questions that are now troubling us. Such a board, then, might be considered an international board of arbitration and therefore our court of last resort.

I am sure that I appreciate and understand the practical workings of the count system, especially as applied to the grading of our students, better than I ever did before, and I think it is a great pity that every teacher who occupies an executive position in a dental college, and every member of the National Examiners' Association could not have been present to listen to both these very valuable essays.

Dr. L. P. BETHEL, Columbus, O. I have enjoyed both of these excellent papers, being especially interested in the address of Dr. Brophy, as it presents ideas that I have for a long time advocated. Making the college course a uniform one is a matter I have urged in the National Association of Dental Faculties for two years, and I was pleased to learn of the adoption of such a course at the recent meeting of the association. When the course of four years of seven months was established there was no mention made of the number of teaching days in the week. I see Dr. Brophy has estimated five and one-half days. A number of colleges have taught only five days in the week, and that has been countenanced by the association. Taking five days a week as the recognized requirement, that would be fifteen days less than Dr. Brophy's estimate, or one hundred and thirty-one days for the year. Now, for the four years of seven months, that would make five hundred and twenty-four teaching days instead of five hundred and eighty-four, as shown on the chart, and five hundred and twenty-four days in four years would be less than the length of course now adopted, three years of thirty teaching weeks, six days a week, for that amounts to five hundred and forty teaching days. So in the present course of three years of thirty weeks we are really teaching sixteen days more per year than in the four years' course of seven months each. As Dr. Brophy says, I do not see that the action has been retrogressive at all. I believe we are progressing. Establishing a uniform course in dentistry is but a just and equitable thing to do.

Dr. H. A. SMITH, Cincinnati, O. Dr. Brophy, in his able address, has given us good reason why the recent action of the National Association of Dental Faculties in changing the minimum course of study in our dental colleges is not necessarily a retrograde step. When we consider, as he has shown, that there is a decided gain in active teaching time over the four years of six months' course, with a strong probability of soon extending the session to at least eight months of actual teaching, it is evident the National Association of Dental Faculties has taken an advanced step in dental education.

This change, together with the proposed adoption of the higher entrance requirement—that of a high-school graduation or its equivalent—should give us the basis of an ideal dental college course for a good number of years to come. It is obvious, I think, from the experiences of the past, that frequent changes in our educational methods are detrimental to that true advancement in dental education that we all hope for.

Dr. JAMES McMANUS, Hartford, Conn. I was pleased with the inclination of the faculties, or a certain portion of them, to give to the students practical and theoretical education and do it in as limited a time as possible. A student knows the hours he will actually get, the teaching that he pays for, and hereafter the board of examiners cannot question, as in the past, whether the student has been given the instruction that he ought to have had. It seems to me that the faculties have their eyes open to the fact that there is something yet to be done by them, and they have made up their minds to do it.

Dr. WILLIAM H. TRUEMAN, Philadelphia, Pa. I feel a keen interest in the question of dental education, and I think Dr. Brophy's suggestion that the dental schools should be made stronger financially is timely and to the point. Very few schools devoted to the higher branches of education are entirely dependent upon their students' fees, as are nearly all the dental schools. This higher education is expensive. Its students require more room, they must be provided with expensive apparatus and appliances, and with talented teachers. All of these things cost money. There is no question that our dental schools would do better work if economy was less considered. The newer methods of education which the dental schools are adopting call for smaller classes and more teachers. The lecturer is giving way to the demonstrator, and training is taking the place of dialectics. The professors are not well paid, and many of the demonstrators serve for but little more than the practice and experience the position gives them, and serve only until their private practice requires all their time. With sufficient funds at command to properly remunerate talent, the colleges could select from available candidates those who had not only ability but the gift of teaching, and build up and retain a staff of well-qualified and experienced teachers and demonstrators.

If the profession wants better schools it can have them by providing the necessary financial support. With all its advances in education, the dental profession in this country has made very little progress on that line. Some of its members have prospered, and dying have left millions, but of their accumulated fortunes very little indeed has been left for the betterment of the profession. In Philadelphia, I know of but two bequests to a dental college; they amounted to about one thousand dollars. An advance in dental education is not so much a question of days and hours as it is a question of dollars and cents. Our dental schools have proved their usefulness and their worthiness. They have done well, exceedingly well, but can do better, and will do better, if furnished with less advice and more cash.

Dr. J. H. KENNERLY, St. Louis, Mo. The subjects presented by Drs. Brophy and Hunt are of vital interest to teachers in the dental schools of the United States. Dr. Trueman has made a remark which brought a thought to my mind, or, rather, it was a reminder of a circumstance of not long ago. I asked the chancellor of the university with which I am connected, for a certain amount of money. He asked: "What do you want it for?" I told him, to buy brains. He said, "I can get all the money you want for buildings but I can't get a cent with which to buy brains." The brains I wanted to buy in this case was the McKellops library. It seems impossible that in the city of St. Louis, which spent $25,000,000 on the World's Fair, it should not be found possible to raise $10,000 to buy such a work as this. Within the World's Fair grounds we have buildings that cost $2,000,000, all given by the generous friends of the university. Men of means in this city or any other city are willing to give money to build large buildings, monuments to their memories, but when you go to a man and ask him to endow a chair it is next to impossible to get him to do it. While Washington University has been teaching in St. Louis for nearly fifty-five years, she has but one endowed chair, and that one was endowed by a brewer. My sole business is to promote the interest of the department of the university which I represent. The medical department of Washington University has several endowments, and small bequests sometimes come to the other departments, but they are very small. There are men here who have millions and could they be persuaded to give us an endow-

ment it would enable us to buy the brains we need.

The subject of the count system has worried me as much as anyone else. There has been a constant interchange of thought with Dr. Hunt in connection with this subject. I have always believed it a good thing, for I don't believe one of the oldest institutions in the country would adopt anything not good. Compare the teaching of today with what was done twenty or thirty or forty years ago and as much difference will be found as in any other branch—if not more. There is one little mistake that the dental profession is making, and that is the claim that we cannot eliminate the money question. It seems to me as though it had been eliminated to a considerable extent. Has it ever occurred to you that you have three or four men teaching the same subject that was formerly taught by a single teacher when you were a student? and yet the cost of tuition remains the same. But you say, We are teaching longer terms. That should make no difference. As an illustration I will give you a little personal experience. When I decided to become a student I secured catalogs from several schools and finally selected the one that seemed the best. It was a two years' course of six months. I had been there but a few days when the demonstrator came to me and told me to get my instruments and put a filling in a certain tooth. I had never filled a tooth, I had never prepared a cavity, but I proceeded to prepare this one as best I could—cleaning out everything that did not seem to belong there. And then I put in the filling, but it wouldn't stay. Every time I put it in it would roll out and I could not understand why the amalgam wouldn't stay in the cavity;

but I later found that it was mercury and not amalgam with which I was attempting to fill the tooth. Now, I guarantee that in the fifty-four schools composing the National Association of Dental Faculties, you will not find a man who, when he enters the operating room, cannot prepare a cavity and introduce a filling better than we could at the end of a two years' course of six months.

There is another question with which we must deal. It is this: The different state boards believe they can best control the dental colleges by examining their students. I believe the schools agree with them. I do, at least. There is a movement on foot to amend the state laws requiring every man who comes into the state to be examined. With four terms of six months these men would be forced to go elsewhere and earn their living during six months of each year. They will forget what they have learned during the first year's work and it will be three years before it is brought back to their memory, and then by the state board, and your men may fail and your work be lost. On the other hand, if we raise the standard and decide that the three years' course of nine months is the better, then we will educate our men so that no man who goes out with our diploma need be afraid of any state board. This is the only solution that I can see.

Dr. BROPHY. I would like to make a comparison of my schedule here with reference to Dr. Bethel's statement. If we take out the Easter holidays and every Saturday, that will add twenty more holidays to the course of seven months, and would make a course of 504 teaching days. We have, consequently, 34 days more in the present course than in the course adopted at Washington.

In conclusion, I thank you for the enthusiasm you have shown.

Dr. HENRY W. MORGAN, Nashville, Tenn. These papers have been so thoroughly discussed that nothing is left for me to do but compliment the two essayists and say that I think they put these two matters before the profession of the United States in a form more concrete and graspable than any papers we have yet had, and I hope to see them soon in print.

Dr. A. O. HUNT (closing the discussion). Just a word or two to get into our mind what is meant by the facts as they have been presented. We talk of years and of months, and when we use the word year in connection with the term of instruction it is always misleading. Of course, we will still be compelled to use it, but in a general sense. Here is the point, 584 days represents a quantity of work done. We must know just how much teaching and what kind of teaching is done in these 584 days, each branch being definitely settled as to the certain number of credits each student must have; then we have the quality. The number of days represents the quantity of work, and the credit or count the quality. These two facts are essential in establishing a permanent basis that everybody will agree is accurate and right. By experience it has been demonstrated, and for more than half a century, that up to this time the count system meets all conditions and is exact.

The subject was passed and the chairman called for the next paper by Dr. CHARLES McMANUS. Hartford, Conn., entitled "International Character of the Early Development of Dentistry in America," which was then read, as follows:

International Character of the Early Development of Dentistry in America.

By CHARLES McMANUS, D.D.S., Hartford, Conn.

IN the few moments at my disposal I desire to touch briefly upon one small feature connected with the early history of our calling in this country. As it concerns a matter of applied sentiment rather than applied science, it seems peculiarly appropriate that we consider it at such a time as this.

The great exposition of which this congress forms a part is not only to display the latest modern achievements of art and science, but to commemorate the great deeds of the past and the men who accomplished them. This proper sentiment is shown most beautifully, in our own case, in the medal struck in honor of this occasion—upon one side of which are inscribed the names of men representing the various nations who have contributed to the upbuilding of the dental profession, while upon the other side it reminds us that we are not only in the city of St. Louis, but are under the patronage of that most distressful lady, St. Apollonia—who seems after all these many many centuries, thanks largely to the gallantry of Professor Peirce, to have come into her own again.

This union of sanctity and science today was many years ago foreshadowed, in a small way, in the person of that accomplished gentleman the Reverend Doctor Solyman Brown, A.M., M.D., D.D., D.D.S., who was not only a dentist but a minister, and could claim in every sense to be a "man of letters."

But, seriously speaking, this inter-national professional spirit of which we have heard so much lately has always been a factor in the development of our profession in this country. There has been a germ of "internationalism in dentistry" from the very beginning of practice in America. As early as 1735 various itinerant Englishmen began to ply their art in a small way, and by 1766 arrived a regularly educated practitioner, Mr. Robert Woofendale, a pupil of the King's dentist, Thomas Berdmore. Two years later John Baker, another Englishman, practiced in Boston, New York, and other towns. About this time several Americans became interested in the subject, notably Isaac Greenwood and Paul Revere in Boston. Later still we find a certain Whitelock or Whitlock, who is kindly spoken of by Dr. Hayden as "a gentleman of polite address and accomplished manners." He is said to have come to this country as one of a company of actors from London; but we must not think any the less of him for that, for if he gave up acting for dentistry, the great French tragedian Talma, the son of a distinguished dentist, forsook dentistry for the stage.

JOSEPH JEAN FRANÇOIS LEMAIRE AND JAMES GARDETTE.

But, whatever place we may be willing to give these early Englishmen, we can safely say that dental science was brought to America by two patriotic young

Frenchmen, toward the close of the Revolutionary war. The first, Joseph Jean François Lemaire, arrived July 12, 1780, as a surgeon of volunteers with the French troops under Rochambeau. Lemaire had studied at the medical school in Paris, giving particular attention to the dental art. The second, James Gardette, was a naval surgeon who had pursued his studies of anatomy and surgery in the Royal Medical School of Paris, afterward removing to the hospitals at Toulon and Bayonne, where he obtained his commission. He had received instruction in dentistry as part of his training as naval surgeon, from M. LeRoy de la Faudignère, a dentist of Paris then in high repute, and had provided himself with the best works extant and with a limited set of dental instruments. He arrived on a warship at Plymouth, Mass., in January 1778.

During the winter of 1781-82, the revolution being then nearly over, the French and American armies were in winter quarters near Providence, R. I., and we find in intimate friendship these two young Frenchmen, and with them a youth of eighteen, Josiah Flagg, destined to be the first native-born American dentist.

"So," Dr. Wm. H. Trueman says, "it needs but little stretch of the imagination to locate the first school for dental instruction in the United States and the first dental meeting for mutual improvement around this revolutionary camp-fire."

Lemaire afterward practiced in New York, Philadelphia, and Baltimore, returning to Paris in 1787, where for many years he continued as a skilful dentist and ready writer.

Gardette having practiced first in Newport, R. I., went to New York, and finally settled in Philadelphia, where he remained for forty-five years, returning to his native land in 1829. He did much in his long and honorable career to make dentistry in Philadelphia what it is to-day.

Josiah Flagg, their pupil, located in Boston in 1783, where he practiced with success until 1812, when his patriotism again got the better of him and he enlisted in the navy, and was captured and taken to England. While on parole he practiced dentistry in London in 1813-15, making the acquaintance of the celebrated surgeon Sir Astley Cooper, frequently attending his lectures and clinics at Guy's Hospital.

In 1803 there came to Philadelphia an Irishman, Edward Hudson, educated at Trinity College, Dublin, and the pupil of his cousin, a talented dentist of that city. Hudson was a remarkable man, a dentist of great skill, and for more than thirty years he occupied a commanding position among the reputable dentists of this country. Dr. Elisha Townsend said of him, "All who knew him intimately, respected and prized him for the exceeding goodness and sincerity which shone so brightly conspicuous in his character. By his patients he was idolized as few of his professional brethren can ever expect to be."

In 1807, at the age of twenty-two, Leonard Koecker, a native of Bremen, Germany, bravely began practice in Baltimore. The chance meeting years before with a kind-hearted traveling Hebrew dentist in Hanover, who had given him some slight instruction and a small outfit of instruments, was the starting-point in the career of this eminent dentist. He went to Philadelphia about 1812, and was very successful, as his practice brought him $8000 in one year, until ill health compelled him to seek rest in Europe in 1822. Upon his arrival in London he decided to locate there. As he carried with him a number of influential letters of introduction he was very successful.

A Frenchman from Paris, A. A. Plantou, introduced porcelain teeth into this country in 1817.

As early as 1817, Dr. Hayden had broached the idea of a national convention of dentists, but as he says, "the pear was not ripe." From time to time he renewed his attempts only to fail. But about 1833 two French empirics, "the Crawcours," arrived in New York with a flourish of trumpets and their "mineral paste," and unwittingly, by their unprofessional conduct, had a good deal to do with forcing the reputable dentists of the day to make their calling a true profession. In the crusade against these men the profession had descried some of the advantages resulting from associated effort. They already had a journal started in June 1839, and a college, a charter for which was granted in the same year. They were now to have a national association.

THE FIRST DENTAL JOURNAL.

Let us consider the journal first. The publishing committee sent a specimen number to every dentist whose name and residence they could obtain in the United States and British provinces of North America. They stated that they had "the promise of assistance from the pens of some of our most talented brethren in England." They announced that "The first dental surgeons of Europe, among whom we are proud to mention the names of Cartwright, Koecker, and Brewster, have in letters written in the kindest and most friendly manner, expressed their

high satisfaction at the efforts we are making to advance, not only in this country, but also in Europe, the interests of the dental art; and no inconsiderable portion of our subscribers are of the most distinguished cities of Great Britain."

Associated with the editors, as collaborators and *ex officio* agents, were Leonard Koecker, M.D.Lond., C. Starr Brewster of Paris, S. Highley of London, and E. Gidney of Manchester, England. Among the early subscribers to the journal outside of this country were twenty-two in England, four in Scotland, two in France, one in Holland, and one each in the West Indies and New Brunswick —nearly ten per cent. of the entire subscription list.

The publication committee also acknowledged with satisfaction the good fortune of receiving from Mr. Eleazer Gidney, dentist, recently from Manchester, Eng., the loan of his dental library, consisting of books and prints collected in France and England with much labor and expense. It was very complete and large for the time—over one hundred volumes—and what became of it heaven only knows, but we can join with the committee in thanking Mr. Gidney in behalf of the profession generally for his liberal encouragement of the efforts to establish an *American Journal of Dental Science*.

THE FIRST NATIONAL DENTAL SOCIETY.

On August 18, 1840, Dr. Horace H. Hayden expressed his desire to make a few remarks before submitting the constitution of the "American Society of Dental Surgeons" to the consideration of the meeting.

He said: "At the present period renewed efforts are making in England, France, and Scotland to place our profession on still higher ground than it has yet attained; and shall we, of these United States of America, remain inactive in this grand endeavor?"

And in the first article of the preamble of the objects of the society, we read: "The objects of this society are to promote union and harmony among all respectable and well-informed dental surgeons; to advance the science by free communication and interchange of sentiments, either written or verbal, between members of the society, both in this and other countries."

The society on August 20, 1840, proceeded to elect honorary members as follows: Samuel Cartwright, London; Robert Nasmyth, Edinburgh; Alexander Nasmyth, London; C. Starr Brewster, Paris; John T. Edmonds, London; James McPherson, Glasgow, Scotland; A. G. Becht, The Hague, Netherlands; Leonard Koecker, London; Thomas Bell, London; C. F. Delabarre, Paris; David Wemyss Jobson, Edinburgh; E. Gidney, Manchester; Joseph Lemaire, Paris.

Lemaire at the time of his election had been deceased about six years. He died in 1834.

In a statement entitled "Information Concerning the American Society of Dental Surgeons," published in the *American Journal of Dental Science*, vol. i, No. vii, Dr. Solyman Brown says: "Among the primary objects kept steadily in view by the projector of this society and his professional coadjutors, may be alleged—first, THE PUBLIC GOOD, resulting from the united efforts of the most distinguished and enterprising dental practitioners in the United States, aided by those of other countries, in settling the best methods of practice in all forms of dental disease."

We have not time to consider further this first national association. It was started on a broad basis, "under the most flattering auspices and with a membership never since surpassed in this country in high professional ability and private reputation, but, through a mistaken course of conduct, obstinately persisted in, it defeated its high objects, and after sixteen years worked its own ruin."

In this brief and hurried way I have endeavored to show that a hundred years ago Englishmen, Frenchmen, Germans, and Irishmen, many of them for their time regularly educated dentists, came to this country and helped lay the foundation for a profession. That over sixty years ago the dentists of a number of the countries of Europe were asked to and did assist in the formation of the first dental journal and dental society. That in the early days many of our best men practiced successfully in other countries—notably Flagg, Koecker, Eleazar Parmly, with others in England; Brewster in France and Russia; the Spooners in Canada.

The history of the pioneers will show that they were honored and respected both professionally and socially. It is true they were comparatively few in numbers, and after a time, particularly about 1833 to 1838, the irregular practitioners who deserved and got little respect increased very rapidly; but we should judge a profession as we would an army, by its advance guard, not by its camp-followers.

I feel that the idea is too generally held by that public—which we sometimes talk about educating—and by some practitioners, that prior to about sixty-five years ago dentists had little or no standing in the community, and that largely because dentistry had laboriously worked itself up from the tinker, the barber, and the blacksmith. Now this is a very pretty little tripod which it seems almost a pity to try to upset. Much can be said with truth about these occupations.

The *tinker*—that primitive trade—the lowest of all the crafts; and yet it has for its own, John Bunyan!

The *barber*—the harmless necessary barber; what an unkempt lot of barbarians we should be without him! Why, one of the sweetest poets France ever produced was a barber. His country honored and his government decorated him, and he wasn't ashamed of his calling.

The *blacksmith*—the village blacksmith—who "looks the whole world in the face, for he owes not any man."

It would ill become us to mock with a disdainful smile their useful toil. They merit our respect and our patronage—when we need them—but they had nothing to do with the evolution of dental surgery.

Why a profession that can look back two centuries and claim as its father the eminent French dental surgeon Pierre Fauchard, and look back two more centuries and justly point to the great French surgeon Ambroise Paré as its foster-father, and which even in this young country has had such an interesting development—the early international character of which I have tried, I am afraid very imperfectly, to show you—why it should seem to search the highways and byways after alleged progenitors, is to me one of the many curiosities of dental literature.

Discussion.

Dr. WILLIAM H. TRUEMAN, Philadelphia, Pa. I congratulate Dr. McManus on having brought to our notice a new phase of dental history, and an interesting one. Science is cosmopolitan; to this, dental science is no exception. Medical knowledge seems to have first crystallized into a science among the Arabians, and the works of their able writers were standard for several centuries. Then Italy took the lead, then France. It was in France that the art and the science of dentistry made a notable and distinct advance by becoming a recognized specialty whose practitioners were known as dental surgeons. When the science reached America it found fallow ground. We were not trammeled by traditions of the past, but were energetic, progressive, and resourceful. New heads and new hands in a new country almost made it a new science. We gathered in the best the nations of the world had to offer, and quickly made it better. We have originated but little, but we have elaborated, improved, and made practical a great deal. Gold foil, especially prepared for dental use, was first made in the United States, where also the best methods and appliances for forming it into tooth-saving fillings originated. Prosthetic dentistry has been remodeled under the magic touch of American ingenuity. Dental education and dental literature owe a great deal to American brains. Although, as Dr. McManus has shown, we owe a great deal to the old world, we have, I think, paid the debt with ample interest. We must not forget, however, a caution Dr. McManus' paper suggests. The nations of the world are all wide awake. Dental science is progressing rapidly on the other side as well as here. If we rest content with having gained a fancied pre-eminence, we may soon become a "once was."

Dr. A. O. HUNT, Omaha, Neb. The reference in the paper to the general belief that we spring from the barber, tinker, and blacksmith is something that I always have resented. We have had these men among us, but they are not the men who have made the history of dentistry. It was not the barber, or the tinker, or the blacksmith, but the educated gentleman who is responsible for the progress and who has held up the profes-sion through the ages and given it dignity and position in spite of the incubus of the barber, tinker, and blacksmith.

The subject was passed, and Dr. S. H. GUILFORD, Philadelphia, Pa., read a paper on "Nomenclature."

The paper was as follows:

Nomenclature.

By S. H. GUILFORD, A.M., D.D.S., Ph.D., Philadelphia, Pa.

IT has frequently been asserted and by many it is believed that a language bears a close relation to the character of the people who originate and employ it. It would be strange if it were not so, inasmuch as anything which man devises is a direct expression of his needs or desires, and could not well be dissociated from his personality in some form.

The Latin races, with their nervous energy and rapidity of speech, employ more words in the expression of their ideas than many other nations. If several simple words are needed to fully express a condition, or state, or object, they are all pronounced and written separately, though fluently spoken.

The Teutons are more slow of speech, more deliberate, more phlegmatic possibly. With them, when an idea needs several single words to express it, they join them into one long, cumbersome word, which may be easy enough for them to comprehend and speak, but which certainly is not so to the foreigner.

The Anglo-Saxons occupy a position between the others. They do not often combine several pure Anglo-Saxon words to form a composite one, but usually employ the single words with such slight ab-breviations as will not impair their value. When a composite word is needed in English, it is constructed from foreign derivatives, sometimes hyphenated but more often not.

Although German is regarded as a language rich in expression and comprehensive in words, neither it nor any other is sufficiently replete to meet the ever-increasing demands of science, art, or philosophy.

Nature is constantly revealing herself to man in so many new ways that his vocabulary fails him in defining or expressing them. He therefore is often driven to the necessity of coining new words or terms, which, while in certain cases they mean nothing in themselves, by association with the idea expressed and with nothing else, are accepted and incorporated into the written and spoken language, where they serve as definite a purpose as others which have a philologic basis.

Thus when the development of electrical science required that certain phenomena should be named so that they could be dealt with in a mathematical, mechanical, and commercial way, it was found that there were no single words in any known language that could be made to serve. New terms therefore had to be coined, and it was happily decided to employ the names of certain persons who, in their day, had been engaged in electrical investigation and had enriched the science by valuable discoveries. In this way the names of Ampère, Volta, and Ohm came to represent the units of electrical volume, force, and resistance, and France, Italy, and Germany were incidentally honored in their selection.

This plan, while serviceable and commendable in certain cases, could not well be followed to any great extent, and in the coining of new words it has been found most convenient to name the new objects or processes after their most prominent characteristics. In many cases it served a better purpose to take the roots from some foreign language and combine them into a single word, thus doing away with the prepositions which would otherwise be necessary in English. The terms photography, biography, etc., were thus created and have proved entirely satisfactory, both on account of their simplicity and their definitive character.

When the new metal radium was discovered, it received its name from the peculiar rays which emanated from it, and when it was found that these rays were capable of affecting a sensitized plate or film and fixing upon it the form and outlines of a given object, the second word radiograph was quickly and scientifically adopted.

So too with the Roentgen ray. It had no previous known place in nature or in the vocabulary and therefore it was given the name of the discoverer. However, as the term Roentgen ray was somewhat cumbersome and as it in itself did not express any characteristic of the peculiar

phenomenon, it was renamed X ray because this algebraic figure, used to denote an unknown thing or quantity, corresponded with the hidden or unknown source of the rays. When it was found that these rays affected a photographic plate much in the same way as sunlight, the impression thus obtained was known as an X-ray photograph. However, these three words seemed unwieldy, and as it was the opaque objects which were impressed upon the sensitive plate and not the transparent ones, as in photography, the term photograph was not scientifically correct. A new term, skiagraph, was therefore coined which exactly described the fact that it was a shadow picture.

Again, when Edison improved and developed the original moving-picture toy into an instrument capable of illustrating on a large scale the motion of men, animals, or other objects, a word was needed. Biograph was at first accepted, but as the word indicated life in the object depicted and as many inanimate objects were equally represented in a state of motion, a more specific term was demanded, and the word kinematograph was substituted, for it signified movement-pictures or illustrations. For the sake of euphony and convenience this term was later abridged to kinetograph.

It will be noticed that in the terms thus far given all are derived from Greek or Latin roots, indeed, all Greek but one. The reason for this is the fact that both are dead languages. Words in a living language often change their meaning through time and custom, but those of a dead language are incapable of it and are thus stable and fixed. We therefore find that the new words introduced into any of the sciences today are

SECTION IX: EDUCATION, NOMENCLATURE, LITERATURE, AND HISTORY. 239

taken from one of these languages or are constructed from their roots.

For this reason it would seem best that in our own science, where single or combined English terms cannot be made to express the idea desired, the new words coined should be taken from the "dead" languages.

Most of the distinctive technical words now found in our text-books are thus derived, many expressing a fine shade of difference, such as the terms anesthesia and analgesia.

Orthodontia expresses, as well as any compound word can, the nature of the condition with which it has to do, while the newly-coined term prosthodontia, while not quite accurate in its derivative meaning, is so convenient and so nearly correct as to sanction its permanent adoption.

The term "autogenous" soldering, as used to denote the union of like metals at a point just short of fusion without the interposition of an alloy to facilitate the process, while not quite correct etymologically, should be considered satisfactory until some more accurate one is devised.

The word odontotechny, while not new by any means, has for some reason never been generally adopted, although it is etymologically correct and comprehensive. By its use, the double word "dental-technics," which is less convenient and is moreover a hybrid, being part Latin and part Greek in origin, would be avoided.

We employ the related words odontology, odontalgia, etc., and so it would seem the part of consistency, at least, to incorporate the word odontotechny into our working vocabulary.

It is a pleasure to notice that many terms adopted hastily, and which answered their purpose for a time, have been discarded because they were not in any way indicative of the condition or part which they were intended to designate. Riggs' disease is a term almost unknown to the younger generation, although the medical profession still retains a few expressions of a similar character, such as Pott's disease, Addison's disease, etc.

Pericementum has supplanted both the inaccurate term periosteum and also the cumbersome one peridental membrane. Resorption has taken the place of absorption when applied to the dissolution or gradual removal of calcareous tissue.

The term "antrum of Highmore" has made way for the more expressive one "maxillary sinus." Both designate a cavity, but the former does not indicate its location, while the latter does. Pyorrhea alveolaris is a cumbersome term and not at all accurate, yet it designates one of the manifestations of a disease and also its location. For this reason and the further one that no other combination of words has appeared that could be readily handled, the former term has thus far refused to be displaced.

In the whole range of dental science, however, no department or specialty is suffering so greatly from a lack of accurate and expressive terminology as orthodontia. Many terms employed in this branch are absolutely incorrect, while others are of very doubtful utility.

Occlusion is a good term when properly used, but it signifies a coming together or contact. Malocclusion is also correct when it is employed to signify that the teeth of one jaw meet those of the opposite one in an incorrect or abnormal manner, but it cannot justly be used to indicate the malposition of teeth. Much less can it be applied to teeth which, owing to their malposition, cannot come into occlusion at all. Thus the terms labial occlusion, lingual occlusion, and infra-occlusion are manifestly incorrect, because they imply conditions which do not and cannot exist.

Protrusion and retrusion as applied to teeth which project beyond their normal arch line or are too far within it, are excellent and expressive terms, while extrusion instead of elevation, and intrusion in place of depression should be adopted because they are equally expressive and derived from the same root-word.

Following this same method of adding prefixes or suffixes to good roots of either Latin or Greek origin would be an intelligent and scientific way of building up a nomenclature both in orthodontia and other branches of the dental art. It may have to be done gradually, for old friends or servants are not readily discarded; but until it *is* done we cannot claim to have a terminology equal to that of other branches of science nor one that can be considered exact in any sense of the word.

Discussion.

Dr. W. C. GOWAN, Creemore, Ont. In an admirable way the essayist has called our attention to the relation between the language and the character of a people. This relation is evident in many ways. It may be perceived in the distinctive language or style of sects, professions, or individuals.

The words peculiar to a sect are often an index of the intellectual character or the extent of knowledge prevailing among its adherents. The language of a profession indicates the scientific culture, exactness of knowledge, love of accuracy, and mental habits of those who devise and use it.

As in the case of Shakespeare the language of an individual may be the only evidence we have of what he was. John Ruskin examining the words of Byron, found in them, among other things, abundant evidence that Byron was not the servant of Lucifer.

Exact and well-chosen terms are evidence of clear thought and scientific habit, if not of exact knowledge. The author points out in a most comprehensive and instructive way what constitutes a good term and also the means whereby a new term may best be devised. In fact, he furnishes us a criterion by which we may know a good name when we get it. Its characteristics are simplicity, brevity, euphony, and definitiveness. A name is satisfactory in proportion as it possesses these qualities. It should be derived from one language only. When the mother tongue fails to furnish it, one or more roots from a dead language may be used in constructing a new term which shall possess so far as may be the four qualities just mentioned.

The most essential of these qualities is definitiveness. The best names define with most exactness the things for which they stand. They are best because they are most easily learned, remembered, and used, thus rendering easier the acquirement and use of knowledge. And since utility is the criterion of beauty, terms having these qualities are the most beautiful.

The improvement of dental nomenclature is a commendable undertaking. For it is desirable, since words are an index of character, that ours should indicate that scientific habit of mind and love of exactness which bring success and honor to the dental profession.

However, proper use of nomenclature now available, could it be successfully urged upon the majority, would be equally advantageous to us. I find in this essay no opinion with which I disagree and no argument that I can refute. The examples chosen to illustrate the author's meaning serve that purpose well. I am delighted to have heard the paper, and if I might fittingly offer congratulations to one so much my senior in experience, I would heartily congratulate the author.

Dr. TRUMAN W. BROPHY, Chicago, Ill. I want to call the attention of the session to some expressions which have been adopted in dentistry which seem to me in conflict with expressions in anatomy. It seems to me that the dental professors are going to have difficulty over these expressions. For instance, take the word for the tooth of the carnivorous animal, now known as the cuspid tooth, anatomists thinking that a better word than the term canine. But we must bear in mind that we have the fossa called for ages the canine fossa because it is above the canine tooth. Anatomists do not call it the cuspid fossa. And in other particulars we find words adopted by dentists which are not accurate in their meaning. The peridental membrane was in my opinion always a cumbersome expression. I agree with Dr. Guilford that the better term is pericementum. Again, we speak of pyorrhea alveolaris when we refer to a condition of pus flowing from the alveoli. A medical man not familiar with the nomenclature of the dentist might think that the pus was flowing from some other tissue, as the alveoli of the lungs, for instance, and he might suppose that it was a pulmonary abscess. Why should we not adopt the expression paralleling other expressions? If we have an inflammation of the membrane covering the tooth we call it a pericementitis and we know just where the inflammation is. We do not state whether it is a chronic, acute, or subacute inflammation. If we wish to convey that information we have to use an adjective in addition. So, if we say we have a dental alveolitis we make it clear that we refer to an inflammation of the membrane of the tooth, which may terminate in a restoration to health or a formation of pus which may flow from the alveoli; but pyorrhea alveolaris is in my opinion very unsatisfactory, for it does not mean anything definite. It has been in use so long that we have become familiar with it and that would be the only reason for continuing its use.

Dr. GUILFORD (closing the discussion). As soon as we get a more satisfactory word I think the profession will accept it, but pyorrhea is more than an alveolitis —it is a pyorrhea.

On motion the meeting adjourned until 2.30 P.M., Wednesday.

SECTION IX—Continued.

THIRD DAY—Wednesday, August 31st.

THE section was called to order at 2.30 P.M. by the chairman, Dr. Truman W. Brophy.

The first paper was that by Mons. B. PLATSCHICK, of Paris, on "The work of Pierre Fauchard," as follows:

L'Oeuvre de Pierre Fauchard dans la Prothèse Dentaire.

Par Mons. B. PLATSCHICK, Paris, France.

C'EST à la France qu'on attribue universellement la gloire d'avoir fondé la prothèse dentaire sur des bases scientifiques; l'Amérique même, qui détient présentement le flambeau du Progrès, avoue l'avoir reçu des mains de la France. Si celle-ci n'avait pas à être fière de quelques-uns de ses maîtres contemporains, elle pourrait du moins s'enorgueillir de ses célébrités du passé. C'est justement ce glorieux passé représenté par le nom de Pierre Fauchard, dont le rôle n'est pas universellement apprécié à sa juste valeur, que j'ai l'intention d'évoquer brièvement à ce congrès.

En analysant l'œuvre de Pierre Fauchard, nous trouverons bien des idées qui se sont développées dans les siècles suivants, de sorte que cet auteur, par la génialité de sa divination, est bien près de nos temps. La mise en lumière de ses travaux a une portée plus haute que de satisfaire une curiosité d'érudit; elle explique historiquement l'évolution de la prothèse dentaire contemporaine.

Je limite mon étude à cette spécialité, il serait trop long et ce n'est pas ma tâche d'embrasser aussi son œuvre de dentiste. Je me borne donc à dire que Pierre Fauchard est aussi grand comme dentiste que comme prothésiste; il a deviné la science comme il a deviné la mécanique dentaire. Sa figure de savant remplit tout son siècle, et son ombre se projette sur le suivant. Après lui, tous les dentistes jusqu'à Delabarre se sont inspirés de son ouvrage

Son nom marque une division très nette et très précise dans l'histoire de la prothèse dentaire; il sépare le moyen âge de l'âge moderne. Avant lui, c'était l'époque des charlatans qui sans aucune idée arrêtée sur la théorie de cette spécialité l'exerçaient chacun à son caprice. Avec lui et après lui, la prothèse dentaire est fondée sur des bases scientifiques. Une trouvaille, une découverte n'est plus cachée jalousement par l'heureux inventeur, comme faisaient ordinairement les charlatans avant Fauchard pour ne pas en faire profiter leurs confrères; mais chaque invention est exposée dans tous ses détails, vulgarisée, livrée au monde scientifique. Les formules empiriques qu'une génération transmettait à la suivante sont remplacées par les principes de la théorie. A l'effort individuel qui finit avec l'individu, se substitue le travail que le livre de la science recueille, et qui se trouve ainsi légué à la postérité. C'est Pierre Fauchard qui a donné l'élan dans ce sens, en exposant le premier à son époque, longuement et clairement, la prothèse dentaire. Il a recueilli dans son traité tout ce que l'on avait fait jusqu'à lui, il y a ajouté ses expériences personnelles, ses efforts, ses inventions. Il y a dans son ouvrage le résumé du passé, il y a aussi la compréhension de l'avenir. Le résumé du passé est dans le choix des matières: dents humaines, hippopotame, cheval matrin, bœuf, cheval, mulet, défenses de vache marine, cœur de l'ivoire. Il faudra attendre encore trente ans avant que Dubois de Chémant fasse la géniale invention de la porcelaine appliquée à l'art dentaire. Le résumé du passé est encore dans la liste des instruments servant à fabriquer les pièces artificielles: le compas, l'étau, la râpe, la lime, la scie, le grattoir et le foret avec son archet. Le résumé du passé est enfin dans quelques procédés de laboratoire. Pierre Fauchard, par exemple, se sert encore du compas comme

guide dans la confection des pièces, la méthode de l'empreinte trouvée vers 1700 par Mathias Purmann de Breslau n'était pas encore parvenue à la connaissance des artistes français.

Mais c'est l'avenir qui commence dans l'invention de la dent à pivot, de la "dent à tenon," comme il l'appelle. Il a étudié cette idée géniale sous tous ses aspects; il l'a appliquée aux cas les plus divers pour restaurations plus ou moins étendues; il en a tiré tous les partis qu'il était possible d'en tirer. Il a utilisé la dent à pivot, même dans les cas où le canal de la racine était trop large. Je ne crois pas trop m'avancer en disant que nous lui devons la dent à pivot avec gaîne, puisqu'il fabriqua un poinçon "qui sert," dit-il, "à percer le plomb introduit dans quelques racines de dents dont le canal est trop délabré pour servir à recevoir un tenon." Avec la dent à tenon, la prothèse cessait d'être un expédient de remplacement de courte durée qu'il fallait renouveler à chaque moment; elle devient un moyen de restauration durable, comme il disait, pendant toute la vie d'un homme. Les dentistes qui viendront après Fauchard ne feront qu'élargir les applications de son invention ingénieuse de la dent à tenon, dont les principes, jetés par le maître ancien, servent en partie aujourd'hui encore dans la pratique courante. Il me parait même justifié d'affirmer que Pierre Fauchard dans un de ses développements de l'idée féconde de la dent à tenon, devina l'avenir et ce qu'est le progrès contemporain de la prothèse dentaire. N'était-il pas un précurseur, lorsqu'il montait une rangée de six dents qui était maintenue en place par deux pivots à vis fixés dans les racines? N'est-il pas permis d'y voir l'embryon d'un bridge rudimentaire? Mr. Geist-Jacobi du reste, dans sa

"Geschichte der Zahnheilkunde," p. 137, n'hésite pas à affirmer que Fauchard a été l'inventeur du pont.

Il y a en Pierre Fauchard bien d'autres idées tout à fait originales, qui ont joué après lui un grand rôle dans la pratique de notre spécialité. Le principe de succion, par exemple, s'il n'a pas été appliqué intégralement à cause de l'imperfection de ses moyens de mensuration, se trouve cependant en embryon dans ces trois essais de dentiers destinés seulement à la mâchoire supérieure, sans ressorts, et qui devaient tenir grâce à leur ajustement parfait sur les gencives, et à la pression exercée par les joues. Nous lui devons également le dentier à ressorts d'acier. Pour faire tenir une pièce à la mâchoire supérieure quand celle-ci était complètement dépourvue de dents, il inventa dit-il, une machine capable de soutenir la pièce du haut. Cette machine était composée de deux lames en or ou en argent, se recourbant sur leur face la plus large pour en faire des espèces de demi-cercles qu'on ajoutait, l'un à la face intérieure, et l'autre à la face extérieure du maxillaire inférieur. Cette armature servait de point d'appui à la pièce supérieure, on la reliait à celle-ci au moyen de ressorts d'acier avec de petites lames de baleine.

Pierre Fauchard a été un véritable artiste doublé d'un savant. Il comprit que le but de la prothèse n'était pas simplement de remplacer les dents tombées, mais de les restaurer artistement, en se rapprochant le plus possible de la nature. Un appareil prothétique devait satisfaire aux exigences de l'hygiène et aussi de l'art; l'artificiel devait être caché sous l'imitation la plus parfaite. Ainsi, comme les matières que Fauchard employait pour la confection des pièces prothétiques étaient dépourvues de l'émail dont sont couvertes les dents naturelles, il éprouva le besoin de mieux les imiter et de conformer leur couleur à celle des dents et des gencives. Il imagina donc, dès 1728, d'y appliquer une couche d'émail. (Vous pourrez apprécier des imitations aussi consciencieuses que possible de quelques appareils de ce genre, dans la collection que l'Ecole Dentaire de Paris, avec une initiative fort louable, a bien voulu envoyer à ce congrès.) Fauchard se mit en rapport avec les plus habiles émailleurs de l'époque, et après bien des essais, il obtint des résultats satisfaisants. Il nous décrit dans son traité sa manière d'opérer : il construisait le dentier en hippopotame comme d'ordinaire, seulement il ne formait pas, il ne sculptait pas les dents. Il appliquait après, sur la face extérieure de la pièce une lame d'or ou d'argent découpée de la largeur et de la longeur de la bande d'ivoire du dentier, il traçait alors sur cette lame avec une lime la figure des dents, et remettait la pièce à l'émailleur. Celui-ci couvrait cette lame d'émail en y formant les dents de la nuance voulue et même la gencive si cela était nécessaire. Il fallait enfin appliquer cette lame sur la pièce, ce que Fauchard faisait au moyen de goupilles rivées.

Je trouve qu'on n'a pas donné à cette dernière idée de Fauchard l'importance qu'elle mérite. Le fait de s'être mis en rapport avec un émailleur pour compléter un travail de laboratoire, d'avoir pensé à une substance qui par certains côtés se rapprochait de la porcelaine pour donner un aspect plus naturel à une pièce, ne marque-t-il pas la première étape vers l'introduction de la céramique dans l'art dentaire? Il n'y a qu'un pas de l'idée de l'application d'un corps cuit dans le four d'émailleur, sur une plaque métallique. à l'idée de l'application d'un autre corps analogue vitrifiable sur un grès sculpté. Il me paraît que ces deux idées se tiennent (voir Delabarre). Si l'on ne peut pas contester le mérite immense de Dubois de Chémant, on doit cependant reconnaître la part de Fauchard dans l'application de la céramique à l'art dentaire, surtout dans la recherche d'un corps brillant pouvant imiter par l'aspect et la couleur les dents et les gencives naturelles. Dubois de Chémant marque le point d'arrivée, mais Fauchard le point de départ.

A côté des voiles et des obturateurs modernes admirables par l'ingéniosité, la praticité, et parfois la simplicité, les appareils analogues de Fauchard, dont j'aurai l'honneur de vous montrer les dessins, vous feront peut-être sourire. Mais si vous vous rappelez l'horreur, infiniment plus grande, des appareils employés avant Fauchard, antihygiéniques, lourds, incommodes, peut-être pires qu'un simple bouchon, vous apprécierez la construction très adroite, basée sur les principes de la mécanique, des appareils de Fauchard qui marquent vraiment un progrès considérable sur tous les précédents. Jusqu'au temps de Fauchard on avait donné la préférence à un obturateur composé d'une plaque et d'une simple tige terminée par une vis sur laquelle on montait un petit écrou, après avoir fait passer la tige à travers une éponge qui couvrait la surface convexe de la plaque. Il en résultait que cet obturateur, bien loin de rester en place, se précipitait et se déplaçait si aisément à cause de son poids et de son inclinaison, qu'il devenait inutile, embarrassant, incommode. Il arrivait à peu près le même inconvénient dans l'application de tous les autres obturateurs que l'on avait imaginés jusqu'alors.

Pour me résumer, je dirai donc que l'œuvre de Pierre Fauchard dans l'art dentaire en général peut se comparer à celle d'Ambroise Paré dans la chirurgie. Ce n'est pas une exagération d'affirmer qu'il a été le créateur de cette branche de notre spécialité. La lutte qu'il soutint contre les charlatans de son époque qui pratiquaient couramment le percement des gencives pour la fixation des pièces artificielles, les nombreux enseignements puisés dans son expérience personnelle et dans sa théorie pour la confection des dentiers, les ingénieuses inventions qu'il trouva en prothèse dentaire, son zèle et son amour pour la science sont autant de titres pour qu'il soit considéré comme le père de cette branche de l'art dentaire. On doit le citer comme ayant fixé le premier les règles scientifiques et pratiques des procédés de laboratoire en usage jusqu'alors, comme celui qui a parlé le premier des dents à pivot, qui a inventé les dentiers à ressorts métalliques, qui a deviné le bridge autant que les matériaux de l'époque le lui permettaient, et qui, par son application du vernis d'émail a ouvert le chemin à Dubois de Chémant pour son heureuse innovation. Toute la prothèse dentaire jusqu'à Delabarre procède de lui. Il a fait l'éducation des dentistes ses contemporains, il a inspiré ceux qui sont venus ensuite. Les Winstow, les Finot, les Helvetius . ., les meilleurs docteurs de son époque accueillent son ouvrage avec les approbations et les encouragements les plus chaleureux et l'étudient avec ferveur. Les Gerauldy, les Lécluse, les Bourdet de la génération suivante l'imitent et le recopient successivement. L'œuvre de Fauchard, dans le texte original dont trois éditions se suivent en soixante ans, et dans la traduction allemande éditée depuis 1733, parcourt le monde et contribue puissamment aux progrès de la prothèse dentaire. Et aujourd'hui encore, c'est sous les auspices de son nom glorieux que Dr. E. C. Kirk le très distingué et infatigable secrétaire general de la Commission d'organisation, a invité les dentistes français à ce congrès avec une phrase heureuse qui lui a valu toute notre gratitude en reconnaissant que "C'est l'art français, l'art de Fauchard, transmis à Lemaire et à Gardette et par eux à Flagg, Greenwood et autres, qui, dans sa dernière évolution est exploité au grandiose congrès de St-Louis."

BIBLIOGRAPHIE.

L'ouvrage original: "Le Chirurgien-Dentiste, ou Traité des dents, par Pierre Fauchard, Chirurgien-Dentiste à Paris. En deux tomes"—a eu trois éditions successives en 1728, en 1746, et en 1786. La première édition a été traduite en allemand sous le titre: "Fauchard—Abhandlung der Zähne, aus dem Französisch. Berlin 1733."

Parmi les analyses je citerai celle de Mr. Lemerle dans sa "Notice sur l'histoire de l'Art dentaire, etc. 1900."

Il serait trop long de citer tous les noms des auteurs Français et étrangers qui mentionnent l'œuvre de Fauchard en prothèse. Nous nous bornerons à citer parmi les Français: Gerauldy, Buron, Lecluse, Bourdet (1750), Aurebbi, et dans le XIXème siècle, tous ceux qui ont écrit sur la prothèse dentaire: Fonsi, Jourdan, Maggiolo, Laforgue Delabarre, etc. Parmi les étrangers citons les auteurs Anglais: Koecker (1835), Robinson (1846), De Loude (1840), etc.

LES PLANCHES.

La présentation de ces tableaux aurait suffi à elle seule à compléter mon petit travail sur Fauchard; je vous demanderai cependant quelques minutes encore pour vous donner certains renseignements qui me paraissent indispensables et que j'ai pu trouver dans l'étude de son œuvre qui par sa rareté ne peut être à la portée de tout le monde.

La planche de l'ouvrage de Fauchard que vous allez voir reproduite par la photographie, éveille sans doute en vous deux sentiments: l'un pénible en comparant l'état ancien avec le progrès accompli, mais aussi, j'espère, celui d'admiration pour l'homme qui le premier porta à la connaissance de ses contemporains tout ce que la prothèse pouvait faire à son époque.

[*Ces planches sont insérées après la page 248.*]

PLANCHE XXIX.

Fauchard veut montrer par cette gravure les deux sortes de limes dont il se servait: celle à queue de rat recourbée, et celle triangulaire. Il y a aussi le compas qui était le seul instrument lui permettant de prendre les mesures nécessaires à la confection de ses appareils.

PLANCHE XXX.

Nous y voyons seulement une sorte de foret à archet que Fauchard appelle "chevalet"; toute description est inutile, on ne peut pas s'empêcher de penser qu'il y a une petite différence entre cet objet et nos tours électriques.

PLANCHE XXXI.

Elle est exclusivement destinée à représenter une scie dont l'arbre ouvragé montre le désir de l'ouvrier de l'époque de posséder des outils ayant un certain cachet.

PLANCHE XXXII.

Deux grattoirs y sont représentés. Fauchard donne une explication très détaillée de ces instruments qui étaient destinés à gratter l'os dans lequel on sculptait les dentiers. Ces grattoirs étaient à différentes faces dont les >iseaux étaient taillés de façon à pouvoir aller de gauche à droite et vice-versa.

PLANCHE XXXIII.

Les figures 1 et 2 représentent les équarissoirs qui servent à préparer les canaux radiculaires, et la figure 3 un instrument très spécial ou "espèce de poinçon," comme l'appelle Fauchard qui était destiné à pratiquer un canal dans le plomb foulé préalablement dans une racine par trop abîmée.

PLANCHE XXXIV.

Vous y voyez une série d'appareils de 1, 2. 3, et 6 dents qui devaient tenir au moyen de deux fils attachés aux extrémités de la pièce. Les dents des appareils jusqu'au No. 4 sont unies entre elles par des goupilles d'or et d'argent. La figure 8 nous montre un perfectionnement avec une pièce inférieure de 6 dents assemblées grâce à un bandeau d'or ou d'argent fixé avec des rivets. Mais ce qui doit le plus attirer notre attention sur cette planche, c'est la dent à tenon, la dent à pivot d'aujourd'hui.

Si je ne craignais pas d'abuser de vos instants, je vous lirais la description qu'en fait Fauchard, non certes pour vous apprendre ce qu'est une dent à pivot, mais pour vous montrer avec quels soins il la préparait et quels bons conseils il donnait à ceux qui voulaient suivre son exemple: limage de la racine, préparation du canal, pose de la dent. précautions spéciales en cas de mauvais état de la racine ou en cas que le pivot fût trop court. En un mot: solidité, hygiène, esthétique, tout est pris en considération.

PLANCHE XXXV

Elle est non moins intéressante que la précédente. Je passerai rapidement sur le No. 5, appareil pour mâchoire inférieure destiné à tenir par son propre poids, ainsi que sur les Nos. 1 et 2 appareils du haut qui devaient être maintenus in situ, l'un par des fils attachés aux molaires postérieures, l'autre également par des fils attachés aux deux

grandes incisives; ces trois appareils n'offrent rien de bien intéressant. Mais c'est sur le No. 4 que je voudrais attirer toute votre attention. Vous conviendrez, je n'en doute pas, que le Fauchard de 1746 nous montre là un bridge tel qu'il serait conçu encore aujourd'hui. avec bien entendu les perfectionnements que les progrès devaient y apporter, mais avec la même idée—mère que nous a léguée Fauchard. Pour celle-là comme pour toutes les autres pièces, cet illustre précurseur donne les détails les plus minutieux, recommandant la direction des pivots, leur fixation, etc.

PLANCHE XXXVI.

Celle-ci nous montre "une pièce ou machine pour la mâchoire supérieure." Fauchard n'était pas satisfait du peu de stabilité des appareils du haut. Il imagina, pour un sujet à qui manquaient seulement les dents du bas, de fixer à la pièce destinée au maxillaire supérieur deux ressorts attachés à deux bandes métalliques dont l'une s'appliquait à la face linguale, l'autre à la face labiale des dents du bas. En pareil cas, avant l'invention de Fauchard, les dentistes de l'époque reliaient l'appareil du haut aux dents de la mâchoire inférieure d'une façon permanente au moyen de deux ressorts de baleine attachés avec des fils.

PLANCHE XXXVII.

Je laisserai de côté les figures 1 et 2 qui représentent le même dentier complet de deux différentes façons, mais j'attirerai votre attention sur la différence énorme qui existe entre les figures 1 et 2 et la figure 3. Celle-ci représente en effet le chef d'œuvre de Fauchard, son fameux dentier émaillé dont vous avez admiré ou vous admirerez, j'espère, le fac-simile dans la collection envoyée par l'École Dentaire de Paris. Vous suppléerez à l'insuffisance d'une simple projection.

PLANCHE XXXVIII.

Voici les deux premiers obturateurs que Fauchard inventa pour remplacer tous les mauvais systèmes employés jusqu'alors: ce ne sont que de simples plaques obturatrices, mais les deux ailes mobiles grâce à la clef figure 10, permettaient d'introduire facilement l'appareil et de le maintenir en place.

PLANCHE XXXIX.

Ici la simple plaque obturatrice est remplacée dans deux cas plus compliqués par un appareil destiné à suppléer aux dents manquantes et à jouer le rôle d'obturateur. Fauchard a déjà amélioré son premier système, et grâce à un mécanisme ingénieux, il parvient à donner une telle satisfaction à ses malades, qu'eux-mêmes en sont surpris. Mais non content des résultats obtenus dans un autre cas, il modifie et perfectionne encore son obturateur et fait construire les appareils de la planche suivante.

PLANCHE XL.

Fauchard aide ses confrères de l'époque non seulement par des dessins, mais aussi par des descriptions très détaillées de ses mécanismes, leur permettant ainsi d'utiliser ses inventions dans les différents cas, car comme dit très justement Fauchard, "Dans ces sortes d'appareils, il est nécessaire d'apporter à chaque cas des modifications plus ou moins importantes." Ainsi la figure 18 nous montre un appareil de 4 dents servant à boucher une simple perforation palatine.

PLANCHE XLI.

Cette planche représente un dentier à ressorts vu de deux côtés différents. Comme vous voyez, les porte-ressorts sont mieux placés que dans les dentiers précédents, et les anses D D constituent aussi une amélioration, car elles couvrent les faces triturantes et latérales des molaires, et servent ainsi à la fois à empêcher l'armature de s'enfoncer et aussi à supporter les ressorts.

Ce dentier fut fabriqué par Fauchard en 1737 pour une dame qui lui fut adressée par un praticien très renommé, M. Caperon, Dentiste du Roi. Ce practicien consciencieux ne sachant pas resoudre ce grave problème, engagea sa malade à aller chez Fauchard, reconnaissant ainsi sa supériorité.

PLANCHE XLII.

Nous constatons ici une petite variante aux dentiers précedemment construits par Fauchard qui n'avait eu à faire qu'à des malades dépourvus de toutes les dents de la mâchoire supérieure, mais possédant toutes les dents du bas. Dans ce cas, il résolut la difficulté de la façon la plus simple et presque semblable à celle suivie par les confrères de nos jours qui voudraient appliquer des ressorts à un dentier dans les mêmes circonstances.

[*Voir les planches suivantes XXIX—XLII (Plates I—XIV).*]

Discussion.

Dr. FRANCISQUE MARTIN, Lyons, France. Je suis heureux d'avoir assisté à la très intéressante communication que je viens d'entendre sur Pierre Fauchard. Trop peu connu en France, presque ignoré à l'étranger, cet homme qui eut tant d'influence sur de l'art dentaire français et mondial vient de nous être révélé par l'éloquente érudition de mon confrère et ami le Dr. Platschick, que je remercie au nom des dentistes français.

Dr. C. N. JOHNSON, Chicago, Ill. This is a volume in itself, and it will be a revelation to many of those who are bringing out patents today. Dr. Platschick has come a long distance to read this paper; he has given a wonderful revelation, and I move that a rising vote of thanks be extended to him.

Motion seconded and carried.

Adjourned until Thursday afternoon.

PLANCHE XXIX.

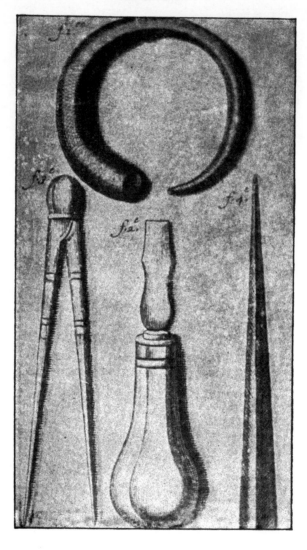

PLANCHE XXX.

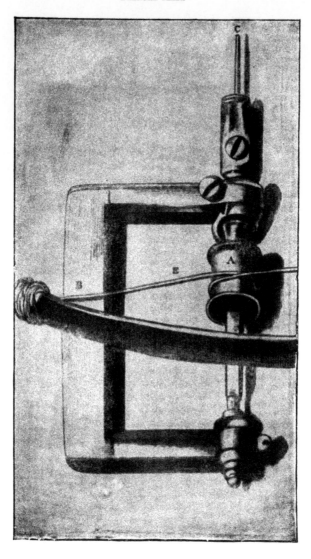

PLANCHE XXXI.

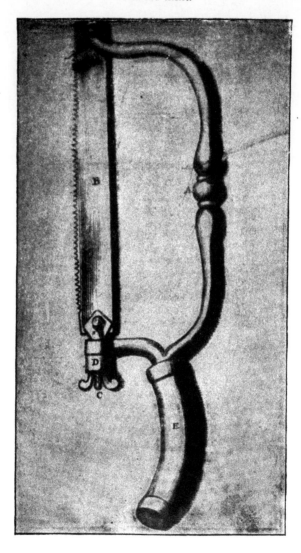

PLANCHE XXXII.

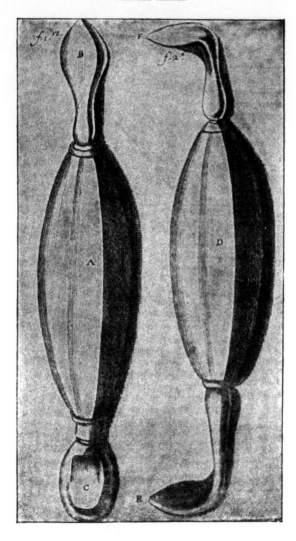

PLANCHE XXXIII.

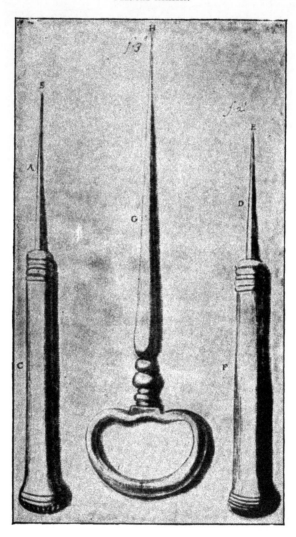

PLANCHE XXXIV.

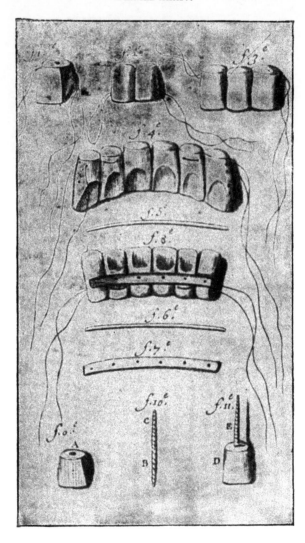

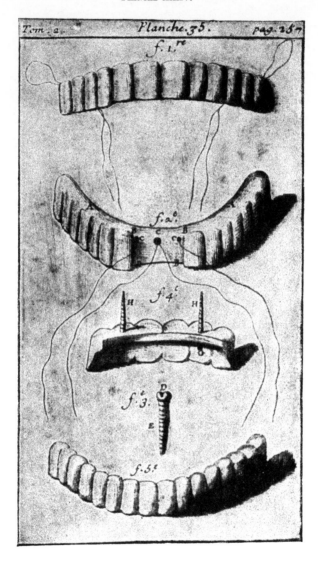

PLANCHE XXXVI.

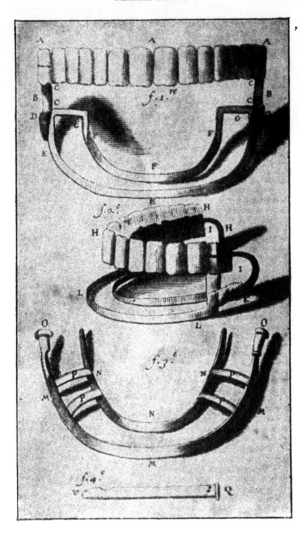

PLANCHE XXXVII.

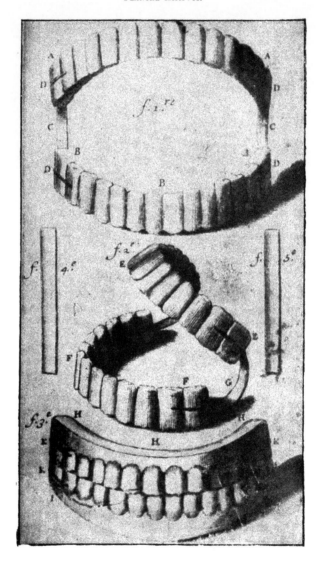

PLANCHE XXXVIII.

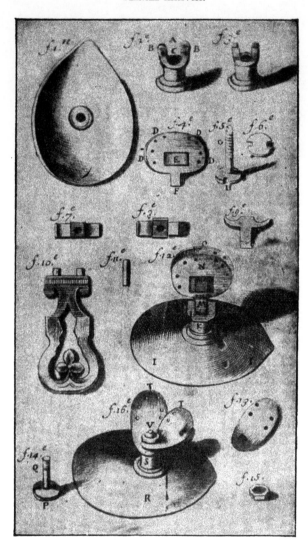

PLANCHE XXXIX.

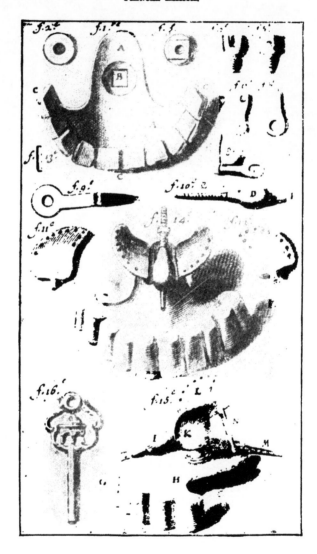

PLANCHE XL.

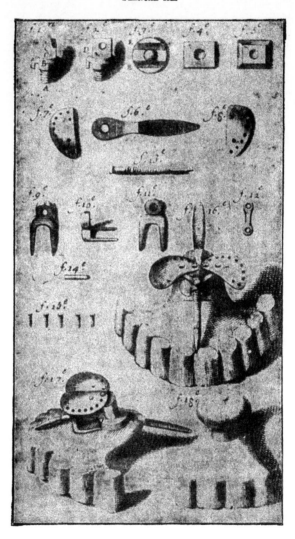

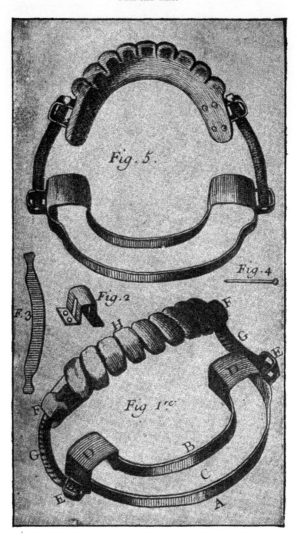

PLANCHE XLII.

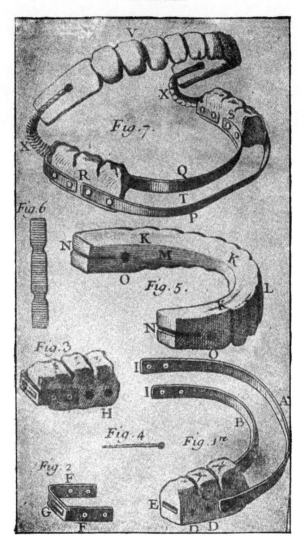

SECTION IX—Continued.

FOURTH DAY—Thursday, September 1st.

THE session was called to order by the chairman at 3 P.M.

The first order of business was the reading of the report of the Committee on Nomenclature, by the chairman, Dr. A. H. THOMPSON of Topeka, Kans., together with the included essays and suggestions, as follows:

Report of the Committee on Nomenclature.

By A. H. THOMPSON, D.D.S., Topeka, Kansas,
CHAIRMAN.

IT was the custom of the old Roman nobility that as one of them proceeded along the way, a slave ran beside the chariot to tell the occupants the names of those whom they met, announcing them as they approached. This slave was called the *nomenclator,* or namer. From this word, and from *nomen,* a name, we obtain the terms that refer to the naming of things, and hence also the science of nomenclature, which has to do with the exact designation of names and their application. Words are thereby made fit things as tools for work. "Nomenclature," the Standard Dictionary says, has reference to a "system of names or of naming, especially to one used in a particular art or science, also a systematic and alphabetic list of technical names." It seems to be a question whether the word "terminology" would

not be better for our use in this sense, as it has a more specific reference to the technical terms in use by a science or an art, *i.e.* the more exact application of terms in work. The distinction might be made that "nomenclature" has reference to the giving of names to things, while "terminology" designates the exact, the refined application of terms and names to things and ideas, to the end of facilitating work.

There ought not to be any argument or question as to the desirability, even the necessity, of a complete and exact terminology for the use of the dental profession. Its position as an acknowledged scientific occupation should warrant the possession of a nomenclature that is scientific, exact, universal and accepted. That this condition does not prevail, is, to say the least, not honorable to a profession claiming to be scientific. To be sure, the great special sciences, as chemistry, zoölogy, botany, and others have but recently put their terminology upon a scientific basis and secured something like harmony. But they have cleared up *their* nomenclature, and it becomes us of the professions which are founded on the special sciences, to clear up *our* terminology and introduce scientific accuracy and harmony. The rank and file of the dental profession are indifferent as to the value of care and exactness in the use of terms, and it unfortunately happens that men in high places, journalists, and writers, are also careless and lacking in the conscientious conception of their duty in this regard. They have a responsibility in the example they set that they should appreciate, and should endeavor to aspire after greater exactness in the selection and the use of terms. A slovenly nomenclature is a great hindrance to work; poor words are like poor tools—good work cannot be performed with them. That this is true has been demonstrated frequently in the history of all the sciences. Not only does confusion arise owing to the use of different terms for the same thing or idea, but the effort wasted in explanation and adjustment of harmony is a distinct waste of brain power—and brain power is the most valuable thing in the world. The great argument for a scientific terminology is economy of brain power, that the world may have the benefit of the highest efficiency of genius, and of trained workers. Nomenclature is, in its last analysis, therefore, an expediency, a means to an end, a tool to work with, that more and better work may be accomplished. But it is a most valuable tool, and therefore deserves the greatest possible consideration and cul-

tivation. Our protest, therefore, is against the indifference of the profession as to the real value of an exact and scientific nomenclature. The arguments have been frequently presented before to the profession, for the subject is not new, but we have failed to impress its members with the fact that an exact terminology in general use and acceptation would be a great economy of time, energy, and brain power, and would inevitably lead to the greater efficiency and usefulness of the dental profession. We would, therefore, urge all of its members, but especially those in high and influential places, to consider their conscientious duty in this regard and to endeavor to bring about a better condition of things in this respect, to the end of advancing the honor of the profession.

On this great occasion, also, when America is honored by the presence of so many of our eminent and respected foreign *confrères,* the subject of a universal terminology for our profession in all European languages must receive our serious consideration. The essays herewith appended by the foreign members of the committee will deal with this branch of the subject. It is the earnest wish of the committee that some steps may be taken toward the ultimate accomplishment of the preparation of a universal terminology that will be understood in all languages. Science is a universal brotherhood and knows no political, linguistic, or geographical boundaries. Scientific men are of one blood, one purpose, one language—and that language should be universal and uniform. Other sciences have such a universal language, and it becomes us as a great and universal profession to prepare a terminology that shall be uniform in all languages, by which the *confrères* of all nations may read each other's literature and learn of each other's work and be enabled to communicate with each other in the common interest of furthering our beloved profession in all lands. To that end it is the earnest desire that steps may be taken at this great meeting to bring about "a consummation so devoutly to be wished." Dr. Chas. Godon speaks of the work of securing an international nomenclature, and it is to be desired that steps should be taken at this congress to further the undertaking.

In America there has been some progress made in the improvement and harmonization of our nomenclature. Committees appointed at the meetings of the American Dental Association through the seventies and eighties, accomplished a perceptible beginning. Old, popular, and unscientific terms were gradually dropped and many of the better names suggested by those committees were adopted and became part of our current literature and general usage. All honor to the workers of those early days, for their task was difficult and thankless, and the obstacles and opposition they encountered were enough to discourage less heroic souls. But they builded wisely and "their works do follow them." The foundations they laid were deep and lasting, and we are today enjoying the benefits of a better nomenclature, owing to the excellent pioneer labors of those early enthusiasts in the field. They found chaos and they left order to a degree that is surprising when we consider the condition of the current terms in common use in the profession. They accomplished wonders in making a beginning, and we cannot but record our appreciation of their labors in first blazing the way for subsequent workers. With their work for a foundation, after-workers have been enabled to accomplish more than they would otherwise have been able to do without the labors of those early pioneers.

The terminology of our profession has been greatly improved since the next initiative made by the committee on nomenclature at the World's Columbian Dental Congress, at Chicago in 1893. Their report was an excellent new starting-point, and from the suggestions then made much good has resulted in the improvement and harmonization of our nomenclature. The problem of the whole subject was so ably discussed in all of its bearings that the arguments do not need to be presented again. It is only necessary to refer to that excellent *résumé* for the exhaustive presentation of the subject in all of its relations. That report undoubtedly exercised a great influence on the profession, and stimulated the appreciation of the necessity for formulating a better nomenclature, and interested students in the investigation of the subject. We may even hope that it assisted at the birth of a conscience on the subject, and that writers and speakers have perhaps better than ever before realized their responsibility to the profession and to the public, for their influence in the use and presentation of a proper terminology. We would like to believe that the suggestions of that committee have been largely adopted by the profession, and that they have been productive of great good. Indeed, we cannot but believe that the impulse there given to the subject eventuated in the next most important step in the evolution of the subject.

At the meeting of the American Dental Association held at Asbury Park in 1895, a committee drew up and presented a considerable list of words which it was hoped would introduce more harmony in the use of terms. This report and list was adopted by the association and was very generally accepted by the profession at large and used to a great degree by text-books and journals. A great step was taken when this list was adopted, for we then had an authoritative list of terms from which to work, and the gradual elimination of duplicate words and inappropriate terms has made some progress since that list was accepted. There has been some conflict of opinion as to the propriety of some few terms, different names for the same thing each having their advocates who upheld their rival claims with great energy, but on the whole there has been less controversy than might have been expected, considering the revolution that the report proposed in the use of names. This was largely due, of course, to the determination of the committee to retain those terms that were most in use and acceptation, and in cases of confusion and controversy giving preference to that term which had the most advocates or was the most scientific.

Perhaps the most difficult task the committee had, or that any reformers of nomenclature will have, is the elimination of so-called popular terms, which, like the popular names of animals and plants, are often local, or confined to sets or classes of persons, and which are varied from place to place or from class to class. This is one difficulty with the rank and file of the profession yet, *i.e.* the use of common, popular terms for things and ideas, that are unscientific and undescriptive. There is an inclination on the part of scientific men also to the use of terms that they consider better and more scientific, as against those proposed by the American Dental

Association committee. Some of these will be noted later.

Right here this committee would make the first recommendation and suggest the first rule for the simplification and harmonization of our nomenclature, viz., *That a spirit of loyalty should pervade the profession that is sufficient to sink all preferences that are not in harmony with acknowledged authority, and to accept their rulings, to the end of securing uniformity.*

The American Dental Association committee was such an authority, duly appointed, and their report and list was formally accepted and adopted. This list, therefore, became the official list of the profession in this country, and as such should be accepted by the profession and its writers and speakers. The terms there proposed should be employed by all until corrected by the National Dental Association as the central authority. That authority is final, and should be so accepted by the profession in a spirit of loyalty for the greatest good to the profession. There is little use of a committee on nomenclature proposing reforms if their authority be not acknowledged and obeyed. To be effective their decisions must be arbitrary if any progress is to be made, and where it is shown they are wrong such errors must be corrected by the central authority. But this committee insists that when terms are adopted by such authority that they should be accepted by the profession, and that the love of harmony and simplicity should be sufficient to warrant the setting aside of all personal preferences in favor of the adopted terms. Otherwise the work of all such committees might as well not be done so far as attaining the ultimate and much desired result of a perfect and uniform terminology.

As a recent writer before the Botanical Section of the American Association for the Advancement of Science, at the recent meeting in St. Louis, said, "Doubtless all will now agree that any rational system of nomenclature must be based strictly on priority. This itself is a long step in advance, for the earlier systematists laid less stress on priority than on the supposed appropriateness of a name. The unfortunate result of their practices we are suffering from now, i.e. that it is impossible to bring their work into harmony with ours without adopting rules and methods that are necessarily more or less arbitrary. Let us, then, nerve our minds to the point of seeing not only many, but if necessary all of our most favored names sacrificed to consistency, and unite in adopting the simplest and most direct code of rules that can be agreed upon." This is the spirit of our sister sciences, and it should be our spirit in the interests of uniformity and of loyalty to the honor and advancement of our beloved profession. Therefore, your committee would make a special appeal to all members of the profession to adopt the terms and names officially decided upon by the committees on nomenclature, to the end of securing a better and more scientific terminology, and that those terms, if they are to be corrected—and they will often need to be corrected, for the committees are but human, and with all their investigations and research will commit errors—that corrections should be made through the regular channels of the nomenclature committees and the national associations. The committee makes this appeal in the interests of harmony and for the honor that would accrue to the profession in having an exact, scientific terminology.

We are now past the discussion of the desirability and advantages that will follow the reformation and improvement of terminology. That part of the subject has been ably presented by various writers and committees on nomenclature, and their conclusions generally accepted and acknowledged. We have now come to the stage attained by most of our sister sciences, i.e. the discussion and if possible the solution of disputed points and terms that are still in controversy. The bulk of the terms in common use are fairly uniform and satisfactory, but there are still many that are in dispute, or duplicate terms applied to the same thing or idea, that require adjustment. All disputed terms should be well considered, especially those which have many friends and supporters, and which are in conflict. Then there is the introduction of new terms for new things or ideas which are new to the profession. The selection of a nomenclature for a new specialty is a very important and delicate matter, and one that needs to be undertaken advisedly. Then there is the increased refinement and differentiation of meanings, by which old terms that were too general and loosely applied were made to cover too much ground and which must be divided and specialized. Therefore, your committee will confine itself to suggestions along those lines, and avoid duplication of previous work as far as possible. The call sent out to persons invited to become members of the committee stipulated that lists of terms were desired as follows: new names for new things, ideas, discoveries, methods, etc., better terms for the correction, elaboration, or displacement of old terms, etc., but that generally adopted and accepted terms should not be listed. In other words, that we would take cognizance only of the advancements made since the adoption of previous reports of special committees on nomenclature. Disputed terms and applications of terms would require attention, of course, and it is an unfortunate fact that several such controversies exist. In regard to some of these disputes the committee reiterates the wish that the disputants would accept the decision of the committee of the American Dental Association of 1895, and tentatively, at least, adopt its rulings in the name of harmony. Many new words have come into use in the new departments, as of porcelain work, which require to be listed and passed upon. It is most imperative that such terms should be harmonized at the beginning of the organization of a new branch, for uniformity can be more easily secured then than later, when varied and diverse terms have come into use in different localities. In such new departments the committee would urge the listing as completely as possible of the terminology and its adoption by the congress, to the end of promulgating the terms widely and giving them the authoritative sanction of this great body. This is one of the most important duties of this committee, and it is to be earnestly hoped that something may be accomplished in all of the new departments. The old question of priority will always be with us, perhaps, as with our sister sciences, and of course all harmony-loving members will accept that which has the best claim. We are not in the quandary of the biologists, however, in having great need of a multiplicity of names and difficulty in finding terms that have not been employed. We have not exhausted the possibilities of ancient and modern languages, and yet some terms are employed in duplication that need to be investigated and the first application decided.

Among disputed terms in controversy, and one of the most prominent, is that of the "cuspid" *versus* the "canine" teeth. It is a curious fact that the disputants are ranged along two lines, *i.e.* the anatomists stand for "canine," and the operators for "cuspid." The American Dental Association committee of 1895, said, "We believe it to be more harmonious and appropriate to use the word 'cuspid' instead of 'canine' to indicate the single-cusped teeth, just as the term bicuspid is applied to their neighbors." Both terms are given in the list offered, and confusion has existed in regard to the terms ever since. A definite decision should be reached by this body, so that there may be harmony. It is a very evident fact that if we are to rank as a scientific profession and have a nomenclature in harmony with other sciences, that we should employ the term "canine," as that term is applied by all odontologists to this particular tooth in all mammals. It is not worth while to discuss the propriety of the word; it has been arbitrarily accepted by zoölogists, and that is reason sufficient for all odontologists accepting it, even in human odontology. It describes the position of these teeth in relation to the other teeth, which is the important thing in anatomy. The more popular name "cuspid" is advocated on the ground that it is a single-cusped tooth, but this is too indefinite. Sometimes other teeth have but one cusp, as in some forms of the lower first bicuspid. Black's "Dental Anatomy" gives the preference to "cuspid." Mr. Chas. Tomes' "Dental Anatomy" says that "The canine is the next tooth behind the intermaxillary suture above, and the lower canine is the tooth which closes in front of the upper canine." It is, of course, modified from the premolar series, and so is distinct from the incisor series. Mr. Tomes says that "It should be borne in mind that its significance is merely equivalent to caniniform premolar." Owen says in "Odontography": "When the tooth which succeeds the incisors, or the first of the upper maxillary bone, is conical pointed and longer than the rest, it is called a 'canine,' as is also its analogue in the lower jaw, which passes in front of it when the mouth is closed." Huxley says ("Anatomy of Vertebrates"): "The distinction between canines and molars is one of form and position in regard to the remaining teeth, the most anterior of the teeth behind the premaxilla-maxillary suture, if it is sharp and projecting, receiving the name of 'canine.' There are never more than four canines." Mr. Jno. Tomes ("Dental Surgery") uses the term "canine." Koecker ("Dental Surgery") employed the term "cuspid," or rather the Latin form "cuspidatus," which so many of the old writers used. Jno. Hunter ("Nat. Hist. of Human Teeth") also employed the Latin "cuspidatus." Thos. Bell ("Diseases of the Teeth") uses "cuspidatus." James Snell ("Operations on the Teeth") used "canine." In the World's Columbian Dental Congress report there is an excellent tabulation of many terms from which, as well as the authorities herewith quoted, it is plainly demonstrated that there has always been, as far back as there has been any mention made of this tooth, great confusion and lack of harmony in the names given to it. Therefore, your committee respectfully urges that this congress should pass upon and decide authoritatively upon a proper term to employ and the profession be urged to adopt that term for the purposes of harmony and uniformity.

Much confusion exists also in regard to the name that should be given to the articulating surfaces of the teeth. The question was exhaustively discussed by the W. D. C. report and the American Dental Association report of 1895. The terms "occlusal" and "moreal" are still in general use. Both words are given in the American Dental Association list, with the preference for "occlusal," in which conclusion the present committee concurs and hopes the congress will put the seal of its approval and that the profession will accept and adopt it. It is the better and preferable word, for many good reasons that are given in the aforesaid reports. But that the term "occlusal" is not really scientific, is well shown by one of the essayists in his observation of the meaning and application of the name. However, as it is in the most general use, it would be best for the congress to adopt it arbitrarily and for the profession to conform for the sake of harmony. Words that have been so long in use, without regard to their appropriateness, should be accepted in the interests of harmony. It is too late to create and introduce new words for such common things and expect them to be accepted and adopted.

A much-disputed term and one that requires to be dealt with by authority, is that of "cast" *versus* "model," as employed in prosthesis. The balance of opinion seems to be in favor of the word "cast," for the reasons best presented by Dr. Geo. H. Wilson of Cleveland, O., in the paper appended. But much confusion still prevails among prosthetists, and it would be well to have a definite decision on this term.

An innovation that the chairman has had in mind for many years and that he now believes should be inaugurated, is the better naming of the parts of the molars to be in harmony with the comparative odontologists. This is especially desired when human odontology is nowadays studied from the comparative standpoint, and with reference to their evolution. The present system is awkward and unscientific, as well as hampering to the student in his studies of general odontology. The change proposed is to adopt the terms employed by all of the comparative anatomists and thereby be in harmony with this great related science.

These terms are briefly as follows:

Protocone. The mesio-lingual cone or cusp of the upper molar.
Paracone. The mesio-buccal cusp or cone.
Metacone. The disto-buccal cusp.
Hypocone. The disto-lingual cone.
Hypoconule. The fifth tubercle (when present).
Protoconid. The mesio-buccal cusp of the lower molar.
Metaconid. The mesio-lingual cusp of the lower molar.
Entoconid. The disto-lingual cusp.
Hypoconid. The medio-buccal cusp of the lower molar.
Hypoconulid. The disto-buccal cusp, or fifth cone.

These terms are as far as we would go at present, leaving the more complicated terms of the bicuspid, or premolar, cones for a later innovation. But your committee would urge the adoption of the terms in preference to the old cumbrous designations of the present compound words; for the sake of simplicity and ease of use; for the history that each name carries of the evolution of the part; for harmony with the terminology of the sister science of comparative odontology on which we are dependent for all that we have of real anatomical science in the study of the human tooth, and finally for the ennobling and uplifting effect that the study of the wonders of nature through the illumination of evolution has upon the human mind. The evolution of the human molars is one of the most beautiful things in the whole realm of nature, and the civilizing effect of such a study upon dental students cannot be overestimated. Hence we urgently request the adoption of this valuable terminology in the description of the human molars.

In conclusion, your committee would recommend the careful selection of a permanent committee on international nomenclature to follow and co-operate with like committees of this and other countries, associations, and congresses to consider and promulgate the idea of an harmonious system of terminology that shall apply to all countries. It is not expected to employ the same words in all languages, but it is to be desired that similar words shall be employed that will be translatable into the same meanings and application. We earnestly recommend this step in the interests of the universal brotherhood of the dental profession and the simplifying of the confusion that now exists in our terminology. It will assist materially in perpetuating the bond that has been created at this great congress between the dentists of all lands, and the obliteration of political, linguistic, and geographical boundaries.

[Forming part of the report were the following essays and suggestions by Dr. Geo. H. Wilson, Cleveland, Ohio; Prof. Dr. Hesse, Leipzig, Germany; Dr. W. T. Reeves, Chicago, Ill.; Dr. W. C. Gowan, Creemore, Ontario, Canada; Dr. Charles Godon, Paris, France, etc.]

Dr. Geo. H. Wilson.

Dr. GEO. H. WILSON, Cleveland, Ohio, contributed the following

REPORT ON PROSTHETIC NOMENCLATURE.

I submit this report for consideration, recognizing that some of the words have been adopted by the lexicographers and many writers; but it seems wise to again bring them to the attention of the profession. When two or more words are used to convey the same idea it is advisable that the best should be adopted and the rest discarded. Some definitions and some words should be given special significance.

The term *prosthesis* should be given the preference over the term prosthodontia.

While "prosthesis" is applicable to the restoration of any lost part, I believe it has now been so associated with the dental profession that we are justified in appropriating it and thus defining it: *Prosthesis*—the art, science, and esthetics of restoring the lost dental organs and their associate parts with an artificial substitute. Art and esthetics are both used because art has a double meaning, and in this definition I would have it mean mechanical perfection, while I would use esthetics to represent the ideal —the harmonizing of the instrument with the associate parts.

If we are justified in using the words "prosthesis" and "prosthetist" as nouns, and not the words "dentistry" and "dentist," then the one strong argument for "prosthodontia" is gone. The Standard Dictionary seems to recognize such use.

"Prosthodontia" is too limited; it refers only to restoring the teeth, and the rest must be inferred.

The term "mechanical dentist" should be limited to the laboratory man, and implies that he does not work directly for the patient but for the "prosthetist" who does all the work at the chair, while the mechanical dentist, as such, never sees the patient. The one implies the "artist," the other the "artisan."

Tray (not cup) for taking impressions.

Impression. A negative likeness of an object or part from which is produced the cast.

Maxillary Surface. Applied to the inner surface of both upper and lower trays and impressions. (Suggested by Dr. Weiss of Minneapolis.)

Cast or *Model.* While there has been much agitation over these words, there is a strong tendency to retain the old and objectionable word "model." "Cast" implies exactness, because it is poured or formed in an impression or mold and is a perfect reproduction of the object. "Model" implies something to be copied or over which a thing is made, as the sculptor's model of clay or staff may be heroic or diminutive; it is to be copied in outline but is not an exact reproduction, only an aid to the creation. The painter uses a model, not for the purpose of exact detail, but as an aid to depict the animation or soul. The dressmaker uses a model over which she forms the garment, which is not designed to fit the human body, but to shape the body to an ideal form. Therefore the accepted use of the word is inappropriate to its general application to dentistry, while "cast" conveys a definite idea. It seems best to limit the word "cast" to plaster and its compounds, and "die" to a metal cast.

Models are used to make dies, and consist of the cast being properly trimmed.

an addition of wax and possibly plaster, and a glaze upon the surface, which is copied exactly. Models are used extensively by students in technic work. In the practice of dentistry casts are never copied or reproduced, but are used to produce the negative likeness.

Denture. Used to designate a completed piece.

Plate. Should be limited in its use to the base-plate upon which the denture is constructed: vulcanite, silver, gold, or platinum.

Contour. Not plumpers.

Porcelain. A solidified suspension of one or more insoluble, infusible substances, in a fusible silicate, which acts as a flux or bond.

Vacuum Chamber. Not air-chamber.

Flasking. Where a piece of work is enclosed in a flask, as vulcanite and cast work.

Invest. When no flask is used, as in solder work.

Rubber. While in a soft state, before the application of heat to the sulfur and caoutchouc.

Vulcanite. After the application of heat to a mixture of sulfur and caoutchouc; may be either soft or hard.

Ferrule (fer'-il). A continuous band about a tooth for sustaining an artificial denture.

Dr. Hesse.

The following terms were recommended for adoption by Prof. Dr. HESSE, Leipzig, Germany:

Corona dentis.
Tubercula (coronæ) dentis.
Collum dentis.
Radix dentis.

Apex radicis dentis.
Facies masticatoria.
Facies labialis (buccalis).
Facies lingualis.
Facies contactus.
Facies medialis. } Dentium incisivorum et
Facies lateralis. }   caninorum.
Facies anterior. } Dentium præmolarium
Facies posterior. }   et molarium.
Cavum dentis.
Pulpa dentis.
Papilla dentis.
Canalis radicis dentis.
Foramen apicis dentis.
Susbstantia eburnea.
Substantia adamantina.
Substantia ossea.
Canaliculi dentales.
Spatia interglobularia.
Prismata adamantina.
Cuticula dentis.
Periosteum alveolari.
Arcus dentalis superior.
Arcus dentalis inferior.
Dentes incisivi.
Dentes canini.
Dentes præmolares.
Dentes molares.
Dens serotinus.
Dentes permanentes.
Dentes decidui.

Dr. W. C. Gowan.

Dr. W. C. GOWAN, Creemore, Ont., Canada, proposed the following fixed definitions:

Drug. Any substance used in the composition of medicine.

Medicine. Anything applied for the cure or lessening of disease or pain.

Remedy. Any medicine, appliance, or treatment which cures disease. The word "remedy" should seldom if ever be used in the plural. For example: "We keep 'drugs' and 'medicines,' but not 'remedies.'" The "remedy" for an alveolar abscess is a course of surgical and medicinal treatment; for a diseased and useless tooth the "remedy" is extraction. Carbolic acid, arsenic, cocain, oil of cloves, are "drugs." When applied to disease they are "medicines."

Treatment. The manner of applying a remedy—which may be surgical, mechanical, or medicinal. The word is not properly used in the plural.

Articulate. To joint.

Articulation. A joining, as of the bones; the parts between the joints.

Occlude. To absorb, as a gas by a metal. (Standard Dictionary.)

Occlusion. A closing of an opening, passage, or cavity; the act of occluding or absorbing.

(It would seem that the relation and contact between the upper and lower teeth is neither "articulation" nor "occlusion." We need a more appropriate term.)

Superior and *inferior* (as of the jaws or teeth). These words, derived as they are from the Latin, are properly used to qualify words of the same derivation, as "maxillary," "dental," etc. But the Anglo-Saxon words "tooth," "jaw," etc., should have the Anglo-Saxon words "upper" and "lower" to qualify them. In English we use the words "superior" and "inferior" in the sense of better and worse, in comparing the quality of one thing with another.

Cuspid and *Canine.* Cuspid is preferable, as it is significant of the thing named, and simplifies the nomenclature, for "cusp" and "bicuspid" are approved and established names for things. "Canine" pertains to the dog. A dog's molar or incisor is really a canine tooth. And besides, the long cuspid is not characteristic of the dog alone, as other mammals have it.

Dr. W. T. Reeves.

Dr. W. T. REEVES, Chicago, Ill, proposed the following terms applying to porcelain work in particular:

Porcelain.	Porcelain restorations.
Bodies.	Porcelain fillings.
High-fusing.	Porcelain crowns.
Low-fusing.	Porcelain bridge-work.
Translucent.	Metal construction.
Opaque.	Platinum solder.
Tense.	Contouring.
Porous.	Carving.
Baking.	Building-up.
Fusing.	Drying-out.
Biscuit.	Popping-off.
Glistening-biscuit.	Checking.
Glazed.	Cooling.
Full-glaze.	Annealing.
Gassed.	Staining.
Gassing.	Mineral stains.
Disintegration.	Oil-paints.
Burned-out.	Cavity preparation.
Developing-color.	Knife-edge margins.
Over-baked.	Joints.
Bulk.	Butt-ended joint.
Feather-edge.	Lap-joint.
Edge-strength.	Saucer-shaped.
Friable.	Seating-form.
Attenuated.	Surface-retention.
Porcelain operative dentistry.	Frictional-retention.

Dr. Blatter.

Dr. GODON presented the following notes, by Dr. Blatter, Chef de Clinique à l'Ecole Dentaire de Paris:

Je propose à la commission de nomenclature différents termes nouveaux pouvant donner une définition vraiment scientifique à certaines affections dentaires, La commission sera seule juge; elle pourra, a son gré, soit accepter, soit rejéter ou modifier les expressions que je soumets à sa haute compétence en dentisterie opératoire.

(1) Pour la dévitalisation pulpaire par l'arsenic et ses dérivés, je propose le terme   .   .   .   .   *Pulpoarséniation.*

(2) Pour la dévitalisation pulpaire soit par le thermo, soit par le galvanocautère (agent physique, la chaleur) je propose les termes   .   .   .   .   .
Thermocautérisation pulpaire ou *Pulpocautérisation.*

(3) Pour la dévitalisation pulpaire par le cocaine et la compression de la pulpe je propose   .   .   .   .   .
Pulpococainisation et compression (Pulpocompression).

(4) Pour définir l'opération consistant dans la résection de la portion apicale d'une racine, atteint d'une lésion du sommet, je propose le mot   .   *Apicectomie.* *

(5) Pour la trépanation ou ouverture alvéolaire je propose le terme   .   .   .
Alvéolotomie.

Par contre la résection de l'alvéole ou d'une de ses parois, cette intervention doit porter la dénomination de   .   .   .
Alvéolectomie. †

(6) La trépanation d'une couronne (cas de mortification pulpaire, etc.) devrait en dentisterie opératoire être définie de la façon suivante   .   .
Coronotomie.
La résection de la couronne   .   .
Coronectomie.

(7) Pour la résection d'une racine ou pratiquerait la   .   .   .   *Racinectomie.*‡

(8) La résection de l'ivoire (préparation d'une cavité, par exemple) serait mieux définie par le terme   .   .   .
soit *Dentinectomie,* soit *Eburnectomie.*§

---

* Pour la formation régulière de ce mot composé il faudrait admettre le néologisme suivante: *Acrectomie* = άκρον du grec = apex.

† Le mot régulier devrait être 1° *Cuttarotomie* = de κύτταρος, grec alvéole; 2° *Cuttarectomie.*

‡ Le mot régulier pour ce dernier terme devrait être *Rhizectomie* de ίζωμα, grec = racine.

§ Ce dernier est le plus régulier.

(9) La résection et le polissage du tissu adamantin (émail) altéré dans le cas d'une carie du premier degré, doit, à mon sens, porter le dénomination   .   .
Adamantectomie.
Pour la régularisation des bords d'une cavité où l'on doit couper dessous l'émail, le terme régulier est   .   .   .
Adamantotomie.

(10) L'amputation de la pulpe (troisième degré) sera   .   la *Pulpectomie.*
L'extirpation des filets radiculaires (des radicules)   .   la *Radiculectomie.*

En Pathologie.

(11) Je propose définir l'inflammation du periodonte de la partie apicale (atteinte du sommet) par le terme   .   .
soit (1°) *Periapiculite;* soit (2°) *Peridontite apicale.*

(12) Le terme pour définir le noircirment des dents devrait être   .   .   .
la *Melanodontie.*

Discussion.

Dr. LOUIS OTTOFY, Manila, P. I. I was intensely interested in the subject of nomenclature while I lived in this country, and I am even more so at the present time, for I realize the great importance of a uniform system as a result of a larger field of experience. In the Philippines the native dentists speak Spanish well, but little English, while the Americans understand but little Spanish. The disadvantage of a lack of uniformity is noticeable in our dental society, in which a common nomenclature would be of great benefit. For instance, the natives still use the terms "approximal," "anterior," "posterior," etc., while "mesial," "distal," "occlusal," etc., are new to them.

Similar valuable papers to the report under discussion, have been presented before, but, so far as I know, no definite and final action has as yet been reached. Whatever terms seem irrevocably satisfactory should be adopted internationally, and not changed, except for the very best of reasons. I have been accustomed to the term "canine," and have barely become well familiarized with the word "cuspid," when I now learn that the former, after all, is the correct one. I trust that through the International Dental Federation definite results may be promulgated in the near future.

Dr. JAMES TRUMAN, Philadelphia, Pa. It seems to me that while I sympathize with the effort to change the terms, yet human nature is human nature, and it is utterly impossible to work out this matter by any resolution or any action of any congress of individuals. It has got to come by a process of evolution. These terms will grow, and their eventual adoption will be effected, but it will take years for this. It is a language itself—practically a new language—one made in the last sixty or seventy years, and in the years to come we will grow into the use of these terms. I believe Dr. Thompson took the position that "canine" should be used in place of "cuspid." I think he is right. I use that term almost exclusively. I think the term "premolar" should be used in place of "bicuspid." That is the term usually used by comparative anatomists. I think Dr. Ottofy was correct in going back to the original terms. I seldom use the terms "mesial" and "distal" for I think "anterior" and "posterior" cover the position very well and they are terms that have been in use very much longer; but this is altogether a matter of taste. But

this effort to create new terms by rule and expect them to be adopted is equivalent to preparing a universal language for the world—doomed to failure from its inception.

Dr. HENRY W. MORGAN, Nashville, Tenn. The question of the adoption of terms in which to express one's thoughts is usually a matter of a man's education. Much depends upon the text-books used when he was a student. In operative dentistry, terms used must be in accord with the terms used by the anatomy studied. In the institution with which I am connected we adopted as a matter of convenience a dental anatomy using the terms "mesial" and "distal." They simplified the matter and relieved us of the necessity of using long descriptive terms. I have for many years discarded the term "canine" because there seems no good reason for its use; the word "cuspid" describes that tooth as well or better than any other that might be given. While the term "occlusal" might be misleading to one unfamiliar with it, it is merely a matter of preference and a question of what a man is used to. One continues to use the terms that he has learned in the early years of college life. Like Dr. Truman, I do not believe there is any possibility of this body, the International Federation, or any other body finally settling these questions, but it does seem to me that they might arrive at some good results if we had a committee to correct the various dental text-books before being published.

Dr. GODON. I was sorry I could not hear the communication of Dr. Thompson. I sent him a little paper on this question of nomenclature. I have mentioned some of the terms that we use in the Dental School of Paris. I do not think that the International Dental Fed-

19

eration could make up a nomenclature of all the terms that we use and the decision be accepted everywhere. Such a committee was named at the meeting in Paris in 1889, and all the words they adopted were not accepted everywhere, but some of them were accepted. I think it would be a good plan for the International Dental Federation to make up a dental nomenclature; it would be a very useful thing. I presented some of the terms that we use in the Dental School of Paris, and I believe Black in his report to the World's Columbian Dental Congress accepted some of these terms, as, for instance, the four degrees of caries. There are also some terms on the preparation of the cavities and the names of the edges of the cavity. I have not attempted to read my paper to you on this question, as it is in French.

The paper here follows:

Quelques Observations sur la Nomenclature Dentaire Internationale.

Par Dr. CHARLES GODON, Paris, France.

UNE des préoccupations principales qui s'imposent à l'esprit des membres de la profession, lorsqu'ils prennent part à un congrès international, est celle qui a pour objet la création d'une nomenclature dentaire internationale.

En effet, en dehors des difficultés déjà grandes que l'on rencontre dans ces réunions où se convient les hommes des différents pays du globe, une autre réside dans l'usage des différentes langues et l'on se prend à souhaiter que l'époque soit prochaine où sera adoptée une langue commune universelle pour faire disparaître cette confusion qui rappelle trop la légende biblique de la Tour de Babel.

Mais si cette langue universelle est encore dans un avenir lointain par suite de difficultés diverses, il est au moins possible d'entrevoir une entente internationale sur les termes employés dans chaque branche de la science humaine.

Cette entente a déjà été réalisée dans nombre de branches où se donne cours l'activité humaine, au grand bénéfice de tous.

Nous ne rappellerons pas toutes les tentatives qui ont déjà été faites dans la science odontologique pour obtenir ce résultat.

Nous signalerons pourtant qu'au premier congrès dentaire international tenu à Paris en 1889, une commission composée de P. Dubois de Paris, de Cunningham de Cambridge, et de Grosheintz de Bâle, fut nommée dans ce but.

Plus tard, au deuxième congrès de Chicago en 1893, il y eut une autre commission de nomenclature dont Black fut rapporteur.

Au congrès de Paris en 1900, quelques propositions furent présentées à ce sujet.

Enfin, en 1902, à la réunion de la Fédération Dentaire Internationale tenue à Stockholm, le Dr. Haderup, de Copenhague présenta un projet intéressant et demanda la nomination d'une commission internationale de nomenclature. Les nombreux travaux qui ont incombé depuis cette époque à la Fédération n'ont pas permis, malgré l'importance de la question, de donner suite au projet du

(I)   *Tableau des onze types de caries simples et composées.*

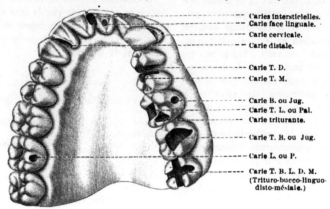

Caries intersticielles.
Carie face linguale.
Carie cervicale.
Carie distale.

Carie T. D.
Carie T. M.

Carie B. ou Jug.
Carie T. L. ou Pal.
Carie triturante.

Carie T. B. ou Jug.

Carie L. ou P.

Carie T. B. L. D. M.
(Trituro-bucco-linguo-
disto-mésiale.)

(II.)   *Les faces, les bords et les angles d'une cavité de carie dentaire.*

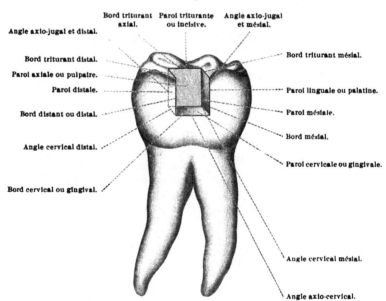

Bord triturant axial.
Paroi triturante ou incisive.
Angle axio-jugal et mésial.
Angle axio-jugal et distal.
Bord triturant distal.
Paroi axiale ou pulpaire.
Paroi distale.
Bord triturant mésial.
Paroi linguale ou palatine.
Paroi mésiale.
Bord distant ou distal.
Bord mésial.
Angle cervical distal.
Paroi cervicale ou gingivale.
Bord cervical ou gingival.
Angle cervical mésial.
Angle axio-cervical.

Dr. Haderup, et de l'adopter. Cette mission a été réservée au Conseil Exécutif de la F. D. I. pendant la deuxième session qui s'étendra entre le quatrième congrès de 1904 et le cinquième congrès.

Cette question de la nomenclature est naturellement très vaste. Les termes sur lesquels il est nécessaire de faire une entente sont si nombreux que l'on ne peut avoir la prétention de résoudre le problème en un seul congrès et qu'une commission internationale permanente serait le moyen le plus pratique de tenir à jour la nomenclature internationale dentaire, d'autant plus que l'évolution de la science apporte chaque année des termes nouveaux qui naissent dans les divers pays du globe.

le Dr. Black au Congrès de Chicago en 1893.

La classification des cavités résultant des caries au point de vue de leur siège, comprenant onze cavités types et divisés en caries simples et caries composées est la suivante :

CARIES SIMPLES.

Caries centrales triturantes (grosses molaires).

Caries latérales interstitielles médianes (incisives centrales).

Caries latérales, interstitielles, distantes (incisives latérales).

Caries latérales jugales (molaires).

Caries latérales palatines ou linguales (molaires).

Caries cervicales (canines).

1er degré.	Altération de l'émail......................	} Carie non pénétrante.
2ème degré.	Altération de l'émail et de l'ivoire..........	
3ème degré.	Altération de la pulpe....................	} Carie pénétrante.
4ème degré. {	Mortification de la pulpe et altération du périodonte........................	

Je terminerai donc ces courtes observations en proposant à la Commission de Nomenclature du quatrième congrès international de Saint Louis d'émettre le vœu qu'il soit créé dans la Fédération Dentaire Internationale une commission internationale permanente de nomenclature.

Chaque école dentaire se créé une nomenclature un peu spéciale. Nous donnons ci-dessous quelques termes employés à l'Ecole dentaire de Paris dans notre enseignement, dans la branche spéciale de la clinique et de la dentisterie opératoires.

Il a été adopté, sur ma proposition et depuis la fondation de l'Ecole dentaire de Paris en 1880, le tableau ci-dessus des classifications des différents degrés de la carie, classification qui a été acceptée par

CARIES COMPLIQUÉES.

Caries médio-triturantes (petites molaires).

Caries disto-triturantes (petites molaires).

Caries jugo-triturantes (molaires).

Caries linguo-triturantes (molaires).

Caries médio-disto-jugo-linguo-cervico-triturantes soit coronales (molaires).

Indication des termes désignant les faces, les bords et les angles d'une cavité de carie dentaire préparée pour l'obturation, est la suivante :

PAROIS.

Paroi mésiale ou médiane.

Paroi cervicale ou gingivale.

Paroi distale ou distante

Paroi triturante ou incisive.

Paroi axiale ou pulpaire.

Paroi linguale ou palatine.

BORDS.

Bord mésial.
Bord cervical.
Bord distal.
Bord triturant distal.
Bord triturant axial.
Bord triturant mésial.

ANGLES.

Angle cervico-mésial.
Angle cervico-axial.
Angle cervico-distal.
Angle axio-distal.
Angle axio-mésial.
Angle axio-triturant.
Angle mésio-triturant.
Angle disto-triturant.

The author concluded his communication by offering the following resolution, which was duly seconded and adopted:

RESOLVED, That an international committee be appointed by the Fédération Dentaire Internationale upon international nomenclature and the preparation of a list of professional terms which shall be interchangeable and translatable into English, German, French, and Spanish; such committee to report at the Fifth International Dental Congress.

On motion of Dr. Thompson this resolution was referred to the committee having the matter in charge, with instructions that it be presented to the congress in general session and its passage recommended.

The subject was passed and the chairman called for the next paper, entitled "Dental Education from the View of Experience," by Dr. JAMES TRUMAN, Philadelphia, Pa., as follows:

Dental Education from the View of Experience.

By JAMES TRUMAN, D.D.S., LL.D., Philadelphia, Pa.

THE following propositions are, in the opinion of the writer, fundamental to a proper realization of ideals in education:

(1) A decided mental tendency, in the individual, in one direction.

(2) This established, training must be to develop these mental tendencies.

(3) Dental education, to be effective, must therefore be developed from these original tendencies, if these are in the direction of its complex character, practical and theoretical.

(4) In this education the *practical* must *precede* the *theoretical*.

Considering these propositions *seriatim* it must be conceded that the mental tendencies of the individual are primarily the most important for the educator to consider. The study of the mental inclinations of youth belongs not alone to the teacher, but is part of the important relations held by parents and guardians. The latter may regard this a difficult problem to solve, belonging more properly to the specialist in psychological manifestations. To reason thus is a fatal error, and one so often made that it has become a very serious evil, forcing young minds in wrong directions and wrecking innumerable lives in vain attempts to acquire, to them, useless knowledge.

The general idea, prevalent not alone among parents but as a part of the general educational thought, is that education to be of value must run along hard and fast lines, and that without variation to meet these special tendencies; in other words, the child is placed, as it were, in a strait-jacket from the time of entering school until the period the diploma is reached. This may be the A.B. of the high school, or of this degree in arts of our universities or colleges. Is it any wonder that the student whose tastes run counter to all this should regard with aversion this iron-clad method? The average teacher, however, holds that to draw out the best in the individual all that is necessary is to force the undeveloped being through the universal educational mill. It is immaterial to this teacher whether the student is to become a mechanic, an architect, minister, lawyer, doctor, dentist, or journalist, in fact any of the varied and useful occupations that go to make up what we term civilization. To merely name this variety stamps the preliminary work, as usually given, as the weak point in the school training of America. They have a far better idea of education in some parts of continental Europe, in that the training is in the direction of the future work of the student, but while this is an advance, it takes but a limited account of the mental tendencies of the individual. It is true that a thorough classical education is of untold value to any individual, and other things being equal, may give to him power and marked advantage over his less fortunate competitor in the race of life. But this will depend so much on natural tendencies and the subsequent use made of these, that no one can wisely prophesy the future of the individual.

Two prominent and very recent illustrations in this country serve to give point to this by no means original idea. One, a graduate in arts from one of the leading colleges of the country, found his acquirements of no practical value in the active world. His training, good as it was for certain purposes, furnished

nothing that would enable him to reach a position consonant with his tastes and necessities. His learning failed to meet the demands of his daily needs, and nothing else offering, he bravely accepted the humble position of a laborer on a railway. The result was that step by step he advanced from this to the position of motorman on an electric street-car. From this, at an early age, to the presidency of the system of street railways in the largest city of the country was the natural result of untiring efforts and original mental training in other directions.

The other began with no such education; in fact his scholastic training was below the average. He started as brakeman on a railroad, and from that, through all grades, became eventually many times a millionaire, a United States senator, and has recently been nominated for the position of vice-president of the United States by one of the great political parties of this country.

The conclusion to be derived from these examples, not at all uncommon, is that the first demonstrates the power of a liberal education when started in the direction of the natural bent of mind in the individual, and the second, that defects in education may be overcome by mental force concentrated on one object.

If then, it be true that a mental tendency in the individual is all-important and must be sought for, when found it becomes of vital importance that the training should be in the direction of these natural tastes. The problem becomes complicated when the individual exhibits no special proclivities, but seems willing to drift along with the world's current. General laws are not for these, however, and the only test for this very large class of young persons is to prove their capacity in some one or more directions. When, however, the tendency is marked, every effort should be made to begin the individual's career properly. If this is in the direction of mechanics, no mistake will be made if, during the impressible period of youth, the muscles are placed in training in schools especially devoted to this work. This experience will be of inestimable value should the youth subsequently prefer the literary training necessary to become a doctor of medicine, minister, or lawyer. Especially will this apply to the surgeon.

Dental education, then, to be effective must be based on an early investigation of the mental tendencies, and those being discovered, the direction which education must take is then plain. Dentistry is a complex study; it begins with the practical and ends with the theoretical, or should so end. From what has already been stated, the necessity for early muscular training in mechanics must be apparent. No other course is left open. Every added year lost in this cultivation is just one year of less ability to overcome mechanical problems.

The idea is often taught, and as often combated, that the theoretical must precede the practical. In other words, the individual must have a special training before he is supposed to be fitted to begin his work in dentistry. The Association of Dental Faculties says the applicant for the degree of Doctor of Dental Surgery must first show, on matriculating, a certificate of entrance to the third year of a high school. Nothing is said as to the character of the training given in the high school. Our universities demand a fixed standard, easily understood, and very much higher than the ordinary routine of studies. What is the result? Our dental colleges are inundated with educated young men who have been sent by those in authority over them to master a calling, a prerequisite to success in which is a taste at least for mechanical work. Nothing in their previous studies leads to a knowledge of this bent of mind, and the results, therefore, are not always satisfactory.

To decide this question of fitness for the proposed study, the practical must precede the theoretical, and any other course, as far as dentistry is concerned, is simply a great wrong perpetrated in the name of higher education. No greater mistake can be made than to place a youth in a medical college as preliminary to his dental training. The time may come, indeed is fast coming, if not already here in some institutions, of carrying the student of medicine and dentistry *pari passu.* This will doubtless lead to the M.D. degree, but a much longer period of probation will be required than the present four years of training to secure separately either of these degrees, that of M.D. or D.D.S. The experience of dental educators has been—and this has been confirmed in the writer's life-work —that the individual who has passed from the higher schools into those of medicine, and then essays the study of dentistry, fails, with few exceptions, in reaching a high degree of skill. The evidences of the truth of this are among the most painful of the writer's experiences as a teacher in dentistry, and this alone would lead him to enter an earnest protest against this, to him, fatal error in the future proposed education of dentists.

There has been a general impression that the higher preliminary education, if it did not increase ability in the two practical branches of dentistry, would at least enable the student to hold his own, and in other respects make him more valuable in the community. This view is partially borne out by the averages taken in the Dental Department of the University of Pennsylvania. The following table illustrates the average standing of the several classes in prosthetics and operative dentistry from the period when the department accepted students upon a grammar-school certificate to the time when a high-school diploma was required:

Certificate.	Mechanical Dentistry.	Operative Dentistry.
Grammar school.......	76.22	84.82
1st year, high school...	81.19	85.91
2d year, high school...	83.13	80.97
Diploma, high school...	75.47	86.54

While averages are somewhat misleading, yet so far as this goes, as the result in one school, it may be taken as an indication that the boy from the grammar school stands an equal chance with the boy with a high-school diploma in mastering the practical work of dentistry. But it is very evident that the higher education has not improved the high-school boy's ability to meet the difficulties of the practical, more than it has the boy of the lower school. It, however, does show that the higher preliminary training enables the one who has it to hold his own in the realm of the practical, and will give him an immense advantage in acquiring the collateral branches peculiar to medicine.

In conclusion, dental education must be first based on mental tendencies, and these proved, then the education should begin with manual-training work. It is immaterial where this is secured. From this, the practical side of dentistry, the prosthetic must be conquered. This will furnish the foundation for the operative branch, and the two constitute the necessary practical basis for the attainment of success in the future professional life-

work of the individual. It must, however, never be forgotten that the old age of manual dexterity begins with maturity, and skill, to be of value and permanent, must be acquired while the mind and the hands are in the impressive period of youth.

Discussion.

Dr. H. A. SMITH, Cincinnati, O. Dr. Truman has given us an interesting paper. Doubtless everyone will agree with him in his main contention, that since dentistry is so largely manipulative all persons seeking entrance to our colleges should show a fondness for or a degree of ability in handicraft. Just how, when, or where this test should be made the essayist does not inform us. Experience shows that parents cannot give a reliable opinion as to their son's fitness to pursue dentistry. A course in the technical school would be out of the question to the majority who apply. Even the old plan of first serving a term in the dentist's laboratory was quite unsatisfactory. As the matter stands today the experienced, able dental teacher is likely to be the best judge of one's fitness to enter upon the study of dentistry.

Dr. Truman has presented some suggestive statistics bearing upon the question of fitness, both natural and acquired, for the study of dentistry. If ultimately it can be shown that students with less education than obtains in a full high-school course excel in prosthetic dentistry, some of us perhaps will have to revise our views in reference to the right educational standard for admission to our dental colleges. Statistics, especially of the kind Dr. Truman gives, are often misleading, but if a systematic, concerted effort was made by our dental colleges to collect statistics bearing upon such subjects as are being discussed before this section today, much aid would be given in the direction of the right education of dentists.

Dr. WILLIAM H. TRUEMAN, Philadelphia, Pa. This question of higher education is very fascinating. It has become a fad. How far it will prove a practical benefit is a serious question. Undoubtedly, a good mental endowment should be possessed by all who seek to enter the more exacting professions. They need, first, sufficient knowledge and sufficient mental training to enable them to understand and appreciate the instruction given in the professional schools. Secondly, and beyond this, they should have sufficient general knowledge to uphold the dignity of their calling. Now, this latter may be carried so far as to unfit one for his chosen vocation. The time comes when the muscles cannot be trained and educated so easily as in early life, and this, to a dentist, is a serious handicap—for to him manual dexterity is a requisite to success. Higher education has entered the dental schools. The curriculum has been so greatly extended that post-graduate schools are springing up all over the land to teach dental graduates practical dentistry. So much time is taken up with teaching prospective dentists the things they ought to know, but have no use for, that the practical side—the things absolutely essential to his daily work—are neglected. Higher education, preparatory and professional, so far as dentistry is concerned, is so recent that we cannot yet judge its results. When we consider that life is short, it hardly seems wise to compel one to defer entering on its work seriously until it is

half spent, as seems to be the trend at the present time, unless it can be shown that better results warrant the sacrifice.

Dr. HENRY W. MORGAN, Nashville, Tenn. I have been very much delighted and greatly interested in this paper and am glad to indorse most of it. I wish Dr. Truman would change the phrase "practical dentistry" to the expression "the art side of dentistry." The sense in which the word practical has for so long been used leads one to think it refers to the work done for the patient at the chair side, while this is not what Dr. Truman means, if I understand it. The art side of dentistry certainly has been neglected in the teaching of many institutions. I believe with Dr. Truman that the training in the two should be carried on *pari passu*. The student should be made to feel that he is doing something from the very first, and not merely that he is getting a theoretical knowledge of what he will have to do in the future.

The reference to the gentleman in the paper who started out with a fine education in the arts, failed utterly in his undertaking and went into the street railroad business, later to become the road's president, reminds me of two dental students in my own experience. One was a college graduate, in personal appearance, dignity of character, and general bearing, all that seemed necessary to make up the ideal student. But just here let me say that the record a man makes in a dental college is no indication of what he will make his professional career. This man graduated second in his class but failed utterly in his profession, and in less than two years had made an application for clerkship in a packing house of a Western state. The other student was not so well prepared and barely got his degree. He seemed an indifferent student, content with only a grade that would pass him, with nothing about him to lead to an expectation of success, and yet about the time the first man was seeking a clerkship the second was found to own his home and office, and had won the confidence of the people in the community in which he resided. As a dentist the man who was barely able to get his degree had made a grand success so far as professional career was concerned.

Someone in the discussion of this paper has asked, Who shall decide? If the boy himself is not able to answer that question then nobody under the sun can answer it for him. We have seen many wrecks where attempts have been made to make something out of a boy who is entirely unfitted for the occupation chosen. I graduated in medicine first and have always contended that it was the one mistake in my dental education. My medical training should have come after I became a dentist.

Dr. CHAS. GODON, Paris, France. I am pleased to add my indorsement to all Dr. Truman has said about dental education. In this education the practical must precede the theoretical. That is the basis at the Dental School of Paris. The student commences with manual training. When making up our program Sir Michael Foster said the time for a man to acquire manual dexterity was when he was young. We must begin very soon. I am pleased that we have that method in our country, and not only in dental education but in general education the same idea begins to prevail. Only last year a report was made by the rector of the University of Paris in which it was stated that the young man must be trained as a woodworker and an ironworker at the same time he takes his university course. This was approved and

I think will soon go into effect. I have been informed by the Commission of Public Education that after October 1904 they will require that dental students take a two-year course in manual training before entering the dental school. They have done this because they believe that practical training should precede theoretical studies. I approve absolutely the principles of Dr. Truman.

Dr. TRUMAN W. BROPHY, Chicago, Ill. While Professor Truman was reading his paper, in speaking of the manipulative skill that must necessarily be acquired when young, I remembered some of the scenes that impressed me when I rambled over Europe years ago, and the place that affected me most was that of Peter the Great, of Russia. When visiting the city of St. Petersburg the tourist is always taken to his room and shown the pieces of mechanism that he made—machinery of wood and iron; almost all the metals are used in the machinery that wonderful man made with his own hands. That he might teach his people the best in mechanics he even went to Holland to learn shipbuilding. I believe that Peter the Great would never have figured in the history of the world as he did had it not been for his mechanical skill. Engineering is only a high development of the skill which comes through manual training. The Massachusetts School of Technology furnishes a most striking example of what men filling the highest places in the United States government can do with their hands. Too much attention cannot be paid to the subject. I think possibly that what I have said on the subject has been due in a measure to what Dr. Truman said many years ago when he was the master and I the boy in school, and had it not been for that kind of teaching in those days, away back in

1870, I doubt if I would ever have accomplished much in manipulative skill. I believe that the high-school training, and university training, while a thing of inestimable value, does not fit the young man in the highest sense for the dental profession. I hold that the students of the future should enter the dental schools as well prepared as we would have them, and when we request that they get this manual training it will guide the members of the profession. The dentists of the world will tell the young men that they must have this kind of training, the young man who has not had this training will get it and he will know how to use the instruments when they are placed in his hands, and instead of pushing the file backward he will draw it forward. I was pleased with Dr. Truman's impressing upon us the importance of that. What is the use of high-school training unless we can get with it manual training? If he has not the manual training, as a dental student he will be a failure.

The next item as announced by the chairman was a paper on educational standards, by Dr. CHAS. GODON, Paris, France, entitled "Le Doctorat Dentaire: Communication à la Commission d'Enseignement," which here follows:

Le Doctorat Dentaire: Communication à la Commission d'Enseignement.

By Dr. CHAS. GODON, Paris, France.

LA commission internationale d'Enseignement de la F. D. I. pendant les trois sessions de Cambridge, de Stockholm et de Madrid a elaboré un programme international d'enseignement dentaire avec le concours des hommes les plus qualifiés dans les principaux pays du monde sur ces questions.

Ce programme qui comprend quatre années d'études théoriques et pratiques, scientifiques, médicales et techniques a pour but de former des praticiens à la hauteur des progrès de la science odontologique moderne et capable de soigner dans les meilleures conditions les patients qui auront besoin de leurs soins.

Mais à cela ne doivent pas se borner les aspirations de l'enseignement odontologique, car ses besoins sont autres.

Elle risquerait en se limitant ainsi de justifier le dédain avec lequel certains hommes de science affectent encore trop souvent de le considérer en disant que le grade de dentiste ne signifie pas des études supérieures, de justifier aussi la recherche d'autres titres scientifiques et surtout médicaux que font qu'un certain nombre de confrères ne sont pas satisfait de leur simple titre professionnel.

La science odontologique a maintenant ses savants spéciaux, ses professeurs, comme les autres sciences, ses cadres universitaires.

Pourquoi n'aurait-elle pas aussi ses études et ses titres universitaires supérieurs, comme toutes les autres branches des connaissances humaines qui forment les diverses sections d'une université?

Ces considérations semblent actuellement répondre à des aspirations professionnelles qui viennent de se former dans certains pays et dont notre grande assemblée internationale doit avoir un écho.

En France, elles ont récemment fait l'objet de discussions dans nos sociétés et de vœux aux pouvoirs publics tendant à la création d'un doctorat scientifique en odontologie dans les universités, à la suite d'un rapport dont m'avait chargé la Fédération dentaire internationale et dont je cite ci-dessous les principaux passages.*

Le seul titre légal qui existe en France pour les dentistes est celui de *chirurgien-dentiste* créé par la loi du 30 novembre 1892 et le décret du 25 juillet 1893. On sait qu'il est délivré, après trois années d'études dans les écoles dentaires, par les Facultés de médecine à la suite de trois examens.

Ce titre, qui s'applique aussi bien à ceux qui se livrent à la pratique de l'art dentaire qu'à ceux qui poursuivent des études scientifiques odontologiques ou font de l'enseignement, ne semble plus répondre à toutes les nécessités de la profession ni à la situation résultant de l'évolution qui s'est accomplie dans cette science spéciale depuis les dix dernières années.

Diverses administrations publiques ont jugé insuffisant ce titre de chirurgien-dentiste pour les postes officiels de dentistes des hôpitaux, d'examinateurs près des Facultés, etc., et ont réclamé le titre de docteur en médecine, que certains dentistes ont cru devoir s'adjoindre.

Quelques jeunes confrères sont allés en Amérique, avant d'exercer, demander aux écoles dentaires des universités des États-Unis le titre de docteur en chirur-

gie dentaire (D.D.S.) pour l'ajouter au titre français de chirurgien-dentiste.

Les Écoles dentaires de Paris et de Lyon, dans une pensée analogue, ont transformé leur diplôme de fin d'études en un grade supérieur à celui de chirurgien-dentiste de l'État, qu'elles ne délivrent qu'après une 4e année d'études et de nouveaux examens.

Ainsi s'est trouvée posée tout naturellement pour les dentistes la question d'un grade supérieur, le *doctorat dentaire*.

On en trouve la première manifestation en 1900 dans une proposition faite au 3e Congrès dentaire international de Paris par MM. Barrié, Loup, etc., et qui fut écartée par la Commission des vœux comme n'ayant pas, à cette époque, un caractère international.

En 1901, nous nous exprimions ainsi à ce sujet dans notre thèse de doctorat en médecine (pages 342 et 343): "Un titre purement scientifique comme celui de docteur en chirurgie dentaire ou en odontologie pourrait être donné en France, avec la législation actuelle, par une décision universitaire analogue à celle qui a été prise récemment pour la pharmacie."*

En 1902, les délégués de l'École dentaire de Paris ont déjà saisi les pouvoirs publics de cette question une première fois, dans leur entrevue avec M. le Recteur de l'Académie de Paris.

Cette première manifestation officielle de l'École dentaire a été confirmée par nous dans le rapport remis au Recteur, au mois de janvier dernier, sur les modifications à apporter aux études dentaires. Ce rapport, qui avait été adopté par le Conseil de direction de l'École, dans sa

* Ce rapport a été présenté à l'Association générale des dentistes de France, le 19 mars 1904, et à la session de la Fédération dentaire nationale, le 9 avril 1904, et a été adopté à l'unanimité par ces deux assemblées.

*Voir "L'Évolution de l'art dentaire, l'École dentaire." Baillière, Paris, 1901.

séance de décembre 1903, contient, parmi diverses revendications, une demande relative au doctorat dentaire.

Le Syndicat des chirurgiens-dentistes de France a étudié cette question dans ses séances de décembre et de janvier après un rapport très étendu de notre collègue M. Loup et a émis un vœu à ce sujet.

L'École dentaire de Lyon nous a informés à la même époque qu'elle approuvait cette revendication.

L'Association générale des dentistes de France, dans son assemblée générale du 19 mars 1904, et le Conseil général du groupement de l'École dentaire de Paris, dans sa séance du 29 du même mois, adoptaient les conclusions que nous leur présentions à ce sujet conclusions que nous reproduisons plus loin.

Enfin, la Fédération dentaire nationale française l'a mise à l'étude pour les séances de la session d'avril à Paris et a adopté le rapport que nous présentions à ce sujet.

Il faut nous féliciter de voir ainsi le doctorat dentaire à l'ordre du jour de nos principales sociétés parce que c'est la conséquence de notre évolution et la conclusion de la réforme odontologique que nous poursuivons.

Nous venons de montrer que cette revendication est actuellement formulée par les sociétés professionnelles françaises. Ajoutons qu'elle est tout à fait justifiée, conforme à notre évolution et qu'elle arrive à son heure. En effet, au point de vue philosophique, cette revendication est le complément nécessaire de la campagne en faveur de l'autonomie de la science et de la profession odontologiques poursuivie par les odontologistes depuis vingt-cinq ans.

Elle établit notamment la différence et l'analogie qui existent entre les plus hauts grades médicaux de docteur en médecine, de docteur en pharmacie, et le plus haut grade en dentisterie, celui de docteur en odontologie ou en chirurgie dentaire, qui existe dans quelques universités dans différents pays.

Elle est conforme à notre évolution scientifique, puisque depuis vingt-cinq ans, nos écoles, nos sociétés odontologiques et nos journaux ont créé une élite de professeurs et de savants en odontologie qui serait digne d'avoir un grade scientifique supérieur à celui de chirurgien-dentiste. Ce dernier n'est qu'un titre de praticien, analogue à celui de pharmacien. Aussi le grade de docteur en odontologie, par exemple, serait-il indiqué par analogie au grade scientifique de docteur en pharmacie.

Si l'on compare les études que l'on fait en France à celles que l'on fait en Amérique, on constate qu'elles sont de même durée et considérées comme équivalentes; les chirurgiens-dentistes français, anglais, allemands, suisses, russes, etc., pourraient, d'abord tout aussi bien que leurs confrères américains, revendiquer le titre de docteur en chirurgie dentaire à la place de celui de chirurgien-dentiste.

La différence de titre crée aux chirurgiens-dentistes européens une infériorité apparente, au moins vis-à-vis des dentistes américains et des docteurs en médecine qui se sont faits dentistes, infériorité que l'on sait professionnellement injustifiée. D'autant plus que par le développement et la perfection de ses études scientifiques, médicales et techniques, par le relèvement graduel de ses études préliminaires jusqu'au baccalauréat, on peut dire que le chirurgien-dentiste européen est aujourd'hui en possession morale du titre de docteur, c'est-à-dire de "maître" dans sa profession, comme le docteur en médecine est "maître" pour la profession médicale.

Il ne s'agit que de transformer cette possession morale en possession effective.

A ces derniers arguments on peut faire deux objections: la première tirée des difficultés pratiques de réalisation; nous l'examinerons plus loin; la deuxième tirée de cette considération que le nouveau titre pourrait accentuer la séparation qui existe entre la profession de dentiste et la profession médicale proprement dite. C'est là l'objection principale; il est nécessaire de l'examiner.

Mais d'abord, en quoi y a-t-il assimilation de la profession dentaire à la médecine et en quoi y a-t-il division?

Il est évident que toutes les sciences partent d'un même tronc commun, filles de la science humaine, et, comme les branches d'un arbre elles se divisent et se ramifient en branches spéciales à mesure qu'elles progressent. L'odontologie est une de ces branches; elle appartient à la grosse division des sciences biologiques, des sciences médicales, comme la pharmacie.

Ceci est le point de vue philosophique, théorique; mais dans les applications, il y aura, dans certains cas, assimilation ou division, suivant les nécessités sociales.

Ainsi, au point de vue de l'exercice, il existe un titre spécial, celui de chirurgien-dentiste avec une profession organisée spécialement; au point de vue juridique, un délit spécial, celui d'exercice illégal de l'art dentaire; au point de vue de l'enseignement, des écoles spéciales dites d'art dentaire, etc., etc.

L'art dentaire n'en appartient pas moins, au point de vue général, à la grande famille médicale, comme les pharmaciens déjà cités. Une transformation du titre de chirurgien-dentiste en celui de docteur en chirurgie dentaire

ou la création d'un grade supérieur en odontologie ne changeront pas plus cette situation pour les dentistes que ne l'ont fait pour les pharmaciens la création du titre de docteur en pharmacie, ou même pour certains médecins, les titres en médecine coloniale, médecine légale, etc., que l'on doit créer.

Enfin, il y a là une aspiration très noble et qui mérite d'être encouragée que celle qui pousse les membres d'une profession à s'élever ainsi davantage dans la hiérarchie scientifique, comme le disait très bien M. Touvet-Fanton. C'est l'émulation d'une élite qui ne peut qu'être profitable aux progrès de l'odontologie en particulier, à ceux de la science en général et par suite à la collectivité tout entière.

Cette élite comprend que noblesse oblige, qu'un titre scientifique plus élevé, s'il donne à ceux qui l'obtiennent plus de considération, réclame des obligations et des garanties nouvelles de savoir, comme l'a très bien fait ressortir M. d'Argent.

En inscrivant aujourd'hui cette revendication du doctorat dans leur programme, les membres de la profession montrent qu'ils comprennent leurs nouveaux devoirs et qu'ainsi ils sont mûrs pour obtenir un titre supérieur qui les place sur un pied d'égalité scientifique et sociale avec les autres professions libérales.

Mais d'abord, pourquoi un doctorat dentaire? Qu'est-ce qu'un docteur? Nous trouvons dans Larousse les deux définitions suivantes:

1° Celui qui enseigne publiquement et par autorisation expresse;

2° Celui qui a obtenu le plus haut des grades d'une Université.

On raconte que la première réception de docteur eut lieu à l'Université de Bologne en 1140, et, peu de temps après, l'Université de Paris adopta ce nouvel usage, cette dénomination remplaçant celle de "maître," que l'on conservait dans la plupart des professions et que l'on retrouve encore dans certaines Universités anglaises, si bien que l'Université de Birmingham créait récemment un titre de *Master in Dental Surgery.*

Nous ne vous parlerons pas de toutes les phases par lesquelles a passé le doctorat, depuis sa création jusqu'au moment de la Révolution française, ni des particularités diverses qui s'attachaient à ce titre. Qu'il nous suffise de rappeler que le doctorat conférait le droit d'enseigner.

Le décret du 17 mars 1898, en établissant la nouvelle Université, avait institué cinq facultés: lettres, sciences, droit, médecine et théologie, chacune avec un doctorat ayant des droits et des règlements particuliers, mais ces doctorats n'en étaient pas moins des doctorats d'État.

Le décret du 27 juillet 1897 a autorisé les quinze Universités à instituer des titres d'ordre exclusivement scientifique, dit doctorats d'Université, qui ne confèrent aucun des droits d'exercice attachés au grade par les lois et règlements.

De cette petite étude historique il résulte qu'il existe, deux doctorats sur lesquels il semble possible de faire porter les revendications:

1° Le doctorat scientifique ou doctorat d'Université appliqué à l'art dentaire; il pourrait constituer un doctorat en odontologie pour ceux qui dans notre profession s'adonnent à la science ou à l'enseignement;

2° Le doctorat diplôme d'État qui pour la médecine, par exemple, tout en étant le plus haut grade, donne le droit d'exercice légal. C'est en même temps un titre scientifique et un titre de praticien pour le médecin et pour le dentiste aux États Unis.

Pour notre profession, le doctorat diplôme d'État pourrait devenir le doctorat en chirurgie dentaire réservé au praticien, à la place du titre de chirurgien-dentiste créé en France par la loi du 30 novembre 1892 et dans les autres pays.

Il reste en troisième lieu le doctorat en médecine que certains voudraient rendre obligatoire pour les dentistes. Je le cite parce qu'on en a parlé; mais il est bien évident, comme l'à déjà dit M. Martinier au Syndicat des chirurgiens-dentistes et à l'Association générale des dentistes de France, qu'il n'est pas en question. Il est en contradiction avec nos principales revendications, puisqu'il ne comprend pas l'étude de la dentisterie dès le début des études professionnelles. C'est un grade en médecine et non un grade en chirurgie dentaire: ce sont, au point de vue de l'exercice légal, deux choses distinctes qui peuvent s'ajouter, mais non se remplacer. Le doctorat en médecine ne constitue ni une preuve ni même une présomption de savoir en dentisterie, par conséquent il ne peut être considéré comme un brevet d'études supérieures en odontologie.

Du reste, lorsque des représentants des pouvoirs publics dans certains pays ont proposé de l'accorder aux dentistes, ce n'a été que par suppression pure et simple de ces derniers.

Dans ce cas, le titre de docteur en médecine, en l'absence de tout grade dentaire, ne saurait être assimilé à un titre supérieur en odontologie que par un sophisme contre lequel les dentistes ont toujours protesté.

Dans quelles conditions est-il possible d'obtenir l'un de ces deux doctorats ou les deux en France?

1° Le grade de docteur en chirurgie dentaire d'État. Pour la création de ce grade donnant droit d'exercer comme aux États Unis et venant remplacer le diplôme de chirurgien-dentiste, partout où il existe il faudrait nécessairement en France une modification de l'article 3 de la loi du 30 novembre 1892, qui ne peut être obtenue que législativement, c'est-à-dire par voie de pétition au gouvernement, par initiative gouvernementale ou parlementaire, la Chambre et le Sénat appelés à en délibérer.

Cela demande beaucoup de temps, beaucoup de démarches et paraît d'une réalisation assez éloignée. Pourtant, avec des circonstances favorables, et les chirurgiens-dentistes s'unissant et faisant masse de toute leur influence près des pouvoirs publics, il ne semble pas impossible de réussir.

2° Le doctorat scientifique. Il faudrait une délibération d'une des quinze universités françaises, l'Université de Paris, par exemple, ou d'une des quatre Universités où existe l'enseignement dentaire: Paris, Lyon, Bordeaux, Nancy.

Il suffirait pour cela de saisir l'une de ces Universités d'un vœu que nous vous proposons plus loin d'émettre et d'examiner avec le Recteur les conditions dans lesquelles ce vœu pourrait être réalisé par le Conseil de l'Université en question.

Cela nécessiterait probablement la création d'un enseignement odontologique supérieur, d'une chaire, par exemple, à la dite Université, et exigerait un décret du Ministre de l'Instruction publique, peut-être une subvention à l'Université par les sociétés et les écoles dentaires.

Cela paraît d'une réalisation possible, étant donné qu'il existe des précédents récents: le doctorat en pharmacie par exemple.

Mais l'Association générale des dentistes de France, dans son assemblée générale du 19 mars 1904, a été d'avis, sur la proposition de M. Bonnard, de limiter d'abord les efforts à celle de ces revendications qui paraissait la plus accessible, le doctorat d'Université, en remettant à une date ultérieure toute revendication nécessitant une modification de la loi du 30 novembre 1892, relative au titre de Docteur du praticien.

En conséquence, la Fédération dentaire nationale française, réunie en assemblée générale à Paris le 9 avril 1904, considérant la nécessité de la création d'un doctorat dentaire, a émis les vœux suivants:

1° Qu'il soit créé un doctorat scientifique d'Université pour l'art dentaire, dit doctorat en odontologie, analogue au doctorat ès pharmacie, accessible seulement à ceux qui possèdent déjà le diplôme de chirurgien-dentiste;

2° Que des dispositions transitoires soient établies pour permettre aux chirurgiens-dentistes actuels d'obtenir le nouveau diplôme, dispositions analogues à celles qui ont été accordées aux officiers de santé pour l'obtention du diplôme de docteur en médecine;

3° Que la Fédération charge son bureau de faire toutes les démarches près des pouvoirs publics et des autorités universitaires, et d'assurer l'entente entre les diverses sociétés et écoles dentaires françaises pour permettre la réalisation de ces vœux. Elle a décidé leur inscription dans sa déclaration de principes adoptée le 8 avril 1902, sous la forme suivante:

Les odontologistes émettent le vœu:

1° Qu'il soit créé un doctorat scientifique d'Université pour l'art dentaire dit doctorat en odontologie, analogue au doctorat ès pharmacie, accessible seulement à ceux qui possèdent le diplôme de chirurgien-dentiste;

2° Des dispositions transitoires devront

être établies pour permettre aux chirurgiens-dentistes actuels d'obtenir le nouveau diplôme, dispositions analogues à celles qui ont été accordées aux officiers de santé pour l'obtention du diplôme de docteur en médecine.

Nous ajouterons, en terminant, en faveur de la réalisation de cette revendication une dernière considération qui était la conclusion de ce rapport.

Il nous semble que la création du nouveau doctorat d'Université serait le meilleur moyen de mettre fin à la division qui règne dans la profession dentaire entre les odontologistes et les stomatologistes.

En effet, elle permettra aux odontologistes de s'élever à un doctorat scientifique supérieur par le perfectionnement réel de leur science spéciale, sans être obligés d'apprendre sans utilité tout ce qu'un médecin doit savoir pour exercer la médecine générale. Elle permettrait aux stomatologistes d'obtenir, après le grade technique de chirurgien-dentiste, un grade scientifique au moins égal au doctorat en médecine, qui serait en même temps la justification de leurs connaissances spéciales en odontologie.

Enfin, pour les administrations publiques, pour les écoles dentaires, le nouveau grade en odontologie sera la garantie cherchée de l'éducation universitaire et spéciale complète du candidat dentiste aux différentes fonctions officielles d'examinateur, d'expert, de dentiste des hôpitaux, de professeur, etc.

Souhaitons donc, pour la réalisation de l'union dans la profession dentaire et les progrès qui doivent en découler, la création prochaine d'un doctorat scientifique en odontologie dans les Universités.

Ces vœux adoptés par la Fédération dentaire française au mois d'avril dernier ont été transmis par le President de la Fédération M. le Dr. E. Sauvez aux pouvoirs publics compétents dans une pétition du mois de juillet 14 dernier signée des représentants des principales sociétés professionnelles françaises.

Nous avons tenu à faire connaître l'état de cette question aux membres du Congrès de St. Louis, persuadés qu'elle peut prendre aujourd'hui un caractère véritablement international et répond aux préoccupations des dentistes du monde entier.

Discussion.

Dr. GODON. Preliminary dental education in France will be modified after this year. The requirement will be a preliminary manual-training course. That will mean that the student, after he has obtained his high-school certificate, will have to take up a systematic course in manual training at a dentist's or at a dental school giving courses in chemistry, physics, mechanics, and metallurgy before he is admitted to the three-year regular course in the dental school. That will give him a five-year course. The examinations will be modified also on the technical side.

We have asked also of the authorities in France that the title given the graduates of the dental school be Doctor of Dental Surgery, as you have it in this country, and I think if this proposition was adopted that it would put your diploma and ours on a similar basis.

Another thing is the question of the scientific degree. We have in the universities of France what we call the scientific diploma. These diplomas obtain for the pharmaceutical course. He who practices pharmacy is called a *pharmacien,* but the higher degree is that of

20

Doctor in Pharmacy. I have given in the paper I presented here a *résumé* of that question. I do not know whether these diplomas are given in your universities, but I feel there must be a difference in degree between the man who wants to practice and the man who wants to do scientific work.

Dr. Jas. Truman, Philadelphia, Pa. it has been a great gratification to me to know of the advance and progress dentistry is making in France. I trust there will in a very short time be such an advance in this country. From present indications here I am very much discouraged in regard to dental education. I feel that the retrogression witnessed in the United States will seriously compromise us in the estimation of the world.

In Europe (Germany, for example) they have divided the people into certain classes, educating them according to the bent of the individual, but in Germany they do not, it seems to me, lead up to the higher standard as they appear to be doing in France. I do not believe it is impossible to know how the individual would need to be educated. The boys and girls do not pretend to know; it is for somebody else to decide that question. The time will come when we will have some standard of work, when we will be enabled to take these young people and lead them in the right direction.

Dr. A. W. Harlan, New York, N. Y. The evidence of the interest that the governments of the world are taking in the training of dentists is being presented to us. In the last ten or a dozen years nearly all high schools in the United States have established manual training; and now France and Germany are insisting that that should be a part of the curriculum. It gives the boy the manual training at the time when he most needs it, as was pointed out by Dr. Truman's paper, in which he laid great stress on the need of practical before theoretical training. We draw many of our students from the agricultural districts, where they now have the steam plow and other modern machinery, so that even farmer boys must know something of mechanics. If they have the training they get in high schools they have a pretty good foundation to begin the study of a profession.

Dr. J. J. Rojo, Mexico City, Mexico. In my country, in the "preparatory school," which it is considered essential to pass before the students enter any professional school, it is necessary to study mathematics, physics, mechanics, cosmography, and drawing, and to my belief that gives the student a knowledge of the requirements of mechanics. As I understand it, the idea in both Europe and America is that the dental student must have a good preparatory mechanical training, and in Mexico that is perfectly recognized and understood.

The next paper on the program was by Dr. A. W. Harlan, New York, entitled "Dental Literature," as follows:

Dental Literature.

By A. W. HARLAN, M.D., D.D.S., New York, N. Y.

THE subject of this paper is large enough for a volume, and the few thoughts which I shall present are simply to treat the subject in a manner different from that in which it has been presented before.

From the earliest ages, some sort of record has been made of the thoughts and discoveries of members of our profession, and at times such records have been made by those who were not of us, and were not even attached to the profession. If we look over the pamphlets and printed books from the fourteenth century to the present day, we find but meager details of the facts then known.

I would therefore suggest that the best method of studying the literature of the profession is to divide it into periods. Before going farther, I would define what I mean by dental literature. "It is the expression of the concrete basis of observed, collected, verified facts, with the necessary deductions to enable the reader to comprehend it, and couched in a language or manner so simple that it may be easily understood."

Before the Christian era (the first period) there is comparatively nothing that is worth recording. From the time of Christ up to the eighteenth century we have such a small showing that I would denominate that as the second period in the history of dentistry. What have we found during that period? No journals, no societies—only a few rambling notices of events which did not foretell even the beginning of societies—simply the observations of one man, too often not clearly expressed. The few books which were produced before 1800 may be found in C. G. Crowley's "Bibliography," but as Crowley was not a dentist many things appear in that volume which can in no sense be considered as of strictly dental origin.

In the translation of F. Maury's work there is an attempt to give a list of dental works and periodicals. "The History of Dental and Oral Science in America," by J. E. Dexter, 1876, has a meager list of books, but it has a complete list of periodicals published in the United States of America, up to that date. In France, England, Holland, Germany, and Italy many essays and monographs had been printed by dentists before 1700, but unfortunately many of them are in the nature of pamphlets for popular distribution. A few are theses for a doctorate, and some are descriptive of methods of practice intended to serve as guides for other practitioners. It cannot be denied that a free and wholly scientific desire to instruct and improve his fellow-man in a professional way did not seize the spirit of the dentist in any country much before the year 1760. After that date the writings of the educated dentist became more valuable, as they delineated methods of practice, discovered new facts in anatomy and pathology, and up to the period of the establishment of the monthly journal, in 1839, pamphlets were all the rage. This was true in other countries as well as in the United

States of America. In the early periods
before 1760, the majority of the practitioners were ignorant even of the scanty
medical and surgical knowledge of the
times. It is true that here and there
may be found a writer of education, general and special, but too many of the
brochures display a superficial knowledge
of the scientific status of the times.

If you would seek to obtain a history
of dental literature, you will have to gain
access to the books written between 1720
and the present day. The late Dr. Patrick of Belleville, Illinois, attempted to
outline a history of dental literature in
periods, but he did not live to finish his
task. Many of the works written in the
years included between 1700 and 1800
have not been translated into English.
Some of these have appeared in French
and German, and a few have been written in Latin. It can be said that more
works written by English-speaking authors have been translated into French,
German, Dutch, and other languages
since 1800, than all others combined.
This is due perhaps to the fact that dental journals and dental societies have
been more numerous in the United States
of America and England than in other
countries. The secrets of the operating
room have been disclosed more rapidly
than in some countries where a general
diffusion of scientific and practical
knowledge was not obtainable through
books and journals.

We may date the third period of dental literature, therefore, from the date
when societies, colleges, and journals
were established. All of these tremendous forces contributed to the dissemination of real scientific knowledge; authors
were encouraged to write books; the
rapid accessions to the profession from
the establishment of all these engines of

advancement furnished a sale for those
works, and many were stimulated to
write, for by so doing they became self-
educated.

If you will look over the transactions
of societies during the years from 1840
to 1880, or the files of the dental journals, or the lists of those who received
honorary degrees during that period, you
will see that many of the authors of
papers and books had, by their studies
and experiments, deserved such honors.
The easy entrance to the profession
caused many men to adopt it—illiterate
but ambitious; so the profession was soon
crowded with them, as may be seen by
reading their productions. The editors
of journals in many instances were not
qualified to judge of the literary merits of
a short paper, and indeed they were only
too anxious to fill their pages to be too
severely critical, if there was a good practical idea in a page of manuscript. You
may conclude that much which the patient reader will have to wade through
is of little value. Look at Taft's "Index
of Dental Literature," to convince yourself of this fact. The pages of the
American Journal of Dental Science,
the *Dental News Letter,* the *Dental Register,* and other journals of that period,
teem with the most elementary and unscientific matter, from 1840 to 1860.
About that time new blood began to be
infused, better-educated men wrote more
frequently, the air was full of invention
and discovery, and the literary quality
of the productions was improved; text-
books and original works on truly scientific subjects began to multiply in this
and other countries, through the influence of such men as Owen, Tomes, Heath,
Salter, Coleman, and Hulme in England; Robin, Magitot, Rottenstein, Le-
gros, Vergne, and others in France;

Waldeyer, Wedl, Brück, Zsigmondy, and Suersen in German-speaking countries; and Harris, Taft, Arthur, Richardson, Watt, Garretson, and a host of others in the United States of America. We began then to find, not exactly a plethora of books, but a sufficient number so that the students in colleges could be taught and be thoroughly grounded in the fundamentals, as well as in advanced professional knowledge.

In all countries journals multiplied, colleges were established, laws governing the exercise of the right to practice were passed, medical congresses established sections of odontology. The dental congress, international in character, was evolved, and now it is a rare thing to find that a dentist is not acquainted with the newest facts in science or practice, no matter where he is located. This is all due to the unstinted development of dental literature and the wide circulation it obtains throughout the civilized world. There is scarcely a country of one-half million inhabitants where there is not already established a dental periodical of some sort, and you will not find a dentist in the most obscure hamlet in any country who does not possess at least a catalog of some dental dealer descriptive of the latest method of producing anesthesia or the baking of a porcelain inlay.

In this very imperfect survey of dental literature, I have only attempted to show some of the reasons for its growth, the immense value it must be to the practitioner, and to say that there can be no limit to the usefulness and value of books and periodicals when carefully written, carefully edited, and conceived in a spirit of broad conservatism added to an exact and definite knowledge of the subject portrayed.

Discussion.

Dr. A. H. THOMPSON, Topeka, Kan. I was very much interested in this paper. Such statistics are very valuable. The prehistoric literature of our profession is of considerable interest, as shown by one of our foreign friends whose exhibit is in the hallway, but of course is of interest only in a curious way. We cannot always presume that everything we have is new. While our literature has improved in quantity I regret that it has not improved in quality, as shown by our journals of the present day. This is very discouraging to the student. We would like to see an improvement, but it seems to me there is no improvement in the last fifty years. The old *American Journal of Dental Science* contained articles better written than those of today. The quality has not improved as it should have done. The writers of today do not study our literature as they should. They bring out as new, ideas that have been passed on years ago. The history of the evolution of our literature is very interesting. The text-books are of better quality than the journals, but even these show a lack of knowledge of what has gone before that is very injurious to the student. All writers should aim to improve the quality of their work, and this paper should tend to a betterment of the literature of the day.

Dr. JAMES TRUMAN, Philadelphia, Pa. I really cannot let my friend's statement go by without objection—that the journals of today are not as good as they were forty or fifty years ago. We certainly have advanced. The better journals (and I am not speaking of those commercial journals that are mediums for advertisements) contain a literature very worthy to be honored. I am speaking of the average papers. I know there is much we are obliged to publish that is of no especial value, but when the work of the present moment is taken as a whole we are in an entirely different age from that of fifty years ago. I do not like to hear members of the dental profession say that there is nothing equal to the old journal that came out with its long lists of translations. Let us be just. Men of science in the dental profession are doing excellent work. The papers that came to me as chairman of the Committee on Prize Essays I think have never been excelled. Take, for instance, Dr. Röse's paper, "Pathology of Lime Salts in Nutrition." There is nothing published that gives a better idea of long and patient endeavor, of four or five years' careful and painstaking research to illustrate a point. Then there are Professor Miller's paper and two or three others. Those who attend regularly the national and local meetings of this country know that the literature is far in advance of that of any other period. Take the text-books—why, there is nothing to compare with them in the past. It would perhaps be out of place to name these, but the students of 1850 will recall the text-books of that period, and will repudiate the idea that the literature of that time was better than this.

Dr. WILLIAM H. TRUEMAN, Philadelphia, Pa. About 1768 a distinguished London dentist, Thomas Berdmore, wrote a treatise upon "The Disorders and Deformities of the Teeth and Gums," and a praiseworthy work it is, except for a few misleading lines in the preface. Excusing himself for avoiding quotations he says, "I could have only quoted a few French authors who have written *to make their names known*, and one or two English who have translated very injudi-

ciously." He would have us understand by this that at the time he wrote, dental literature did not amount to much. This work was republished in 1844 by the American Association of Dental Surgeons as part of the American Library of Dental Science, and the profession in this country seems to have "caught on" to this misstatement and are fond of repeating it. The old dental pioneers are usually credited with a well-thumbed copy of "Hunter on the Teeth," the only dental work extant a hundred years ago, and the reminiscences now and again appearing in the dental journals invariably recite the stereotyped phrase, "There were very few dental books when they began practice, 'way back in the thirties or forties." Now when the American Association of Dental Surgeons proposed, about 1840, to republish some of the old dental works, an English dentist very kindly placed at their disposal his dental library of some one hundred separate titles from which to make selection. It was a choice collection, containing many of the more notable works published up to that time; it was, however, far, very far, from being complete. So you see dental books were not so very scarce fifty or sixty years ago. As to the character of these old dental works, I refer you to that of Eustachius, published in 1563, to that of Hemard, dated a few years later, to the works of Fauchard, Mouton, Lecluse, Bourdet, Jourdain, Gariot, and Joseph Fox, as samples of the dental literature extant a hundred years ago.

It is true, prior to 1839 there were no dental journals. There were, however, a large number of medical and scientific journals through which practitioners of dental surgery made known to the world their observations and discoveries, and they were freely used. I have recently photographed a collection of daily newspapers published more than a century ago, containing many items of dental interest that would now be sent to dental journals.

Dental literature of the past is worthy of far more attention than it has yet received. The more we look into it the more we find, and the more we find to appreciate and admire in those who made it. The time was when its study would have been of much profit. Take, for instance, the use of arsenic for devitalizing exposed pulps. What a wonderful help it has been of itself, and by that which it has prompted, in tooth-saving. Had it been generally known to dental surgeons that this potent remedy was in constant use by the old Arabian physicians of more than a thousand years ago, as a last resort in persistent tooth-pain, would not this fact have suggested its use in conservative dentistry long before the time of John Spooner? Fauchard, in the first edition of his work, notes the invention of a machine for separating teeth and preparing cavities of decay for filling; later, Jourdain and Bourdet discuss its advantages and its failings; these works, with their useful suggestion, became "back numbers;" they were forgotten, and the advent of the indispensable dental engine was delayed more than a century. Mouton, in 1746, suggested the gold shell crown for restoring to usefulness badly broken-down teeth. He even suggested that when these are placed upon conspicuous front teeth they should be enameled so as to resemble in color the teeth on either side. While this suggestion was not entirely forgotten, it was but little used until a comparatively few years ago. It is not just to compare the work of these old writers with that of

today, or to disparage their theories or their methods because they seem in the light of the present, vague or crude.

For the early dental journals I have a high regard. The first twenty volumes of the *American Journal of Dental Science,* in my judgment, stand today without a peer. The journal was practical in the fullest sense of the word. Its contents, for the most part, were well written, they were helpful to its readers, and thoroughly up to date. Its editors were earnest, thoughtful, scholarly men; they gave to the world a dignified professional journal, and set up a standard of which we have every reason to be proud. There were other journals of which so much cannot be said, notwithstanding, however, they doubtless served a useful purpose, and have helped in the upbuilding of the profession. When we remember that our professional brethren are many, that they have varied tastes and varied needs, it seems a good thing that there are so many dental journals, and that they are not all alike. They are all doing a good work, and we wish them God-speed.

Dr. Harlan (closing the discussion). I have a copy of Fauchard and I do not underestimate its value and his knowledge of the times. But I said that from that period dated a practically better knowledge than any previous period. The knowledge his predecessors possessed was not demonstrated, for the books were not translated, and many of them were written in Latin and were not even translated into French; 1789 to 1860 gave us many articles of absolute merit; but I was taking a survey of all that we called dental literature. In many of the dental journals there were articles that could not gain entrance in a dental journal now, unless it was one of those we have already mentioned as advertising mediums, and while we are numerically much stronger, the dental literature produced from 1860 to the present time is of greater value to the world through the essence of what it presents than all that was presented prior to that time. I do not want to decry or underestimate the work that was done by these men; but of all the works Dr. Trueman mentioned none was published in a larger edition than from 100 to 150 copies, therefore they never had a wide circulation, and though of extreme value they

had no effect upon the formation of the dental thought of the time. Many of these works I have collected during my trips to Europe and I am familiar with them and many others, but it was to give a kind of *résumé* of the three periods that I tried to make clear in my paper, not to undervalue that which was good.

On motion the following paper by Dr. LOUIS OTTOFY, Manila, P. I., "History of Dentistry in the Philippine Islands," was read by title and ordered to be incorporated in the proceedings:

History of Dentistry in the Philippine Islands.

By LOUIS OTTOFY, D.D.S., Manila, P. I.

THE history of dentistry in the Philippine Islands is very brief. In 1900 I wrote a history of dental legislation* in which I covered the field to that date. A brief *résumé* of that article shows that prior to 1853 some legislation relating to dentists had been enacted, but as dentists were included with phlebotomists and midwives, and as there were no dentists in practice here at that time, I apprehend that the term dentist was included in the following way: It was customary with Spain to issue "royal decrees" and "royal orders" for her colonies. These orders and decrees were practically copies of laws then in force in Spain; and in case some regulation as to midwives, for instance, was necessary, the specific decree or order was sent out to the governors of the various colonies as copied from the home laws. Thus

a regulation was put in force here, governing dentists, before any were engaged in that calling.

The Royal Decree of September 22, 1853, provided that in order to practice dentistry it was required that one should prove that he had practiced at least three years under the tutelage of a practitioner who was designated by the term "professor." Those who were able to prove this could enter the University, and after passing an examination and paying a fee, were admitted to practice. The next enactment was the Royal Decree of June 4, 1875, which practically embodied all the essential features of the law as it was in force at the time of the American occupation. It provided, briefly: Dentistry constitutes a profession under the name of dental surgery; special certificate necessary; requires dentists to devote themselves only to the diseases of the mouth and teeth; the possession of certain theoretical and prac-

---

* *Dental Review*, vol. xiv, August 1900, p. 579.

tical knowledge must be shown; three medical and two dental practitioners compose the board of examiners; certificate of dental surgeon issued to successful candidates; examination fee, fifty pesetas, certificate fee, two hundred pesetas; dentists practicing, if considered worthy, may continue.

A Royal Order of May 28, 1876, one of December 6, 1881, and one of February 11, 1886, modify the previously issued decrees in minor details, as to method of enforcement, etc., and require all to register, while another order of May 1, 1890, places the examination under the charge of the rector of the University. Under the military government of the United States an order was issued in August 1899 requiring all dentists to register with the Board of Health, and this was the condition up to the passage of the present law, on January 10, 1903, which is hereafter referred to.

I am unable to secure any infallible data in regard to the practice of dentistry until the time the natives were brought under the influence of foreign dental practitioners. I invite your attention to an article signed "A Returned Soldier," published in a dental journal,* in which the soldier describes and illustrates primitive dentistry, and some of the tools used. I am unable to verify the correctness of the statements made, but in any event the practice and the instruments are evidently based on recent methods of, and modern appliances used by, dentists. In another magazine† one signing himself "A Regular" describes and illustrates some of the practices of

* *Dental Brief*, vol. vii, February 1902, p. 318.

† *Dental Review*, vol. xviii, April 1904, p. 318.

the "head-hunters" of Mindanao, showing the disfiguring practices of those people, as well as the tools used for filling the teeth, inserting pearls, etc. I am also unable to confirm the statements made in that article.

Like all semi-civilized people, the Filipinos also possessed some methods for relieving pain. One superstition was that if a piece of bamboo was whittled to a sharp point, ignited and charred, and then thrust into the skin on some part of the body, preferably the hand, the pain would cease. The old Chinese practice of "extracting the worms" from the teeth by holding the open mouth over a steaming vessel of hot water, was also practiced. From the shell of the cocoanut they also obtained substances giving relief. Into a half shell some water was placed and heated from underneath, thus practically boiling the water in the shell. By this process some principle was extracted from the shell, resembling creasote; this was then placed in the cavity. From careful inquiry from men who have lived here all their lives, and much of the time in the provinces, I am unable to gather anything reliable as to any practice worthy of note on this point, and it seems to me certain that practically nothing was done from a dental standpoint until about 1860.

In that year, or 1861, an American dentist, named Pettengill, visited the Islands, and entered into a lucrative practice among the few foreigners who were engaged in business in Manila; he was also patronized by the better-educated and wealthy natives. He employed as an assistant and student a native, José Arévalo, now eighty years of age, and justly entitled to be known as the "father of dentistry" in the Philippines. Since then his sons, a daughter, grandson, and other relatives have entered the profession. At the present time five of that family name are practicing in these Islands. Pettengill left and said that he would return, leaving his chair and instruments with Señor Arévalo, who continued in practice. Some time later Pettengill returned, and soon drew a handsome prize in the lottery, after which he disappeared from the Islands. With that beginning, Arévalo entered into practice, and did the best he could. A Frenchman, Mons. Petlere, also practiced here for a while. Dr. Melanchthon Stout, formerly of Chicago, now of Marlinton, West Virginia, visited the Islands some thirty years ago, and Dr. Eastlake, who practiced in Japan, is also said to have made visits to the Islands about that time, while others from the China coast made occasional visits to Manila, sometimes also going to Iloilo and Cebú. In 1888 a Cuban dentist, Señor Villa Raza, and about the same time Señor Conrado Martel Arandes, and other Spanish dentists, located in Manila. From the nucleus of Pettengill's visit, and with what could be gathered from other Americans and Spaniards, the native dentists picked up what they could. One Spanish lady and one of the native dentists tried to improve their education by a visit to Japan, while one native is a graduate of one of the schools in Philadelphia. Under these circumstances it is no wonder that but little progress has been made, and such as it is was made under difficulties.

Prior to the American occupation these men secured some medical instruction in the College of San José, a medical school affiliated with the University of Santo Tomás. This led to a certificate of a "Cirujano Ministrante" (Ministering Surgeon) at the end of a two years'

course. For four or five years preceding the insurrection of 1896 (soon after which the school was closed for several years) some attempt was made to teach extracting, treatment of teeth, etc., but no effort at the establishment of a regular dental course was ever made. Nor has there ever been any dental journal published here, or any regular dental supply house established.

When the Americans entered Manila in 1898 there were not to exceed twelve dentists practicing in the Islands. With the exception of one American and a few Spaniards they were all Filipinos, and nearly all of them were located in Manila. By reason of the disturbed conditions prior to the capitulation of the city, August 13, 1898, the only American dentist located in Manila had taken refuge in Hong-Kong, and therefore no American dentists were engaged in practice in Manila in September 1898. With the volunteer troops several dentists came out, and at least one was assigned by the military authorities to the troops; this was done by a detail to the Hospital Corps, and by permission being granted to the man so detailed to render dental services to the soldiers. Since then, not to exceed twenty American dentists have located in the Islands at various times, of whom not more than six are still in practice in the Islands.

On February 4, 1900, the Manila Dental Society was organized with a charter membership list of nine. During that year the society met with fair regularity and several papers were read and discussed. The unsettled condition of the Islands as well as the constantly changing personnel of the profession and the desire to confine the membership to those who understood English, resulted in apathy, which continued during the years .

1901, 1902, and 1903. At the annual meeting in February 1904, and since then, new members having been admitted, the drawback as regards the language is partially removed, Americans having acquired some knowledge of Spanish, while some of the Filipinos have become acquainted with English. The society has since that time met regularly, and several interesting papers have been read and discussed. Probably the first paper ever read in the Spanish language in the Islands by a native was read at the meeting in April of this year. The Filipinos are eager to learn, and the usefulness of the society henceforth seems assured.

In the fall of 1900 the Manila Dental College was organized, modeled on the basis of the advanced position of dental education in the United States. After one successful session the school had to be abandoned. The course laid out was entirely too advanced for Filipinos, while the changing character of the American population would have prevented the drawing of classes from among the Americans. Furthermore, by reason of the prevailing insurrection at that time, the conditions were unfavorable for the maintenance and growth of a dental school, or for that matter of any school, except those long established and connected with the monastic orders. Six or seven matriculated, of whom three American gentlemen, all connected with the Hospital Corps of the United States army, completed the full course. At least two of these gentlemen have since then completed their dental education in the United States, and both of them with honors.

During the summer and fall of 1901, the dentists appointed for the United States army, under the act of February 2d of that year, began to arrive in the Islands, and a base dental hospital and supply depot was established in connection with the First Reserve (military) Hospital in Manila. The members of the dental corps in the Islands until recently averaged about fifteen men, distributed at the various military posts in the Islands, and visiting outlying districts where troops are quartered. I am unable to give any report of the extensive and valuable services of the corps, and presume that such information will reach the congress through other sources.

An Act to Regulate the Practice of Dentistry in the Philippine Islands was passed by the Philippine Commission on January 10, 1903, a copy of which in English and Spanish I have transmitted to the Section on Dental Legislation of this congress. Under this act a number of members of the Army Dental Corps have registered, some of whom have since been transferred to the United States, while those still remaining, by the nature of their duties cannot be reckoned as resident dentists of the Islands. The register of the dental board contains a total of less than forty-five names (inclusive of temporary licenses and undergraduates) of whom not to exceed twenty-five are engaged in the *bona fide* practice of dentistry. Of this number nineteen are located in Manila, and on June 19, 1904, an effort was made to secure a group photograph of all those engaged in practice in this city, with the result that fifteen out of a possible nineteen responded to the call. I take pleasure in transmitting with this paper a copy of the photograph, which is representative. In the center of the foreground is José Arévalo, above referred to, as the "father of dentistry" in the Philippines, who is now eighty years of age, and retired. The group gives some idea of the polygenic population in the Orient. There are seven Filipinos, five Spaniards, one British subject, and two Americans represented in the group.

While a history deals only with the past, it may not be out of place at this time to look somewhat into the future. It should be remembered that the Philippine Islands have recently passed through a critical period, which has materially affected the economic welfare of the Islands and their inhabitants. The insurrection, which broke out in 1896, was followed by the war with Spain, and succeeded by another insurrection. In the meanwhile the Islands passed through a pestilence of plague and cholera, while the draft animals were decimated by such diseases as surra, glanders, the rinderpest, etc. Nor did the various crops escape unscathed, being often totally destroyed by a plague of locusts, and by various insects attacking the coffee plant and other vegetation. Happily, the Islands are now practically free from these scourges, and very little is now feared, except possibly from the locusts. It is not too optimistic to predict that the Islands are now entering on an era of prosperity.

It has been seen that the number of dentists in proportion to the population, which is over 6,000,000, and of whom many are educated, while a larger number are prosperous (or can be, under normal conditions) is very small. As a matter of fact, outside of the city of Manila, dentistry is a sealed book, and first of all the general education of people along the lines of dentistry is essential to create a demand for dental services. In another paper which I have contributed to this congress I have conclusively shown that caries and tooth-de-

struction is just as prevalent here as in the United States and elsewhere. In this large city of Manila, containing as it does a native and Chinese population of about a quarter of a million, there is no place where the poor may get relief except a small free dental clinic which I established last January and have since maintained in connection with St. Luke's Hospital. The mass of the people absolutely know nothing of dentistry.

One of the most important needs of the Islands is the establishment of a dental school, and that is now under consideration. The law is extremely favorable toward native young men who desire to make a beginning in this direction, contemplating a brief course of instruction, looking toward the giving of relief in remote sections of the country, the introduction of simple fillings, and substitution of the teeth when lost. It is believed that a small beginning will have to be made, and the course of instruction increased as the education of the people creates the demand for the higher class of service made possible by the advance made by the profession. Natives thus educated would be enabled to render services within the means of the people, being able to live inexpensively and subsist on less expensive food than foreigners. And in this lies the answer to the question, why there are practically no desirable locations for Americans or foreigners outside of Manila. Aside from this fact, it should be borne in mind that comparatively few foreigners are located in the Islands, that few natives speak Spanish, and that the knowledge of some native dialect is essential to enable one to get along with the people.

I hope in the near future to see such

steps inaugurated as will ultimately extend to these people the beneficent advantages accruing from the intelligent exercise of our profession.

On motion, Dr. WM. H. TRUEMAN'S paper, "Report of the Committee on the History of Dentistry," was read without discussion. It here follows:

Report of Committee on the History of Dentistry.

By WILLIAM H. TRUEMAN, D.D.S., Philadelphia, Pa.,
CHAIRMAN.

YOUR Committee on Dental History beg leave to report that after a careful survey of the field it was deemed wise to confine their efforts to one object, the history of dental educational institutions. They regret that, although this choice of subject was approved, they failed, except in one instance, to secure the co-operation of their *confrères* in other lands.

From Dr. Vincenzo Guerini of Naples, Italy, they have received an excellent paper entitled "Italian Writers on Dental Science and Their Works."* This subject is quite new in dental history, and, coming from so capable and careful a writer, is a notable addition to dental history.

Dr. William Simon of Baltimore, a member of its faculty, has contributed an exhaustive history of the Baltimore College of Dental Surgery, the first dental school in the world's history.

Dr. Wm. L. J. Griffin of Philadelphia has contributed an interesting history of the Philadelphia College of Dental Surgery, the first dental school in Philadelphia, and of its successor, the Pennsylvania College of Dental Surgery. He has also contributed histories of the Dental Department of the University of Pennsylvania and the Dental Depart-

ment of the Medico-Chirurgical College of Philadelphia.

From Dr. Charles McManus of Hartford, Conn., we have histories of Tufts College Dental School and of the Dental Department of Harvard University.

From Dr. Burton Lee Thorpe of St. Louis, Mo., a list of the Western dental colleges, accompanied, where data could be obtained, by a brief sketch of their rise and progress.

Your committee has found great difficulty in obtaining accurate data for this work. Apathy in some cases, and loss of original records owing to changes in location or management, or from accident, in others, has greatly hampered their efforts.

As in all research work, so in this, results are not always commensurate with the labor expended, although that labor may not be in vain. As an instance of this, Dr. Clarence J. Grieves of Baltimore, a member of your committee, spent several months endeavoring to ascertain what had been done in this country toward systematic dental education prior to the advent of dental colleges. After patiently exhausting every available clue, while he found much that was suggestive and that might be true, he found nothing sufficiently authenticated to be considered "history." In this case, a synopsis of

---

* See Vol. I, page 73.

lectures by Dr. Hayden upon dental science, which would have proved valuable in determining this question, was, it was ascertained, destroyed by a fire which a few years ago annihilated the library in which they were deposited. No one has so far been found who could say positively when or where they were delivered; nor can this be determined by any trustworthy record.

Many of the early records of the first college in Philadelphia met a like fate, and are irretrievably lost.

These two instances emphasize the importance of promptly placing on record well-authenticated histories of all our professional institutions.

Your committee desires to acknowledge historic information received from Dr. Erastus Wilson of Havana, Cuba, regretting, however, that owing to the limited time at their disposal, they have been unable to present it to the present congress.

Respectfully submitted,
WILLIAM H. TRUEMAN,
Chairman.

VINCENZO GUERINI,
WILLIAM SIMON,
W. L. J. GRIFFIN,
BURTON LEE THORPE,
CLARENCE J. GRIEVES,
Members.

———

Following are printed the several papers (1-VIII) accompanying the report of the Committee on the History of Dentistry. The first paper is by Dr. WILLIAM SIMON of Baltimore, Md., as follows:

I.

History of the Baltimore College of Dental Surgery.

By WILLIAM SIMON, Ph.D., M.D., Baltimore, Md.

I. INTRODUCTORY.

THE progress of civilization has been due chiefly to the labors of those few men who through their greater ability, intellectuality, and energy occupied positions often far ahead of their contemporaries. This statement, while applicable in every sphere of human activity, finds special corroboration when we apply it to the conditions existing in the dental practice of former periods. For hundreds, yes for thousands of years, the care-taking of diseased teeth had been very largely in the hands of ignorant, uneducated, and unscrupulous persons. It was often the barber and watchmaker, the shepherd and blacksmith, if not the quack and charlatan, to whom the people applied in times of sadly needed dental aid. Yet during all this period we find men who through their superior skill, their painstaking care, and intelligent interpretation of existing conditions stood far above the average dental manipulator of those days.

If we consider for a moment the conditions as they existed in the first quarter of the last century, we find that both in this country and in Europe fairly good, and at times even very good, dental work was done by a limited number of practitioners. Some of them had laid the foundation for their dental knowledge under the tutorship of other practitioners, while most of them were self-taught, there being neither schools nor much readily accessible literature to assist any-

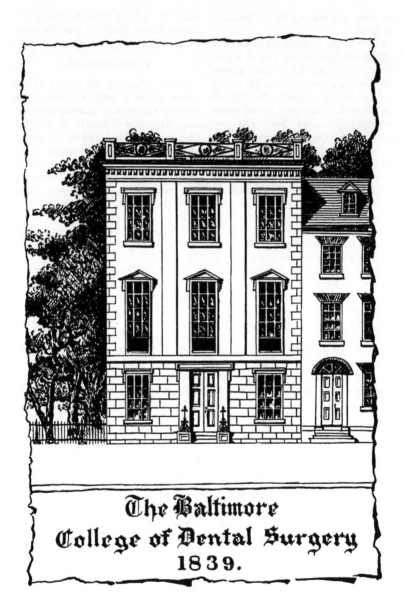

The Baltimore
College of Dental Surgery
1839.

one desiring to take up the profession of the dentist.

Although the study of the diseases of teeth should have formed part of a physician's education, the medical schools gave practically no instruction pertaining to this subject. Indeed, the medical practitioners of those days looked rather contemptuously upon those who performed any kind of dental operations.

These sad conditions were fully understood by those few prominent men who recognized that much good might be accomplished by proper dissemination of dental knowledge through the three principal channels open to us, viz: (1) Through personal contact of the parties engaged in the common field of labor, i.e. through exchange of thoughts and experience in association meetings; (2) through literature, especially when in the form of periodical journals; (3) through proper theoretical and practical instruction given at well-appointed institutions.

The thought that these means should be employed no doubt had been in the minds of many, and indeed a few isolated efforts were made here and there to bring about the desired result; but it was not until the fourth decade of the nineteenth century that the first institution giving instruction in the science and art of dentistry was founded, and that almost simultaneously the first dental journal and the first dental association were established. It is not without significance that the founders of the first institution for teaching dentistry were also instrumental in calling into life the first journal and the first association devoted to the exclusive benefit of the dental practitioner.

It is to the history of this first dental school in the world, chartered in 1840

under the title of "The Baltimore College of Dental Surgery," that this paper is devoted.

II. THE FOUNDERS.

Before taking up the history of the college it may be well to introduce the two men who were its founders and creators. They were Horace H. Hayden and Chapin A. Harris, to whom the dental profession, as well as the people of the whole civilized world, owe everlasting gratitude. They stand out prominently and conspicuously as intelligent, energetic, far-sighted, and unselfish men, willing and ready to give freely to others their knowledge and experience, and to do so cheerfully even at a personal sacrifice.

Horace H. Hayden was born October 13, 1769, at Windsor, Conn. One of his ancestors was William Hayden, who distinguished himself in the Pequot War of 1637 to such an extent that he received from the colony of Connecticut a tract of land for gallantry in battle. That land, granted in 1642, is still in possession of the family, which has owned it for 262 years. Many of the descendants of William Hayden occupied prominent positions as members of the General Court of Connecticut, or as officers in the Colonial service, participating in the French and Indian Wars. The father of Dr. Hayden served with distinction in the Revolutionary War for seven years. When the war ended he returned to his home and took up his profession, which was that of architect and builder. The mother of Dr. Hayden, a Miss Abigail Parsons, was descended "from one of the brainiest families in New England." It is thus seen that Dr. Hayden had the advantage of distinguished and intellectual ancestry.

Being a boy during the Revolution, he and his mother took care of the farm, while all the men were in the army, the mother giving him also his first training in elementary schooling. At the age of ten years he began the study of ancient languages, in which he became quite proficient. It is said that during his boyhood he exhibited a remarkable liking for natural history, often surprising his friends by his ingenuity and success in discovering objects of interest while rambling in the woods.

His schooling was interrupted by two trips to the West Indies in a brig on which he served as a cabin boy. At the age of sixteen he learned the trade of carpenter and architect from his father. Even at this early stage of his career he showed that mere mechanical work did not satisfy him and that his mind had to take an active part in his duties. To satisfy this desire he procured such books on modern and ancient architecture as were obtainable, and the combined results of his studies and practical experience were laid down in a number of drawings and writings.

The charms of the West Indies must have left quite an impression on the boy, because he sailed twice (at the age of twenty-one and at twenty-two) to the islands with the view of locating there permanently. Fortunately, attacks of fever drove him back to the States, and for several years he followed his vocation as architect; also teaching school near Hartford for one winter.

Then (in 1795) an incident occurred which became the turning-point in Hayden's life-work. Requiring the professional service of a dentist he called on Mr. John Greenwood of New York, and so deeply was he impressed with the skill of this dentist and with the possibilities of the art that he concluded to adopt dentistry as his calling. He at once procured such books and essays as were available for his purpose, and with the energy that was so characteristic of him commenced the study of dentistry.

When thirty-one years old, i.e. in the year 1800 or 1801, Hayden came to Baltimore, rented a room, and made known that his services as dentist were at the command of the public. He soon made a success as a dental practitioner, the people quickly appreciating his skill and painstaking work.

Realizing that an intelligent treatment of diseases of the teeth depended largely on a thorough knowledge of the human system, he studied anatomy, physiology, and, to some extent, other medical branches. Indeed, we find him as an investigator of physiological and pathological conditions, his researches in this field being concerned in the functions of the thyroid, salivary, lacrymal, and other glands of the human system.

That his scientific attainments were recognized by the medical profession is best shown by the fact that in 1837 the honorary degree of Doctor of Medicine was conferred on him by both the Jefferson College of Medicine of Philadelphia and the University of Maryland.

In 1814 the blood of his martial ancestors running through his veins compelled Hayden to take an active part in the battle of North Point. He first enlisted in Captain Warner's company of militia, but later was appointed assistant surgeon in the hospital.

While from the time of his taking up dentistry his profession and its promotion were nearest to his heart, yet his versatile mind was not satisfied to work in one direction only. His love for nature, developed in his boyhood days on the banks of the Connecticut river, remained during his life. Indeed, he devoted much

21

of his time to botany, to geology, and to the culture of silkworms. He wrote on these subjects, and his "Geological Essays," a book of 400 pages, published in 1821, was the first general work on geology printed in the United States. A new mineral which he discovered was named "Haydenite" in his honor.

In 1818 Hayden took an active part in the founding of the Baltimore Physical Association, for the promotion of natural science, of which society he became the first secretary. This society was the forerunner of the Maryland Academy of Sciences.

The thought of forming a national dental association had been in Hayden's mind long before this society became a reality. As early as 1817 he advocated a union of dental practitioners, but apparently the time and conditions were as yet not ripe for the undertaking.

Years later he visited Boston and other Eastern cities and found his professional brethren more willing and ready to co-operate with him in any practical scheme to elevate the profession. It was, however, not until August 18, 1840, that a number of prominent dentists assembled in New York city and founded the "American Society of Dental Surgeons," of which Hayden was chosen first president, continuing in that office until his death. Most justifiably does Dr. Burton Lee Thorpe, in his excellent biographical sketch of Hayden,* call him the "father of the American Society of Dental Surgeons."

At the birth of this society Hayden expressed his great satisfaction in the progress dentistry had made during the previous forty years. He himself, he said, had seen the development of the pro-

fession from the days when the name of dentist was a reproach and a byword, to the time when men of learning, worth, and genius had been added to its ranks.

Continuing, Dr. Hayden spoke as follows: "At the present period renewed efforts are making in England France, and Scotland to place our profession on still higher ground than it has yet attained; and shall we of these United States of America remain inactive in this grand endeavor? If, like the Jews, we are scattered and despised, may we not, like that persecuted people, at least hope for a day of restoration to our promised land? There are indeed many obstacles still to overcome! A new race of Canaanites must be expelled from our borders. Many errors must be exploded and much ignorance must be dispelled before the light of truth will beam clearly upon our path; but with diligence, zeal, and perseverance we are certain of ultimate success. Let us, therefore, go forward in the good cause, unintimidated by the skepticism of the faithless, the fears of the timid, or the apathy of the selfish. If there are some who prefer to plod onward in the path of private enterprise, let us unite our efforts in one great social endeavor to elevate our profession from the degraded condition to which it has sunk and in which it must ever remain until the high-minded and well-educated amongst its practitioners shall unitedly arise and shake themselves from the dust."

Almost simultaneously with the founding of the first* dental association came the publication of the *American Journal of Dental Science*. Although Hayden's

* *Dental Review*, Sept. 15, 1902.

* Several local societies preceded it, but they were short-lived and left no impress upon the profession.

name neither appears as a member of the publishing committee nor as one of the editors, yet he was instrumental in organizing the journal. Dr. Wm. H. Trueman* justly remarks: "It is generally recognized that Horace H. Hayden's was the master mind pushing forward the movement which was rapidly bringing about important results for the advancement of the dental profession."

Most of the great men whose minds bring out new ideas and whose work creates new conditions, seem to be compelled to share with others the fruits of their labors; they must give vent to their overcrowded minds, brim-full with new impressions, new facts, new theories, new discoveries.

What should be more natural than that these men become not only the leaders but the instructors and teachers of others. And Hayden was a teacher *par excellence*. Almost from the time when he began the practice of his profession in Baltimore he was accustomed to hold classes in dentistry in his office at night, with no light but the tallow dip. He continued this work until the college was decided upon. Elisha Townsend, the founder of the first dental college in Philadelphia, was one of the men who thus received his education; and indeed, Townsend remarked in later years that "all he ever knew of dentistry was the result of Dr. Hayden's instruction."

That dentists should be educated like other professional men in schools and colleges was a thought often brought out by Hayden in his conversations, and as he always looked upon dentistry as a branch of medicine his desire was to obtain a foothold for dentistry in medical schools.

Having discussed this matter with some of his friends who were members of the medical faculty of the University of Maryland, this institution invited him to give a course of lectures before the medical class in the session 1837-38. This most likely was the first attempt to introduce dentistry as a branch of medical education. The lectures were not a success from the students' point of view. We learn this best from a letter* by Dr. H. Willis Baxley, who writes: "Dr. H. H. Hayden delivered to a few medical students of the University of Maryland some lectures on dental physiology and pathology. I was one of his class, and found the lectures very speculative and unsatisfactory. Certain it is that those engaged in tooth-pulling, filing, and filling, which then seemed the sole business of the craft, took no interest in Dr. Hayden's attempt to enlighten them. Nevertheless he is entitled to credit for an effort, however unsuccessful, to give dentistry better claims to public confidence."

One can now readily understand that Hayden's scientific treatment of his subject did not meet with the approval of medical students, who most likely would have preferred some demonstration in practical work. However, there can be no doubt that Hayden's attempt to teach scientific dentistry by a course of lectures was the starting-point for the founding of the college a few years later.

Dr. Hayden married February 23, 1805, at Baltimore, Marie Antoinette Robinson, daughter of Lieutenant Daniel Robinson, a United States revenue officer. He died January 26, 1844, when seventy-five years old, and was buried in the family vault in Greenmount cemetery.

---

*American Journal of Dental Science, June 1903.

* This letter, dated London, Sept. 29, 1874, is in the archives of the Baltimore College of Dental Surgery.

Chapin A. Harris was born at Pompey, Onondaga county, N. Y., in 1806. He commenced his medical studies when quite young and began practice in Ohio. His attention was called to dentistry by his brother, John Harris, but he gave little attention to the subject until he moved to Baltimore, where he became a pupil of Hayden. Under the guidance and influence of Hayden's master mind Harris soon became imbued with his teacher's views regarding the problems requisite for the elevation of the dental profession. Being young, aggressive, ambitious, full of energy, and thoroughly equipped mentally, he grasped the situation and succeeded in accomplishing results where others might have failed. He brought order out of the chaotic state of dental knowledge and published his results in the first dental text-book, "Harris' Principles and Practice of Dentistry," and in the first "Dental Dictionary."

From the second year of the founding of the *American Journal of Dental Science, i.e.* from 1840, Dr. Harris was one of the editors, and retained this position until 1850, when the journal passed into his hands, and he continued to be both its owner and editor until his death.

Harris was one of the founders of the American Society of Dental Surgeons, and president in 1844. He was also editor of the *Guardian of Health*, a publication which appeared in 1841. After the death of Hayden he was elected president of the college and retained this position until his death, September 29, 1860.

In the founding of the college Harris took a most active part; indeed, it was he who pushed matters. He solicited signatures from influential citizens to the application to the legislature for a charter, and looked after many other details.

He thus relieved Hayden of a great deal of work which at the high age of seventy would have been a burden to him. Thus brought into the foreground, Harris was looked upon as the originator of the plan of founding the college by those who did not understand the situation and did not know that the driving force back of Harris was Hayden.

The question has been repeatedly asked to which of the two men is the greater honor due, and specially, in whose mind was born the thought of establishing a dental school. Indeed, there has been a period when this question was hotly contested by opposing parties taking sides for one or the other of the two founders. This time, fortunately, has passed, and we may now judge more calmly and impartially of the share each one has taken in the establishment of the institution.

It appears to the writer that neither of these men alone would have succeeded. In many respects they supplemented one another admirably, and thus through exchange of thought and through combining their forces the creation of the college was made possible.

The respective merits of each that have a bearing on the question may be briefly summarized thus:

Hayden was fond of teaching, as shown by the fact that he delivered lectures at the university and gave evening classes at his office; that he strongly believed in and labored for the advancement of scientific pursuits in general, and that of dentistry more especially; he was imbued with the idea that only through proper dissemination of knowledge and through the combined action of the workers existing conditions could be improved. But to some extent Hayden's great intellectuality overshadowed his practical endowments, and here it was that Harris supplied the lacking force. Harris was not only a man of science, but also of the practical affairs of the world. Just as it was in him to create order out of the chaos of diffused dental knowledge when writing his great text-book, so he possessed the power of systematizing and

man—and found him in Harris—to show the way for carrying out his lofty ideas, to take the necessary steps in matters of detail, such as securing a charter, forming a faculty, creating a board of visitors, etc.

The plans were perfected and details arranged at Dr Hayden's office, where

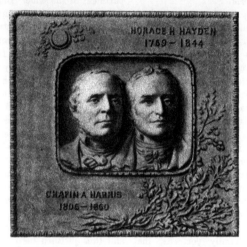

FOUNDERS OF THE BALTIMORE COLLEGE OF DENTISTRY.

(Excellent portraits of Drs. Hayden and Harris are also presented in the paper entitled "A Biographical Review of the Careers of Hayden and Harris," by Dr. Burton Lee Thorpe. See pages 414 and 415.)

organizing other affairs or of solving problems of a practical nature.

Even in the respective chairs occupied by the two men this difference in their powers is brought out. Hayden lectured on dental pathology and physiology, branches which at that time were largely of a theoretical, if not of a hypothetical nature. Harris was professor of practical dentistry, and as such had to deal with facts and actualities. Now, while dental education was uppermost in the mind of Hayden, yet he needed the

the two men were closeted together night after night for many weeks prior to the establishment of the college.

That Dr. Hayden was the moving spirit in the undertaking may be inferred from the fact that he was made and remained to his death the president of the college. That the institution from the day of its birth was a complete success seems to have been largely due to the efficiency, tact, organizing power, and untiring labors of Dr. Harris.

Surely there is honor enough to divide,

and we may well apply the answer of Goethe which he gave when told that there was a doubt in the minds of many whether he or Schiller was the greatest poet of the times. Said Goethe, "What use to discuss this matter? the people ought to be glad that two such men as we are in this world."

Thus, not only the dental profession, but the people generally ought to be glad and grateful that two such men as Hayden and Harris existed and laid the foundation for an institution which was destined to exercise a vast influence upon the practice of dentistry in the whole civilized world.

That to the two men, Hayden and Harris, who had labored so faithfully and successfully in elevating dentistry, some lasting memorial was due by the profession was recognized a few years ago when a committee was formed to take up the matter. As a result of the agitation Mr. Ernest W. Keyser, the talented sculptor, was employed to model in relief, after family portraits, the heads of the two men, showing them life size, in the prime of life. Two of these beautiful mural tablets, cast in bronze, were dedicated with appropriate ceremonies in the winter of 1902-03, one at the Baltimore College of Dental Surgery, and one in the Dental Department of the University of Maryland. (See page 297.)

III. THE CHARTER.

Ever since Dr. Hayden had delivered dental lectures in the medical department of the University of Maryland during the winter of 1837, his mind was occupied with the thought of supplying means for a thorough dental education. It appears that both he and Dr. Harris made efforts to induce the University of Maryland to add dental instruction to their medical course.

Dr. Eugene F. Cordell,* the acknowledged authority on the medical history of Maryland, speaks thus: "The founders of the school first endeavored to engraft it upon the university as a separate department of the same. Being unsuccessful in this, doubtless owing to the unsettled condition of the latter, which had shortly before this been rent in twain and was but just emerging from a nearly fatal lawsuit, they boldly launched out upon the untried sea, with an independent school. Their immediate and marked success shows that this effort was opportune and that they supplied a real want."

That both men, Hayden and Harris, worked together in their efforts to obtain favorable action by the University of Maryland is shown by the fact that the faculty of the university addressed to Dr. Harris the letter rejecting the proposition, giving as an excuse, "that the subject of dentistry was of little consequence, and thus justified their unfavorable action."

The plan having failed, the independent college was decided upon. As stated before, Harris for many weeks prior to the obtaining of the charter spent night after night at the office of Dr. Hayden, and here it was that the plans were laid out and gradually perfected. Here no doubt it was, where the degree of "Doctor of Dental Surgery" was decided upon, and it is needless to ask by which one of the two men this degree was proposed. As often happens in such cases, it might have been difficult for Hayden and Harris themselves to say positively who created the title, which most likely was the outcome of many deliberations.

* "The Medical Annals of Maryland," page 105.

All preliminary matter for the establishment of the college having been finally arranged, a charter was applied for and granted by the legislature in session at Annapolis. The document is of sufficient interest to find at least in part a place here. It reads:

AN ACT INCORPORATING THE BALTIMORE COLLEGE OF DENTAL SURGERY.

Passed February 1, 1840.

SECTION I. Be it enacted by the General Assembly of Maryland, that a College of Dentistry be, and the same is hereby established in the city of Baltimore, to be known and designated by the name and style of THE BALTIMORE COLLEGE OF DENTAL SURGERY.

SEC. II. And be it enacted, that the following persons be and are hereby appointed and constituted the Professors of said College, to wit: Horace H. Hayden, M.D., to be Professor of Dental Pathology and Physiology; Chapin A. Harris, M.D., to be Professor of Practical Dentistry; Thomas E. Bond, Jr., M.D., to be Professor of Special Dental Pathology and Therapeutics, and H. Willis Baxley, M.D., to be Professor of Special Dental Anatomy and Physiology.

SEC. III. And be it enacted, that the said Professors and their successors shall be, and are hereby declared to be a Corporation and body politic, to be perpetuated under the name of The Baltimore College of Dental Surgery.

Sections IV to VI refer to legal rights and obligations, to the election of officers, filling of vacancies, holding of meetings, etc.

Section VII states that the professors and their successors shall hold at least one term in every year, for the period of four months, for the purpose of delivering lectures and instruction in the different branches of dental science, for which they are empowered to charge such fees as they may deem proper.

SEC. VIII. And be it enacted, that R. S. Stewart, M.D.; Joshua T. Cohen, M.D.; Thomas E. Bond, M.D.; Thomas C. Risteau, M.D.; Rev. John G. Morris, Rev. Beverly Waugh, John H. Briscoe, M.D.; Samuel Chew, M.D.; Rev. George C. M. Roberts, M.D.; John James Graves, M.D.; Rev. Dr. J. P. K. Henshaw, Rev. James G. Hamner, John Fonerden, M.D.; Leonard Mackall, M.D., and Enoch Noyes, be appointed a Board of Visitors, to be styled the Board of Visitors of the Baltimore College of Dental Surgery, who shall be empowered to examine into the state and condition of the Institution, and see that the requirements of this Charter are fulfilled.

Sections IX and X contain provisions for conferring the degree of Doctor of Dental Surgery on students having been found worthy of it after an examination, and of conferring the same honorary degree on any dentist who may have rendered service to the science, or distinguished himself otherwise in his profession.

Sections XI to XIII contain merely formal legal matters of no interest here.

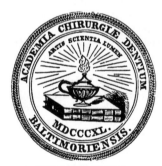

SEAL OF THE COLLEGE.

The charter seems to have been modeled after the charters of medical schools and contains all essential provisions for carrying on the work of such institutions.

Of interest is the long list of members of the Board of Visitors, embodying a number of the most prominent scientific Baltimoreans of that time.

We also find in the document the

names of Drs. Thomas E. Bond and H. Willis Baxley, who with Drs. Hayden and Harris formed the faculty, as also the incorporators of the college. That all four members of the faculty were entitled to affix M.D. to their names shows that the best of dentists of these times fully appreciated the advantage of a medical education for the dental practitioner.

IV. THE FIRST COLLEGE YEAR.

The charter having been granted on February 1, two days later the first official faculty meeting was held and is reported in the "Record of the Proceedings of the Faculty of the Baltimore College of Dental Surgery," thus:

"A meeting of the faculty of this institution was held February the 3d, at half-past seven o'clock P.M., at the house of Dr. H. H. Hayden, with a view to its organization by the election of a president and dean.

"On motion, Dr. H. H. Hayden was appointed chairman and Dr. C. A. Harris secretary. A motion was then made that the faculty proceed to the election of the officers above named; whereupon Dr. H. H. Hayden was nominated and elected president and Dr. C. A. Harris dean. There being no other business before the faculty, it adjourned."

It is somewhat significant that neither Dr. Bond nor Dr. Baxley is mentioned in the above minutes, though it must be supposed that they were present at this, the first faculty meeting. The omission shows, like all data at the writer's disposal, that the chief work was done by Hayden and Harris, the other two men having been invited to become members of the faculty in order to have their co-operation chiefly as teachers.

The next task of the faculty was to secure students for the first session, and of this Dr. Baxley wrote in a letter: "The practical inauguration of the new college presented a difficulty well known in America, where professors often outnumbered students. At length five legitimate students of dentistry were found to covet the honor of the new title D.D.S., and the first course of instruction was given in the winter of 1840-41. The didactic lectures were delivered in a small room, publicly situated, but the teaching of practical anatomy demanded privacy; other prudential considerations also suggested the use for that purpose of a secluded stable loft.

That efforts were made to let the world know that a school for dental instruction had been established, is shown by the action taken in the second faculty meeting held May 15, 1840. It was then decided upon to insert a proper advertisement in the following journals or newspapers: *National Intelligencer, Globe, Philadelphia U. S. Gazette, Louisville Journal, American Journal of Dental Science, American Journal of Medical Sciences, Maryland Medical and Surgical Journal, Baltimore American, Patriot, Charleston Courier,* and *Baltimore Pilot.*

Besides thus advertising the institution, an "Annual Announcement of the Board of Visitors" was issued, and as this publication contains many points of interest it may be best to present it here in full:

ANNUAL ANNOUNCEMENT.

In announcing the incorporation of a college, organized with particular reference to instruction in Dental Science, the Board of Visitors deem it proper to state the considerations which have prompted its projectors to engage in the enterprise, and also to make known the general plan of instruction which it is proposed to pursue, and the requisitions to be complied with by candidates for the honors of the Institution.

It is well known to all that the wants of society resulting from diseases and distortions of the teeth, and the morbid conditions of collateral structures, are multiplied and great; but it is only those who have made it a subject of particular inquiry who are aware of the fact that the number of those professing to control these diseases, and correct these distortions, who are competently educated dentists is small in proportion to the many engaged in the practice of this profession. It has been ascertained that there are about 1200 professing dentists in the United States; of these but a few have enjoyed the advantages of collegiate instruction in this science. Some, it is true, have overcome the difficulties encountered in the commencement of their studies, and by the persevering application of rare abilities in the pursuit of knowledge, have contributed to enlarge the boundaries of usefulness, and established for themselves just claims to distinction. But the greater number of those engaged in the active duties of the profession—most of whom would gladly have availed themselves of suitable means of instruction, could such have been commanded —have enjoyed but limited opportunities for acquiring information, neither do they possess the original power of investigation, acuteness of observation, and discriminating judgment, which fall to the lot of but few, and which are indispensable to supply the deficiencies of education.

It is also a fact that many totally incompetent individuals from the humbler occupations of life, influenced either by mercenary or aspiring feelings, have, without any kind of preparation, assumed the title of Dentists, and engaged in the practice of Dental Surgery, and thus the science has been unjustly disparaged, and the profession has sustained unmerited reproach. Charlatanism has been too often successful in imposing upon the credulity of society, who, in the absence of all testimonials of competency, have unfortunately been unable to demand what the opportunity should be afforded to them to require, viz: a professional credential, in the absence of all knowledge of persons, a necessary *prima facie* evidence of qualifications. And thus imposture has been emboldened to occupy a position, arrogate pretensions, and engage in a practice to the detriment of the community, and the injury of the deserving cultivators of this department of science.

Regarding, then, the necessity of providing means of instruction, suited to the improved condition of this science, and also of securing to the public a guaranty against the impositions of the unqualified, the Legislature of Maryland have entrusted to the Faculty already named, the duty of executing its purposes in relation thereto.

In the performance of this duty, the Faculty propose to extend their scheme of instruction, so as to embrace all divisions of knowledge necessary to constitute an enlightened practitioner. The authorized agents of the State in founding the first School of Dentistry in this country, the Faculty are resolved that no censure shall rest upon them for establishing a reduced standard of qualification; but appreciating justly the importance of the profession as well as the responsibility of their trust, it is their purpose, as we doubt not it will be their effort, by furnishing ample facilities for acquiring knowledge, and exacting from candidates for the honors of the College, evidence of thorough qualification, to elevate the character of the profession, and secure for it the just confidence of the public.

Professor Baxley, already well known as a Professor of Anatomy and Physiology, is in possession of a valuable anatomical cabinet, and thus will be enabled to adopt without delay that demonstrative course of instruction so important to those who are to engage in the pursuit of a profession consisting mostly of practical details.

A valuable cabinet of pathological specimens, collected during many years of extensive practice by Professor Hayden, will also enable that gentleman to illustrate fully the course of instruction which has been assigned to him.

The Operations of Dentistry will be described, and exhibited in minute detail, by Professor Harris—a gentleman well known both as a dental practitioner and author.

The subject of General Pathology and Therapeutics, as allied to dentistry, has been committed to the care of Professor Bond, whose character as a practitioner of medicine and whose general acquaintance with medical literature will enable him to give all information upon these subjects necessary to constitute an enlightened dentist.

A course of lectures will be delivered in each year, commencing on the first Monday in November and terminating on the last of February.

Candidates for graduation who have attended two full courses of lectures in this college, or one course in some respectable medical college, and one in this institution, will be subjected to a critical examination by the Faculty, and be required to defend a thesis on some subject connected with dental science; they will also be required to present one or more specimens of mechanical skill in preparing and setting artificial teeth, and likewise be expected to perform certain dental operations in evidence of practical qualification; and on being found competent, they shall receive the degree of Doctor of Dental Surgery.

The charge for attending each professor, for each session, will be $30. Diploma fee $30. Matriculation fee $5.

In presenting this brief exposition, the Board of Visitors admit their earnest desire to have the claims of this Institution to particular patronage justly understood. Interested as all are in the advancement of science, they would have none insensible to the merit which projected this novel and highly commendable scheme for elevating the character of a most useful profession and promoting the general good, and they therefore ask for the enterprise the liberal support of the medical profession and the public.

That the medical profession looked favorably on the new undertaking we learn best from an editorial in the *Maryland Medical Journal,** from which this may be quoted:

"We hail with no ordinary pleasure this effort to carry out the observations made in the preceding number of this journal on this important subject. We feel confident that under the direction of the talented gentlemen in the several chairs, it will prove a lasting benefit to that branch of the profession whose immediate interests it contemplates. We have understood that the prospect for a large class is much more flattering than its warmest friends have anticipated. We wish it the greatest possible success, and hope sincerely that nothing may arise to dim the prospect of its rising influence."

The efforts made to advertise the college by issuing the foregoing announcement, and by placing notices in journals and newspapers, resulted in the matriculation of five students for the first session.

* April 1840, vol. i, page 280.

The names of these students were: J. Washington Clowes of New York city; Thomas Payne of New York city; Robert Arthur of Baltimore; Joseph Lavier of Norfolk, Va.; R. Covington Mackall of Baltimore.

The introductory lecture was delivered by Dr. Harris on November 3, 1840. Some of the thoughts in the mind of Dr. Harris at that time should find a place here:

No credential or evidence of competency having been looked for or required, the profession has become crowded with individuals ignorant alike of its theory and practice; and hence its character for respectability and usefulness has suffered in public estimation, and a reproach has been brought upon it which it would not otherwise have deserved.

The community is at present unable to discriminate between the well-educated and skilful practitioner and the merest pretender —and until it shall be able to do this, more or less of the reproach that is brought upon the pursuit by the latter will be visited upon the former.

Accessible as has been the calling of the dentist to all that were disposed to engage in it, and that, too, without regard to qualification, it has been resorted to by the ignorant and illiterate, and, I am sorry to say, in too many instances, by unprincipled individuals, until it now numbers in the United States about twelve hundred, and of which I think it may be safely asserted that not more than one-sixth possess any just claims to a correct or thorough knowledge of the pursuit. That, under such circumstances, it should occupy a place in the world's estimation inferior to that to which it would otherwise be entitled, is not a subject of wonder.

Of the qualifications necessary to be possessed by a dental practitioner, and the time required for their acquisition, few seem to be aware. On this subject an erroneous opinion seems pretty generally to prevail. A little mechanical tact or dexterity is thought by some to be all that is requisite to a practitioner of dental surgery, and that this could be obtained in, at most, a few weeks. The prevalence of this belief has given countenance to the assumption of the profession by individuals totally disqualified to take upon themselves the exercise of its complicated and difficult duties. But it is to be hoped that the day is not remote when it will be required of those to whom this department of surgery shall be intrusted to be educated men, and well instructed in its theoretical and practical principles. Elevate the standard of the qualifications of the dental surgeon to a level with those of a medical practitioner and the results of his practice will be always beneficial, which at present are frequently the reverse. Require of the practitioner of dental surgery to be educated in the collateral sciences of anatomy and physiology, surgery, pathology, and therapeutics, and the sphere of his usefulness and his respectability will be increased.

Aware of the responsibility that rests upon them, the faculty will spare no efforts to make it creditable to the state that created it and beneficial to the public. Conscious that its claims to respectability and usefulness will depend upon the manner in which they shall discharge their duties, it will be their constant endeavor to impart not only correct, but thorough, theoretical and practical information; persuaded that without this it is impossible for any to practice the art with credit to themselves or for the benefit of their employers, they are resolved to admit none to the honors of the institution except such as possess it. In short, they are determined that no reproach shall rest upon them for fixing a standard of qualification that shall not at once be respectable, and entitle those coming up to it to the confidence of an enlightened community.

These words require no comment; they speak for themselves; they clearly show the bold and intelligent spirit with which the new enterprise was launched on its road to success.

The writer cannot do better than to repeat here the words of Dr. B. J. Cigrand,* who says: "Thus a system of education was initiated which immediately placed the practitioners of dentistry upon an equal footing with other liberal professions. All hail the banner of the old Baltimore College of Dental Surgery! the progenitor of much good and the alma mater of alma maters, claiming

* "The Rise, Fall, and Revival of Dental Prosthesis." By B. J. Cigrand, B.S., D.D.S. Second edition, page 211.

among her collegiate alumni your own adopted mother."

Lectures were delivered and practical instruction given to the class from November 3, 1840, to the latter part of February 1841. The minutes show that two of the students, according to the provision of the charter, were entitled to come up for graduation after having attended but one session. These two candidates were Robert Arthur and R. Covington Mackall, of whom we learn that "each having defended a thesis and sustained a satisfactory examination, the faculty resolved to admit them to the degree of Doctor of Dental Surgery."

This degree was conferred by Dr. Hayden at the first commencement, held on March 9, 1841, at the Assembly Rooms. The valedictory address was delivered by Professor Bond, and some passages of his address are of sufficient interest to find a place here:

You have been taught that dental surgery is not a mere art separate from, and independent of, general medicine; but that it is an important branch of the science of cure. Your knowledge has been based on extensive and accurate anatomical investigation. You have seen and traced out the exquisitely beautiful machinery by which the organism is everywhere knit together. You have learned the secrets of nervous communication, and studied the simple, yet admirable, arrangement by which nutrition is drawn by each part from the common receptacle of strength. You have also carefully examined the phenomena of health and disease, as they are manifested in the dental arch, its connections and relations. Your attention has been particularly directed to the effect of irritation on the general health, and you have seen how readily organs apparently unconnected and independent, may be involved in mutual disease. You have been taught to regard the human body as a complete whole, united in all its parts, and pervaded everywhere by strong and active sympathies; and your principles of practice have been carefully formed on a sound knowledge of general medicine.

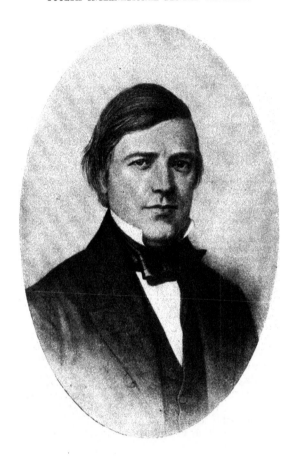

With the commencement exercises the first session of the college closed successfully.

V. THE YEARS 1841 TO 1852.

The development of the college, and the work done by the faculty during the first decade of its existence, may be followed up from the minutes of the faculty meetings. These meetings were held chiefly at the office of Dr. Hayden, and after his death either at the residence of Dr. Harris or in the lecture hall.

Conferring of degrees. One of the

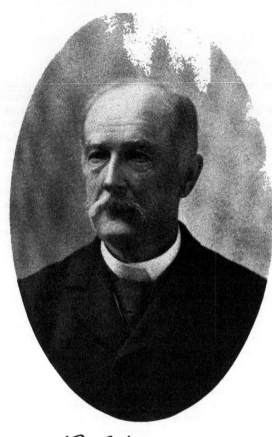

R. C. Marshall

first official functions of the faculty after the close of the first session was the conferring of the honorary degree of D.D.S. on a number of prominent dentists at home and abroad. Diplomas were sent to Canada, England, Scotland, and France. In later years applications for this honorary degree were often made to the faculty either by the dentists themselves or through friends. In a few cases the requests were granted at once, in others it was necessary to inquire into the professional standing of the applicants, while in yet others the applications were laid on the table and never acted on.

As according to the charter, any reputable dentist could apply for an examination even without having been a student in the college, many practitioners who could not obtain the honorary degree availed themselves of this opportunity to secure the much-desired title of D.D.S. All candidates had to present a thesis and specimens of their mechanical work; they also had to demonstrate their operative skill on a patient, and were finally examined orally by all members of the faculty.

Most of the applicants gave satisfactory evidence of their proficiency and received a diploma, but this was by no means always the case. Thus we read in the minutes: "Dr. S., a practitioner of dentistry of fourteen years, was admitted to examination for the degree of D.D.S., and rejected as altogether unworthy of the honor, as he showed no acquaintance whatever with the science of dentistry, being nothing but a dental mechanic."

Mode of instruction. While from the beginning both theoretical and practical instruction was given, the facilities for the latter were rather limited until in 1846 the college found a better home in a building situated in Lexington street, near Calvert street. Here the first dental infirmary was established, which gave at once better opportunities for the teaching of operative dentistry. As early as 1843 a demonstrator of mechanical dentistry had been employed, and now (in 1846) a demonstrator of operative dentistry was added to the staff.

Originally but one chair had been founded for "practical dentistry." In 1852 the desirability of dividing this de-partment was recognized, and accordingly two separate chairs of mechanical and operative dentistry were created.

All these facts show that the faculty was wide awake, laboring faithfully in making the course of instruction more complete and more thorough. That these efforts were fully appreciated is best shown by the constantly increasing number of students enrolled. While in 1841 but two, and a year later only three, men were graduated, the number of graduates increased rapidly, so that in 1851 eighteen students received their diploma at the commencement exercises.

That the efforts of the faculty to bring dentistry into closer touch with medicine were also successful is best shown by the fact that, beginning with the year 1848, members of the faculty were appointed annually as delegates to the meetings of the American Medical Association.

Thus, after a decade of toil and labor, dental college education had been firmly established on a sound basis; it was recognized as an important factor by the dental and medical professions.

Indeed, the Baltimore school exerted, largely through its alumni, a remarkable influence on the progress of dentistry; it was the forerunner and prototype of other dental schools which were gradually established in other American cities. Aided and supported by these younger sister institutions the old Baltimore College of Dental Surgery has continued to this day to do good and noble work in the education of the young dentist, and for the elevation of the dental profession; it has contributed its full share in the establishment, through its alumni, of a place of honor all over the civilized world for the words "American Dentist."

VI. THE FACULTY.

The success of any institution of learning depends chiefly on the corps of teachers and instructors, and for this reason it is of interest to the historian to become acquainted with the men who formed the faculty and conducted the affairs of the college. In the following table are enumerated the more important officers and men who held a chair of one of the principal branches taught at the college, but it does not give the names of all the many teachers who, for a shorter or longer period, held positions as lecturers, instructors, and demonstrators.

Provost.

1847-1852.† Eleazar Parmly, M.D., D.D.S.

Presidents.

1840-1844.* Horace H. Hayden, M.D.
1844-1860.* Chapin A. Harris, M.D., D.D.S.

Deans.

1840-1841.† Chapin A. Harris, M.D., D.D.S.
1841-1842.† Thomas E. Bond, M.D.
1842-1853.† Washington R. Handy, M.D.
1853-1865.† Philip H. Austen, M.D., D.D.S.
1865-1882.† Ferdinand J. S. Gorgas, M.D., D.D.S.
1882-1894.* Richard B. Winder, M.D., D.D.S.
1894——. M. Whilldin Foster, M.D., D.D.S.

Professors of Principles of Dental Science.

1840-1844.* Horace H. Hayden, M.D.
1844-1860.* Chapin A. Harris, M.D., D.D.S.
1860-1875.† Philip H. Austen, M.D., D.D.S.
1875-1882.† Ferdinand J. S. Gorgas, M.D., D.D.S.
1882-1894.* Richard B. Winder, M.D., D.D.S.
1894——. B. Holly Smith, M.D., D.D.S.

Professors of Theory and Practice of Dental Surgery.

1840-1846.† Chapin A. Harris, M.D., D.D.S.
1846-1849.† Amos Westcott, M.D., D.D.S.
1849-1852.† Cyrenius O. Cone, M.D., D.D.S.
1852-1856.† Alfred A. Blandy, M.D., D.D.S.
1856-1857.† Edward Maynard, M.D., D.D.S.
1857-1860.* Chapin A. Harris, M.D., D.D.S.
1860-1882.† Ferdinand J. S. Gorgas, M.D., D.D.S.
1882-1894.* Richard B. Winder, M.D., D.D.S.
1894——. B. Holly Smith, M.D., D.D.S.

Professors of Theory and Practice of Dental Mechanism and Metallurgy.

1840-1846.† Chapin A. Harris, M.D., D.D.S.
1846-1849.† Amos Westcott, M.D., D.D.S.
1849-1852.† Cyrenius O. Cone, M.D., D.D.S.
1852-1873.† Philip H. Austen, M.D., D.D.S.
1873-1888.† James B. Hodgkin, D.D.S.
1888——. William B. Finney, D.D.S.

Professors of Pathology and Therapeutics.

1840-1872.* Thomas E. Bond, M.D.
1872-1875.† Henry Reginald Noel, M.D.
1875-1882.† Ferdinand J. S. Gorgas, M.D., D.D.S.
1882——. M. Whilldin Foster, M.D., D.D.S.

Professors of Anatomy.

1840-1841.† H. Willis Baxley, M.D.
1841-1858.* Washington R. Handy, M.D.
1858-1861.† A. Snowden Piggot, M.D.
1861-1864.† Philip H. Austen, M.D., D.D.S.
1864-1865.† Ferdinand J. S. Gorgas, M.D., D.D.S.
1865-1869.† Russell Murdoch, M.D.
1869-1875.† E. Lloyd Howard, M.D.
1875-1889.† Thomas S. Latimer, M.D.

*Died.   †Resigned.

U of M

1889-1894.† B. Holly Smith, M.D., D.D.S.
1894-1903.* W. F. Smith, A.B., M.D.
1903——.   Standish McCleary, M.D.

Professors of Physiology.

1840-1841.† H. Willis Baxley, M.D.
1841-1858.* Washington R. Handy, M.D.
1858-1861.† A. Snowden Piggot, M.D.
1861-1865.† Philip H. Austen, M.D.,
D.D.S.
1865-1878.* Henry Reginald Noel, M.D.
1878——.   Thomas S. Latimer, M.D.

Professors of Chemistry.

1849-1852.† Philip H. Austen, M.D.,
D.D.S.
1852-1862.† Reginald N. Wright, M.D.
1862-1865.† Alfred Mayer, A.M.
1865-1870.* A. Snowden Piggot, M.D.
1870-1873.† M. J. De Rosset, M.D.
1873-1875.† Philip H. Austen, M.D.,
D.D.S.
1875-1881.* E. Lloyd Howard, M.D.
1881-1891.* James E. Lindsay, M.D.
1891——.   W. Simon, Ph.D., M.D.

Miscellaneous Branches.

1856-1864.† Christopher Johnston, M.D.,
Professor of Microscopical and Comparative
Anatomy.
1872-1882.† James H. Harris, D.D.S.,
Professor of Clinical Dentistry.
1894-1897.† R. Bayley Winder, Ph.G.,
D.D.S., Lecturer on Materia Medica.
1894——.   Edward Hoffmeister, A.B.,
Ph.G., D.D.S., Lecturer on Materia Medica.
1900-1903.* W. F. Smith, A.B., M.D., Lecturer on Bacteriology.
1903——.   Standish McCleary, M.D.,
Lecturer on Bacteriology.

While the large number of professors who were connected with the college excludes the advisability of giving in an article of this kind a life sketch of each one of them, yet some of the more prominent teachers should be at least briefly

* Died.   † Resigned.

considered. · As the biography of the founders of the college, Hayden and Harris, has been given in a previous section, they need not be considered here. The founders had associated with them as incorporators and members of the faculty two men who deserve special mention. They were Thomas Emerson Bond, Jr., M.D., and Henry Willis Baxley, M.D.

Thomas Emerson Bond, Jr., was born in Harford Co., Md., November 1813. He graduated at the University of Maryland in 1834, and practiced in Baltimore for fifteen years. Besides holding the chair of pathology and therapeutics in the dental college for thirty-two years he was also professor of materia medica and hygiene in Washington University, Baltimore. He translated the "Treatise on First Dentition" (from the French of M. Baumes), New York, 1841; he was author of a "Treatise on Dental Science," 1845, and "Treatise on Dental Medicine," Philadelphia, 1851-52. He was joint editor of the *Guardian of Health,* 1841; editor of the *Baltimore Christian Advocate* and of the *Episcopal Methodist.* He died August 19, 1872.

Henry Willis Baxley was born in Baltimore in 1803, graduated at the University of Maryland in 1824, was professor of anatomy and physiology, University of Maryland, 1837-39; professor of anatomy in the Baltimore College of Dental Surgery, 1840-41; professor of surgery in the Washington University, Baltimore, 1842-47; professor of anatomy and surgery in the Medical College of Ohio; government inspector of hospitals, 1865. He traveled extensively in southern Europe and in the Pacific, and wrote books describing those regions. His connection with the dental college lasted but one year. He died in 1875.

Amos Westcott, B.S., C.E., M.D., D.D.S., who occupied the chair of operative and prosthetic dentistry from 1846 to 1849, was born at Newport, Herkimer county, New York, April 28, 1815. His early education was that of the common school; but he manifested, as a boy, a desire to obtain an education beyond the ability of his parents to provide. They yielded to his wish and allowed him to educate himself, which he did by teaching district school in the winter, beginning at the age of seventeen. He attended the academy at Truxton during the summer months. His favorite studies were mathematics and astronomy. In the winter of 1834 he entered Rensselaer Polytechnic Institute at Troy, where he manifested interest in botany and mineralogy, and received the degree of Bachelor of Natural Science, and in 1835 he graduated as a civil engineer from the same institution. His fondness for minerals continued through life, and he made a large collection of rare specimens.

From 1836 to 1838 he was a teacher in the famous Pompey Academy, giving special attention to lectures on chemistry. At the same time he pursued the study of medicine with Dr. Jehiel Stearns, immediately thereafter attending a course of lectures at the medical college at Geneva, New York, and at the Albany Medical College, where he was tutored by the celebrated Dr. Aden S. March, and graduating from that institution in medicine and surgery in the spring of 1840.

In March, 1852, he obtained a charter and founded the New York College of Dental Surgery at Syracuse, the third dental college in the world, of which he was dean and professor of theory and practice of dental surgery and dental technology. Owing to lack of support this

college closed in 1855, the buildings having been destroyed by fire. He was an early member of the American Society of Dental Surgeons, the American Dental Convention and the American Dental Association.

He was elected first president of the Dental Society of the State of New York, and was one of its active organizers. He was also a member of the Fifth District Dental Society of New York, of the Onondaga Medical Society and of the Onondaga Historical Association. From 1844 to 1850 he was associated with Dr. Chapin Harris as associate editor of the *American Journal of Dental Science.*

Dr. Westcott was a vigorous and interesting writer, and was the author of numerous valuable contributions to dental science. His essays were on "Amalgam Fillings," "Arsenic for Destroying Nerves," "Sulphuric Ether," "Forceps," "Extraction Key," "Gold Foil," "Irregularity of the Teeth," "Exposed Nerves," "Operative Dentistry," "Teeth Destroyed by Saleratus," "Transplantation of Teeth." He was author of a "Dissertation on Dental Caries," in which he proved by experiment that caries of the teeth is produced by external chemical agents. This paper and several of his appliances gave him reputation both at home and abroad. He was bitterly opposed to the use of amalgam from its introduction, but of later years seceded from his former belief and admitted its place in dentistry. Westcott was the first to discover and utilize the principle of cohesion of gold at ordinary temperature. It is said he ordered a book of gold, the paper being removed to save the postage, and when it arrived the sheets were welded together Westcott vigorously contested with Dr. Robert Arthur the discovery of the welding properties of gold. Dr. James Leslie

22

also claimed the credit, but as Arthur immediately made his discovery known, and the others did not do so until after Arthur had repeatedly demonstrated it, the credit belongs to the latter.

He invented many instruments and introduced to the dental profession many methods and processes of merit. He was also the inventor of agricultural and other implements of practical value. The Westcott jack-screw for regulating teeth, now made and patented by others, was one of his inventions.

He took a deep interest in the town in which he lived and was elected republican mayor of Syracuse in 1860, which position he filled with great satisfaction. In 1871 he went to Europe on account of his health, and was received with respect by the most distinguished dentists in all the cities he visited. The return of health did not come, as he had hoped, and for three years previous to his death his mind weakened, and on July 6, 1873, in a fit of temporary aberration, he ended his life, with a pistol, at the age of fifty-eight. He received the honorary degree of D.D.S. from the Baltimore College of Dental Surgery in 1843.

Washington R. Handy, M.D., the successor to Professor Baxley in the chair of anatomy, was born in Somerset county, Md., 1811. After having obtained his preliminary education at the Classical Academy in Newark, Delaware, he went to West Point as a cadet. A severe indisposition incapacitated him for the rigid discipline of that institution and necessitated a long rest. Upon his recovery he studied medicine at the Washington Medical College of Baltimore, from which he was graduated with honors in 1834, and was appointed demonstrator of anatomy in that school.

Professor Handy was an excellent teacher; convinced that the ordinary methods of instruction in anatomy, as used at that time, left much to be desired, he created a method of his own and published it in "A Text-book of Anatomy and Guide to Dissection," Philadelphia (two editions, 1854 and 1856). The book was used in all dental colleges and in many of the medical schools.

Dr. Handy taught at the college from 1842 until shortly before his death, January 4, 1858.

Philip H. Austin, M.D., D.D.S., was born in Baltimore, 1822. After having obtained his degree of A.M. from Yale, he studied medicine at the University of Maryland, graduating in 1845. He then took up dentistry, obtaining his degree of D.D.S. from the Baltimore College of Dental Surgery in 1849.

During twenty-two years, *i.e.* from 1853 to 1875, Dr. Austin occupied different chairs in the college, giving great satisfaction in every branch he taught. He revised, in 1871, the tenth edition of Chapin A. Harris' "Principles and Practice of Dentistry," and was the translator of "Diseases and Surgical Operations of the Mouth," from the French of Jourdain, Philadelphia, 1851. He died October 28, 1878.

Edward Maynard, A.M., M.D., D.D.S., was elected professor of theory and practice of dental surgery in 1856. He was born at Madison, N. Y., April 26, 1813, was educated at Hamilton Academy, and entered the military academy at West Point in 1831. On account of his health he resigned, and gave his attention to civil engineering and the study of architecture. He settled in Washington in 1836, and with occasional absences practiced dentistry there up to March 1890.

Dr. Maynard made a number of inventions in instruments, contributed valuable papers to dental literature, and introduced and described methods of practice, some of which have been generally adopted. He called the attention of the Baltimore College of Dental Surgery, in 1846, to the diversity of situation, form, and capacity of the maxillary antra, and asserted the existence of dentinal fibrils, before their discovery by the aid of the microscope.

In 1845, he was employed as court dentist to the imperial family of Russia, and was offered a permanent position of title with rank of major, and to be attached to the imperial court, on condition of his remaining ten years in Russia. The offer was declined.

In 1858, he accepted the chair of theory and practice in the faculty of the National University at Washington. His *clientèle* included presidents, cabinet officers, etc.

Dr. Maynard invented and patented from 1845 to 1886 many devices relating to rifles and muskets, including a breech-loading rifle known as the Maynard rifle.

He died in Washington, May 4, 1891, in the seventy-ninth year of his age.

R. B. Winder, M.D., D.D.S., was dean and professor of theory and practice of dental surgery from 1882 to 1894. He was born at Eastville, Northampton county, Va., July 17, 1828, was a student at the University of Virginia and at Princeton, but did not study dentistry until after the civil war, graduating from the Baltimore College of Dental Surgery in 1869. Later he became a member of the faculty and dean of the Maryland Dental College, an institution which was merged into the Baltimore College of Dental Surgery in 1879. On becoming a member of the faculty of this school he was elected dean, filling the office most creditably to the time of his death, July 18, 1894.

Dr. Winder was perhaps the first one who conceived the idea of uniting more closely the different dental schools of the country, and to his long-continued efforts was due the ultimate formation of "The National Association of Dental Faculties" in 1882. Dr. Winder's energy was also instrumental in causing the Census Bureau to assign dentistry to the list of professions.

The formation of the "Maryland and District of Columbia Dental Association" was largely Dr. Winder's work. He was a member of the American and Southern Dental Association and labored for a consolidation of the two societies, a task which was not accomplished until several years after his death.

As teacher and instructor of young men, Dr. Winder occupied a high position, as can be testified to by those who came under his supervision and personal companionship while they were students.

Christopher Johnston, M.D., occupied the chair of microscopical and comparative anatomy from 1856 to 1864. He was born in Baltimore in 1822, graduated from the University of Maryland in 1844, visited Europe, and on his return to Baltimore became a practitioner of medicine, until his death in 1891.

Dr. Johnston was for many years one of the principal leaders in his profession, and more especially in surgery. In his alma mater he occupied successively the chairs of physiology, microscopy, anatomy, and surgery. He was founder and president of pathological and clinical societies, president of the Baltimore Medical Association, consulting surgeon to the Johns Hopkins Hospital, etc.

He was a frequent contributor to scientific, medical, and dental journals, many of his writings having been translated into other languages. His contributions to dental literature appear chiefly

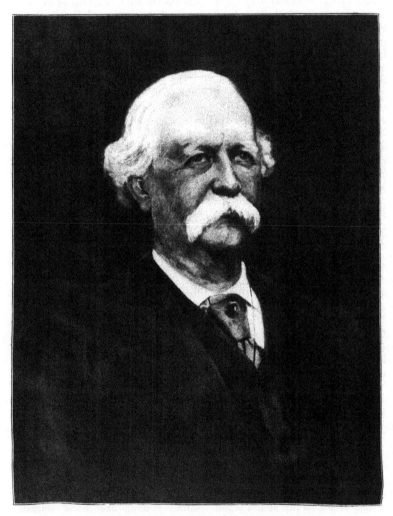

RICHARD BAYLEY WINDER, M.D., D.D.S.

in the *British Journal of Dental Science*. Dr. Johnston was an accomplished gentleman, a thorough scientist, an able teacher, an expert artist and microscopist and a skilful surgeon.

A. Snowden Piggot, M.D., was connected with the college from 1858 to 1870, first as professor of anatomy and then of chemistry. He was born at Philadelphia in 1822, graduated from Yale in 1841 and from the University of Maryland in 1845. He became professor of anatomy and physiology in the Washington University, Baltimore. in 1845; was surgeon C. S. A. 1862-65; co-editor of the *American Journal of Dental Science* in 1856 and 1867-69. In 1854 he published his "Dental Chemistry and Metallurgy," and four years later, "Art of Mining and Preparing Ores." He died February 13, 1869.

Henry Reginald Noel, M.D., occupied the chair of physiology from 1865 to 1878. He was born in Essex county, Va. in 1836, and graduated in medicine from the University of Virginia in 1858. During the civil war he was surgeon in the Sixtieth Virginia Infantry, and in 1866 settled in Baltimore. Besides his professorship in the dental college, he also occupied the chair of physiology in the College of Physicians and Surgeons, Baltimore.

Dr. Noel was a frequent contributor to dental and medical journals. He died January 23, 1878.

The consideration of the men who form the present faculty, or of those who occupied chairs in the college and are yet among the living, must be left to the historian of the future.

VII. THE ALUMNI.

No less than 2358 men and women have graduated from the college. have scattered all over the world, making in most cases a reputation for themselves and incidently for their alma mater. It is with a feeling of justifiable pride that the college looks upon the large number of its alumni who have become prominent in the profession not only as successful practitioners, but also as teachers, examiners, on state boards, authors, inventors, investigators, officers of dental societies, etc.

The time has not arrived when the historian has to consider in detail the work done and being done by those who are yet among the living, but it is proper to speak of the alumni who became more prominent, aided in the elevation of the profession, and have now passed into the great beyond.

Robert Arthur, M.D., D.D.S., was the first one upon whom the degree of D.D.S. was ever conferred, the honorary degree of M.D. being given him in later years by the Washington University of Baltimore. He was born in Baltimore county, Maryland, in 1819, received his early education in private schools, became a pupil of Dr. Chapin Harris, entered the first class of the college as one of the five matriculates, receiving his diploma on March 9, 1841.

Dr. Arthur practiced dentistry with great success successively in Washington, Philadelphia. and Baltimore. He was largely instrumental in the organization of the Philadelphia College of Dental Surgery, which was established in 1852, and in which he filled the chair of principles of dental surgery, becoming also dean in 1855. The Board of Incorporators insisting upon the right of conferring honorary degrees, regardless of the wishes of the faculty, and upon men who were unworthy of that distinction, he and his colleagues resigned. and organized the

Pennsylvania College of Dental Surgery. From this school he resigned in 1857, and removed to Baltimore, where he died in 1880.

At different times Dr. Arthur wrote small works upon dental subjects, viz, "Popular Treatise on the Teeth," 1845; "Professional Patents," (about) 1850; "Treatment of Dental Caries Complicated with Disorders of the Dental Pulp;" translation of Delabarre's "Second Dentition," 1854; "Treatment of the Dental Pulp," "Nature and Treatment of the Decay of the Teeth," 1871 and 1879; "On the Use of Adhesive Foil," 1857. The last-named publication is of special interest as being the first treatise ever written on cohesive gold.

On account of his active interest in every step and improvement of his profession, he was a frequent contributor to its current literature, writing usually with force and clearness. His most marked articles were those in support of the position he defended in the treatise on "Treatment of Dental Caries Complicated with Disorders of the Dental Pulp," in which he maintained that dental caries was not self-propagating, and that under certain circumstances it was allowable to permit a certain portion of caries to remain. His lectures were distinguished by excellent arrangement, energetic language, and simple logic, and will keep remembrance of him fresh in the minds of those who had the opportunity to hear him.

Dr. Arthur's early experience was concurrent with those important movements in the dental profession which were at their climax about the time of the establishment of the first dental college. They had much influence upon him, and he became alive to the value of everything calculated to enhance the interests of den-

tal surgery. His interest in dental education was constant and paramount, and his efforts toward improvement in that direction were unremitting. His views, however, were in advance of the general demands of the public and ahead of the average sentiment of his fellows.

The subject which he made the principal work of the later years of his life was the prevention and treatment of decay of the teeth by peculiar methods of separating them. The principles underlying his methods, and the manner of performance, he advocated and practiced from 1862 until his death. So strong were his convictions of the value of this system that he pursued it unswervingly, notwithstanding that it produced injurious results upon his pecuniary interests, on account of the prejudices excited against him by those opposed to his system of operating.

His most distinguishing moral characteristics were his strict integrity and conscientiousness, as it was impossible for him to admit, or even tacitly acquiesce in any act tainted with the least suspicion of dishonor.

It must be conceded that wherever the influence of dental literature has extended, the moral force and views of Dr. Arthur have commanded consideration and respect, and that his suggestions have modified the practice of dentistry to no inconsiderable degree.

W. W. H. Thackston, D.D.S., class of 1842, was born in Charlotte county, Va., February 29, 1820, and died at Farmville, Va., December 8, 1899. At the time of his death he was the oldest graduate in dentistry in the world, and in the recollection of the younger men he stood forth as a master of his profession, and also as the always graceful expression of the old-time gentleman of the

Washington type. He was an active member of the Virginia State and the Southern Dental Association, and for a number of years was the mayor of Farmville.

John McCalla, D.D.S., class of 1848, was born in the Province of Ulster, Ireland, November 21, 1814; came with his parents to Philadelphia in 1821. He was apprenticed to the tailoring business and followed it in Philadelphia and Baltimore until 1846, when he commenced the study of dentistry in the Baltimore College of Dental Surgery, being also a special student of Dr. C. A. Harris.

He was one of the petitioners for the charter of the Pennsylvania College of Dental Surgery, one of the organizers of the Odontographic Society of Pennsylvania, and one of the founders and first presidents of the Harris Dental Association. He ranked among the pioneers of progressive dentistry, and was considered skilful in his profession. He practiced in Lancaster until 1877, when he retired from active practice.

W. H. Morgan, D.D.S., class of 1848, was born in Logan county, Ky., February 22, 1818. As a boy he was an industrious student, and after having graduated in dentistry, commenced practice in Russellville, Ky., but in 1849 removed to Nashville, Tenn. He was elected a member of the board of trustees of the Ohio Dental College in 1865, and was later elected president, which position he resigned in 1879 to accept the chair of clinical dentistry in Vanderbilt University. He organized the dental department of the university and held the position of dean until his advanced age caused him to resign.

He was one of the oldest dentists in the South at the time of his death. He became a member of the American Dental Association in 1865 and in 1870 was elected its president. His contributions to dental literature were frequent and important, and his labors have been a great factor in the elevation of his profession.

In 1885 he was appointed to the Indian Commission by President Cleveland.

Frank P. Abbot, D.D.S., class of 1851, was born in Maine and after graduation left for Berlin, thus becoming one of the pioneers of American dentistry in Europe. He drew into his professional life the teachings of Harris, and never in the long course of his extensive practice seemed to lose that influence. He was a combination of the liberal with a good share of conservative feeling in a professional sense. While he seemed to be opposed to innovations, yet his courage was equal to any change that coincided with his judgment, though it might be in opposition to established rule. This was manifest in his faithful advocacy of tin and gold foils combined in one filling. He disclaimed any originality in this, but accepted it, and it was through his persistent effort that this was recognized as a valuable addition to practice. He died near Dresden, Germany.

Samuel J. Cockerille, D.D.S., class of 1853, practiced for many years in Washington, D. C., and was known as being perhaps the most unique and clever operator with non-cohesive gold. He worked on each separate operation as if it were to be a finished jewel.

F. H. Rehwinkle, M.D., D.D.S., class of 1854, was born at Celle, Hanover, Germany, June 15, 1825. He received his medical education at a German university, came to this country in 1849, commenced a medical practice at Natchez, Tenn., and subsequently was associated with Dr. J. H. Pulte, in Cincinnati, Ohio. In 1850, he removed to Chillicothe, and about the year 1853 turned his attention to dentistry, attending college in the session 1853-54. He practiced dentistry continuously, with the exception of the years 1861 and 1862, when he was with the Union army. After a period of severe service, he went home on sick leave, and was about to rejoin his regiment when he met with an accident which compelled him to leave the army.

Dr. Rehwinkle was an industrious member of the state and national medical and dental associations. He was president of the Ohio State Dental Society, Mississippi Valley Dental Association, secretary of the Dental Section of the Ninth International Medical Congress, chairman of the Section of Oral and Dental Surgery of the American Medical Association. His contributions to dental literature have been considerable and an intimate acquaintance with European dentists of eminence enabled him to introduce them and their works to the profession in America. He was always modestly prominent in the meetings of every dental society which he would attend and he held the confidence and attention of his medical brethren.

He died at Chillicothe, Ohio, June 8, 1889, and the high esteem in which he was held was shown by the large and distinguished gathering of men at his funeral, including the governor of the state.

Henry Hobart Keech, D.D.S., class of 1857, was born January 25, 1831, in Harford county, Maryland. He received his early education partly from his father's instruction, and partly from a district school. He entered the Baltimore College of Dental Surgery in 1855, and after graduation engaged at once in the practice of dentistry, at first in several counties of Maryland, and then in Baltimore, where he quickly acquired a good reputation.

In 1861, Dr. Keech was elected demonstrator of operative dentistry in the Baltimore College of Dental Surgery. In 1873, he was appointed professor of anatomy in the Maryland Dental College, then organized. In 1874, he received the degree of M.D., from the Washington University, Baltimore. Subsequently, for four years, he occupied the chair of dental pathology and therapeutics in the Maryland Dental College, but he resigned to devote more of his time and attention to mission work.

Henry Bliss Noble, D.D.S., class of 1857, was born in Blandford, Mass., began the study of dentistry with his brother Lester, then attended college, and immediately after graduation began the practice of dentistry in Washington. He was a member of the District of Columbia Dental Society, of which he was twice president; he was a member of the District of Columbia Board of Examiners from the date of its organization to the day of his death; he was also a member of the National Dental Association, and an honorary member of several societies.

While a general practitioner of dentistry, he in a measure made a specialty of orthodontia, and was quite successful in correcting the irregularities of the teeth. He was a special lecturer in the Baltimore College of Dental Surgery, and also in the Dental Department of Columbian University. He died March 5, 1902.

Benjamin H. Catching, D.D.S., class of 1870, was born at Georgetown, Miss., June 28, 1848. He was a great-grandson of Benjamin Catching of Georgia, a delegate to the original Constitutional convention.

He began the study of dentistry in the office of Dr. J. S. Knapp of New Orleans, and commenced his professional career in Canton, Miss., but removed to Atlanta in 1881, where he remained until his death.

Dr. Catching was one of the most prominent men in his profession in the South. In addition to his large practice, he devoted a great deal of time to his literary pursuits. He founded the *Southern Dental Journal,* and edited it for about eight years. Upon retiring from this journal, he commenced the publication of "Catching's Compendium of Practical Dentistry," which had a worldwide circulation. He continued this valuable volume for five years, when his health broke down from overwork and he was obliged to discontinue it. After a lapse of two years, he established the *American Dental Weekly,* which was published but one year owing to the enormous amount of work involved. He was a member of all the leading dental societies of the South, and of the National Dental Association. He died in November 1899.

John C. Story, M.D., D.D.S., class of 1869, practiced dentistry in Texas, was a member of the Dental State Board of Examiners, and was repeatedly elected president of local and other dental societies.

In order to show the influence exerted on matters relating to the profession of dentistry by the alumni of the college it may be justifiable to enumerate very briefly the graduates who now hold positions of importance, or became prominent in the profession. This list is far from complete and the writer apologizes to the many alumni whose names should, but do not, appear here.

Adelbert J. Volck, class of 1852, Baltimore, Md., has the distinction of being the oldest living Doctor of Dental Surgery in the world. He started to practice at a time when the dentist had to cut

the artificial teeth in ivory; he was the first worker in porcelain in Maryland; was president of the Maryland State Dental Association, etc.

Benjamin F. Arrington, class of 1853, North Carolina. Prolific writer; able exponent; wrote treatise on pyorrhea, and clinics.

Ferdinand J. S. Gorgas, class of 1855, Baltimore, Md. Formerly dean and professor of principles of dental science in the Baltimore College of Dental Surgery; holds now same position in the Dental Department of the University of Maryland. Writer and author.

Vines Edmund Turner, class of 1858, Raleigh, N. C. For years an examiner on the state board; a Nestor of his profession; an officer of, and contributor to, local and national associations.

J. Smith Dodge, Jr., class of 1858, New York. A name which means respectability and standing to any association.

James H. Harris, class of 1861, Baltimore, Md. Formerly professor in the Baltimore College of Dental Surgery, now professor of operative dentistry in the Dental Department of the University of Maryland.

James B. Littig, class of 1861, New York. Professor of prosthetic dentistry in the New York College of Dentistry. Writer and clinician.

Luther D. Shepard, class of 1861, Boston, Mass. President of Columbian Dental Congress, Chicago, 1893. Contributor to and worker in dental associations. Distinguished in Massachusetts and nationally.

W. W. Evans, class of 1863, Washington, D. C. Large contributor to society proceedings, author and inventor of cleft-palate specialties and prosthetic appliances.

E. P. Keech, class of 1864, Baltimore,

Md. Late professor in Maryland Dental College; member of the Maryland State Examining Board; writer and exemplar of the dental profession; former president of the Maryland State Dental Association.

Thomas Sollers Waters, class of 1865, Baltimore, Md. Clinical instructor in the Baltimore College of Dental Surgery; president of local societies, etc.

John C. Uhler, class of 1867, Baltimore, Md. For years demonstrator in the Baltimore College of Dental Surgery; later held same position in the Dental Department of the University of Maryland.

B. M. Wilkerson, class of 1868, Baltimore, Md. Patentee of Wilkerson chair, etc.

Charles Gray Edwards, class of 1868, Louisville, Ky. Late professor of orthodontia and prosthetic dentistry in the Louisville College of Dentistry; ex-president of the Association of Dental Examiners; ex-president of the Kentucky State Board of Dental Examiners.

George F. Keesee, class of 1869, Richmond, Va. State board examiner and active worker in dental societies.

Judson B. Wood, class of 1869, Amarillo, Texas. Examiner and teacher.

George H. Winkler, class of 1869, New York. Prominent in the affairs of dental societies.

James B. Hodgkin, class of 1869, Manassas, Va. Late professor of prosthetic dentistry in the Baltimore College of Dental Surgery and in the National University, Washington, D. C. Writer of essays and stories.

Alexander D. Cobey, class of 1870, Washington, D. C. Professor of prosthetic dentistry in the National University, Washington, D. C.

John H. Coyle, class of 1870, Thomas-

ville, Ga. Late associate professor in the Baltimore College of Dental Surgery; state board examiner, and officer in local and other societies.

Oscar E. M. Salomon, class of 1870, New Orleans, La. Ex-secretary of the Louisiana state board examiners.

E. L. Hunter, class of 1871, Fayetteville, N. C. Examiner, officer, and leader in dental societies.

William A. Mills, class of 1871, Baltimore, Md. President of local society; contributor to journal and society proceedings (local anesthetics); lecturer in the Dental Department of the Baltimore Medical College.

Thomas H. Parramore, class of 1871, Hampton, Va. Writer on dental subjects and clinician.

Henry Cabell Jones, class of 1871, Richmond, Va. Professor of operative dentistry in the Virginia School of Dentistry of the Medical College of Virginia.

Robert B. Adair, class of 1872, Atlanta, Ga. Clinician and writer.

William B. Finney, class of 1874, Baltimore, Md. Professor of dental mechanism and metallurgy in the Baltimore College of Dental Surgery.

Alfred D. Eubank, class of 1874, Birmingham, Ala. Professor of orthodontia in the Birmingham Dental College; member of the State Board of Dental Examiners; one of the organizers and former presidents of the Alabama Dental Association.

John A. Chapple, class of 1874, Atlanta, Ga. Professor of oral surgery and general pathology in the Atlanta Dental College; writer and president of the Georgia State Dental Society.

Charles T. Dursh, class of 1874, Baltimore, Md. Ex-president of the Maryland State Board of Dental Examiners.

F. F. Drew, class of 1875, Baltimore.

Md. Secretary of the Maryland State Board of Dental Examiners.

Alexander C. McCurdy, class of 1878, Towson, Md. President of the Maryland State Board of Dental Examiners; vice-president of the National Association of Dental Examiners.

J. Hall Lewis, class of 1879, Washington, D. C. Professor of dental prosthetics and dean of Columbian University, Dental Department; formerly president of the District of Columbia Dental Society, and member of the Dental Examining Board.

Louis C. F. Hugo, class of 1880, Washington, D. C. Poet and writer.

B. Holly Smith. class of 1881, Baltimore, Md. Professor of dental surgery and operative dentistry, Baltimore College of Dental Surgery. Former president of the Maryland State Dental Association, the Southern Dental Association, the National Association of Dental Faculties, and the National Dental Association.

William G. Foster, class of 1881, Baltimore, Md. Demonstrator of operative dentistry in the Baltimore College of Dental Surgery; president of the Maryland State Dental Association. Chairman of the organization committee of Maryland for the Fourth International Dental Congress, St. Louis, 1904.

James H. Grant, class of 1881, Texas. Member of the Texas State Board of Dental Examiners; ex-president of the Texas Dental Society.

Thomas J. Welch, class of 1882, Pensacola, Fla. Member of the Florida State Board of Dental Examiners.

Norman J. Roberts, class of 1882, Waukegan, Ill. Professor of Oral Surgery in the Northwestern Dental College, Chicago; clinical professor of anesthetics in the Chicago College of Dental Surgery.

Charles L. Alexander, class of 1882,

Charlotte, N. C. President of the Southern Branch National Dental Association; inventor and writer.

M. G. Sykes, class of 1882, Ellicott City, Md. Member of the Maryland State Board of Dental Examiners.

Charles A. Meeker, class of 1884, Newark, N. J. Secretary to the National Association of Dental Examiners; secretary of New Jersey State Dental Society for twenty-six years; founder and treasurer of the Central Dental Association of New Jersey.

W. W. Walker, class of 1884, New York. President of the New York Odontological Society; dental organizer and society worker.

W. A. Montell, class of 1884, Baltimore, Md. Professor and late dean in the Baltimore Medical College, Dental Department.

Price Cheaney, class of 1884, Dallas, Texas. Formerly dean and professor of prosthetic dentistry in the Northwestern College of Dental Surgery, and in the Columbian Dental College.

William T. Kelley, class of 1884, Easton, Md. Member of the Maryland State Board of Dental Examiners.

J. F. Dowsley, class of 1884, Boston, Mass. President of the Massachusetts Board of Registration; ex-president of the National Board of Dental Examiners, the Northeastern Dental Association, and the Massachusetts Dental Society.

William Crenshaw, class of 1884, Atlanta, Ga. Professor of operative dentistry in the Atlanta Dental College; inventor and writer.

J. E. Orrison, class of 1886, Baltimore, Md. Professor in the Dental Department of the Baltimore Medical College.

H. Herbert Johnson, class of 1886, Macon, Ga. Professor of prosthetic dentistry and metallurgy in the Southern Dental College; ex-president of the Georgia State Society.

Emory A. Bryant, class of 1886, Washington, D. C. Clinical instructor; inventor of prosthetic specialties.

Frank W. Stiff, class of 1886, Virginia. Professor of prosthetic dentistry in the School of Dentistry of the Medical College of Virginia.

Elmer E. Cruzen, class of 1887, Baltimore, Md. Professor of porcelain dental art in the Baltimore Medical College, Dental Department.

M. N. Mixon, class of 1887, Atlanta, Ga. Ex-president of the Georgia State Dental Association.

Jules J. Sarrazin, class of 1887, New Orleans, La. Ex-president and professor of operative dentistry in the New Orleans College of Dentistry; ex-president of the New Orleans Academy of Stomatology and of the Louisiana State Dental Association.

G. E. Hardy, class of 1888, Baltimore, Md. Demonstrator of mechanical dentistry in the Baltimore College of Dental Surgery.

J. Rowland Walton, class of 1888, Washington, D. C. Dean and professor in the National University, Washington, D. C.

W. W. Dunbracco, class of 1888, Baltimore, Md. Member of the Maryland State Board of Dental Examiners. Formerly demonstrator in the Baltimore College of Dental Surgery.

James H. Crossland, class of 1888, Montgomery, Ala. Recording secretary of the Southern Branch of the National Dental Association.

J. W. Smith, class of 1888, Baltimore, Md. Dean and professor of prosthetic dentistry in the Dental Department of the Baltimore Medical College.

Joseph W. Penberthy, class of 1889, Minneapolis, Minn. President of the Minneapolis Dental Society.

William E. Walker, class of 1889, New Orleans, La. Ex-dean and professor of orthodontia in the New Orleans College of Dentistry; prolific writer; author of many original treatises on mechanism of articulation of the human jaw.

H. J. Burkhart, class of 1890, Batavia, N. Y. Late president of the National Dental Association; chairman of the Committee of Organization and president of the Fourth International Dental Congress, St. Louis, 1904; mayor of Batavia. N. Y.

J. H. London, class of 1890, Washington, D. C. President of the Board of Dental Examiners.

L. D. Archinard, class of 1891, New Orleans, La. Professor of oral pathology and therapeutics in the New Orleans College of dentistry; ex-president of the Louisiana State Dental Society and New Orleans Academy of Stomatology.

G. V. Milholland, class of 1891, Baltimore, Md. Demonstrator in the Baltimore College of Dental Surgery.

Josiah G. Fife, class of 1891, Dallas, Texas. Editor *Texas Dental Journal*.

J. W. David, class of 1891, Corsicana, Texas. Clinical instructor in the Baltimore College of Dental Surgery; ex-president of the Texas State Dental Association; member of the Committee of Organization of the Fourth International Dental Congress, St. Louis, 1904.

P. E. Sasscer, class of 1892, La Plata, Md. Member of the Maryland State Board of Dental Examiners.

J. T. Stuart, class of 1892, Milwaukee. Wis. Dean and professor of clinical dentistry in the Dental Department of the Wisconsin College of Physicians and Surgeons.

C. N. *Guyer,* class of 1892, Denver, Col. Former professor of oral surgery in the Denver College of Dentistry, ex-secretary of the State Board of Dental Examiners of Colorado.

Charles A. Bland, class of 1892, Charlotte, N. C. Member of State Board of Dental Examiners for North Carolina.

Edward Hoffmeister, class of 1894, Baltimore, Md. Lecturer and demon-. strator of materia medica and chemistry in the Baltimore College of Dental Surgery.

Carroll H. Frink, class of 1895, Fernandina, Florida. Charter member and corresponding secretary of the Southern Branch, National Dental Association.

Harry E. Kelsey, class of 1896, Baltimore, Md. Demonstrator in the Baltimore College of Dental Surgery.

Chaplain H. Carson, class of 1897, ex-president of the Southwest Virginia Dental Society.

Howard Merritt, class of 1898, Maine. Formerly president of the Maine Dental Society, and of the Section of Stomatology of the Maine Academy of Medicine and Science.

J. H. Schlinkmann, class of 1901, Baltimore, Md. Demonstrator in the Baltimore College of Dental Surgery.

VIII. THE MUSEUM.

The museum of the college is justly renowned, as it contains many objects of historic interest and specimens valuable from the viewpoint of dental manipulative skill, and from their pathological import and rarity. The catalog of the contents of the museum is a lengthy one and shows the accumulation of many years.

Collection of prosthetic specimens. Here are found artificial dentures representing the various successive stages through which this branch of the profes-

sion has progressed up to the comparative perfection of the present day. Of specimens of particular interest may be mentioned: a lower denture made in France with the eight posterior teeth carved in ivory, and the other eight (natural) teeth attached to the plate by means of wooden pivots; a full upper and lower carved in ivory, the plate and teeth being continuous; an old lower set from England, carved in ivory, with holes for riveting the teeth; partial uppers carved in ivory; a full upper denture, the plate and six posterior teeth carved in ivory, the other teeth, porcelain, mounted by means of gold pins and cylinders.

Pathological collection. Specimens indicative of pathological conditions; abnormalities and malformations are numerous. Some of the former are: molars with ossified pulps; molars with exostosed roots; inferior molars showing ill effect of administration of tincture of chlorid of iron; syphilitic teeth with process attached; molars showing pulp-nodules; specimens showing the result of mercurial salivation; exceedingly large piece of salivary calculus, with molar encased; specimens of tumors, etc.

Among the specimens showing abnormal conditions we find: irregularly shaped teeth in clusters, removed from the antrum; inferior canine with two roots; teeth erupted at birth and extracted at the age of six weeks; abnormally shaped superior molar with inverted third molar in bifurcation of roots; specimens showing osseous union of crowns and roots of various teeth; bicuspid of the third dentition; supernumerary molars, each having four roots; inferior molar with three roots, etc.

Graduation specimens. As it is one of the requirements for graduation for candidates to submit specimens showing the

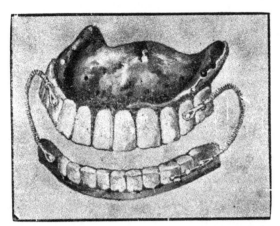

George Washington's ivory carved teeth, made by John Greenwood, the
first American dentist.

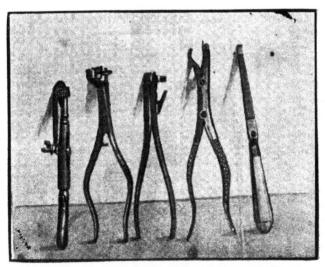

Dental instruments in the museum of the Baltimore College of Dental Surgery.

mechanical or operative skill, an extensive collection of over a thousand of such specimens is found in the museum. They show all possible varieties of gold fillings in natural teeth, porcelain substitutes, partial and full artificial dentures, etc.

Anatomical exhibit. Of special interest to the dentist is the large number of crania showing the various stages of eruption of the temporary and permanent teeth. The collection of the skulls with the teeth *in situ* of a great number of animals, facilitates the study of comparative dental anatomy.

Of *historic interest* is a collection of some of the instruments used a century ago in dental surgery. Among them is a group of "keys," the forerunners of the modern forceps. One huge specimen resembles a corkscrew, with a large wooden handle, made especially with a view of getting a good purchase or leverage on the resisting tooth.

There is also a molar, extracted from the mouth of Amadeus I, King of Spain, and presented to the college by J. C. Gardiner, D.D.S., of London. Another molar, which evidently caused King George IV discomfort until relieved by Robert Wooffendale of London.

Of no small interest is the collection of death masks of famous or notorious people. Here are found the masks of Benjamin Franklin; of Sir Isaac Newton; of King George III; of Willis the painter; of Roberts the engraver; of Zip, Barnum's "What-is-it" of the circus days gone by, and many others.

George Washington's artificial teeth. The "Encyclopedia Britannica" in the article on George Washington says: "It has always been a subject of curious speculation to some minds how much of the calm and benign expression of the face was due to the shape of Washington's false teeth." To this the American editor of the "Britannica" adds in a footnote: "This 'curious speculation' must be that of a curious sort of mind. These ivory carved teeth, however, made by John Greenwood, the first American dentist, are now in the museum of the oldest of all dental colleges, which is in Baltimore, Md."

This highly prized specimen was presented to the college by Dr. John Allen, who obtained it from a grandson of Dr. Greenwood. It is the full upper and lower denture carved in ivory and mounted on gold, with springs for holding them in position. The specimen demonstrates also a method of repair in vogue at that time; an iron plate having been utilized as a means of uniting the fractured parts.

Collection of portraits. Quite a number of the pioneers in dentistry are represented in the gallery. Here are found excellent portraits of the founders of the college, Hayden and Harris; of Greenwood, George Washington's dentist; of many of the former members of the faculty; of Drs. Robert Arthur and R. C. Mackall, the first graduates in dental surgery, as also of men who, while not directly connected with the college, assisted in the advancement of the profession.

II.

History of the Philadelphia College of Dental Surgery, the First Dental College in Pennsylvania.

By WM. L. J. GRIFFIN, D.D.S., Philadelphia, Pa.

THE closing years of the fourth and the beginning of the fifth decade of the last century witnessed an important and far-reaching event in the history of dental science in the United States. Among the more progressive dental practitioners there was a growing desire to uplift the science to a position entitling it to the same respect the community accorded to its kindred callings. While they themselves had no reason to complain—their personal worth and professional standing being unquestioned in the community, among their professional compeers, and their associates in other scientific and learned vocations—they recognized that the entrance door of the dental profession was not as clearly defined nor as well guarded as it should be. Furthermore, while there was much to learn, and the accumulated knowledge of the past had been properly recorded, there was no way provided by which the constant and ever-increasing additions to this knowledge could be quickly disseminated among practitioners; nor yet was there any provision for imparting, systematically, needed information to those about to enter the ranks. The best opportunity offered to a student desiring to qualify for dental practice was a strictly medical course in a medical college, supplemented in some cases by a few desultory lectures upon dental science or by a longer or shorter pupilage with a dental practitioner. Neither of these was at all satisfactory. In too many cases, indeed, they were one and all entirely ignored. Inasmuch as there was no recognized standard of qualification, no recognized method of instruction, and the self-assumed title of "Surgeon-Dentist" was used alike by the thoroughly qualified and by ignorant pretenders, it naturally followed that the title itself commanded but little respect in the community.

The first effort of those who had this matter at heart was to enlarge the facilities for acquiring a dental education offered by a few medical schools. To many enthusiastic advocates of professional advancement this seemed the only proper course. Those practically engaged in teaching, however, soon recognized its utter impracticability. The faculties of the medical schools were not convinced that the movement was of sufficient importance to warrant the great change in their methods of instruction and the increased facilities required by dental students. They fully appreciated that to the dental student opportunity for practical work was of equal importance to the dictum from the lecture table, and they realized the difficulty of providing for this in a medical school. Several attempts to combine the two were abandoned after a short but fair trial.

Drs. Hayden and Harris of Baltimore, the Parmly brothers, and other prominent dentists of New York who had been prime movers in these attempts, seeing no other way determined to found a school for the express purpose of teaching *dental science*. To this end they secured a charter from the state of Maryland and organized the Baltimore College of Dental Surgery early in 1840. Concurrent with this event, under the same auspices, the publication of the *American Journal of Dental Science* provided a much-needed medium for the interchange of thoughts and ideas; this was followed by the organization of the American Association of Dental Surgeons. These three notable events established the dental profession in the United States upon a firmer and broader foundation than it ever before had occupied. That the time was ripe for some such movement is evidenced by these events following each other so quickly, and by the further fact that within a very short time dental schools, dental journals, and dental societies rapidly multiplied.

Members of the dental profession in Philadelphia had not been idle during this time. Philadelphia was then the recognized center of medical education in the United States; its two larger colleges enjoyed a well-deserved world-wide reputation. Members of the dental profession residing in Philadelphia had taken an active part in the organization of the American Association of Dental Surgeons, and in promoting the dental journal; in furtherance of these two projects they worked earnestly and in harmony. Regarding the educational movement, however, trouble quickly developed. The more prominent dental practitioners possessed the medical degree, and were not inclined to favor the new idea. The prompt indorsement of the Baltimore College by the American Association was resented by those who were earnestly hoping to make the medical school the proper entrance to the dental profession. A marked conservatism and difference of opinion that at times was expressed with much bitterness, seriously hampered those who were diligently working for better things.

About this time Dr. J. F. B. Flagg, the younger son of Josiah Flagg, the first native-born American dentist, arrived in Philadelphia. He had previously practiced in Providence, Rhode Island, and brought with him to Philadelphia a reputation that at once gave him a standing among his professional brethren. He was aggressive, yet tactful. He was thoroughly imbued with the true professional spirit, and had but little patience with the exclusiveness which led so many to regard the teachings of experience as trade secrets. His personal magnetism and genial manners made him a welcome addition to a little circle of those who like himself were willing to communicate and anxious to learn. Among the more active members of this little group who met now and again for social and professional intercourse at each others' office or laboratory were John D. White, Stephen T. Beale, Robert Arthur, and J. F. B. Flagg. While Dr. Arthur was not at this time a resident of Philadelphia, on account of close family ties he was a frequent visitor, and took a keen interest in all that was going on. This beginning of that which has done so much for professional advancement was emphatically a "young men's" movement; it interested mainly the younger and more ambitious element of the profession. While not discouraged, it received but little assistance from the older members of the profession.

It was not long before the establishment in Philadelphia of a counterpart of the Baltimore College of Dental Surgery was broached. It was realized that in order to make such an enterprise successful it was necessary to first cultivate and inspire among the dentists of Philadelphia a healthy professional sentiment. In October 1845, a meeting was called of dentists resident in Philadelphia, at which it was determined to invite all reputable dental practitioners in the state of Pennsylvania interested in educational matters to a convention, to consider the propriety of forming a state dental society. In response to this invitation the convention met December 15, 1845, in the lecture room of the Philadelphia Museum, then situated at the northeast corner of Ninth and Sansom streets, Philadelphia, and on the following day, December 16, 1845, the Pennsylvania Association of Dental Surgeons was organized.

In an address at the golden anniversary of this association, held December 16, 1895, Dr. William H. Trueman said: "The association was organized for a specific purpose. It was the outcome of an earnest desire of the progressive dentists of Philadelphia to establish in Philadelphia a dental college having a strong state dental society at its back."

A short time after the formation of the association a committee was appointed to apply to the legislature of the state for an act of incorporation. The bill was referred to a committee of the legislature, but was returned negatived. The reasons given by the chairman were that it was "inexpedient, impracticable, unnecessary, and without the sanction of the majority of the dentists." While this was discouraging, it did not dishearten the friends of dental education.

On December 13, 1847, a letter was read before the association from Dr. Samuel Fleming of Harrisburg, in which he said: "Ever since the organization of this association I have felt a deep interest in its welfare, for, although our profession has been rapidly emerging from the trammels and darkness of empiricism into the bright sunlight of science, and its requirements may be said even now to rank side by side with those of medicine, yet we, in Pennsylvania, have been without an institution or association of any kind. We speak with pride, and justly so, of our medical schools and colleges, and yet we are behind some of our sister states in moving for the promotion of dental science. Can there be a question then as to the utility of this association, or a single doubt as to its ultimate success? I tell you, gentlemen, that public sentiment demands such an institution for the suppression of imposture and quackery, and your efforts will be hailed with joy by thousands who have experienced the evil effects of ignorance and pretense. In these days of reform no argument is needed to prove the necessity of united efforts for the promotion of public improvement. The public know where to look for it, and are expecting such a movement from the high-minded and honorable of our profession. Go on then, gentlemen, and like the American Society, let your standard be high, and rest assured your efforts and your self-denial will one day be rewarded."

From the letters of Dr. Fleming to the association, to Dr. J. D. White, and to others interested in the proposed dental college, it is evident he was an earnest advocate of the enterprise. While the association as a body was keenly interested in the project and fairly well represented the profession, the opposition of those who looked with disfavor upon dental colleges was a serious hindrance. They were in a minority, but they were men of standing and influence. The labor of overcoming this opposition and organizing the first dental college in Pennsylvania was assumed by Drs. J. D. White and Stephen T. Beale of Philadelphia, and Dr. Ely Parry of Lancaster, Pa. Dr. J. D. White was a dentist of marked ability, he had a large practice, and being a close observer and studious, had learned much that was new and valuable. He was ever ready to impart to others, and had a well-deserved reputation as a dental preceptor. Dr. Stephen T. Beale had an excellent reputation as a skilful dentist. As a relaxation from the cares of a large practice, he now and again taught music of evenings. As his reputation as a dentist became known, he was solicited to give instruction in matters pertaining to his profession by dental students and dental practitioners who desired to improve, and gave up his music teaching in order to devote the time to dental instruction. He organized classes which he taught in his office and laboratory. Realizing that there was much more needed by a properly qualified dentist than skill in mere mechanical manipulations, in anticipation of becoming a teacher in the new dental college, he attended medical lectures in the Jefferson Medical College, the University of Pennsylvania, and in a summer medical school. The strain, however, proved too much; his health gave way, and when the time came he was unable to take the place for which he was so well qualified in the faculty of the college he had done so much to make possible. These three men had a personal interest in the enterprise in so far as they expected to occupy positions in the faculty; nevertheless, they were prompted not by selfish motives, but by earnest and unselfish devotion to their profession's best interests.

There are extant several letters to and from those actively engaged in pushing forward this enterprise that give an insight into the difficulties they encountered. They were unfamiliar with the methods of procedure for obtaining grants from state legislatures; in the beginning, at least, they did not appreciate that the authority of such an institution as that which they contemplated should be lodged in a corporate body separate and distinct from its teaching faculty. Their inexperience in these matters caused a long delay in properly formulating their intentions and desires, in seeking and endeavoring to overcome an occult supposed adverse influence, and in securing for their scheme an interested sponsor to present it to the state legislature. A carefully prepared bill providing for a dental college and defining its powers and privileges was prepared, and accompanied by a numerously signed petition* was pre-

---

*"PETITION PRESENTED TO THE LEGISLATURE OF PENNSYLVANIA FOR A CHARTER FOR A DENTAL COLLEGE."

"To the Honorable, the Senate and House of Representatives of the Commonwealth of Pennsylvania in General Assembly met:

"The Petition of the subscribers, Citizens of the Commonwealth aforesaid, respectfully showeth; that

"Whereas, The Science of Dentistry is continually improving and requires facilities for a peculiar attention and study which the General College of Medicine, wisely established by your Honorable Body, fails to afford; and

"Whereas, It is a distinct profession, demanding great skill and undivided application of the practitioner, who, in order to guard the community from imposition and pretence in what not only concerns comfort, but even health and life, should be thoroughly

sented and read before the state legislature at the session of 1851; but it went no further. Much to the surprise of those having the matter in charge it was then learned that a charter for a dental college had been granted to the Hon. Jesse R. Burden, a member of the legislature from Philadelphia and an influential political leader, at the previous session, under date

of May 13, 1851. His influence was sufficiently potent to prevent any further action at that time, so, in order to avoid further vexatious delay it was determined to secure the advantages a charter would afford by an amicable arrangement with the holder of the act of incorporation already in force. Accordingly the Pennsylvania association appointed a commit-

conversant with its principles and practice. We, therefore, feeling its great importance, ask your Honorable Body to take into favorable consideration this prayer of your petitioners and grant them the accompaning Act of Incorporation, that they may in conformity with its provisions establish a College for Dentists, as has been done in neighboring States, where they may be taught the correct principles of their profession, and that thus they may obtain the knowledge of a useful and constantly improving science; and your petitioners, as in duty bound, will ever pray, etc."

This petition was signed by seventy-five dentists, and also by many medical practitioners.

The bill sent with the petition read:

"BE IT ENACTED by the Senate and House of Representatives of the Comonwealth of Pennsylvania in General Assembly met; and it is hereby enacted by the authority of the same, that Eli K. Price . . . and their associates and successors (provided, however, that their number shall at no time exceed eleven members) be, and they are hereby made and created a body politic and corporate in law and in fact of the name and style of the Trustees of the Philadelphia College of Dental Surgery and under that name shall· be perpetual succession, and may sue and be sued, have a common seal, purchase, hold and convey all lands and tenants. money, goods, chattels and effects (provided, however, that said corporation shall hold no more real estate than the buildings and fixtures necessary for a full course of dental instruction) and to make all rules and by-laws necessary for their government, not contrary to the laws and Constitution of this Commonwealth.

"Three members of the Board of Trustees shall constitute a quorum to transact any business except the appointment or removal of a trustee or a professor, when a majority of the whole Board of Trustees shall be required to form a quorum to act.

"The Board of Trustees shall, within . . . months after the passage of this Act, meet and organize by the appointment of a president and a secretary, and elect five or more professors competent to teach dental surgery in all its branches, who shall constitute the faculty of the college, to whom, as a body, shall be committed the immediate regulations and government of the school, subject to the rules and by-laws of the trustees.

"A professor may be removed by the trustees for incompetency, neglect of duty, or misconduct, when the removal is recommended by all the other members of the Faculty. When a professor is to be appointed to fill a vacancy in the Faculty, the candidate shall be recommended by the remaining members of the Faculty, when, if the Board of Trustees approve of the candidate they shall appoint him.

"The Faculty shall have the power to determine the course of instruction, and the necessary qualification for any degree of Doctor of Dental Surgery to be conferred.

"They shall examine the candidates for graduation, and if they are found qualified, recommend them to the Board of Trustees as worthy of the degree of Doctor of Dental Surgery, when, if the recommendation is approved of by them. they shall have power to confer the degree or cause it to be conferred as recommended, provided said trustees shall have no power to confer any degree except that of Doctor of Dental Surgery."

tee to confer with Mr. Burden, and to arrange plans by which the desired dental college could be established. After much negotiation an agreement was reached providing that the association should select the faculty and Mr. Burden name the trustees.

The Association named as the faculty: Drs. J. D. White, Ely Parry, Robert Arthur, Elisha Townsend, and T. L. Buckingham. The trustees named were: Eli K. Price, George L. Busby, Washington L. Atlee, M.D., T. S. Arthur, George Truman, M.D., William G. Alexander, Joseph B. Smith, William Vogdes, Hon. Jesse R. Burden, E. C. Dale, Hon. James Hepburn, Charles Townsend, Lewis E. Reading, Gillingham Fell, Alexander Gaw, William Craig, and Benjamin Malone.

During the summer of 1852, rooms over Jones, White & McCurdy's Dental Depot, No. 116 (now 528) Arch street, were secured, fitted up and furnished as lecture room, operating room, and laboratory. The faculty organized by electing Dr. Elisha Townsend to the deanship, and instituting the following chairs: J. D. White, M.D., D.D.S., professor of anatomy and physiology; Ely Parry, M.D., D.D.S., professor of chemistry, materia medica, and special therapeutics; Robert Arthur, D.D.S., professor of principles of dental surgery; Elisha Townsend, M.D., D.D.S., professor of operative dental surgery; T. L. Buckingham, M. D., professor of mechanical dentistry; L. P. Whipple, M.D., demonstrator of surgical and mechanical dentistry. Fees, each professor, $15; demonstrator, $10; diploma, $30.

The first dental college in Pennsylvania, the Philadelphia College of Dental Surgery, was now fully organized and promptly issued its first announcement, from which we make the following extracts:

"The Philadelphia College of Dental Surgery takes its legal existence under a charter from the Pennsylvania Legislature conferring upon it collegiate powers and privileges, corresponding to those ordinarily granted to the schools of general medicine and surgery; the faculty is regularly and effectively organized, and the institution stands prepared to fulfil the duties it is designed to perform in the service of dental medicine and surgery.

"Twelve years ago the first dental college in the world was founded in the city of Baltimore. The history of that noble pioneer in this department of the educational system of our profession fully justifies the highest hopes of its founders and friends.

"It is entitled to the credit of contributing much in demonstrating the advantage and hastening the establishment of its successors. Two or three other schools answering to the rapidly growing demand have since been established in our country, and now the same impulse has thrust the Philadelphia College into existence.

"The faculty feel no necessity to argue the right or the propriety of their enterprise, or to vindicate its policy or its prospects. They feel that they are but yielding to a necessity of their position and performing a duty which their relation to the profession and the public renders imperative. Public opinion has decided all the questions fundamental to the general enterprise of collegiate instruction in Dentistry, and it remains only for the profession, wherever favorably situated, to provide the ways and means to meet the requirements. Philadelphia is the acknowledged metropolis of medical learning in the United States, and must sooner or later take her position in the great work of dental education. In the judgment of those who have now undertaken it, the time has fully come for such active exertions as they are able to make in the furtherance of the movement.

"This city has now six medical colleges and a number of private institutions of the highest character, in which more than twelve hundred pupils from all parts of the continent are annually receiving instruction, and a museum, libraries, hospitals, dispensa-

ries, and other educational advantages connected with these schools and open to their
pupils, are of unsurpassed excellence.

"All the collateral aids to systematic instruction in our department of surgical
science will be fully at the command of our
pupils. The professors and directors of these
institutions give us an hospitable welcome
to the field of our proper work. These superior advantages obtained by our city and
the prospects of success which they promise.
stimulating the zeal and sustaining the efforts of the faculty, will be felt throughout the
country as a pledge of such prosperity to our
new institution as renders it worthy of the
best support and reliable for the best results
in the advancement of its pupils and in the
general prosperity of the profession. The professors are all practicing dentistry, therefore
the course of instruction will not only be
theoretical but practical.

"A clinical department especially arranged
to afford the pupils actual practice in all the
branches of treatment will be provided, and
opportunities will be so ample that the intelligent and industrious student may attain
greater skill and familiarity with dental practice than is usually acquired in the first four
years of professional life."

The first matriculate was Louis Jack,
who registered September 2, 1852. C.
Newlin Peirce matriculated shortly afterward. Both of these gentlemen have
earned honored positions in their profession; the former, not only as a skilful
practitioner, but also by his earnest and
well-directed efforts for professional advancement; the latter, as a student and
writer, and by his long service as professor in the Pennsylvania College of
Dental Surgery.

Thirty-three students matriculated for
the first session, which began on the first
Monday in November 1852. Dr. Elisha
Townsend delivered the opening address.
In the course of his remarks he said:
"The city in which our school is located
holds, above all dispute, the position of
medical metropolis to the American con-

tinent. Its libraries, museums, hospitals, and colleges are inferior to none in
the world in excellence and adaptation to
the purpose of professional education.
The attendance of over twelve hundred
students at every session of collegiate lectures is ample proof of the eminent rank
which Philadelphia has sustained in this
respect, and it is a circumstance of material importance also to the prosperity of
our enterprise."

The first meeting of the faculty after
they had commenced practical work was
held November 22, 1852. Dr. J. D.
White occupied the chair and Dr. Elisha
Townsend officiated as secretary. It
was an important meeting, as many details concerning the college and its management which had not been reached
owing to press of business incident to organizing the college and furnishing its
lecture and workrooms remained to be
considered.

Dr. Robert Arthur presented a form
of diploma to be used by the college.
This departed from the usual custom in
that it was in English instead of Latin.
This being an important matter it was
laid over to be considered at a future
time.

On motion of Dr. Parry it was decided
that candidates for graduation should
prepare and present to the dean on or before the first of February, accompanied
by the graduation fee, a thesis upon some
subject connected with the science of dentistry, the said thesis to be at least twelve
pages of thesis paper in length.

On motion of Dr. T. L. Buckingham,
each candidate for graduation was required to construct and leave with the
college one piece of mechanical work,
upon which his capability for practice
should be judged.

On motion of Dr. Arthur, each candidate for graduation must also exhibit to the faculty, in further proof of his capability for practice, a patient whose mouth has been put in thorough order according to his own judgment and discretion. It was also decided to exact the graduation fee from all gentlemen upon whom the honorary degree is conferred.

Of other faculty meetings no record has been found until that of January 6, 1854.

During the session of 1852-53, fifteen lectures were delivered each week, and a clinical lecture by one of the professors on Saturdays. The forenoon was devoted to mechanical work in the laboratory and clinic room, and the afternoon to operating.

The first annual commencement was held in Sansom Street Hall, Sansom street below Seventh, February 28, 1853. The rules of the college required that a student should attend two sessions to be eligible for graduation. It was provided, however, that three years' previous actual practice would be considered equivalent to the first session. Under this latter provision the degree of Doctor of Dental Surgery was conferred by the dean upon the following seven regular graduates:

S. Townsend Brown, Phœnixville, Pa.
George W. Emerson, Washington, D. C.
James S. Gilliams, M.D., Philadelphia, Pa.
Henry Garrett, Wilmington, Del.
R. Allison Miller, Huntingdon, Pa.
Arthur B. Williams, Washington, D. C.
John Scott, Connecticut.

The honorary degree was conferred upon the following twenty-two:

William Bradley, M.D.
J. F. B. Flagg, M.D.
James M. Harris, M.D.
Daniel Neall.
Charles Townsend, Jr.
Samuel Stockton White.
Thomas W. Evans, Paris, France.
James Fleming, Harrisburg, Pa.
William R. Webster, Richmond, Indiana.
Stephen T. Beale, M.D.
William W. Fouche.
John H. McQuillen, M.D.
Frederick Reinstein.
D. B. Whipple, M.D.
J. F. Flagg, M.D., Boston, Mass.
O. R. Post, Brattleboro, Vermont.
S. Dillingham.
Jacob Gilliams, M.D.
S. L. Mintzer.
Edward Townsend.
C. C. Williams.

Dr. Townsend, after announcing the names of those receiving the honorary degree, said: "In conferring these degrees the faculty was governed by considerations which have ample warrant in the peculiar circumstances of the college and the profession.

"Many gentlemen who now adorn the profession entered it when the opportunities for collegiate instruction and collegiate honors were not within their reach. They have earned from the public and from their brethren at least equal rank with those who now by official position have legal power to certify to their worthiness, and it was felt to be but just and decorous to accord the claim.

"The effort which the college is making to establish a formal standard of character in the profession, while it owes this justice to deserving men, and could not without invidiousness withhold it, will also be greatly forwarded by the frank acceptance of this distinction of the schools, on the part of men of acknowledged merit."*

The valedictory address was delivered by Prof. J. D. White. In the opening

* *Dental News Letter*, vol. vi, pages 186 and 187.

paragraphs he said: "Gentlemen, the period must come, by the mutations of time, when the nearest and dearest friends and relatives must say farewell; that period has come to us, and, in the name of the trustees and faculty of your alma mater, I am entrusted with the pleasing duty to convey to you our warmest congratulations on the successful completion of the course of studies which were arranged for you to pursue, and also to tender to you such sentiments of encouragement as may stimulate you to exertion, when the trials of the new life which this epoch opens before you would threaten to crush the spirit in its legitimate and arduous exertions. Today witnesses the going into the world of the first graduates of the only dental college in this state, and is of course a period from which will date the working of an influence, for good or for evil, in our beloved profession, proportionately as you impress the communities which hereafter shall be the field of your duties."

He reminded the graduates that the good name of their calling was in their hands, and expressed the hope that the educational advantages they had enjoyed would return a profit in valuable improvements in the art, and in winning for the profession a more honorable place in the community. He then referred to the rise and progress of the dental educational movement in Philadelphia which had culminated in the organization of the college now sending forth its first graduating class. He referred to the extensive field covered by medicine, and how useless it was to expect that with so much to contend with medical instructors can properly instruct dentists. He defended dentistry as a specialty of medicine, and the dental college in its special teaching, contending that it is not necessary for a mer-

chant to learn the details of every branch of business before being considered competent to enter any one branch. "Dentistry," he declared, "will form a very broad specialty—sufficiently broad to require the largest capacities to fully comprehend."*

The closing prayer was then offered by the Rev. Dr. Howe.

In the evening a banquet was tendered the graduates by the faculty and about fifty-five guests sat down to a strictly temperance repast, the toasts being drunk in water.

The demonstrator, Dr. L. P. Whipple, in a note to the *Dental News Letter* (vol. vii, October 1853, page 39), gives the following record of clinical operations during the session, which began the first Monday of November 1852, and terminated on the first of March 1853:

Fillings	273
Treatment of the nerve	26
Treatment of the nerve, which proved successful	22
Extractions	191
Pivot teeth set	5
Superficial caries removed by filing and polishing	9
Removal of calculi	10
Entire sets inserted	1
Partial sets inserted	3
Obturator, constructed and inserted	1
Treatment of irregularities	ι

In making this report he calls attention to the variety of operations performed, and to the value of this opportunity of seeing and doing so much practically at the dental chair, an opportunity a student who relies exclusively upon his preceptor for practical instruction is not likely to enjoy.

The second course of lectures began on

---

*Dental News Letter, vol. vi, page 129.

the first Monday of November 1853. Thirty-three students matriculated. The session closed February 28, 1854, when the annual commencement was held in Musical Fund Hall, on Locust street above Eighth. At this commencement the degree of D.D.S. was conferred upon the following nineteen regular graduates by Prof. Ely Parry, in the absence of the president of the college, the Hon. Eli K. Price:

Horton Bailey, Pennsylvania.
William Calvert, Pennsylvania.
Firman Coar, Pennsylvania.
Alexander G. Coffin, Massachusetts.
E. G. Cogburn, Mississippi.
Benjamin Cohen, Germany.
Samuel W. Frazer, Pennsylvania.
William Gorges, Pennsylvania.
Eli W. Haines, Delaware.
W. Storer How, Maine.
Louis Jack, Pennsylvania.
Bernard J. Loughlin, Pennsylvania.
C. Newlin Peirce, Pennsylvania.
Isaiah Price, Pennsylvania.
David Roberts, Pennsylvania.
John M. Rothrock, North Carolina.
John R. Rubencame, Pennsylvania.
Thomas H. Shaw, Alabama.
James Truman, Pennsylvania.

The honorary degree was conferred upon the following seven gentlemen:

John Tomes, London, England.
J. G. Koehler, Schuylkill Haven, Pa.
Paul Beck Goddard, M.D., Philadelphia, Pa.
Chapin A. Harris, M.D., Baltimore, Md.
F. M. Dixon, Philadelphia, Pa.
Charles Moore, Pottstown, Pa.
John R. McCurdy, Philadelphia, Pa.

Prof. Elisha Townsend delivered the valedictory address, as follows:

Gentlemen:—The ceremonial of this evening formally admits you to the honors of the Doctorate in Dentistry. The term of your pupilage is closed; your diploma certifies your right legitimately to practice and teach your profession, and the duties and authority of the faculty which has conferred your well-earned degrees terminates with the act which places the pupil in the rank of technical equality with his teacher. In the name of the faculty and of the profession, I bid you welcome, and exchange with you the cordial embrace of professional fraternity.

Suppressing the expressions of those personal regrets that necessarily attend the severance of ties which have bound us together in our collegiate relations, as much because they do not admit of adequate utterance as because they are compensated by the pleasures of those still higher and worthier, though less intimate connections, which are now established between us, allow me to address you these, our last lingering words, in the altered tone of the new functions and responsibilities which you this evening assume to the profession and to the world.

Of that second, *self*-education now to commence with you, I have little to say. The instructions already delivered from the several chairs upon which you have attended, must serve both for communicating what we had to teach and directing you in the method of what you still have to learn. Systematic education in dentistry does not terminate in confessions and apologies for incapability to effect its intentions. It does not frustrate its own design by cramming its graduates with a chaos of theories to the suffocation of the intellect. It does not crowd the science of half a dozen professions into the program of a single novitiate. Nor does it so sever the discipline of practice from the study of principles as to leave the alumni of its schools in the helplessness of utter inexperience at the outset of their independent career. Fortunately for you, the change from the preparatory study to that of responsible practice, under our method, is as nothing compared with the compound profession of medicine and surgery, into which the degree of Doctor of Medicine plunges the untrained disciple of the general healing art. Having finished our professional prelections and ascertained your proficiency by tests that are not mere abstractions, and cannot be illusory, we can in the strictest justice of application say to you, when we send you out to the warfare of life, "Walk by the same rule, and mind the same things whereto you have already attained."

Our specialty in the healing art has such

balance, adjustment and relation among its elements, and so happily illustrates and verifies its theory and its practice throughout the whole period of study, that we are not obliged to adopt the fashionable valedictory warning which announces to the terrified graduates that "they are now only indoctrinated to the facts and principles of their study, and cannot be said to have fairly commenced to learn their profession until they have entered its practice." You, gentlemen, in your public study, as well as under your private preceptors, have been trained and instructed to a fair, practical proficiency in every department of the calling which your diplomas declare you competent to undertake. We need, therefore, at the moment of parting, say to you nothing but—go forward in the work of self-development. Whether in the conduct of your continued studies, or in the fulfilment of the varied duties before you, we have but one word to utter—persevere. As we have hitherto so far conducted you, so we for the future direct you. We know of nothing before you that need surprise you. We know of nothing lying in wait for you that is not fully provided for in the teachings already imparted. We take leave to say that we have not turned you out of our hands Doctors of Parchment—dentists in expectancy, or peradventure, but we pronounce you dentists now —worthy of the title and ready for use. I do not say that the growth of manhood and old age does not lie out in long-drawn prospective before you, but I do say that you have reached your professional majority in the qualifications of your art; in a word, that you are not so many collegiate grubs, waiting for your wings till they are grown by the tedious and painful metamorphosis of future experience. Your system of study, both in method and appliances, is an actual matter-of-fact anticipation of future practice, and if any of you have the slough of chrysalis yet to cast, it is either because you or we, or both, have been delinquent in our duty; it is not an intrinsic fault in the policy of dental education. The method of study, the direction of principles and the drill of practice, you will bear us witness, have run current with, and been incorporated in, all our teachings in such interdependence that you are well assured today of the pathway that will lead you onward to the attainment of your future aims,

and guide you safely to their eventful achievement. Nothing less than this would answer the promise and the trust implied in the contract entered into between us. You carry with you from these halls the certificate of the faculty that you have well and honorably performed your part of the engagement, and, we trust you very confidently to demonstrate to the world the fulfilment of the pledge on our part. Yesterday, gentlemen, you were our pupils, but today you take rank and fellowship with us in our common profession; and laying aside the claims, with the duties and relations of preceptor and pupil, let us turn together for a moment to the consideration of some of those interests and responsibilities which have now become our mutual and equal concern as members of the profession.

Dentistry is usually spoken of as a branch of the great healing art, but in point of fact it has grown not out of the stem but up from the root of the tree of remedial science, and as it has not sprung from, so it does not depend upon the older trunk, but stands beside it, drawing its separate nourishment from the same soil indeed, yet by the independent energies of its own vitality. Hitherto, in fact, it has been indebted rather for shadow than sunshine to the elder-born growth. A thrifty sapling it has proved, with roots and branches of its own; distinct in its vital economy, though kindred in origin; distinct, also, in its fortunes and necessarily so in the conditions and policy of its culture. Moreover, it has already so far matured that it is full time for it to be set out by itself for larger room to grow and ripen its proper fruits.

Doctor of Dental Surgery is a comparatively new patent of nobility in the heraldry of science, and necessarily institutes the relations and duties of a new order in the diplomatic ranks. To this service we have pledged a generous devotion. We have enlisted in the regular army of advance, and the consciousness that its fortunes must be vitally affected by our conduct in the field, cannot fail to fire the zeal and steady the fidelity due to the cause. What does it ask at our hands, and how shall we best answer its great demands?

Very rapidly and successfully, but still very recently, our profession has advanced from a sheer chaos of empiricism to the form and order of a regular systematic art; so founded upon principles, and so justified by experience as entitles it to the character of an integral science. It has also richly provided itself with the apparatus and methods of future growth and progressive achievement. Already we are in possession of elementary treatises on every department of the study. We have an able periodical literature, and colleges for thorough and comprehensive education are springing up with a rapidity and a capability almost equal to the demands of the times. We have so well advanced in the transition stage of our progress, if not quite passed it, that the elements of a permanent order are rapidly arranging themselves into the most efficient forms. Our duties are determined by these favorable conditions, and our obligations proportionately enhanced by the resulting facility of their performance. The duties before us, it seems to me, may be best understood by dividing them into two concurrent but distinct branches. The first and most direct is the improvement of the profession by all the aid it is in our power to contribute; and the second, the equal obligation which lies upon us to repress and eradicate the remaining irregularity and unworthiness that still attaches to the fraternity. The duties under the first division, which I have placed first because they lie nearest home, and are first in rank and importance to the objects aimed at, fall for the most part within the regular range of that self-culture and self-improvement which concerns our individual interests most narrowly considered.

Whatever we can do to render our art most helpful to our patients will best serve to enhance the character of the profession and raise the standard of its public estimation. In the proportion that we illustrate its dignity and demonstrate its utility in our practice and conduct, we will have advanced the requirements that the public will make upon all who in our own neighborhood make claims of proficiency in our science. To the extent that we shall be able to indicate a clear superiority, we will have established a reforming criticism over the pretensions and a correcting influence over the practice of inferior men. The legitimate, the best mode of exposing the darkness around you is by the brightness of the light you shed into it, and

the happy advantage of this method is, that while it exposes it also dispels it. But besides this, and a little beyond it, there is the duty we owe to the profession at large, of contributing by word and deed, by care and service, to the efficiency and success of all the means that are available, especially all those that are already provided for the liberal education of the men who are hereafter to fill our places. The responsibility resting upon you in this behalf embraces several important particulars. I can only glance at them now, and commend them to the fuller consideration which they deserve from you. The private education of pupils in dentistry is a high and responsible trust necessarily incident to the doctorate of the profession. Upon every capable practitioner in the country this duty rests with imposing force; but you, by all your commitments, are especially pledged to its worthiest performance. Collegiate faculties are not the only nor even the most important agents in this function. Doctors of Dentistry literally means teachers of the art, and you are in your private capacities the primary, and by no means the least important functionaries of the educational faculty. You are aware that the college whose honors you have won insists upon an adequate private preceptorship as a condition of graduation. Its importance to the individual you understand too well to need any enforcement from me; but I cannot let this opportunity pass without pressing upon you the expectation that you will in this matter fully second and zealously forward the general effort to elevate the standard of regular study, and generously devote yourselves to the discharge of your share of this honorable service. In your judgment there is no question of the indispensable necessity of a thorough preliminary study in the principles of the profession. There results from this conviction, therefore, the corresponding duty of indoctrinating all those within your influence, who propose to enter the profession, with the soundest views of its requirements, and for providing for your own pupils all the facilities and devoting to them all the care that are necessary to the fullest requirements.

Your office and workroom, your library of elementary books, and your supply of our periodical publications should be provided with liberal completeness, and your personal instructions must be fully and conscientiously afforded. The applicant depends upon your judgment for the knowledge of his proper qualifications. Be faithful to him and to the profession in this. See that he has the mind and the general education that qualifies him for the study. See that habits of study as well as application to practical operations are justly regarded. Let the idea that the profession is a learned and liberal one rule the conduct of the pupil, and your conduct towards him. Keep steadily before him the connection of all the departments of physical and remedial science which our own involves and depends upon for its completeness and for its further progress. Allow me to say to you in the most emphatic manner, that we look to you for the best service you can render to the cause of preparatory education with a solicitude and confidence second to none that we have in any of the agencies in existence for the reformation and development of our noble profession; and we charge you, by every consideration of duty, honor, and ambition, that you fail us not in this grand hope of our enterprise. The preceptor engaged in the onerous duties of his practice is under great temptation of convenience and of interest to slight his duty to his pupil; nay, it is only at considerable sacrifice that he can fully perform it. But this, for its importance to the common interests of the faculty and of the community, is exactly the service that is exacted from him. Perform it in the spirit of your calling; perform it in the fulfilment of your pledge punctiliously, effectually, religiously, and your reward will be the consciousness that you have well deserved the rank you have assumed in a liberal fraternity; neglect it, and the reproach of delinquency of the highest trust will outweigh all the pleasure and pride of the largest selfish success.

The standard and periodical publications devoted to our art have unquestionable claims upon our support. Every dentist worthy of the name should consider himself an agent for their circulation, and a contributor by implied contract to their stores of information. Every liberal profession, as much as that of religion, has, besides its sanctity to be guarded, its interests and usefulness to be promoted. The lawyer, the physician, the naturalist, the dentist, is a sort of priest of his order, and owes to it the required fidelity, sacrifice, and service. The philosophers of Greece exacted a sacramental vow from the disciples whom they initiated into the mysteries of their schools. Hippocrates administered an oath to the adepts of the healing art. I will read it to you, both for the curiosity and the instructive suggestions it contains:

"I swear by Apollo the Physician, by Æsculapius, by Hygeia, by Panacea, and all the gods and goddesses, calling them witness, that I will religiously, according to the best of my power and judgment, keep the solemn promise and the written bond which I now do make: I will honor as my parents the master who has taught me this art, and endeavor to minister to all his necessities; I will consider his children as my brothers, and will teach them my profession should they express a desire to follow it, without remuneration or written bond. I will admit to my lessons, my discourses, and all my other methods of teaching, my own sons, and those of my tutors, and those who have been inscribed as pupils and have taken the medical oath, and no one else. I will prescribe such a course of medicine as may be best suited to the constitution of my patients, according to the best of my power and judgment, seeking to preserve them from anything that might prove injurious. No inducement shall ever lead me to administer poison, nor will I be the author of such advice. I will maintain religiously the purity and integrity both of my conduct and of my art. Into whatever dwellings I may go I will enter them with the sole view of succoring the sick. If, during my attendance, or even unprofessionally in common life I happen to hear of circumstances which should not be revealed, I will consider them a profound secret, and observe on the subject a religious silence. May I, if I religiously observe this my oath, and do not break it, enjoy good success in life and in the practice of my art, and obtain general esteem forever. Should I transgress and become a perjurer, may the reverse be my lot."

Now, whatever the altered circumstances of the times have made obsolete and inapplicable in this grand summary of professional obligations, the principles which it recognizes are of perpetual obligation; none of them could be better presented, and some of them I might not have chosen to express; but there is a parity of conditions which will not fail to warrant their application to ourselves, our relations to each other, to our calling, to our patients and to the public. But especially are the sanctity and the devotedness of the order to which these principles of conduct and these sentiments of fraternity apply, as well in our case as in any other, well worthy of acceptance and observance. Our young profession demands of us equal ardor of service and equal zealousy of defense, as medicine did in the age of its early infancy. Above all things it needs the spirit and corporate enthusiasm and priestly purity, the sacredness of dedication that corresponds to its divine origin and beneficent aims. The idea I would enforce here must be obvious enough, and sufficiently warranted by its practical results, but I am tempted to strike the thought still deeper to the grand principle upon which it rests. History testifies that every upward movement among men has been effected through the spirit of corporate association.

The orders of nobility, knighthood, priesthood, medicine, law, fellowship in liberal learning, and the less formal but equivalent etiquette of rank in social life, teach unmistakably that the policy of distinction in degrees is inseparable from culture and progress. That labor, which in itself is as honorable as any other, but is still degraded, dependent, and oppressed, is so simply because it lacks the organization and the protective sacredness of fraternity and corporate enthusiasm. Every function by which the world's interests are served, is equally honorable intrinsically, but none becomes free, efficient, and honored, till its members recognize their unity, interchange sympathies, support its common interests and defend its distinctive rights and honors. I do not need to say to you that I recommend no selfish conspiracy, no supercilious exclusiveness of cast, with a monopoly of honors and emoluments for its aims, and invidious means for their attainment. It is not the maintenance of a party, but the promotion of progress, that is intended as the object of your ambition; and only such measures, offensive and defensive, as comport with the most generous public ends, and are compelled by liberal and enlightened policy. Such conduct, in a word, in everything as makes a prudent man better

and wiser by the observance, and operates by replacing abuse with general benefits. These motives will direct us most wisely and worthily in our dealings with the empiricism or quackery which still deforms the profession, and with the public opinions and prejudices which sustain it. I do not like the word empiric, and would be very cautious in its application. Literally, the word signifies no more than one who makes experiments; by custom it is applied to one who enters the medical profession without a systematic education, and relies solely upon the teachings of his own experience. The censure which the term is intended to convey is certainly not deserved by a practitioner of our art who, in default of all opportunity for regular and best methods of professional study, has depended upon his own industry and talent for such qualifications as he could thereby attain to. We stand too near the time when dentists must have been self-made or not made at all, and we have too many examples among us of honorable and enviable distinction thus acquired to be rash in applying the reproach which a better order of things now leaves without excuse. The honorary degrees conferred by our young dental colleges upon a large number of gentlemen in the profession have been induced by a sentiment of simple justice, strengthened also by our modesty in the doctorate itself, which could not bear its own titular honors easily in contrast with equally deserving men who could not formally, but have equitably earned them. In these circumstances, therefore, gentlemen, it is not your parchments simply but your attainments which should be your pride, and this apprehension will dictate the consideration and delicacy due to the deserving. An empiric may, nevertheless, be a proficient in his art, and a graduate with all the honors may, also, be a mere sciolist.

A man is to be measured by his merits, notwithstanding that a diploma is *prima facie* evidence, and a worthy distinction, of character and standing, still it is your duty to repress and discredit unfounded pretension by all the means fairly and effectually in your power. This in general will be best accomplished by fully and decidedly answering to every claim of the accomplished and regular professors of our art, and by us as decidedly refusing to admit those of the unworthy and incapable. A great advantage—an indispensable one—of the corporate organization which we have already urged is, that its honorable reciprocities withheld will act as distinctions and penalties upon groundless pretension. Just as the disciples of Hippocrates were sworn to admit to the fraternity "those who had been inscribed as pupils, had taken the medical oath, and no one else," so we are bound to refuse fraternity to the irregulars who repudiate the essential obligations of the profession and discredit its name. We do not expect and I do not think we desire quack laws of the legislature to repress abuse, but we require quack tests established by ourselves, and well received by the community, by which they may be speedily and certainly extirpated. This is our proper duty, and we must address ourselves to it, and the means within our command are, in general terms, the improvement of the system now fast rising into confidence among us; the liberal encouragement of our periodical publications, the organization of efficient dental associations among practitioners for their mutual improvement and protection in every district where such parliaments of progress are practicable, and also the decided establishment of all those distinctions which serve to certify character and standing among ourselves and instruct the public judgment in deciding upon professional pretensions. These things, and all which they include, we would press upon your consideration and commend to your hearty observance. The profession, to adopt the battle orders of Lord Nelson, "expects every man to do his duty." To you is assigned the post of honor, and we will not allow ourselves to doubt your worthiness of the trust, or your fidelity or efficiency in performing. There is a moral chivalry, nobler in tone, pitch and purpose, because more beneficent than that of arms. Are you baptized by its spirit, capable of its service, devoted to its achievements? Then you will exert its energies and secure and enjoy its victories.

I began by bidding you welcome to your professional honors. I close by committing you to the divine care in your public duties and personal destiny. Farewell.*

---

*Dental News Letter, vol. vii, April 1854, page 129.

The demonstrator reported that 471 patients, 55 male and 416 female, had been treated, and the following operations performed:

Fillings	385
Treatment of pulp by extirpation	29
Extractions	231
Pivot teeth set	4
Treatment of superficial caries	9
Removal of salivary calculus	19
Insertion of entire sets	3
Partial sets	2
Treatment of irregularities	7
Total	689

The third session opened on the first Monday of November 1854, with thirty-four matriculates. The teaching staff was increased by appointing Dr. Whipple, who heretofore had been the only demonstrator, to be demonstrator of operative dental surgery, and Dr. William Calvert demonstrator of mechanical dentistry.

During the session Dr. Townsend resigned owing to sickness, and Dr. J. D. White was appointed, temporarily, to the deanship. J. F. B. Flagg, M.D., D.D.S., was appointed to fill the vacancy in the faculty. The division of subjects taught was also changed by appointing Prof. J. D. White professor of operative dental surgery and special dental physiology, Dr. Flagg taking the subjects formerly taught by Professor White. At the close of the session Dr. Whipple resigned and Dr. Louis Jack was appointed demonstrator of operative dentistry in his place.

Matters were not harmonious during this session. Trouble between the Board of Corporators, or trustees, and the faculty had been brewing for some time in regard to conferring honorary degrees.

It was a custom with the early dental colleges to confer this degree upon worthy members of the profession who had been long in practice, and had established an unquestioned reputation. It was thought wise to do so in order that the community might the sooner recognize the broad distinction between competent and incompetent practitioners. It was in many cases, however, really a misnomer. As the applicants were required to pay at least the usual graduating fee, it was really a degree conferred *sine curriculum*. Inasmuch as the degrees were conferred by the board, the Board of Corporators contended that they were competent to name and decide upon whom these degrees should be conferred. The faculty on the other hand contended that as these degrees placed the recipient on an equal standing with a student who received his degree in regular course after having proved his worthiness by an examination before them, it was their right to be satisfied that the applicant for the honorary degrees was fully competent, and that the application should be first submitted to them and have their approval. The quarrel soon became a bitter one. Other matters, more personal in their nature, and now happily forgotten, tended to make the quarrel more acrimonious. Toward the latter part of the year 1854, in an effort to set this matter right, the faculty met and formulated a series of rules for the government of the college designed to define clearly and unmistakable the requirements for its degree, and the relations which should subsist between the board and the faculty. After the matter had been fully discussed, Professor Parry was delegated to put in proper form the conclusions reached.

At a meeting of the faculty December 16, 1854, Professor Parry presented his report, which was accepted and adopted. Professor Parry was then delegated to present his report to the Board of Corporators. (A copy of this report cannot now be found, and it is supposed to have been destroyed in a fire a few years ago, with many other college records.)

At a meeting of the faculty held January 17, 1855, Professor Parry reported that, as requested, he had presented to Eli K. Price, president of the Board of Corporators, the rules for the government of the college which they had adopted. After Mr. Price had examined them, he proposed that they be drawn up in legal form, and Thomas Hood, Esq., was selected for that purpose. The rules as revised by that gentleman were submitted to the Board of Corporators at a meeting held in the college building January 3, 1855. The attendance at the meeting was small, and the rules were thrown aside as unnecessary. At this same meeting the board formulated a series of rules as evidenced by the following communication sent to the dean of the faculty:

PHILADELPHIA, January 8, 1855.

Dear Doctor:—At a meeting of the corporators of the Philadelphia College of Dental Surgery, held on last Wednesday, 3d inst., it was resolved—

First, That the degrees conferred at the last commencement be sanctioned and ratified by the corporators.

Second, That the present arrangement of the faculty as in the announcement be approved.

Third, That the dean be required to pay one dollar for every diploma signed by the secretary for the use of the corporators.

Fourth, That all articles presented to the college shall be in charge of the dean, who shall furnish a list of the same to the secretary of the college in order to have it entered in the minutes.

Fifth, That the faculty shall furnish the secretary with a list of the students who have passed examinations for degrees, one week before the stated meeting of the corporators.

Very respectfully,

CHARLES A. DuBouchet,
Secretary B. C. P. O. D. S.

While the candidates were being examined for graduation during this session, J. C. Harris, a student, became sick and left the city. The secretary of the Board of Corporators proposed that the faculty graduate this man. The faculty refused to do this, as they were not satisfied that he was qualified. The board then sent word to the faculty authorizing them to confer the degree; this the faculty refused to do.

The third annual commencement was held in Musical Fund Hall, Wednesday evening, February 28, 1855. The regular degree was conferred upon the following fifteen graduates:

D. S. Hutchinson, Pennsylvania.
Jeremiah Hayhurst, Pennsylvania.
Samuel Walton, Pennsylvania.
Vinecome Shinn, Pennsylvania.
John Levering, Jr., Pennsylvania.
Jethro J. Griffith, Pennsylvania.
Joseph P. Cornett, Pennsylvania.
W. H. Freeman, M.D., Pennsylvania.
E. G. Cummings, New Hampshire.
James Bayson, Tennessee.
James A. Butner, North Carolina.
David W. Hogue, M.D., Scotland.
Daniel McFarlan, Washington, D. C.
Jacob S. Simmerman, New Jersey.
Aurelio Letamendi, Cuba.

The honorary degree was conferred upon Hudson S. Burr, M.D., of Philadelphia. The valedictory address was delivered by Prof. Robert Arthur.*

---

*Dental News Letter, vol. viii, April 1855.

Prior to the opening of the fourth annual session, Dr. Whipple presented his resignation, which was accepted, the faculty directing the dean to express to him their acknowledgment and appreciation of his faithful services as demonstrator. Dr. Louis Jack was appointed demonstrator of operative dental surgery in his place. Dr. Robert Arthur was elected dean, to succeed Dr. White, who had served temporarily since the resignation of Dr. Townsend. Among other changes the time of actual practice to be considered equivalent to the first course was increased from three years to five years. The case of Mr. Harris was finally decided by the faculty announcing that the only way by which he could obtain a legitimate degree was to come forward at such time as might be convenient to him and submit to an examination. They also demanded that the secretary of the board, who had used disrespectful language when this case was under discussion, be removed from his position.

The advertisement of the fourth annual session contains the following emphatic clause:

The profession throughout the country may rest assured that the interests of this faculty are too intimately associated with those of the dental profession, even if they were influenced by no higher motive, to permit them to do anything tending to lower the standard of qualification, or in any way to detract from the present honorable character of their calling. They refer, with confidence, to their past course for confirmation of this statement. So far from desiring to increase the size of their classes, by promising facility in passing through the school, they wish it distinctly understood by those who propose to place themselves under their instruction, that a thorough knowledge of what is taught in it will be demanded of everyone who becomes a candidate for a degree which this college is empowered to confer.

Conditions of graduation as set forth in the fourth annual announcement read as follows:

The candidate must be twenty-one years of age, and of good moral character. He must have studied under a private preceptor at least two years, including his course of instruction at the college. Attendance on two full courses of lectures in this institution will be required of all, but satisfactory evidence of having attended one full course of lectures in any respectable dental or medical school will be considered equivalent to the first course of lectures in this college; three years' practice, inclusive of the term of pupilage, will also be considered equivalent to the first course of lectures. The candidate for graduation must prepare and defend a thesis upon some subject connected with the theory or practice of dentistry. He must treat thoroughly some patient requiring all the usual dental operations, and bring such patient before the professor of operative dental surgery. He must also prepare a piece of artificial work, and show its adaptation to the mouth; such operations and such work to be done at the college building. He must also undergo an examination by the faculty, when, if found qualified, he shall receive the degree of Doctor of Dental Surgery.

Fees.

Fees for the course, demonstrator's ticket
included $85
Matriculation (paid but once) 5
Diploma fee 30

The college so far had been remarkably successful, the classes had yearly increased, and had necessitated increasing the facilities of the clinic room and the laboratory.

The fourth, and as it proved, the last session, commenced on the first Monday of November 1855. Forty-four students matriculated, one of them Mr. Martin DeCastro, a native of Porto Rico, who was presented with a ticket for the course, in recognition of his services rendered the citizens of Norfolk, Va., during the severe epidemic of yellow fever in that section.

The fourth annual commencement was held at Musical Fund Hall, February 29, 1856. The degree of Doctor of Dental Surgery was conferred upon twenty-two graduates, as follows:

J. Canning Allen. Jr., Philadelphia, Pa.
J. Foster Flagg, Philadelphia, Pa.
James E. Garretson, Philadelphia, Pa.
Charles Neil, M.D., Philadelphia, Pa.
W. Bartling Robbins, Philadelphia, Pa.
Robert McClellan, Pennsylvania.
James K. Whiteside, Pennsylvania.
Henry B. Parry, Lancaster, Pa.
Alan W. Read, Norristown, Pa.
William T. Arrington, Tennessee.
James P. Broun, Virginia.
Charles H. Burr, Maine.
Louis Martin y DeCastro, Porto Rico.
José G. Lopez, Porto Rico.
Antonio L. Coopat, Cuba.
Francis Field, Massachusetts.
William Grimes, Indiana.
John W. Hunter, North Carolina.
Samuel Martin, M.D., North Carolina.
A. F. McLain, Louisiana.
R. Woodward Robinson, New York.
John Z. Stranger, New Jersey.

After these degrees had been conferred, and the graduates had resumed their seats, the president announced that the honorary degree had been conferred upon two persons, whose names and addresses are not given in any account of the transaction available. This was done against a most earnest protest of the faculty, as the parties were not known as dentists.

The valedictory address was delivered by Professor Flagg.

Dr. Louis Jack, demonstrator of operative dental surgery, made the following report:

Fillings 562
Treatment of the nerve 84
Extractions 723
Superficial caries removed............ 2
Removal of salivary calculus.......... 27
Pivot teeth set...................... 7
                                      ————
    Total operations 1405

24

Dr. Calvert, demonstrator of mechanical dentistry reported as follows:

Entire sets of teeth.................... 3
Partial sets of teeth.................. 16
Total number of teeth inserted........ 163

At a banquet following the commencement exercises, Dr. Arthur in a frank and manly address protested publicly against the action of the Board of Corporators in conferring a degree against the protest of the faculty. His remarks were received with applause and an enthusiasm which evidenced most satisfactorily that the sympathies of the dental profession were on the side of the faculty.

The unpleasant relations between the board and the faculty had become intensified during the session. The board demanded that the faculty confer the degree upon whom they wished; the faculty were not willing to submit to this. The faculty contended that they had done everything to establish the college except to procure the charter. They had rented and furnished the rooms occupied by the college at their own expense, and had borne all the expenses of the college without asking the board for a dollar. Furthermore, they were the only parties known to the profession and were by the profession held responsible for the acts of the college. The action of the president of the board at the last commencement evinced a determination on their part to consult no longer with the faculty before conferring honorary degrees, and quickly brought the matter to a crisis.

A meeting of the faculty was held the Monday evening following the commencement. On this occasion they carefully reviewed the situation and reached the conclusion that they could not honorably continue to work with the Board of Cor-

porators, and therefore decided to disband.

In anticipation of an effort to reorganize the college, the following announcement was issued:

FIFTH ANNUAL COURSE OF THE PENNSYLVANIA COLLEGE OF DENTISTRY.

The Corporators of the Philadelphia College of Dentistry respectfully inform the dental profession that the fifth annual course in this flourishing institution will begin on the first Monday of November next.

The regular announcement, which will shortly be published, will present several additional features and contain the names of the faculty, which the corporators have every reason to believe will meet with the entire approval of the profession.

WILLIAM VODGES, LL.D.,
                                          President.
CHAS. A. DuBOUCHET, M.D., D.D.S.,
                                          Secretary.

CORPORATORS: William G. Alexander, William Craig, Hon. Benjamin Malone, M.D.; E. C. Dale, Joseph B. Smith, J. A. Phillips, Esq., J. Gillingham Fell, Isaac Meyer, George L. Buzby, Charles Townsend, A. M. Burden, M.D.; T. L. Arthur, Alexander G. Gaw, Joseph R. Mitchel, Hon. J. R. Burden, M.D.; W. L. Atlee, M.D.; Lewis E. Reading, Charles A. DuBouchet, M.D., D.D.S.

From the well-known character of the gentlemen comprising the Board of Corporators we feel assured that the faculty selected by them will combine all the essential elements to impart a thorough dental education.

They feel sanguine that the wholesale resignation of the late faculty will not seriously embarrass them, or affect the prosperity of the college.

No serious effort, however, was made to continue the college. The causes which led to the disbanding of the faculty were well known throughout the profession, and their decisive action met general and hearty approval. The Pennsylvania Association of Dental Surgeons, which held a commanding position, not only in Philadelphia but throughout the country, promptly took action toward establishing a dental institution free from the embarrassing complications of their first effort. The course of the Board of Corporators was universally condemned, and the effort to secure a new faculty proved, to the honor and credit of the profession, a failure.

Of the sixty-three graduates of the four sessions of the Philadelphia College of Dental Surgery, many achieved success as dental operators at home and abroad, or have served their profession with credit as instructors, investigators, and inventors; pre-eminently among these may be named Drs. Louis Jack, C. Newlin Peirce, James Truman, J. Foster Flagg, and James E. Garretson, as gentlemen who have reached a well-earned position of prominence in their profession to which but few attain.*

III.

History of the Pennsylvania College of Dental Surgery.

By WM. L. J. GRIFFIN, A.B., D.D.S., Philadelphia, Pa.

THE Pennsylvania College of Dental Surgery is practically a continuation of its predecessor, the Philadelphia College of Dental Surgery. When the faculty of the latter institution determined that they could not honorably continue in harmony with a Board of Corporators who arrogated to themselves the right of granting degrees upon whomsoever they would, regardless of the candidates' fitness, and insisted upon the degree being conferred upon one whom they had not as yet examined, and of whose qualification's they were not satisfied, they immediately took measures to organize an institution that could be trusted to properly safeguard the honor and dignity of a dental diploma. They realized that the charter under which they had organized the college was not in the hands of those who had the good of the profession at heart; they furthermore realized that the question at issue was not one that could be compromised. The charter under which they had been working was obtained by one not at all identified with the dental profession, from a legislature which had rejected their request, and which they felt sure would treat with the same scant courtesy a second request, then pending before it. They had entered into negotiations with the political leader who held the charter, to avoid further prolonging a disheartening delay, and finally agreed to permit him to select the legal head of the institution (the Board of Corporators) on finding these the best terms they could make. Four years' experience had demonstrated that the profession in Philadelphia would support a dental college.

*[To Professors C. N. Peirce, Edward C. Kirk, Albert P. Brubaker, and to Drs. William H. Trueman, Thomas W. Buckingham, J. D. White, Jr., and J. Clarence Salvas, I am indebted for many of the records from which this history is compiled, for many valuable suggestions, their goodwill, and kind assistance.—WILLIAM L. J. GRIFFIN.]

They had demonstrated their ability as dental teachers, the usefulness of the dental college was now fully recognized, and they felt sure that no state legislature would again say of a dental college that "it was inexpedient, impracticable, unnecessary, and without the sanction of a majority of dentists." That time had passed. They had learned how such an institution should be organized, and had become sufficiently versed in political affairs to know how to approach a law-making body.

Dr. J. D. White affiliated with the board, and took no part in the new venture. Dr. Townsend, although still far from well, promptly took his place, and with Drs. Arthur, Parry, Flagg, and Buckingham, formulated the necessary legal measures to obtain a charter for a college to be known as the Pennsylvania College of Dental Surgery. Dr. Townsend was delegated to go to Harrisburg and present the matter to the state legislature, then in session. This he did. Being unable to remain until action could be taken upon the application, he left the matter in the hands of Mr. Charles Hamilton of Philadelphia. Mr. Hamilton was a gentleman of means, retired from business, and while not a politician, was a man with influence at the state capital. He took a keen interest in dental educational matters, and so well managed the business that the following act was passed by both houses, and signed by Governor James Pollock, on Thursday, April 3, 1856.

AN ACT

To Incorporate the Pennsylvania College of Dental Surgery.

Section 1. Be it enacted by the Senate and House of Representatives of the Commonwealth of Pennsylvania in General Assembly met, and it is hereby enacted by the authority of the same, that Henry C. Carey, William Elder, Washington L. Atlee, Elisha Townsend, George Truman, Benjamin Malone, Alfred Stillé, Daniel Neall, Thomas Wood, William W. Fouché, John R. McCurdy, and T. S. Arthur, and their associates shall be a body corporate with perpetual succession under the name of the Pennsylvania College of Dental Surgery, to be located in Philadelphia, and as such may sue and be sued, have a common seal and purchase and convey real and personal estate not exceeding in annual income two thousand dollars beyond the building to be occupied by said College: Provided, That said corporators shall not at any time be more than fifteen nor less than ten without the vacancies being filled. *[marginal note: Corporators. Amount of property allowed to hold. Number of Trustees.]*

Sec. 2. That the said corporators shall have power to make by-laws for their own government, and that of the Faculty, not contrary to the laws of this State or of the United States; to establish a college for lectureships, and to confer the degree of "Doctor of Dental Surgery" upon persons duly qualified to receive the same. *[marginal note: Corporators make by-laws for themselves and faculty confers the degree.]*

Sec. 3. That the corporators shall have power to elect five or more professors, skilled in dentistry, to constitute the Faculty of said College, who shall deliver the lectures and control the course of instruction therein; and no degree shall be conferred, whether honorary or upon the qualified students of the College, without the written request of said Faculty. *[marginal note: Number of professors: their qualifications and duties. Degrees.]*

RICHARDSON WRIGHT,
Speaker of the House of Representatives.

WM. M. PIATT,
Speaker of the Senate.

Approved, the third day of April, *Anno Domini,* one thousand eight hundred and fifty-six.

JAMES POLLOCK.

It will be observed that this act is very explicit in confining the selection of those who shall receive its collegiate honors to the faculty alone. The corporators cannot designate the candidates, they can exercise their right to confer degrees only at the written request of the faculty. Controversy on this point cannot arise under this charter. The Board of Corporators named in the act were men of influence in the community, and well known and respected by the profession. Hon. Henry C. Carey was one of Philadelphia's most distinguished citizens, Thomas Wood was a merchant, John R. McCurdy was of the firm of Jones, White & McCurdy, predecessors of the present S. S. White Dental Manufacturing Co., and editor of the *Dental News Letter*, T. S. Arthur, the brother of Prof. Robert Arthur, was a distinguished writer, then at the height of his popularity. These were the lay element in the board. The medical profession was represented by Drs. Elder, Atlee, Stillé, and Malone; and the dental profession by Drs. Daniel Neall, W. W. Fouché, Elisha Townsend, and George Truman. Than these, a more acceptable selection could not have been made.

At the first meeting of this board, April 6, 1856, they organized by electing Hon. Henry C. Carey president, and Mr. Thos. Wood secretary. Dr. Townsend and Mr. McCurdy retired. It is worthy of note that of the ten composing the board, four, Mr. Arthur, Drs. Atlee, Malone, and Truman, had been members of the board of the Philadelphia College during its entire existence. They had evidently proved worthy and acceptable to the members of the faculty, and they so continued to their successors, remaining faithful and active members of the board until removed by death. The faculty was composed as follows:

Elisha Townsend, D.D.S., M.D., professor of operative dental surgery; Ely Parry, D.D.S., M.D., professor of chemistry, materia medica, and therapeutics; Robert Arthur, D.D.S., M.D., professor of the principles of dental surgery; J. F. B. Flagg, D.D.S., M.D., professor of anatomy and physiology; T. L. Buckingham, D.D.S., M.D., professor of mechanical dentistry.

The first meeting of the faculty was held April 23, 1856, when Dr. Robert Arthur was elected dean, and Dr. Louis Jack and Dr. William Calvert were appointed demonstrators of operative dental surgery and mechanical dentistry, the same positions they held in the former college. The organization of the new college was now complete; the rooms they had furnished at their own expense at 528 Arch street were engaged, and the first annual announcement of the Pennsylvania College of Dental Surgery was forthwith issued for the session of 1856-57.

Not quite two months elapsed between the resignation of the faculty of the Philadelphia College of Dental Surgery and the organization of the new college at the same stand, with the same teaching staff except one, under decidedly more favorable auspices. The session of 1855-56 ended the old one and the session of 1856-57 inaugurated its successor. The following explanation of this is found on the last page of the first announcement:

It seems proper that the faculty of this school, with the exception of one of its members, should make some explanation of the fact that, after having been for several years connected with another institution, which met with unprecedented success, they should suddenly cease to hold connection with it and attach themselves to a new one.

The history of this matter is a brief one.

The Trustees of the "Philadelphia College of Dentistry"—the institution above referred to—claimed the right of conferring honorary degrees independently of the faculty, and, in spite of the unanimous protest of the faculty against the act, did, at the last commencement, confer this degree upon two individuals, who, so far from being distinguished members of the dental profession, were not even generally known as belonging to it.

It is not necessary to occupy any space to show that such a practice was unjust to the faculty, who could not escape from the responsibility of the conferring of such degrees, and that it would have led to the most injurious consequences to the college and to the profession. Believing this to be the case there was but one course left, and the faculty determined to disband. This was done.

Finding that the faculty of the Philadelphia College had disbanded and feeling satisfied that no faculty who could command the confidence of the profession would consent to work under the same auspices, an application was made to the Legislature for a new charter, containing a clause expressly prohibiting the Board of Trustees from conferring any degree, regular or honorary, except at the written request of the faculty of the college. The charter was granted and a new faculty formed. Such members of the present faculty as were formerly connected with the Philadelphia College, and refused to work under the charter and board of that school, felt no hesitation in accepting a place in this institution.

The conditions for graduation were substantially the same as had formerly ruled, and required the candidate to have studied at least two years under a private preceptor, including his course of instruction at the college. He must attend upon two full courses of lectures, but satisfactory evidence of having attended one full course in any respectable dental or medical school, or five years' practice, were considered equivalent to the first course. The candidate was also required to treat thoroughly some patient requiring all the usual dental operations, to prepare a piece of artificial work, and show its adaptation to the mouth; this practical work to be done at the college building. In addition he was required to pass a satisfactory examination by the faculty.

The fees were twenty dollars for each professor's ticket, and seven dollars and a half for each demonstrator, making one hundred and fifteen dollars for the course. Matriculation fee (paid but once), five dollars, and diploma fee, thirty dollars.

The session began on Monday, November 3, 1856, precisely as it would have done had no change in the school taken place. Thirty-three students matriculated for this session; the first was Henry Winterbottom, who had taken his first course in the former school.

During the session Professor Townsend's health broke down, and his friends realized that he was approaching the close of his career. Such duties as he was unable to perform were assumed by the other members of the faculty.

On Tuesday, February 26, 1857, the first commencement was held in Musical Fund Hall, Locust street below Eighth, at which thirteen students received the degree of Doctor of Dental Surgery. The valedictory address was delivered by Professor Townsend; it proved to be his last appearance before the profession, his death occurring the following year.

At a meeting of the faculty held March 15th, Professor Townsend tendered his resignation, his health having become so far impaired that he was no longer able to fill the position. In accepting his resignation the faculty unanimously recommended Dr. Townsend to the Board of Corporators as worthy of the appointment of emeritus professor, a suggestion that was promptly acted upon. Dr. Townsend's retirement was deeply regretted by teachers and students. His reputation as a skilful operator and close observer, his affability, earnestness as a teacher, and scholastic attainments were highly appreciated. This, with his unselfish devotion to the best interests of the patient and the profession, caused him to be looked upon, deservedly, as a model professional gentleman. At this same meeting Dr. John H. McQuillen was elected to fill the vacancy.

On Tuesday, March 24th, Drs. Arthur and Parry resigned because the faculty proposed to make a change in the chair of operative dentistry of which they disapproved. The faculty recommended to the Board of Corporators, Drs. William Calvert and J. Hayhurst to fill the vacancies. This having been approved, Professor Buckingham was transferred to the chair of chemistry, materia medica and therapeutics, Dr. Calvert was appointed professor of mechanical dentistry, and Dr. Thomas W. Walker was appointed demonstrator of mechanical dentistry. On Tuesday, June 23, 1857, Professor Buckingham was elected dean. Beginning with the second session, the fee for the course was one hundred dollars, including the demonstrators' fees, thus reducing the fee for the course fifteen dollars.

The second session commenced November 2, 1857. For this session forty-eight students matriculated. Of these, fifteen graduated at the ensuing commencement. Those connected with the college thought all were working in harmony, but Prof. J. F. B. Flagg, in connection with his son, established a "dental academy"; this the faculty believed would lessen the interest of Professor Flagg in the college, or would retard the progress of the college in public favor and recognition. Dr. Flagg was requested to close his dental academy, but preferred to resign his chair in the college.

At the close of the session Professor Hayhurst resigned his chair, and Dr. Jack resigned as demonstrator. July 1858, Dr. Walker, demonstrator of mechanical dentistry, died. Drs. C. Newlin Peirce of Philadelphia, and J. L. Suesserott of Chambersburg, Pa., were elected to the vacancies in the faculty. Professor McQuillen was transferred to the chair formerly occupied by Professor Flagg (anatomy and physiology), Dr. Peirce taking his place as professor of dental physiology and operative dentistry. Dr. Suesserott became professor of principles of dental surgery and therapeutics, and Professor Buckingham's chair was entitled chemistry and metallurgy. Dr. D. H. Goodwillie was appointed demonstrator of operative dentistry, and Dr. J. J. Griffith demonstrator of mechanical dentistry. Dr. Walker's death was a serious loss. He was a young man of bright promise, an apt teacher, a skilful dental mechanic, and particularly expert as an artistic block-carver.

During the third session, which commenced November 1, 1858, the faculty changed the manner of voting for candidates for graduation. The ball system heretofore used, which gave to each professor but one vote, was discarded, and a rule, which gave to each five votes, adopted in its place. Sixteen votes were required to "pass" a candidate, this being later raised to nineteen. The new method was more favorable to the student. On February 26, 1859, Professor Calvert was elected dean, and Professor Peirce treasurer.

Fifty-one students matriculated for the fourth session, 1859-60. Of these twenty-one received the degree of Doctor of Dental Surgery at the commencement held February 28, 1860. During this session vulcanized rubber was introduced into the college as a base for artificial teeth.

The fifth session opened with sixty-three matriculates, of which thirty-six graduated when the session closed.

On June 13, 1862, Professor Calvert resigned, as he was about to remove permanently to California. Dr. E. Wildman was elected to fill his chair, and Professor Peirce · took his place as dean. September 26, 1862, Professor Suesserott resigned. This resignation coming so near the opening of the session was embarrassing to the faculty. After canvassing the matter, being unable to agree upon a candidate to recommend for his place, they requested the Board of Corporators to make a selection. Two applicants appeared for the place, Dr. Geo. T. Barker, who had recently succeeded Dr. Goodwillie as demonstrator of operative dentistry, and Dr. J. Foster Flagg, son of former Professor Flagg. The board elected Dr. George T. Barker. Professor McQuillen was dissatisfied with this choice and immediately resigned. W. S. Forbes, M.D., was elected his successor. Dr. James Truman was appointed demonstrator of operative dentistry, and Dr. E. N. Bailey demonstrator of mechanical dentistry, positions vacated by the promotion of Dr. Barker and the resignation of Dr. Griffith.

Notwithstanding adverse circumstances, the session was fairly successful. At its close the honorary degree of D.D.S. was conferred upon Professor Forbes, and Dr. J. D. White was elected emeritus professor.

The changes in the ·teaching staff just before the opening of the session had been happily adjusted, but other impending troubles for a time threatened the existence of the institution. The faculty was notified that the rooms they occupied would be required at the close of the session to accommodate the increasing business of the owners of the building.

A charter had been obtained for a new dental college, and under the leadership of Dr. J. H. McQuillen the Philadelphia Dental College was organized. Dr. McQuillen was the editor of the *Dental Cosmos,* and the publishers of this journal refused to issue, as heretofore, the announcements of or to advertise the Pennsylvania College of Dental Surgery, but gave its influence and sympathy to the new enterprise. The faculty of the old college were refused, also, the use of the mailing list that previously had been at their disposal. These events seriously hampered them. The faculty, however, were thoroughly in earnest, and in perfect harmony. They secured a lease of the premises at the southeast corner of Tenth and Arch streets, and fitted up the second, third, and fourth floors for the use of the college. The location was more central than the former one, and the building much better suited to their purpose. To restore their mailing list, they sent a printed circular to the postmaster of every county in the United States, requesting a list of dentists in their locality. These were generally responded to; and by this means, and the directories of the larger cities, the names and addresses of over four thousand dentists were thereby obtained. They also established a quarterly dental journal, the *Dental Times,* edited by the faculty, which for ten years held an honorable place among dental periodicals. The crisis was successfully passed, and the opening of the session of 1863-64 found the college far better located, better housed, more independent, and with brighter prospects than ever before.

Dr. Edward N. Bailey, demonstrator of mechanical dentistry, died June 18, 1864, and Dr. J. M. Barstow was appointed in his place.

At the close of the session of 1864-65, Professor Peirce resigned, and Dr. James Truman was appointed in his place, Dr. E. T. Darby, who had just graduated, taking his place as demonstrator of operative dentistry.

At a meeting held December 22, 1865, the faculty decided to confer the degree of Doctor of Dental Surgery upon dentists who had been in practice before 1852, and who had established a professional reputation as good operators, without requiring their attendance at lectures. Under this rule about thirty-six received a diploma during the years this rule was in force, stating the conditions under which it was granted. This condition was first published in the announcement of the eleventh session, 1866-67,* and reads as follows:

Candidates for Graduation Who Have Not Attended Lectures.

Dentists who have been in continued practice since 1852 are eligible to be candidates for graduation without attendance on lectures. The candidate for graduation must present satisfactory evidence of his having been in practice for the allotted time, also of his good standing in the profession; he must prepare a thesis upon some subject connected with the theory or practice of dentistry. He must present specimens of his workmanship. He must undergo a satisfactory examination by the faculty, when, if qualified, he shall be recommended to the Board of Trustees, and if approved by them shall receive the degree of Doctor of Dental Surgery.

* *Dental Times,* vol. iv, July 1866, page 351.

The first graduates under this rule were John B. Wheeler of New York, A. Lawrence of Massachusetts, and W. G. A. Bonwill of Delaware; these received the degree at the tenth annual commencement, March 1, 1866, just before the rule was published. This rule was advertised for the last time in the annual announcement for the fourteenth session of 1869-70. About thirty-six received diplomas under these conditions, the last being Theodore F. Chupein, then of Charleston, S. C., but later of Philadelphia, in 1872, and W. T. Smith of Maryland, in 1879. Candidates for graduation under this rule paid the matriculation and diploma fees only. Referring to the reason for its adoption, Prof. James Truman, in the *Dental Times,* vol. iv, April 1867, page 163, has this to say:

By resolution of the faculty of the college all who have been in the reputable practice of dentistry since 1852 have the privilege of matriculating and submitting to an examination without attending lectures. But in order to receive the diploma of this institution they must not only be satisfactory to the faculty, but they must produce evidence of practical ability in operative and mechanical dentistry. The object of this rule is to endeavor to separate all truly worthy members of the profession from the unworthy, with the belief that it will materially hasten the time when, by the moral force of the community, if not by legal enactment, all will be obliged to possess a certificate of ability to practice. In accordance with this rule our readers will observe a large number of names under the appropriate heading, of those who voluntarily came forward to comply with the requisitions of this rule. To many the diploma may be of trifling value in a pecuniary sense; but the effort to obtain it will, as an example to younger men, be of immense value, and will do much, in our judgment, to elevate the profession. The action of this college in granting these degrees may be open to criticism in some respects, yet we still regard it as the only means to bring the profession to a common level. All proper means have been and will continue to be adopted, to guard with jealous care the rights of students and the honor of the profession.

The growth of the college is well shown by the report at the close of the session of 1864-65. There were fifty-six matriculates and twenty-nine graduates. During the session two thousand six hundred patients visited the clinic room, and three thousand six hundred and seventy-seven operations were performed in the operative clinic, and two thousand and nine artificial teeth mounted in the mechanical clinic. At the ninth annual commencement held at the close of this session, February 25, 1865, the honorary degree was conferred upon Theodore S. Evans of Paris, France, J. M. Barstow and Mahlon Kirk of Philadelphia, Jesse C. Green, West Chester, Pa., and J. D. Wingate, Bellefonte, Pa.

During the session of 1866-67 the faculty decided to charge patients for the material used in the mechanical clinic. Previous to this all work was done gratis. For this session there were one hundred matriculates, twenty-six regular graduates and twenty-three who had been in practice prior to 1852 and who passed a satisfactory examination.

During May 1867, Dr. Henry Hartshorn at the recommendation of the faculty was added to the teaching staff, which now consisted of six active professors and two demonstrators, as follows: J. D. White, M.D., D.D.S., emeritus professor; T. L. Buckingham, M.D., D.D.S., professor of chemistry; E. Wildman, M.D,. D.D.S., professor of mechanical dentistry and metallurgy; G. T. Barker, M.D., D.D.S., professor of dental pathology, materia medica, and therapeutics; W. S. Forbes, M.D., D.D.S., professor of anatomy and physiology; James Truman, D.D.S., professor of dental histology and operative dentistry; Henry Hartshorn, M.D., professor of physiology and hygiene; Edwin T. Darby, D.D.S., demonstrator of operative dentistry; J. M. Barstow, D.D.S., demonstrator of mechanical dentistry.

The session of 1867-68 was made notable by the admission of the first woman matriculate, Mrs. Henriette Hirschfeld of Berlin, Germany. She was the first woman dental student in Philadelphia, and the second in the United States. To her credit, be it said, as a student she carried herself well; by her earnestness and thorough devotion to her college duties she did much to overcome the professional prejudice to co-education that was strongly expressed at the time, and gained the respect of her classmates. Her subsequent career and that of the many others who have followed her example, has demonstrated the futility of the many learned arguments to prove the unfitness of her sex for dental practice. Over one hundred women have since then gone out from this college alone, and they seem to have found in this vocation a promising field of usefulness.

The action of this college in making special provision, and offering inducements for the older practitioners to acquire the dental degree, did not meet the approval of other colleges. Notwithstanding that it applied to a class of men who in the course of nature would not increase, and that it required from them all that was required from regular students except attendance upon lectures and the practical work of the clinic room, and that it tended to more quickly bring about the universal requirement of the dental degree as a prerequisite to entering upon dental practice—the profession, ever sensitive and quick to resent any attempt to make this distinction accessible by any other than a proper college course, looked upon it with distrust.

Prior to this, the dental colleges throughout the country had formed a union with the laudable desire to, as far as possible, unify the course of instruction, and by united effort raise the standard of professional requirements. Delegates from the several colleges in furtherance of this met at stated times to discuss matters of mutual interest. At a meeting of such delegates held in Philadelphia, March 20, 1867, this matter was brought up and fully discussed. It was finally resolved, "That no dental college should be permitted to grant a diploma to any practitioner unless he attended the regular course of lectures, or had made himself eminent by valuable contributions to the science." This action was resisted by the representatives of the Pennsylvania College. They contended that their course in recognizing merit in those who, entering the profession before collegiate opportunities were generally available, had by their own efforts sufficiently advanced to pass the same tests as required of a regular student, was right and proper, and that their requirements for this class of applicants were sufficiently stringent to properly safeguard the dignity of the dental degree. Considering the resolution a censure upon the past and prospective course of the Pennsylvania College of Dental Surgery, its faculty withdrew from the organization.

Prof. Geo. T. Barker referred to this in an editorial in the *Dental Times* (vol. iv, April 1867, page 166), entitled

THE REASON WHY.

A meeting of the Association of the Colleges of Dentistry was held at Philadelphia, March 20, 1867. Delegates were present from the following institutions: Baltimore College of Dental Surgery, Pennsylvania College of Dental Surgery, Ohio College of Dental Surgery, Philadelphia Dental College and New York College of Dentistry. The principal business was the adoption of rules acted upon at the former preliminary session. This was proceeded with in harmony, and was characterized by the desire to work together for the general good. At the evening session a resolution was introduced by Professor Weisse, of the New York College of Dentistry, the character of which was to prohibit any institution from granting a diploma to any practitioner unless he should attend the regular course of lectures, under the rules previously adopted by the Association, except only to those who have made themselves eminent by valuable contributions. This resolution was modified by Professor Austin of the Baltimore College, so that instead of a prohibition the Association would disapprove of the conferrence of the degree. The introduction of these resolutions was avowedly designed by their authors and supporters to strike at the following rule, which was in force in the Pennsylvania College of Dental Surgery.

Professor Barker, after quoting the rule published in the eleventh annual announcement, 1866-67, already given, further says:

The passage of the amended resolution was resisted by the faculty of the Pennsylvania College, as they believed it was the province of colleges not only to teach but to recognize and reward the merits of men who had by their labors contributed to the advancement of the interests of dentistry. That the indiscriminate granting of degrees was not desired; but that as far as they were concerned, they would abide by the judgment of the profession on the character, reputation, and ability of those thus graduating. These and many other reasons which space will not at present allow us to give, were offered for the non-passage of the resolution; but on a vote by colleges it was adopted. As this resolution was considered a censure on the past and prospective course of the Pennsylvania College of Dental Surgery, the faculty unanimously severed their connection with the Association.

On February 22, 1870, Professor Hartshorn resigned. On April 30th, Professor Forbes also resigned. On May 9th, Dr. James Tyson and Dr. J. Ewing Mears were elected to fill the vacancies. Professor Tyson's chair was entitled the chair of physiology and microscopic anatomy. Professor Mears of the chair of anatomy and surgery, was an adept in surgery, and had given special attention to surgery of the mouth and adjacent parts. Oral surgery was beginning to attract professional attention, and in his desire to make his services to the college as useful as possible, Professor Mears instituted a surgical clinic in connection with his chair. The following announcement appeared in the *Dental Times* (vol. viii, page 86):

We would announce to our friends that it is the desire of Professor Mears to hold a surgical clinic every Wednesday from 10 to 12 noon, during the session of the Pennsylvania College of Dental Surgery. At the clinics diseases of the oral cavity and all adjacent parts will receive particular attention. We respectfully request our friends to assist in obtaining cases, and all operations will be performed gratuitously.

This was very much appreciated by the students, and the clinic was continued during his thirty years' service as professor of these branches in this college.

No matters of special interest occurred in the college until the session of 1872-73, when the co-education question was finally settled. For several years it had been freely discussed, at time with much warmth. It had been brought to the notice of the board, who decided that there was no legal reason for excluding women from the school, but they recognized that it was the right of the faculty to decide who they would and who they would not admit. At a meeting of the board held June 26, 1871, after a free discussion of the subject the following resolution was adopted:

RESOLVED, That the advancing spirit of the age and the just right of women require that they shall be admitted to medical and dental education, and that the faculty of this college be requested to admit women as matriculants to the college at as early a period as they may deem advisable.

Several women had been admitted to the session of 1872-73, and on account of objection being made to their presence in the class their exclusion from the following session was suggested. The matter was carried to the board, which after having heard both sides of the question referred it to a special committee. This committee reported at a meeting of the board held March 31, 1873. Their report, which is quite long and which fully covered the whole matter, held that the act of matriculation was a contract between the school and the student of such a nature that while the student was under no obligation to attend a second course, the faculty were obligated to permit him to do so if he desired, and to continue his studies in the school as long as he continued to pay the fees and to conduct himself properly. That there was nothing in the charter of the institution prohibiting the entrance of women. That while the faculty had perfect liberty to matriculate or to refuse to matriculate anyone whom they chose, having once matriculated a student and accepted the customary fees they were obliged to permit that student to attend the full course, and to graduate if found qualified and no specific charges were brought against him. In taking the action they did, the whole faculty disclaimed any intention of excluding women from practicing dentistry, but objected to the education of the two sexes together in the same class.

In March 1873, the faculty decided to add a spring course of lectures, supplemental to the regular course, beginning on the first Monday in April 1873, and continuing until the last of June. During this session each one of the faculty was to deliver one lecture each week. The mechanical clinic was open from 9 to 12 noon, and the operative clinic from 2 to 4 P.M. A demonstrator was appointed for each clinic. They also decided to discontinue the *Dental Times* with the April number, when it would complete its tenth volume, the cause which brought it into being having ceased to exist.*

Another innovation introduced at this time was a corps of clinical lecturers, selecting for this position gentlemen who were specially skilful in some department of practice and were willing to now and again operate before the class or demonstrate some operative or mechanical procedure. This was inaugurated by appointing the following seven clinical lecturers: Drs. A. L. Northrop of New York city, C. A. Marvin of Brooklyn, C.

---

*The following announcement was published in the *Dental Times*, vol. x, April 1873:

"At a recent meeting of the faculty it was decided to suspend, for the present at least, the publication of the *Times* with the issue of this number, which completes volume x. The *Times*, which is, therefore, ten years old, was started at a period when the formation of energetic rival schools and the editorial relations held by the management of some of them required that our college should have an organ. The necessity seems now no longer to exist, and the faculty deem that they now, without detriment to the interests of the school, may relinquish the onerous duties of editors and publishers—how onerous they only know who have actually encountered them."

Palmer of Ohio, E. T. Darby, Robert Huey, and William H. Trueman of Philadelphia.

At a meeting of the board held September 5, 1876, the death of Professor Wildman was announced, and at the same meeting Professor Truman tendered his resignation. He was then in Germany, and finding that his business arrangements required his presence there for an indefinite period, decided to resign, which he did in a kindly note addressed to the board. Drs. Charles J. Essig and Edwin T. Darby were elected to fill the vacancies.

The session of 1877-78 was especially successful. The matriculates numbered one hundred and fifty-seven, and taxed to the utmost the accommodations afforded by the building then occupied. The advances in dental education required a large increase in the teaching staff; in addition to the professors it was deemed desirable to increase the number of demonstrators, and to make other changes looking to a more thorough training of the students.

About this time the University of Pennsylvania decided to organize a dental department in connection with its medical school, and made overtures to the faculty of the college suggesting the adoption of the college as a dental department of the University. At a meeting of the faculty of the Pennsylvania College of Dental Surgery, held December 17, 1877, the following communication was received and thoughtfully considered:

UNIVERSITY OF PENNSYLVANIA,
MEDICAL DEPARTMENT,
PHILADELPHIA, Dec. 10, 1877.
DR. CHAS. J. ESSIG, Dean of Pennsylvania College of Dental Surgery.
MY DEAR SIR: At a special meeting of the medical faculty held this evening, it was, on

motion, "Resolved that this faculty make overtures to the faculty of the Pennsylvania College of Dental Surgery with the view to a union of the latter college with the University of Pennsylvania as its Dental Department."

And on motion it was further "Resolved, that Professors Joseph Leidy and William Pepper be appointed a committee from this faculty to confer with the faculty of the Pennsylvania College of Dental Surgery at such time as may be appointed for the purpose."

Respectfully yours,
JAMES TYSON,
Sec'y of the Medical Faculty.

On motion of Dr. Barker it was resolved that a committee of the faculty as a whole be appointed to meet the committee .of the medical faculty on Wednesday evening, December 19, 1877, at the residence of Prof. James Tyson, 1506 Spruce street.

Thursday, December 27th, a special meeting of the faculty was held to consider the proposition of the University of Pennsylvania for a union of the two institutions by which the Pennsylvania College of Dental Surgery would become the Dental Department of the University of Pennsylvania. After much discussion a vote was taken with the result that four voted in favor of and two against the proposition.

The dean was directed to send to Prof. Joseph Leidy, chairman of the committee representing the faculty of the Medical Department of the University of Pennsylvania, the following answer:

To the Committee appointed by the Medical Faculty of the University of Pennsylvania.

DEAR SIRS: The faculty of the Pennsylvania College of Dental Surgery would respectfully state that they have carefully considered the proposition to unite the two institutions.

Drs. Essig, Barker, Tyson, and Darby would agree to unite under such regulations as might be agreed upon, provided it could be satisfactorily shown to them that such a fusion would tend directly to the advancement and good of the dental profession.

Drs. Mears and Buckingham object to the union on the ground that in their opinion such a coalition does not offer a promise of any advantage over the teachings of a well-appointed dental college.

CHARLES J. ESSIG,
Dean.

As it required the unanimous consent of the faculty to authorize the union, and this could not be obtained, the project was abandoned.

Toward the close of the session Professor Barker died, at the age of forty-two years. As the subjects he taught could be covered by the other chairs, the faculty, with the consent of the board, decided to permit his chair to remain vacant.

At the close of the session, Professors Essig, Tyson, and Darby, resigned to accept positions in a projected dental department of the University of Pennsylvania. Thus a second time in its history the faculty was compelled to reorganize.

Drs. C. N. Peirce, Wilbur F. Litch, and Henry C. Chapman were elected to fill the vacancies.

In order to increase the facilities of the college, the faculty secured a much larger building at the northwest corner of Twelfth and Filbert streets, leasing the second, third, fourth, and fifth floors. This location was quite as desirable as the one vacated, and the building was not only much larger but better adapted to the purpose. The windows were large and more numerous, and the entrance so situated as to permit a much more convenient arrangement of rooms. Among the more notable improvements introduced was a chemical laboratory properly fitted with desks for the individual use of students and well stocked with supplies and apparatus for the practical study of this science. Another was a dissecting room, properly fitted for this branch of anatomical study. This was placed in charge of Dr. Percival E. Loder, who was appointed demonstrator of anatomy. Heretofore dental students were compelled to seek conveniences for the practical study of anatomy outside of the dental school, and under teachers not conversant with their special needs. The lecture rooms were large, with high ceilings, provided with comfortable seats so disposed around the lecture table that the speaker could be heard and his demonstrations seen to the best advantage. Drs. Robert Huey and F. M. Dixon of Philadelphia, and Dr. J. N. Farrar of New York, were appointed lecturers on operative dentistry. These gentlemen delivered a short course of practical lectures during the session upon subjects with which they were especially familiar. These, with a staff of seven demonstrators in daily attendance at the clinics and thirteen clinical instructors who lectured occasionally or demonstrated practical operations or processes, made an imposing teaching staff. They also lengthened the term from four to five months. This with the fall and spring course made it possible for the student to spend nine months of each year under instruction in the theory and practice of dental surgery. So thorough, indeed, was the course, that with the first session in the new building the faculty were able to announce that owing to the increase in the length of term of the regular session and the great advances they had made in their methods of instruction, they had been able to make an arrangement with the Jefferson Medical College, through which such students as might desire to do so could, if found qualified, obtain the two degrees, in dentistry and medicine, in three instead of four years as heretofore.

Nothing of special interest occurred in the history of the college for several years. It was constantly progressing. The classes were large, and the staff of demonstrators and lecturers were from time to time increased.

Professor Buckingham died in the fall of 1883, and Dr. Henry Leffman was elected to fill the vacancy. March 20, 1885, Professor Chapman resigned the chair of physiology and general pathology, and on the same date Dr. Albert P. Brubaker was elected to fill the vacancy.

Constantly increasing classes demanding increased accommodations for practical work, and important extensions of the college curriculum requiring a substantial increase in the number of demonstrators, and in the auxiliary teaching staff, again prompted the faculty to look for better accommodations. A property at the northeast corner of Eleventh and Clinton streets was purchased. This location, in a residential section of the city, was especially desirable. Of the buildings already on the property, a portion was torn down to make way for new erections and the remaining part remodeled, making when completed a commodious and convenient college building. When the improvements were complete, the title to the property was transferred to the Board of Corporators, so that it will be for all time held in trust as an institution for the education of students in dentistry and the advancement of dental science. This building was occupied by the college for the first time at the beginning of the spring term, 1893.

During the following decade the dental colleges throughout the country experienced a season of great prosperity. Notwithstanding that dental colleges had increased in number from three, when this college was first organized, to nearly one hundred, and that the requirements were becoming more and more exacting, and that all "short cuts" to the dental degree were by united action of the colleges discontinued, the classes increased so rapidly that the capacity of the colleges was taxed to accommodate them. Of this the Pennsylvania College of Dental Surgery had a full share. To meet this, and to provide teachers for the new studies added to the dental curriculum, the staff of auxiliary instructors was largely increased. The introduction of a graded course, and the division of the matriculates into classes, each pursuing its own special course, and the further division of these into small groups for the purpose of individual instruction, made this necessary, and made necessary also a greater number of class and workrooms. It was not long before the entire building was fully occupied.

At a meeting of the board, May 15, 1898, it was decided to establish two additional chairs, to be entitled respectively dental anatomy, dental histology, and prosthetic technics, and clinical dentistry and oral pathology. I. Norman Broomell, D.D.S., was elected to the former and George W. Warren, A.M., D.D.S., to the latter. On March 2, 1899, Professor Mears tendered his resignation, which was accepted, and Dr. Loder, demonstrator of anatomy, was appointed to complete Professor Mears' course, and later was elected his successor. A new chair was created, W. J. Roe, M.D., D.D.S., being elected professor of surgical pathology and oral surgery.

This college is the third oldest now in existence, and at the close of its last session, 1903-04, had graduated over 2600. Its teaching staff, as announced for the coming session of 1904-05, is composed as follows:

FACULTY.

Wilbur F. Litch, M.D., D.D.S., Dean; Geo. W. Warren, A.M., D.D.S., Secretary; C. N. Peirce, D.D.S., emeritus professor of principles and practice of operative dentistry; Henry Leffman, A.M., M.D., D.D.S., emeritus professor of chemistry; Wilbur F. Litch, M.D., D.D.S., professor of materia medica, therapeutics and principles of prosthetic dentistry; Albert P. Brubaker, M.D., D.D.S., professor of physiology, general pathology and bacteriology; I. Norman Broomell, D.D.S., professor of dental anatomy, dental histology and prosthetic technics; George W. Warren, A.M., D.D.S., professor of principles and practice of operative dentistry; Percival E. Loder, M.D., D.D.S., professor of anatomy; W. J. Roe, M.D., D.D.S., professor of surgical pathology and oral surgery; J. Bird Moyer, B.S., Ph.D., professor of chemistry and metallurgy.

AUXILIARY INSTRUCTORS.

Instructors in Operative Dentistry.—E. Rowland Hearn, D.D.S., chief instructor; J. T. Yoder, D.D.S.; Louis Britton, D.D.S.; J. W. Adams, D.D.S.; Morris Lowenstein, D.D.S.; Frank G. Ritter, D.D.S., extracting and anesthetics.

Instructors in Prosthetic Dentistry.— Rupert G. Beale, D.D.S.; Frederick R. Brunet, D.D.S.; E. A. Kretschman, D.D.S.; S. E. Conley, D.D.S.; W. T. Herbst, D.D.S.

Instructor in Chemistry.—H. H. Shepler, B.S.

Instructor in Metallurgy.—E. E. Huber, D.D.S.

Instructor in Anatomy.—A. Grant Loder, A.M., M.D.; Justin E. Nyce, D.D.S., assistant.

Instructor in Surgery and Bandaging.—W. R. Roe, D.D.S.

SPECIAL INSTRUCTORS.

William B. Warren, D.D.S., instructor in crown and bridge work; H. L. Cragin, D.D.S., instructor in microscopy, dental histology and ceramics; F. P. Rutherford, Ph.G., D.D.S., instructor in bacteriology and pharmacology; Rupert G. Beale, D.D.S., instructor in appliances for cleft-palate deformities and maxillary fractures; W. K. Thorpe, D.D.S., instructor in operative technics.

Clinical Assistants.—Chair of anatomy: Samuel S. Peck, D.D.S.; Leroy W. Swartz, D.D.S.; Geo. B. Irvine. Chair of oral surgery: Edgar S. Coulter, D.D.S.; Anna M. Sellors, D.D.S.

CLINICAL INSTRUCTORS.

Dr. C. Palmer, Dr. Charles F. Bonsall, Dr. W. R. Millard, Dr. W. H. Trueman, Dr. R. Hollenback, Dr. A. B. Abell, Dr. H. Newton Young, Dr. J. Howard Gaskill, A. L. Orr, D.D.S., Dr. G. L. S. Jameson, Dr. H. C. Register.

DEANS.

The following professors of the College have filled the office of dean:
1856-57. Robert Arthur. 1857-60. T. L. Buckingham. 1860-62. William Calvert. 1862-65. C. N. Peirce. 1865-71. T. L. Buckingham. 1871-76. E. Wildman. 1876-77. George T. Barker. 1877-78. Charles J. Essig. 1878-99. C. N. Peirce. 1899-—. W. F. Litch.

SECRETARY.

1898—. G. W. Warren.

THE BOARD OF CORPORATORS.

The first Board of Corporators organized April 6, 1856, by electing Hon. Henry C. Carey president, and Mr. Thomas Wood secretary. Mr. Carey continued to serve as president, taking a keen interest in the welfare of the college until his death, which was announced at a meeting of the board, February 24, 1880. He left to the college by his will securities to the value of one thousand dollars. Notwithstanding that this legacy was legally void on account of his death taking place within thirty days of the date of his will, his residuary legatee promptly informed the board that his intentions would be respected, and in due time the

legacy was placed in the treasurer's hands.

February 24, 1880, Samuel D. Gross, M.D., L.L.D., D.C.L.Oxon., the distinguished surgeon, was elected his successor, and continued to serve until his death, in the latter part of 1884. December 2, 1884, S. W. Gross, M.D., was elected president, continuing in office until his death, which was announced at a meeting of the board held May 13, 1889. On this date I. Minis Hays, M.D., the present incumbent, was elected. Dr. Hays was elected a member of the board, March 20, 1885, and as a member of the board, and as its president, has ever shown a keen interest in the progress of the college and in efforts looking to a higher standard of professional education.

Mr. Thomas Wood, the first secretary, resigned that office in 1860; he continued, however, a member of the board until his death, May 27, 1880. Until near the close of his long and useful life he was a regular attendant at its meetings, and took an active part in the business of the board.

He was succeeded by Mr. Charles Hamilton, in 1860. Mr. Hamilton first interested himself in the college when the application for a charter was made to the legislature; he was elected to the board in 1857. For many years he was a constant visitor at the college clinics, and took a keen interest in the students' work. He was ever ready with a kind, encouraging word for a student, and quick to notice and praise a successful effort. Unobtrusive, and with tact just at the right time, he was ever ready with a helpful, practical suggestion to the inexperienced student, or with a soothing word to a restless patient; and now and again, when the working hour was over he was fond of a social chat with the "boys." He

25

died in 1872, leaving a legacy to the college. As his will was made within a short time of his death, this was legally void; no advantage, however, was taken of this, and in due time the college received an equitable share of his estate.

W. W. Fouché, D.D.S., was elected secretary February 25, 1873. Dr. Fouché, a member of the original board, was one of Philadelphia's prominent and skilful dentists, and took an active part in the educational movement which led to the organization of the first dental college in Philadelphia. He resigned the office of secretary February 24, 1880, but continued an active member of the board until, feeling the burden of advancing years, he resigned February 23, 1886.

David Roberts, D.D.S., was elected secretary February 24, 1880. Dr. David Roberts was elected a member of the board, February 23, 1875. Although he had been in practice several years before it was organized, he entered the first class of the Philadelphia College of Dental surgery, and was graduated from that institution at its second commencement, February 28, 1854. He continued to acceptably fill the office of secretary until his death, in the latter part of 1891.

His successor, Joseph Pettit, M.D., D.D.S., the present incumbent, was elected secretary February 26, 1892. He became a member of the board February 23, 1886.

G. R. Morehouse, M.D., the present treasurer, became a member of the board in 1857, and was shortly after elected treasurer. For nearly half a century he has taken an active part in the business of the board, and has faithfully performed the duties of the office he so acceptably fills.

Of the original members of the board, all have passed to the great beyond; some

died in harness, others resigned when feeling the burden of advancing years. Mr. T. S. Arthur left the board in 1862. Dr. Washington L. Atlee was a regular attendant at the meetings until his death, which was announced at the meeting held February 25, 1879. Dr. Daniel Neall resigned in 1863, was again elected February 26, 1878, and resigned on account of impaired health February 22, 1887. Dr. William Elder resigned in 1858. Dr. Stillé resigned in 1857. Dr. Benjamin Malone took an active part in all the work of the board, seldom missing a meeting, and was present at the one held immediately preceding that at which his death was announced. He died December 28, 1871, aged sixty-five years. Dr. George Truman was another faithful member of the board who died in harness. His death occurred November 21, 1877, in his seventy-ninth year.

The following were elected members of the board after its organization, April 6, 1856:

Elleslie Wallace, M.D., elected 1857. His death was announced at a meeting held March 20, 1885.

S. Dillingham, D.D.S., elected 1857. His death was announced at a meeting held February 28, 1882. Dr. Dillingham was a prominent member of the profession.

Mr. John R. McCurdy, elected 1862. He was of the firm of Jones, White & McCurdy, and edited for some time the *Dental News Letter*. While not a practitioner, his business brought him in close touch with the profession, and he took a keen interest in all that concerned its advancement. His death was announced at a meeting held February 26, 1867.

J. D. White, M.D., D.D.S., elected May 22, 1867. Dr. J. D. White entered the profession before the advent of dental colleges, and quickly made his mark as a skilful operator. He was a rapid workman, his office hours were long, and his practice extensive. He was studious, a close observer, and early appreciated the advantages to be derived by a mutual interchange of ideas between members of a common profession. He was energetic, a born leader, generous, and companionable. He took an active part in organizing the first dental association in Philadelphia, and the first dental college, and for many years as editor of the *Dental News Letter* and the *Dental Cosmos* he was one of the best-known dentists of Philadelphia, and his influence in advancing professional interests was widespread and lasting. Although a member of the faculty of the Philadelphia College of Dental Surgery, he was not in accord with those who disbanded, and took no part in organizing its successor. From that time his influence rapidly declined, and later he took no part in professional work. As a member of the board, until quite advanced in years, he took a fairly active part. He was still a member of the board when he died, Christmas Day, 1895. The dental association he did much to found celebrated its fiftieth anniversary a few days after his death.

Hon. William S. Peirce, elected May 22, 1867. Judge William S. Peirce, a highly esteemed member of the bar, proved a useful member of the board, as he freely gave of his legal talent in solving the vexed questions that now and again came before it. He took an active part in all its work until he resigned, May 20, 1885.

S. Weir Mitchell, M.D., elected February 27, 1872. Resigned Feb. 22, 1876.

James Aitken Meigs, M.D., elected February 26, 1879. Died the following year.

Prof. T. L. Buckingham, elected February 21, 1883; died September 4th in the same year.

Albert Pancoast, Esq., elected February 27, 1883. Resigned January 26, 1892.

Edward Hopper, Esq., elected February 27, 1883. Resigned February 21, 1891.

T. Morris Perot, elected December 2, 1884. Mr. Perot was a very faithful member of the board, and a useful one. His large experience in other like institutions gave weight to his counsel, and enabled him to quickly reach just conclusions. He was always present, even after he was stricken with blindness and had to be led to and from the meeting-place and his home. His death was announced to the board April 27, 1903.

Henry C. Gibson, elected February 28, 1888. His death was announced at the meeting held February 25, 1892.

Joseph M. Wilson, elected March 6, 1894. His death was announced April 27, 1903.

N. B. Crenshaw, elected March 2, 1895; died 1903.

THE PRESENT BOARD.

President, I. Minis Hays, M.D.; *Secretary,* Joseph Pettit, M.D., D.D.S.; *Treasurer,* George R. Morehouse, M.D.; John H. Brinton, M.D., LL.D., elected February 23, 1886; William W. Keen, M.D., F.R.C.S. (Lond.), elected May 13, 1889; William H. Trueman, D.D.S., elected February 25, 1892; Emlen Hutchinson, Esq., elected February 25, 1892; Hon. Samuel Gustine Thompson, elected February 25, 1892; W. Atlee Burpee, Esq., elected February 24, 1893; Charles F. Bonsall, D.D.S., elected March 2, 1895; C. N. Peirce, D.D.S., elected May 4, 1903; G. C. Purves, Esq., elected May 4, 1903.

IV.

History of the Dental Department of the University of Pennsylvania.

By WM. L. J. GRIFFIN, D.D.S., Philadelphia, Pa.

SHORTLY after its removal in the early seventies from the building on Ninth street between Chestnut and Walnut (which had been its home since 1802) to West Philadelphia, the University of Pennsylvania under the energetic and able leadership of the late Dr. William Pepper, entered upon an era of extension and increased usefulness made possible by its new location and the liberality of its friends. As part of this, its trustees decided to establish in connection with its medical department a department of dentistry. In furtherance of this, after an informal discussion of the project with those interested, a formal offer, inviting it to become the dental department of the University, was made to the faculty of the Pennsylvania College of Dental Surgery in the following communication, presented and read at a meeting of the said faculty December 17, 1877:

UNIVERSITY OF PENNSYLVANIA,
MEDICAL DEPARTMENT,
PHILADELPHIA, Dec. 10, 1877.

DR. CHAS. J. ESSIG, Dean of the Pennsylvania College of Dental Surgery.

My dear Sir,—At a special meeting of the Medical Faculty held this evening, it was, on motion, "Resolved, that this Faculty make overtures to the Faculty of the Pennsylvania College of Dental Surgery, with a view to the union of the latter College with the University of Pennsylvania as its Dental Department."

And on motion it was further "Resolved, that Professors Joseph Leidy and William Pepper be appointed a committee from this Faculty to confer with the Faculty of the Pennsylvania College of Dental Surgery at such time as may be appointed for the purpose."

Respectfully yours,

JAMES TYSON,
Sec'y of the Medical Faculty.

On motion of Dr. Barker it was "Resolved that the faculty as a whole be appointed a committee to meet the committee of the medical faculty on Wednesday evening, December 19th, at the residence of Professor Tyson, 1506 Spruce street." At the time and place named, the two committees met in conference.

On Thursday, December 27th, a special meeting of the faculty of the Pennsylvania College of Dental Surgery was held to consider the proposition of the medical faculty of the University. After a full discussion a vote was taken, four voting in favor of the proposed union and two against it.

The dean was directed to communicate to Prof. Joseph Leidy, chairman of the committee representing the faculty of the Medical Department of the University, the result of their deliberation, which he did in the following note:

To the Committee appointed by the Faculty of the Medical Department of the University of Pennsylvania.

Dear Sirs,—The Faculty of the Pennsylvania College of Dental Surgery would respectfully state that they have carefully considered the proposition to unite the two institutions. Drs. Essig, Barker, Tyson, and Darby would agree to unite under such regulations as might be agreed upon, provided it could be satisfactorily shown to them that such a fusion would tend directly to the advancement and good of the dental profession. Drs. Mears and Buckingham object to the union on the grounds that in their opinion such a coalition does not offer or promise any advantage over the teachings of a well-appointed dental college.

CHARLES J. ESSIG,
Dean.

As the unanimous consent of the faculty was necessary to a union, and this could not be obtained, the University proceeded to organize a dental department. Drs. Essig, Barker, Tyson, and Darby being favorable to the project, they resigned from the Pennsylvania College of Dental Surgery in order to take part in the new enterprise.

On March 6, 1878, the trustees of the University adopted the following resolutions:

RESOLVED, That there be a Dental Department of the University of Pennsylvania.

RESOLVED, That this department be under the government of a faculty of dentistry, subject to the general rules of the Board of Trustees.

RESOLVED, That the Faculty consist of the following professors: (a) Professor of mechanical dentistry and metallurgy; (b) Professor of operative dentistry and dental histology; (c) Professor of anatomy; (d) Professor of physiology; (e) Professor of chemistry; (f) Professor of materia medica; (g) Professor of general pathology. That the chairs of anatomy, chemistry, physiology, materia medica, and general pathology be filled *ex officio* by the corresponding professors of the medical faculty.

RESOLVED, That the lectures be delivered in the Medical Hall, and that the practical instruction be given in the proposed laboratory building.

Dr. Tyson, while holding a professorship in the Pennsylvania College of Dental Surgery was also a member of the medical faculty of the University. The burden of organizing the new department fell upon Drs. Essig and Darby; Dr. Barker, who entered upon the work with much enthusiasm, was not destined to take part in its active work, his death, January 10, 1878, in his forty-second year, cutting short a useful and promising career.

The organization of the new department was completed February 15, 1878, with the following professors appointed as its first faculty:

Charles J. Stillé, LL.D., provost of the University, and *ex officio* president of the faculty.

Charles J. Essig, M.D., D.D.S., professor of mechanical dentistry and metallurgy.

Edwin T. Darby, D.D.S., professor of operative dentistry, dental histology, and dental pathology.

Joseph Leidy, M.D., LL.D., professor of anatomy.

Horatio C. Wood, M.D., professor of materia medica, pharmacy, and general therapeutics.

James Tyson, M.D., professor of physiology, *ad interim*.

Theodore G. Wormley, M.D., LL.D., professor of chemistry.

Marshall H. Webb, D.D.S., and Robert Huey, D.D.S., lecturers on operative dentistry.

Clinical Instructors—Drs. Louis Jack, S. H. Guilford, H. C. Register, W. R. Millard, J. A. Woodward, R. H. Shoemaker, and George W. Klump.

H. C. Longnecker, D.D.S., demonstrator of operative dentistry.

H. K. Leech, D.D.S., assistant demonstrator of operative dentistry.

William Diehl, D.D.S., assistant demonstrator of operative dentistry.

A. H. Scofield, assistant demonstrator of operative dentistry.

E. C. Kirk, D.D.S., assistant demonstrator of mechanical dentistry.

Robert J. Nickell, assistant demonstrator of mechanical dentistry.

H. Lenox Hodge, M.D., demonstrator of anatomy.

Griffith E. Abbott, Ph.G., demonstrator of practical chemistry.

At a meeting of the faculty held March 15th, Dr. Charles J. Essig was elected secretary of the faculty. At this same meeting Drs. Tyson, Essig, and Darby were appointed a committee to arrange a curriculum. The furnishing of the operating room and laboratory, issuing of announcements, and other business matters were considered.

Shortly thereafter, Dr. Essig, as secretary of the faculty, announced to the provost of the University that the dental department was fully organized.

The first spring session began April 1, 1878. The lectures were delivered in the lecture rooms of the medical department, the operative and mechanical clinics were temporarily provided for in an adjoining building. The trustees of the University provided liberally for this new department, and at once ordered the erection of a new building for its special accommodation. The plans for the new structure provided on the first floor an operating room, 140 feet in length by 40 feet in width, lighted by windows on all sides, thus affording 360 feet of window frontage, giving ample light for a large number of chairs. It also provided for this

room stationary washstands, and other conveniences and appliances for comfort and use.

The upper floors accommodated the chemical and other laboratories, used jointly by dental and medical students. The prosthetic laboratory and the lecture rooms were located in an adjoining building.

The first matriculate was Dr. Edward C. Kirk, who had just graduated from the Pennsylvania College of Dental Surgery. The first to enter as a regular full-course student was Mr. R. B. Martin of Rocky Mount, Louisiana, who graduated March 15, 1881.

The first session of the Dental Department of the University of Pennsylvania was very encouraging. The matriculates numbered fifty-three. The clinics were well attended; more patients presented than could be accommodated. The session was closed March 1, 1879, by a public commencement at the Academy of Music, when the degree of Doctor of Dental Surgery was conferred upon the following twenty-five students:

Walter La T. Graves, California.
Stephen L. Wiggins, Canada.
Alfred H. Scofield, Connecticut.
Henry J. Garrett, Jr., Delaware.
George C. Brown, Iowa.
Edwin C. Timerman, Illinois.
William J. O'Doherty, Ireland.
George H. Van Meter, Italy.
Henry C. Aldrich, Minnesota.
Lactance A. Brodeur, M.D., Michigan.
Wayland W. Hayden, Massachusetts.
Alfred J. Nims, Massachusetts.
Levi W. Johnson, New Jersey.
Willoughby D. Miller, Ohio.
J. Dorrance Dow, Pennsylvania.
Charles G. Joy, Pennsylvania.
Frank Morton Long, Pennsylvania.
William H. Masser, Pennsylvania.
Louis DeL. Moss, Pennsylvania.
Robert J. Nickell, Pennsylvania.

John Ramsden, Pennsylvania.
Charles C. Walker, Pennsylvania.
Alexander McG. Denham, Scotland.
Fritz Hroch, Saxony.
Adolf Wetzel, Switzerland.

The new building was completed and furnished in time for the second annual session. No change was made in the faculty, and but little in the teaching staff.

The matriculates numbered seventy-seven, a notable increase; and at the second commencement, held March 15, 1880, the degree D.D.S. was conferred upon twenty graduates.

The third session opened with one hundred and ten matriculates and at its close, March 15, 1881, the graduates numbered forty-seven.

At the close of this session Dr. Horatio C. Wood withdrew from the dental faculty. To fill this vacancy, Dr. William Pepper, provost of the University, suggested to the dental faculty that they forward to the trustees a formal request for the establishment of a chair of dental therapeutics, materia medica, and pathology, thus enlarging and strengthening the distinctive dental faculty. He also suggested the appointment of Dr. James Truman, as lecturer on this subject. This suggestion meeting the approval of the dental faculty was promptly acted upon, and at their request the trustees established the new chair, and elected Dr. Truman, a former member of the faculty of the Pennsylvania College of Dental Surgery, to this new position, as suggested by Dr. Pepper.

At a meeting of the faculty of the Dental Department held December 20, 1881, the following resolution was adopted:

Whereas, considerable numbers of females come to this country from Europe for the purpose of studying dentistry, and

Whereas, there are no dental schools for females in which young women can obtain the desired learning, the dental faculty favoring the admission of females to the department of dentistry: therefore, be it

RESOLVED, That the Honorable Board of Trustees be requested to give the matter concerning female matriculates in the dental department early consideration.

No action was, however, taken.

The matriculates of the fourth session numbered eighty-eight, and the graduates forty-one.

On September 26, 1882, Prof. Chas. J. Essig resigned the secretaryship, owing to the demands of a large practice. He had held this position from the organization of the department, and had labored unceasingly to promote its welfare. His resignation was accepted, and at a meeting of the faculty held May 22, 1883, Prof. James Truman was chosen his successor.

The matriculates for the fifth session numbered seventy-nine, and the graduates thirty-four.

During the session of 1885-86, Professor Truman called the attention of the faculty to the fact that the diploma of the Dental Department was not recognized in Europe, and that an opportunity was then open to bring the subject before the British General Medical Council. To further this, Professor Truman was instructed to communicate with that body. This he did. A reply to his communication was read at a meeting of the faculty held February 16, 1886, in which the General Medical Council declined to recognize the dental qualification of the University of Pennsylvania. This action was taken in pursuance of a policy adopted by the General Medical Council of Great Britain to upbuild their own dental schools by refusing to recognize those of foreign countries.

The question of admitting female matriculates was again brought up at a meeting of the faculty held May 17, 1887, when letters were read from several female dental students attending other schools, who desired to complete their course at the University. These were referred to the provost, Dr. William Pepper, who returned to Professor Truman, secretary of the faculty, the following reply:

DEAR PROFESSOR TRUMAN:

I have carefully considered your note. There is no objection to allow female students to work in the operating department only, it being understood that they do not become regular students, but are only taking a special course. On the other hand, according to the prevailing views, it would be entirely wrong to admit Mrs. N. or any other woman as a regular student in the Department of Dentistry.

Yours respectfully,

WILLIAM PEPPER.

Prior to this a few minor changes had been made in the teaching staff. At the opening of the session of 1881-82, Dr. Ambler Tees was appointed lecturer on mechanical dentistry, a position he held only for that session. Dr. Marshall H. Webb, who had acceptably filled the position of lecturer on operative dentistry from the foundation of the department, died January 1, 1883; the vacancy was not immediately filled.

Dr. Harrison Allen resigned from the chair of physiology the latter part of 1885, and Dr. Edward T. Reichert was elected to his place.

At the beginning of the session of 1886-87, Dr. Louis Jack was appointed lecturer on operative dentistry, a position he held for several years.

No further changes were made until the session of 1889-90, when Dr. George A. Piersol was elected professor of his-

tology; Dr. Edward C. Kirk appointed lecturer on operative dentistry, and Dr. John D. Thomas lecturer on nitrous oxid anesthesia.

The following session Dr. John Marshall was elected assistant professor of chemistry.

The session of 1891-92 witnessed a decided advance in dental education. In accordance with a resolution of the National Association of Dental Faculties the dental course in all the colleges was extended from two to three years, and in addition to this, more attention was given the preliminary educational requirements. During the few years the Dental Department of the University had been in existence its teaching staff had been gradually increased from sixteen until at this period it numbered twenty-six, fifteen of that number being demonstrators, an important teaching body from the fact that they are in frequent and prolonged personal contact with the students, and are in a measure depended upon for instruction in manipulative work. The curriculum of the department has been enlarged, and every effort made to teach more of the collateral sciences closely associated with dental surgery, and to teach more thoroughly its technics, which form so important a part of dental practice. The addition of another year was warmly welcomed, giving as it did a wished-for opportunity of doing better work. In view of this, Dr. Pepper suggested renewed effort to secure foreign recognition for its diploma. The authorities abroad, however, were inflexible.

At the beginning of the session of 1894-95, Dr. Norman Sturges Essig was appointed lecturer on mechanical dentistry, and Dr. Meyer L. Rhein of New York, lecturer on dental pathology.

During the year 1895, Dr. William

Pepper resigned as provost of the University. The cares of his large medical practice and his ceaseless energy in molding and directing the business affairs of the University, and in providing for its maintenance on broad and generous lines, proved a severe strain upon his well-endowed physique. His indomitable will long held this in check, but the time came, nevertheless, when he was compelled to seek rest and to leave the work so well begun in other hands. A few years later, while reading, and alone, he quietly passed to the great beyond; so quietly indeed, that he still sat, apparently absorbed in his book, long after life had ceased. It may truly be said of Dr. Pepper that he made the University what it was, and opened to it possibilities yet to be realized.

He was succeeded as provost by Charles Custis Harrison, LL.D.

During this year Dr. Edward C. Kirk was elected to the newly created chair of clinical dentistry, and at the same time elected dean of the faculty, vice Professor Truman, who had held the position a number of years.

During the session of 1896-97, Dr. Wormley having died, Dr. John Marshall was elected to his place as professor of chemistry; Dr. Matthew H. Cryer was elected assistant professor of oral surgery; Dr. Safford G. Perry of New York was appointed lecturer on operative dentistry, and Dr. Fred. A. Peeso lecturer on crown and bridge work.

The building erected for the accommodation of the Dental Department at its organization proved quite satisfactory for a number of years. As time passed, however, larger classes, changes in the curriculum and in methods of instruction, required more room than this building afforded. The equipments of operating room and laboratories, while well up to date when installed, no longer met modern requirements.

To remedy this, the trustees of the University proceeded to erect a more modern building for the exclusive use of the Dental Department.

The plans were carefully drawn under the supervision of the dental faculty after a critical examination of the more modern structures occupied by dental schools. This building was completed, furnished, and ready for occupancy in October 1897, and was used in the session of 1897-98.

It provided a large operating room 180 by 50 feet, lighted by windows on all sides; this was furnished with one hundred operating chairs and other appliances of modern pattern. In addition to this a number of smaller rooms, suitably furnished, provide accommodation and equipment for the performance of various prosthetic operations, and for special clinics. A large prosthetic laboratory fitted with the latest and the best appliances for the construction of all kinds of dentures and dental appliances, laboratories for instruction in metallurgy, porcelain work, etc., lecture and class rooms, museum, library, offices, etc., provide ample and convenient facilities for teaching and for conducting the business affairs of the school.

In the latter part of 1898 Dr. George C. Milliken was elected assistant professor of operative technics.

After the close of the session 1898-99, Dr. Robert Huey resigned as lecturer on operative dentistry, a position he had held continuously since the department was organized, in order to fill his appointment as a member of the State Board of Dental Examiners of Pennsylvania.

Beginning with the session 1900-01, Dr. Cryer was promoted to the full professorship of oral surgery, and Dr. Alexander C. Abbott was elected professor of bacteriology.

About the time the session of 1901-02 opened, Dr. Essig resigned the chair of mechanical dentistry and metallurgy. On December 2, 1901, he died after a brief illness from pneumonia, in his sixty-first year. Dr. Essig was skilful in his profession, and particularly expert in all that pertains to the subjects he taught; he was also a fluent speaker. He had the happy faculty of clearly expressing ideas, and was an artist in blackboard illustrations. Dignified, yet approachable, he commanded the respect and attracted the attention of his pupils. As one of the organizers of the Dental Department of the University, his experience, his zeal, his clear comprehension of present and prospective needs did much to place the new school upon a firm foundation; his ability, his wise counsel and untiring devotion to its interests contributed much to its success. His chair remained vacant during that session.

Near the close of the session, Dr. Julio Endelman was appointed instructor in materia medica.

At the opening of the session of 1902-03, Dr. Charles R. Turner, an alumnus of the school, was elected to the chair made vacant by the resignation of Dr. Essig.

Preparatory to the session of 1903-04, several changes were made in the teaching staff. Dr. Milliken was elected assistant professor of operative technics; Dr. R. Hamill D. Swing assistant professor of oral surgery and anesthesia; and Dr. A. DeWitt Gritman assistant professor of prosthetic dentistry.

For the coming session of 1904-05 two new names are added to the faculty: Dr. Elisha H. Gregory, Jr., assistant profes-

sor of anatomy; and Dr. David H. Bergey, assistant professor of bacteriology.

The following list of the full staff for this session, embracing as it does the names of forty-six instructors, each of whom have a stated part in the course, and of five clinical instructors who render an occasional service, compared with that of the first session is a striking exhibit of the progress made in dental instruction, and of the growth of the institution. The students at the first session numbered fifty-three; at the last, three hundred and sixty-two.

FACULTY.

Charles C. Harrison, LL.D., provost; Edgar F. Smith, Ph.D., Sc.D., vice-provost; Edwin T. Darby, D.D.S., M.D., professor of operative dentistry and dental histology; James Truman, D.D.S., professor of dental pathology, therapeutics and materia medica; Edward C. Kirk, D.D.S., Sc.D., professor of clinical dentistry, and dean of the Faculty; Matthew H. Cryer, D.D.S., M.D., professor of oral surgery; Charles R. Turner, D.D.S., M.D., professor of mechanical dentistry and metallurgy; Edward T. Reichert, M.D., professor of physiology; George A. Piersol, M.D., professor of anatomy; John Marshall, M.D., Nat. Sc.D., LL.D., professor of chemistry and toxicology; *Alexander C. Abbott, M.D., professor of bacteriology; George G. Milliken, D.D.S., M.D., assistant professor of operative technics; R. Hamill D. Swing, D.D.S., assistant professor of oral surgery and anesthesia; A. DeWitt Gritman, D.D.S., assistant professor of mechanical dentistry; Elisha H. Gregory, Jr., M.D., assistant professor of anatomy: David H. Bergey, A.M., M.D., assistant professor of bacteriology.

LECTURERS.

John D. Thomas, D.D.S., lecturer on nitrous oxid; Meyer L. Rhein, D.D.S., M.D., lecturer on dental pathology; Safford G. Perry, D.D.S., lecturer on operative dentistry; Julio Endelman, D.D.S., lecturer on materia medica.

*Absent on public business.

DEMONSTRATORS.

William Diehl, D.D.S., demonstrator of operative dentistry; James G. Lane, D.D.S., demonstrator of mechanical dentistry; Ambler Tees, D.D.S., demonstrator of dental ceramics; Frederick Amend, Jr., D.D.S., demonstrator of mechanical dentistry; Milton N. Keim, Jr., D.D.S., demonstrator of mechanical dentistry; J. Edward Dunwoody, D.D.S., demonstrator of crown and bridge work; Robert J. Seymour, D.D.S., demonstrator of mechanical dentistry; A. Swanton Burke, D.D.S., demonstrator of mechanical dentistry; William C. Marsh, D.D.S., demonstrator of operative dentistry; James A. Dowden, D.D.S., demonstrator of mechanical dentistry; Wilson Zerfing, D.D.S., demonstrator of operative dentistry; G. Janvier Paynter, D.D.S., demonstrator of tooth-modeling; Frederick W. Allen, D.D.S., demonstrator of operative technics; John A. McClain, D.D.S., demonstrator of operative dentistry; Robert Formad, M.D., demonstrator of normal histology; George H. Chambers, M.D., assistant demonstrator of normal histology; Augustus O. Koenig, B.S., M.D., demonstrator of dental metallurgy and assistant demonstrator of normal histology; John M. Swan, M.D., demonstrator of osteology; Daniel W. Fetterolf, M.D., demonstrator of chemistry; S. Merrill Weeks, D.D.S., demonstrator of orthodontia; Walter W. McKay, D.D.S., demonstrator of porcelain inlay work; Albert W. Jarman, D.D.S., demonstrator of mechanical dentistry; Jehu T. Gore, D.D.S., demonstrator of operative dentistry; Edward Lodholz, M.D., demonstrator of physiology; J. Garrett Hickey, D.D.S., assistant demonstrator of physiology; George O. Jarvis, M.D., assistant demonstrator of applied anatomy; Charles H. Jaco, D.D.S., demonstrator of operative dentistry; Alfred P. Lee, D.D.S., demonstrator of operative dentistry.

CLINICAL INSTRUCTORS.

Dr. C. S. Beck, Dr. Edward I. Keffer, Dr. Daniel N. McQuillen, Dr. H. C. Register, Dr. John R. Yorks.

V.

History of the Boston Dental College.

By H. H. PIPER, D.D.S., Somerville, Mass.

WHEN, soon after the close of the war of the States, men began to turn their attention from the devastation of contending armies to the arts of peace, a new impulse and a new effort became manifest in almost all the activities of life. Dental education was no exception to the rule. Hitherto in New England there had been no systematic instruction in the theory and practice of dentistry. There had been two methods by which skill might be acquired in this profession: one by means of a medical education with such other help as could be obtained by a greater or less amount of time spent in a dental office; the other through an apprenticeship in a dental office chiefly, and often with very little supplemental aid from books and lectures. It was largely a matter of emphasis—in one instance on the theoretical side, in the other on the practical—and occasionally the two methods were happily blended.

It is not strange then, under these conditions, that though the impulse was one, and in the same place, the outcome should have been divided. Two dental schools came into existence in the city of Boston at practically the same time, each graduating its first students in the year

1869. The former, the Harvard Dental School, was founded in 1867, and was a continuation of the instruction given to dental students in the Harvard Medical School supplemented by clinical and mechanical departments and definite lectures along dental lines. The latter school, The Boston Dental College, was founded in 1868. Two students with one year each of previous medical education were graduated the following year. This school was a continuation (for everything grows out of something gone before) of the best elements and best traditions of the dental office, with the addition of a full quota of lectures in theory and practice. Here then were two schools—one allied to an older institution, the other independent; one laying emphasis rather on the theoretical side, the other on the practical—each with its ideals and its place to fill in the development of dental education. So much of previous history it has been necessary to give that the antecedents and the true place of the Boston Dental College might appear in clearer outline.

Confining our attention now to the one school, it must appear at a glance that in the beginning it had elements both of strength and weakness: strength in its practical efficiency which has never been seriously called in question, in its independence and open-mindedness toward new methods and new truth; weakness along lines of administration, where much was to be learned through experience, through the lack of funds and the inability to secure those varied helps which are to be found in an alliance with an old and well-endowed institution. The men who took charge of the school at the beginning were many of them among the most prominent and skilful in their profession. Some of them were possessed of

decided executive ability, but they had never been called to manage the affairs of an educational institution. Those early years, it was needless to add, were more or less stormy; disaffection and discouragement were not unknown; but there were also present elements of devotion and self-sacrifice, and there was constantly reappearing a vital energy which would not allow an institution with so evident a mission to languish and die. At the end of ten years the school had become favorably known beyond the borders of New England. During the second decade the membership of the classes increased rapidly and the average membership of the graduating classes for this period was twenty; during the third decade the average number graduated each year was thirty-eight; and at the time of the union with Tufts College it was nearly fifty. The total number of students who received a degree was seven hundred. The course of instruction, at first two years, was extended to three years after 1884.

Changes in the location of the school were at first frequent; later they became less frequent and were usually for the purpose of securing ampler accommodations. The first home of the school was at 4 Hamilton place. The stay here was brief, and a change was made to rooms in Tremont Temple. A second removal was to a building on the corner of Dover street and Shawmut avenue, the whole building being occupied above the first floor. A fourth home was at 485 Tremont street, where, as before, a whole building above the first floor was utilized. The very rapid growth of the school at this period (1890) soon necessitated another change, and very much enlarged quarters were found at 563 Tremont street. This latest home soon became inadequate for the nearly two hundred students in attendance, but no further change was made till the occupancy of rooms in the new medical and dental building of Tufts College on Huntington avenue.

As is many times the case with young and unendowed institutions, the school was often sorely in need of funds. Again and again those who had its interests at heart came to its rescue. Gradually, however, this difficulty was overcome, a fund was accumulated for building purposes, and when by an act of the legislature the school came under a new management, it was able to make over to Tufts College the sum of forty-two thousand nine hundred and fifty dollars.

In an article of this length it is impossible to enter into the details of the thirty-two years of the school's independent life. It grew as a young man grows, through storm and stress, through difficulty and failure, through the joy of success and realized hope, into an ever-deepening knowledge of its powers, its

needs and its mission. Its life was singularly one: it had practically but one administration. Two men whose names appear in the list of incorporators, and who were vitally connected with the school at the beginning, were as vitally connected with it thirty-two years later: Dr. I. J. Wetherbee, president of the board of trustees for nearly the entire period, and Dr. J. A. Follett, a member of the faculty and for many years the dean.

It would be very pleasant to give some idea of the men eminent in their various callings who gave the school a standing and contributed to its success; to select for special mention some of the graduates of the school who by their success in the best sense have made its name honorable; but space forbids. It can only be added that good work never dies, and growth never ceases; and that the Boston Dental College, itself a growth out of the past, will live on worthily under another name, and never cease to exert an influence for good.

VI.

The Harvard Dental School.*

By L. D. SHEPARD, D.D.S., Boston, Mass.

BRIEFLY told, the history of Harvard Dental School is as follows: The annual address to the Massachusetts Dental Society in 1865 was delivered by its president, the late Dr. Nathan Cooley Keep.

He gave expression to a feeling which existed in New England, that students in dentistry should not be required to go to distant states for their education, by suggesting the inquiry "whether Harvard University might not appoint professors of dentistry and confer upon proper candidates the degree of Doctor of Dental Surgery."

On March 6, 1865, the society voted:

*[From Anniversary Address, with Historical Reminiscences, by Dr. L. D. Shepard. Delivered March 11, 1889; published, Boston, 1890.]

That a committee of three be appointed to take under advisement the subject of the establishment of a chair of dentistry in the Harvard Medical College, in accordance with the recommendation of the president in his annual address.

A committee was appointed consisting of Drs. Nathan C. Keep, I. J. Wetherbee, and T. H. Chandler. The records of the society contain no other reference to the subject until March 5, 1866, when, upon a report from Dr. Keep, a new committee was appointed to confer with the officers of the medical college. This committee consisted of the late N. C. Keep, M.D., the late E. C. Rolfe, M.D., and L. D. Shepard, D.D.S.

The medical faculty appointed as a committee to meet this committee was Drs. Henry I. Bowditch, Henry J. Bigelow, and Calvin Ellis. Conferences were held, the subject discussed, and at the request of the medical committee, the dental committee drew up a plan for the formation of a dental school. This plan was the basis of a report by the medical committee to the medical faculty, March 29, 1867, favoring the project.

Among the reasons given by the medical committee were the following:

Dentistry has become within the past quarter of a century a most important art, a knowledge of which supposes not only mechanical skill but a thorough acquaintance with the processes of dentition physiologically and pathologically considered. Hence arises the necessity for a knowledge of the general principles of anatomy, physiology, surgery, chemistry, and materia medica, to which should be added some knowledge of the theory and the practice of medicine. A medical school already established is therefore the best place at which these various studies can be attended to. It is all-important that the art should be cultivated by all the means in our power, in order that the crowd of dentists that will hereafter be in this city may not be of a lower quality than their predecessors. . . . .

With such facts and others that might be named, can there be any doubt that some dental college should be established in Boston?

To this report was appended the following resolution, which was unanimously adopted by the medical faculty:

RESOLVED, That the dean be directed to petition the Corporation of Harvard College to establish a dental school, according to the terms proposed in the second report of the committee of the Massachusetts Dental Society.

The corporation, after full investigation, voted, on July 17, 1867, to establish the dental school, and that the faculty consist of the professors of anatomy and physiology, chemistry, and surgery in the medical school and of three new professors—of dental pathology and therapeutics, of operative dentistry, and of mechanical dentistry. In this vote the Board of Overseers afterward concurred.

It will be noticed that the committee of the dental society consisted of two M.D.'s and one D.D.S. The committee of the medical faculty insisted with firmness upon one condition, that in the dental school all the professors, dental as well as medical, should be graduates in medicine. The one D.D.S. found himself not only in a minority, but that, if he opposed this condition too vehemently, the whole project might fall through. He felt that the cordial and hearty support of the medical faculty was necessary to establish such a dental school as the committee had planned. He accepted the situation for himself and for all the dental graduates whom he represented, and the two committees were thus unanimous.*

_____

*At a later date October 16, 1871 the corporation, in justice to its own dental graduates, removed the restriction which required that the dental professors be graduates in medicine.

During these thirteen months of deliberation and conference the dental committee made no report to the dental society; but at a meeting on April 1, 1867, Dr. Keep reported:

That the committee had attended to its duties; had held several meetings with the committee of the medical faculty, consisting of Drs. Bowditch, Bigelow, and Ellis; that a plan had been agreed upon which was satisfactory to each committee, and had already been unanimously adopted by the medical faculty.

A report was made also of the plan of the school, and with these reports the work of the committee was ended.

The provision that the dental professors should be graduates in medicine caused dissatisfaction and disappointment on the part of many. This soon after culminated in the organization of the Boston Dental Institute, and the following winter a charter was secured from the legislature for another dental college in Boston. It is also worthy of notice that earnest efforts made at the same time to induce a university in a neighboring state to establish a similar school were unsuccessful, because that institution demanded as a preliminary a large endowment as a pecuniary safeguard against loss. The expression of President Hill in this connection should be recorded: "In whatever direction there is a demand for liberal culture, Harvard should be ready and willing to furnish the means." The first appointments were made on November 30, 1867, that of Daniel Harwood, M.D., to the chair of dental pathology and therapeutics, and of N. C. Keep, M.D., to the chair of mechanical dentistry.

It was not till four months after these appointments, March 19, 1868, that the first faculty meeting was held. At this meeting Dr. Keep was elected dean and there were present President Hill, Drs. Bigelow, Holmes, Bacon, Harwood, and Keep.

A second meeting was held April 8, 1868. At the third meeting, May 28, 1868, the resignation of Dr. Harwood was announced. Notwithstanding his eminent abilities the appointment of Dr. Harwood was a mistake. He had not been in sympathy with the movement from the beginning, and he continued to hold rigidly to his view that the dental student should be educated both in medicine and dentistry in the medical school by adding to that school a chair of dentistry, rather than in a separate dental school. Thus, six months were lost in vain efforts to organize with such discordant elements. At this meeting, May 28, 1868, it was unanimously voted:

That in the event of the acceptance of the resignation of Daniel Harwood, M.D., by the corporation, the name of Thomas Barnes Hitchcock, M.D., be suggested to fill the chair of dental pathology and therapeutics made vacant by the resignation of Dr. Harwood; that the name of George T. Moffatt, M.D., be suggested as a suitable person to fill the chair of operative dentistry; and that L. D. Shepard, D.D.S., be suggested as a suitable person for adjunct professor of operative dentistry.

On June 5, 1868, the corporation made the above appointments. The faculty thus constituted proved harmonious and united, and at once began preparations for a session the following autumn.

A little incident which happened at the commencement of the first course of instruction illustrates the spirit of that first faculty. A young man had written from his home in Washington to the dean of a dental college and had been accepted, by letter, as a student, but when he arrived and presented himself for matriculation he was informed that he could not be received since it would jeopardize the success of the college to admit one of his race as a student. He next applied to the dean of another college in the same city and met a like repulse. He came to Boston, called upon our dean, Dr. Keep, and asked to be received. The faculty decided that the Dental School of Harvard University should consider right and justice above expediency, and know no distinction of nativity or color, and among the six who received the dental doctorate, Robert Tanner Freeman was the peer of any as a student and a gentleman. His name stands upon the records as the earliest of our alumni to be starred, and in history will remain as the first of his race to receive dental collegiate honors.

The first session commenced at the usual date of all the dental colleges, the first Wednesday in November. There were sixteen matriculated, of whom six had been in practice from five to twelve years. The dental students received instruction in common with the medical students in anatomy, physiology, surgery, and chemistry.

The Massachusetts General Hospital, with great liberality gave to the school the free use of its out-patients' department as an infirmary for clinical operations and instruction, and for lectures on operative dentistry. This assistance from the hospital authorities should ever be held in grateful remembrance. The close connection of the school and the hospital continued for many years and was of inestimable assistance to the school in its youth and poverty.

At a faculty meeting on February 16, 1869, it was voted: "That Dentariæ Medicinæ Doctor (D.M.D.) be recommended to the Board of Government of Harvard University as the title for the degree to be conferred upon the graduates of the dental department"; and on February 27th the corporation established this degree.

Considerable criticism, some of it harsh and ungenerous, has resulted from the introduction of a new degree in place of the old D.D.S. It was not thought necessary at the time to explain the reasons for the change. These reasons, however, were very simple. It was the original expectation of the faculty to confer the old degree. The writing of a diploma was committed to Professor Lane, the head of the Latin department. Upon investigation it was found that a degree had never been conferred upon dentists by a classical institution. From a classical standpoint the question was thus a new one. It was also found that the dental college which had originated the degree of D.D.S. (the Baltimore College of Dental Surgery) had written its diploma in Latin, and that the degree which it had always given was "Chirurgiæ Dentium Doctor," the proper initials of which would give a C instead of an S with the two D's. It was first proposed to make the degree "Scientiæ Dentium Doctor," so that the initials would remain unchanged; but this would be liable to the same charge of being a new degree; and, moreover, dentistry was not properly a science. It was decided, finally, to qualify the old degree of "Medicinæ Doctor" by the prefix "Dentariæ," and thus at the same time meet the classical requirements and give what seemed a proper and distinctive title. There was no thought of arrogating to the institution any special superiority or claim of exclusiveness. Further, it was expected that the new degree would approve itself to other universities which might have dental departments and thus gradually become the accepted degree.

On March 6, 1869, was held at the old Harvard Medical College the examination of the candidates for the degree. This was an oral examination, since at that time the examinations for the medical degree were also oral. On March 10th occurred the commencement. Prof. Edward H. Clark, M.D., delivered the address; Prof. Henry J. Bigelow, M.D., conferred the degrees upon six successful candidates.

The following year there were twenty-seven matriculates and twelve graduates. This year is noticeable for the addition to the faculty on October 26, 1869, of Dr. Thomas H. Chandler as adjunct professor of mechanical dentistry.

The third session, 1870-71, there were thirty-three matriculates and six graduates.

In the fall of 1870 the house No. 50 Allen street was bought with borrowed money and altered to adapt it for lectures, and for general headquarters for the school, and furnished with a large and complete mechanical laboratory. The debt caused by its purchase proved a great burden to the school for many years.

Thus far the Harvard School had pursued a course similar to the other dental colleges. It had steadily gained in reputation and was year after year attracting an increasing number of students. The outlook was brilliant and promised larger and larger classes.

But in the fall of 1871, upon the recommendation of the faculty, the corporation voted to abolish the custom which was universal with the dental colleges of allowing a practice of five years to be equivalent to the first course of study, and of permitting the graduation of stu-dents after attending one course at the school. This was the most important innovation ever made, and its influence upon the profession and the colleges was excellent. It was equally disastrous in its effects, pecuniarily considered, upon the school. The faculty felt that this custom had been a great hindrance to progress, that its effect had been to hold out to young students an inducement to wait till their five years' experimenting upon patients enabled them to graduate after one short course, rather than to prepare for practice by a proper, thorough course of preliminary study.

The Harvard School was the first, and for many years the only one, to establish the principle, at great expense to itself, that the college was designed to educate the young men just entering the profession, and not simply to confer the doctorate upon the more or less skilled handiworkers who had practiced without a degree for five or more years. Boldly living up to its convictions, it maintained unassisted for years this higher standard, and thus cut itself off from the support of a very large class of practitioners, throughout New England especially, who, having no degree and wishing one, would otherwise have attended its instruction and enrolled themselves among its alumni.

On November 13, 1871, owing to ill health, Dr. Keep resigned his professorship, and was succeeded by the adjunct professor, Dr. Chandler. The name of Dr. Nathan Cooley Keep should be cherished above that of any other dentist who has ever lived in Boston. He alone of the older, more experienced, and celebrated dentists of the day united with the younger and less-known class in forming the Massachusetts Dental Society. The others stood aloof and held

26

themselves above such association. He, in his age, was as young as the youngest. He was earnest in investigation, generous in opening the storehouse of his extended experience, prudent and wise in counsel, and indefatigable in every good dental work. The starting of the Harvard Dental School was mainly the result of his efforts. It is doubtful if success would have followed other leadership. Until compelled to retire he was devoted to the school, and in the feebleness of advanced age these extra labors and anxieties undertaken undoubtedly hastened his breaking down which soon followed. Let us remember him ever as the Harvard Dental School's father, great friend, and first martyr.

In the year 1872 several important changes were made. Dr. Hitchcock was elected dean. Written examinations were substituted for oral, and the candidate was required to pass successfully in each subject instead of in a majority of them, as had been the custom.

In their draft of a plan for the school, the committee of the Dental Society proposed that, "besides the winter session, there should be established, as soon as practicable, a summer session for recitations from approved text-books and lectures, and demonstrations illustrating the use of the microscope and microscopic anatomy."

This early recognition that the ordinary terms of study and discipline were too short properly to prepare the students for practice, resulted in another innovation upon the custom of other dental schools, viz, the establishment of a summer course lasting four months, immediately following the winter session, and designed to take the place of a private pupilage for the same length of time. In this the school was soon followed by nearly all the schools of the country. The summer course was a success, was well attended, and prepared the way for the greater change which took place three years later.

At a faculty meeting, February 8, 1872, it was voted "To request the Corporation of Harvard University to assume the management of the financial affairs of the Dental School."

Up to this time this had been attended to by the dean and the faculty.

In 1874, the school suffered its greatest loss in the death of the professor and dean, Thomas Barnes Hitchcock. When appointed to his professorship on the organization of the school he was but little known outside of the narrow circle of the Massachusetts Dental Society. In a sense the school made Dr. Hitchcock and Dr. Hitchcock made the school. He put his whole soul into his work. The school engrossed his attention by day and his labor far into the night. His enthusiasm was marvelous and contagious. Equally strong in his likes and dislikes, he sometimes made enemies and tried the patience of his friends; but no man ever doubted that he was conscientious and honest in every detail of his daily practice in the office, cherishing his profession as a noble and honorable vocation, and giving himself up without reservation to his professorship as his highest duty and most important work. He impressed his personality upon every student. It was always a positive force. He was a partisan, but always zealous for the school and its interests. He was warm-hearted and affectionate to his friends. He was bold and outspoken in opposing what he considered wrong. He was not always right, but he aimed to be and thought he was. He took blows unflinchingly as well as gave them. He knew no fatigue, no hesitancy, no thought of failure in reaching after his ideal. When weakened by disease he gave no heed to the warning of his friends, but kept right on working, often late into the morning, until the fell stroke came and he was prostrated never to rise again. He was a martyr to the Harvard School, to professional education, and to dental progress. Viewed in years his life was short, but in achievement long and honorable.

At a faculty meeting, July 8, 1874, Dr. T. H. Chandler was elected dean as Dr. Hitchcock's successor.

While the changes and advances which have been mentioned had placed Harvard in the van, the faculty still felt that more was required to bring the methods nearer to their ideal. After much study and consideration the faculty voted, February 14, 1875, to recommend an entire change in the curriculum. Their plan was adopted by the corporation March 1, 1875. The new scheme embodied:

First. A consolidation of the winter course with the heretofore optional summer course into one school year extending from the last of September to the last of June.

Second. A progressive course of instruction extending over two years, the teaching of one year not being repeated in the next.

Third. An examination at the end of the first year in anatomy, including dissection, physiology, and general chemistry. Unless the student successfully passes two of these examinations he is not admitted to the studies of the second year.

Fourth. At the end of the second year an examination in dental pathology, dental materia medica and therapeutics, oral surgery and surgical pathology, operative and mechanical dentistry.

Fifth. That the candidate must have passed a satisfactory examination in all of the above-mentioned subjects.

Sixth. All the examinations to be conducted in writing. This scheme adopted in 1875 has been in operation ever since, but few slight modifications having from time to time been considered necessary. It has resulted in securing fine scholarship and excellent skill. It has been found sufficiently difficult, as is shown by the fact that a great proportion of the students find it necessary to spend three years in the school to pass all the examinations.

The entrance examination was not originated by the Harvard Dental School. It was, however, adopted by it, not from a feeling of its need, but because it seemed a good rule for all dental colleges. Harvard has never been selected by the ignorant any more than by the indolent. In fact, there have been none so simple as not to know that Harvard was no place for those who were deficient in a fair amount of brain tissue of proper color.

The invaluable assistance of the medical faculty in the origin of the school has been spoken of. The same generous spirit has marked all the succeeding years, resulting not only in moral support, but in valuable pecuniary assistance. The school could not have been carried on without this aid unless money had come from some other source. Under the old plan the medical professors had no stated salaries, but received more or less remuneration according to the number of the students. The dental students added to the total number to be taught and examined by them, and so to their labors, but the fees for medical instruction in the dental school were paid directly to the dental school. The medical professors generously waived their claims to any of these fees, and the money which would otherwise have gone to them was spent in carrying on the dental school. These professors, as members of the dental faculty, have always been as constant and prompt in attending faculty meetings and as active and earnest as the dental professors.

Upon the completion of the new medical building, the medical faculty added still further to the obligation of the dental school to them by giving to the school the free use of the old medical building on North Grove street. In this building all the work of the second and third years of the dental school was carried on, both the didactic teaching and the practical operations, infirmary teaching and practice. This generous aid from the medical faculty rendered unnecessary the further carrying of the load of debt and expense connected with the house No. 50 Allen street. This house was sold at a loss and a part of the debt of the school incurred in its purchase extinguished.

This school, and that of the University of Michigan founded in 1875 upon the same plan, received, without solicitation or previous knowledge, a distinguished mark of approbation from the General Medical Council of Great Britain. Their diplomas alone of the American dental colleges exempted the holders from examination for registration and license to practice in Great Britain. This privilege was enjoyed until May 1893 when it was by resolution of the General Medical Council of Great Britain rescinded.

When one remembers the longer period of attendance which the Harvard School demands of its students, the very thorough medical training of its first year, and its exacting examinations, one will not be surprised that it failed to attract students in as large numbers as the other schools in which the requirements and discipline were less severe. As a result its receipts from students' fees have been

smaller, but the faculty have preferred to maintain this higher course rather than lower the standard to obtain more students. The true principle was ably expressed by President Elliot in one of his annual reports: "The University should be more concerned to have a very good school than a very large one."

The public are hardly aware of the work which the school has quietly done during the past years in providing skilled dentists.

With the exception of certain subordinate assistants, who could not afford to give their services, and of some who in recent years have received small salaries, the gentlemen who have devoted so much of their time and labors to the school have done so gratuitously. All the fees from students were needed for current expenses. This has been no small tax upon busy men, taking about one-twelfth of their productive hours from October to July.

Is it then strange that the temptation should be strong to release themselves from this extra labor? For be it remembered that the same qualities which make a man valuable as a teacher also cause his professional services to be sought by the public. The instructors, past and present, can truly claim that the work which has been accomplished by the Harvard Dental School—its great charity to the suffering poor, its elevating effect upon professional training everywhere, and the higher standard of professional skill in Boston today—is their own work and at their own expense.

This school has a double claim upon the public: first, as a trustworthy place of education for a profession which is now recognized as indispensable; and secondly, as a charity which, like hospitals, infirmaries, and dispensaries, ministers to the suffering poor.

VII

History of the Department of Dentistry of the Medico-Chirurgical College of Philadelphia.

By WM. L. J. GRIFFIN, D.D.S., Philadelphia, Pa.

THE Medico-Chirurgical College of Philadelphia had its inception as a society or permanent association of physicians May 13, 1848, soon after the founding of the American Medical Association, and was granted its first primary charter by the State Legislature of Pennsylvania on February 12, 1850. Later, this charter was amended by the act of April 10, 1867, and the organization was transformed into a regular medical college, with the additional privilege of granting degrees in the different special branches of medicine and surgery. The first course of lectures was given in 1881, but the institution had a comparatively slow and uneventful growth during the succeeding four or five years. About 1885 new life was infused into the enterprise, and it has since become a progressive and prosperous institution. As a medical school, it was first located at the southwest corner of Market and Broad streets.

In 1888 it joined the Philadelphia Dental College in the erection of new buildings for joint occupancy on Cherry street, between Seventeenth and Eighteenth streets, each organization, however, remaining distinct, each having certain portions of the buildings for its own special use, and using other portions jointly. This proved for a number of years a satisfactory and economical arrangement, giving to each college better accommodations than either could have otherwise obtained. As time passed, the Medico-Chirurgical College having prospered and requiring for the accommodation of its own classes and its hospital the entire plot, it bought out the interests of the Philadelphia Dental College, and that institution purchased a location and erected buildings of its own at Eighteenth and Buttonwood streets.

For a number of years the former made no effort to extend its domain beyond medicine and surgery, but when it had acquired larger facilities the time seemed ripe for utilizing the provision of its charter empowering it to "grant degrees in the different special branches of medicine and surgery," by establishing a department of dentistry. This right was contested in the interests of the Philadelphia Dental College, with which it had been so closely associated. After legal argument, which was carried to the Supreme Court of the state, the right of the Medico-Chirurgical College to establish a department of dentistry under its charter was confirmed.

The Dental Department of the Medico-Chirurgical College of Philadelphia, the youngest dental school in that city, began its career in the building formerly occupied by the Philadelphia Dental College, on Cherry street above Seventeenth, in the fall of 1897, with the following faculty:

R. Walter Starr, D.D.S., dean and professor of operative dentistry, crown and bridge work; Robert H. Nones, D.D.S., professor of prosthetic dentistry and metallurgy; Charles R. Jefferies, D.D.S., professor of dental pathology, therapeutics, materia medica, and clinical dentistry; Ernest Laplace, M.D., D.D.S., professor of oral surgery; Isaac Ott, A.M., M.D., professor of physiology; G. H. Meeker, B.A., M.S., professor of physics, chemistry, and metallurgy; John C. Heisler, M.D., professor of anatomy.

The first session closed on May 21, 1898, when the first annual commencement was held at the Academy of Music, and the degree of Doctor of Dental Surgery was conferred upon the following four gentlemen: Frederick G. Davis and Frank G. Hawksworth of Pennsylvania, S. Leigh Frawley of Canada, J. E. McConnell of Washington, D. C.

In June 1898, Professor Starr resigned as professor and dean. Professor Jefferies also resigned, and Drs. Walter H. Neall and James D. Price were elected to fill the vacancies. The faculty for the second session was as follows:

Robert H. Nones, D.D.S., dean and professor of prosthetic dentistry, dental metallurgy, crown and bridge work; Walter H. Neall, D.D.S., professor of operative dentistry; James D. Price, D.D.S., professor of dental pathology, therapeutics, and materia medica; John V. Shoemaker, M.D., LL.D., professor of anesthesia and anesthetics; Ernest Laplace, M.D., LL.D., professor of oral surgery; Isaac Ott, A.M., M.D., professor of physiology; Joseph McFarland, M.D., professor of pathology and bacteriology; John C. Heisler, M.D., professor of anatomy; George H. Meeker, M.S., Ph.D., professor of physics, chemistry, and metallurgy; Charles L. Furbush, M.D., professor of histology.

The second session brought an increased number of students, and when the second annual commencement was held at the Academy of Music, May 20, 1899, the degree was conferred upon twenty-one graduates, as follows:

Canada—Robert C. Bain, Edgar C. Hoskins, T. G. Turcot.
Germany—Jacob Bingle.
Indiana—August P. Graf, Samuel M. Wharton.
Louisiana—Emerson A. Dunbar.
New York—George G. Lawyer.
Pennsylvania—Van Cola D. Burgess, James M. Cornyn, Charles M. Frantz, V.M.D., Condy C. Gallagher, H. G. Hadley, Ph.G., John L. Hughes, G. Middleton, Michael C. Ryan, M.D., George O. Reed, Ph.G., John J. Stetzer, A. F. Wehr, Charles L. Zimmerman.
Tennessee—H. L. Samelson.

The third session began October 2, 1899. Since the last session Professor Price resigned and Dr. Geo. W. Cupit was elected to the vacancy.

The third annual commencement was held at the Academy of Music May 19, 1900, when the D.D.S. degree was conferred upon the following twenty-two graduates:

New Jersey—Raymond S. Miller.
New York—Joseph H. Gallagher, Fred. K. Grandy.
Maine—Bert Doyle.
Massachusetts—James F. Spencer.
Pennsylvania—Harley Ackerman, F. E. Buch, J. C. Dougherty, Robert M. Ewing, Irvin F. Fegley, Leon Gismore, John B. Jones, Charles E. Koehler, Mark Marcus, William Meter, Charles F. Pierce, Joseph L. Rutter, R. R. Robinson, Chester T. Starr, Harry Truitt, Alanson U. Welch.
Rhode Island—Henri E. Gobeille.

The fourth session began October 1, 1900, with no change in the faculty. It ended with the annual commencement May 25, 1901, when the degree was conferred upon twenty-five graduates, as follows:

Austria—Michael Shapiro.
Delaware—Charles M. Hollis, Cahall Sipple.
England—Arthur R. Dray, Wm. H. Gwinnutt.
Louisiana—Maxie J. Becnel, Louis J. Gelpi,
Minnesota—Charles T. Searle.
New Jersey—Sam. I. Callahan, Stanley A. Ireland.
Pennsylvania—E. Armstrong, James C. Attix, Wm. E. Davis, R. B. Gillars, Edw. C. Hughes, Robert Kirshner, David M. Sanders, Joseph Scott, R. M. Schaffer, Richard D. Steim, Edgar D. Urich, John T. Woolfe, Pascal Yearsley.
Russia—Morris H. Chann.
Syria—Iskander Hajjar.

With the faculty the same as before, the fifth session began October 1, 1901. At the annual commencement held May 24, 1902, the degree was conferred upon the following thirty-two graduates:

Canada—Ernest C. Halliday.
Connecticut—Joseph J. Ryle.
Germany—David Epstein, M.D.
Massachusetts—Joseph F. Langlois.
Maryland—Albion C. Tollinger.
New Jersey—H. T. Birkinshaw, William Hayday, Imly Sharpe.
New York—Edw. J. Mead, Marcus D. Powers, L. J. Vanderpool.
Pennsylvania—Charles C. Bristow, John K. Brallier, F. B. Campbell, Howard E. Cupit, Charles F. Dull, Elmer E. Henry, James D. Husted, Martial W. Hayes, Edward Lloyd, Burdette G. Love, Peter A. McAneny, A. E. Muchnic, John J. Russel, J. F. Sanderson, Samuel S. Smith, Wallace B. Stewart, Warren H. Stover, C. J. Weisenburn.
Russia—Wildimir Lutz, Jacob C. Field, Jacob L. Zimmerman.

The sixth session opened on October 6, 1902. During the summer Professor

Neall resigned. Professor Cupit was transferred to the chair of operative dentistry, and Dr. Earle C. Rice was appointed professor of the branches previously taught by Professor Cupit.

At the annual commencement held May 23, 1903, the degree was conferred upon the following twenty-five graduates:

Canada—H. A. Harvey.
Connecticut—George F. Lancaster.
Louisiana—Oliver J. Reiss.
Massachusetts—M. M. Dunphy.
New Jersey—H. C. Davis, Arthur M. Knight.
New York—S. J. Clark.
Pennsylvania—Robert Adams, Jr., Clarence H. Crist, Peter E. Costello, R. Z. Clemmer, Louis Englander, B. B. Filer, O. K. Hoppes, E. E. Howerter, D. D. Hyman, Wm. J. McKinley, Charles A. Miller, Frank W. Miller, Albert F. Seip, Richard Souder, Raymond W. Wilson, Edwin K. Wood.
South Africa—N. Fox.
South America—S. B. Harris, M.D.

The seventh session began October 5, 1903, the faculty remaining the same as the previous year.

At the annual commencement held May 28, 1904, the degree was conferred upon the following twenty-one graduates:

Canada—Garnet C. Cowan, Arthur T. Mackay.
North Carolina—R. McIver Wilbur.
New Jersey—David T. Davies.
New York—J. B. Arrowsmith, Arthur Adams, Samuel Freeman.
Pennsylvania—George H. Grim, David E. Hahn, John H. Hart, Frank J. Hawley, Wm. Henderson, Ben Ira Herr, Wm. Hoppman, Kenneth G. Lenhart, Joseph A. Moran, John A. Orwig, Russel Rudolph, Ira H. Spangler, Fred. L. Wallace, Isaac H. Whyte.

The session of 1903-04 has been marked by small classes in nearly all the dental colleges throughout the country, caused in part probably by the proposed increase of the term to four years, and in part by prevailing industrial conditions. This college had seventy-two matriculates. Its classes have been small compared with those of the other Philadelphia schools, but, nevertheless, considering that it is the youngest, and that the large number of dental schools in the United States tends year by year to narrow the field and localize the patronage of each, it has done remarkably well. From first to last its dental professors have been men inexperienced as teachers, and of local reputation only. They have, however, done their work well, as tested by the record of their graduates before the examining boards. The facilities offered by this college for acquiring a thorough, practical dental education may be judged by the following list of instructors, and of the branches taught, taken from the announcement for 1904-05:

FACULTY.

Robert H. Nones, D.D.S., dean, professor of prosthetic dentistry, dental metallurgy, crown and bridge, and clinical dentistry; George W. Cupit. D.D.S., professor of operative dentistry; Earle C. Rice. D.D.S., professor of dental pathology and therapeutics; John V. Shoemaker, M.D., LL.D., professor of anesthesia and materia medica; Ernest Laplace, M.D., LL.D., professor of oral surgery; Isaac Ott, A.M., M.D., professor of physiology; Joseph McFarland, M.D., professor of pathology and bacteriology; John C. Heisler, M.D., professor of anatomy; George H. Meeker, M.S., Ph.D., professor of physics, chemistry, and metallurgy.

AUXILIARY FACULTY.

Seneca Egbert. A.M., M.D., professor of hygiene; A. C. Buckley, A.M., M.D., associate professor of histology; Matthew Beardwood, Jr., A. M., M.D., adjunct professor of clinical chemistry; Herbert J. Smith, Ph.D., M.D., assistant professor of materia medica and anesthesia; John M. Fogg, D.D.S., lecturer on clinical dentistry; Thomas J. Clemens, M.D., D.D.S., lecturer on materia medica; John R. Yorks, D.D.S., lecturer on operative dentistry; W. A. Borden, D.D.S., lecturer on nitrous oxid and extraction of teeth; C. F. Horgan, D.D.S., lecturer on oral hygiene; G. E. Pfahler, M.D., lecturer on physical diagnosis and skiagrapher.

CLINICAL INSTRUCTORS.

S. Eldred Gilbert, D.D.S.; Henry A. Ickes, D.D.S.; S. Blair Luckie, D.D.S.; R. H. John. D.D.S.; J. D. Peters, D.D.S.; John M. Fogg, D.D.S.; Harman Yerkes, D.D.S.; Thomas D. Sinclair, D.D.S.; Hayes A. Clement, D.D.S.; Frank L. Bassett, D.D.S.; C. H. S. Littleton, D.D.S.; George F. Root, D.D.S.; Frank D. Focht, D.D.S.; Lewis Martin, D.D.S.

CHIEFS, DEMONSTRATORS, INSTRUCTORS, AND ASSISTANT DEMONSTRATORS.

Arthur R. Dray, D.D.S., chief of clinics; Henry B. Nones, D.D.S., chief of prosthetic department; Thomas J. Byrne, D.D.S., demonstrator of clinical prosthetic dentistry; H. Woodrow, D.D.S., demonstrator of crown and bridge work; R. H. Calely, D.D.S., assistant demonstrator of operative dentistry; P. E. Costello, D.D.S., assistant demonstrator of prosthetic dentistry and demonstrator of operative technic; R. R. Robinson, D.D.S., assistant demonstrator of operative dentistry; L. J. Vanderpool, D.D.S., assistant demonstrator of operative dentistry; D. T. Davies, Jr., D.D.S., assistant demonstrator of operative dentistry; Frank S. Bowman, M.D., demonstrator of anatomy; Mitchell P. Warmuth, M.D., demonstrator of operative surgery; William H. Good, A.M., M.D., instructor in physiology; Joseph F. Ulman, M.D., assistant demonstrator of physiology; Frank S. Bowman, M.D., instructor in oral surgery; R. J. Adams, D.D.S., demonstrator of pathology and bacteriology; H. D. Jordan, M.D., assistant demonstrator of histology; H. D. Senior, M.D., J. Gilbride, M.D., G. Mill, M.D., Van Duyne A. Sutliffe, M.D., assistant demonstrators of anatomy.

VIII

The Progress of the Western Dental Education.

By BURTON LEE THORPE, M.D., D.D.S., St. Louis, Mo.

THE progress of dental collegiate education west of the Mississippi river has been a marked factor for the betterment of the profession, as is shown by the following compilation of facts furnished by the various deans of the institutions herein mentioned.

The oldest landmark of dental education in the West is the

Missouri Dental College,

DENTAL DEPARTMENT OF WASHINGTON UNIVERSITY, ST. LOUIS.

At the first annual meeting of the Missouri State Dental Society, held in June 1866, a committee was appointed to consider a proposition to form a dental college under the auspices of the society, with power to take such action as in their judgment the interests of the profession and of the public required.

The committee, after patient investigation of the subject, decided that the prospects of establishing a college in St. Louis were so encouraging at this time (the faculties of two medical schools having proffered the most liberal co-operation) that they decided to apply for a charter.

Under the general laws passed by the legislature of 1865-66 to govern the issue of such charters, it was found necessary to form an association. This corporate body consisted of the following members:

Homer Judd,
H. E. Peebles,
E. Hale, Jr.,
Wm. N. Morrison.

W. H. Eames,
G. W. Crawford,
A. M. Leslie,
Isaiah Forbes,
H. J. McKellops,
M. Westermann,
Isaac Comstock,
Alix. Dienst,
Wm. A. Cornelius,
W. A. Jones,
C. Knower,
John P. Hibler,
Edgar Park.
Henry Barron.

This done, the members petitioned for a charter, which was granted. Under the charter the association appointed a board of trustees, as follows:

Isaiah Forbes, D.D.S., president.
A. M. Leslie, D.D.S., secretary.
H. E. Peebles, D.D.S., treasurer.
Charles A. Pope, M.D.,
J. S. Clark, D.D.S.,
S. H. Anderson.
J. L. Knapp.
W. O. Kulp.
W. H. Eames, D.D.S.,
M. McCoy, M.D.,
Edwin Hale, Jr.,
C. W. Rivers,
J. B. Johnson. M.D.

To this board was confided the appointment of professors and other instructors and power to make such changes in the teachers or the curriculum as the interests of the profession demanded. Also to hold all property of the association.

The facilities for establishing a dental school in St. Louis were peculiarly encouraging. The faculty of the St. Louis Medical College had shown such a liberal spirit in offering the association the use of their lecture rooms and the advantages of their established museum and hospitals that the trustees cannot but here acknowledge the obligation of the profession. The trustees feel

assured in declaring that if the dental profession of the Mississippi Valley take hold
of this new enterprise in as broad and liberal
a spirit we will soon have established here an
institution which will reflect honor on our
profession and prove a powerful lever in its
elevation by the diffusion of science pertaining to dentistry.

As a result of the foregoing action, the
Missouri Dental College, now the Dental
Department of Washington University,
was chartered on September 16, 1866,
the charter being issued to Homer Judd,
H. E. Peebles, Isaac Comstock, and
others. The first regular meeting of the
faculty took place on September 24,
1866, at the office of Dr. Judd, corner
of Sixth and Pine streets, St. Louis. A.
Litton was called to the chair. The business meeting resulted in the election of
Homer Judd as dean and Frank White
as secretary. The only other business
done at this meeting was to appoint Dr.
Judd a committee of one to formulate a
constitution and by-laws for the governing of the school. The first course of
lectures began on Monday, October 1,
1866, and closed on February 22, 1867,
the course at that time being five months.

The first faculty was composed of Homer Judd, M.D., dean, professor of the institutes of dental science; C. W. Stevens,
M.D., professor of general descriptive
and surgical anatomy; A. Litton, M.D.,
professor of chemistry and pharmacy; J.
T. Hodgen, M.D., professor of physiology
and medical jurisprudence; F. W. White,
M.D., professor of materia medica and
therapeutics; E. H. Gregory, M.D.,
demonstrator of anatomy; H. E. Peebles,
D.D.S., professor of surgical and operative dentistry; W. H. Eames, D.D.S.,
professor of artificial dentistry; L. Winkler, curator.

The first annual commencement was
held on February 22, 1867, in O'Fallon

Hall, Dr. Judd, dean of the faculty, delivering the valedictory on the subject of
"The History and Progress of Dental
Science." There is no doubt that this
paper would be interesting reading now
after thirty-eight years have added their
history to the profession. The following
named gentlemen who were of that class
are still living: A. W. Franch of Spring-
field, Ill., and Geo. A. Bowman of St.
Louis.

At the second annual meeting of the
faculty J. S. B. Alleyne succeeded Dr.
White as professor of materia medica and
therapeutics, and retained the chair from
1867 until 1891. He was also made secretary of the faculty at the same time.
At this meeting it was decided that the
course in the Missouri Dental College
should close at the same time as that of
the St. Louis Medical College, and that
the commencements should be held
jointly, an agreement which was continued for twenty-six years, up to and including 1900, at which time the first dental commencement was held alone, at
Memorial Hall, Nineteenth and Locust
streets, St. Louis. It might be well to
note here that the Missouri Dental College was the first one in the United States
to deliver the greater portion of its lectures jointly with the medical students.
At the second annual commencement
there were three graduates, all of whom
have since passed away.

At the third annual meeting John T.
Hodgen was made professor of anatomy;
Ellsworth F. Smith, professor of physiol-
ogy; H. S. Chase, professor of surgical
and operative dentistry; John T. Mc-
Dowell, demonstrator of anatomy; Wm.
N. Morrison, demonstrator of mechani-
cal dentistry. At this meeting E. H.
Gregory was elected professor of the prin-
ciples and practice of surgery, and his

name has been in every catalog issued since that time, he having been made emeritus professor of surgery in 1900.

During the year 1872 A. H. Fuller was made demonstrator of surgical and operative dentistry. He was elected secretary of the faculty in 1873 and filled that office continuously until the death of H. H. Mudd in 1899, when he succeeded to the office of dean, Geo. A. Bowman being at that time adjunct professor of mechanical dentistry, and Dr. Eames filling the chair as professor of the same.

On February 11, 1874, the entire faculty of the Missouri Dental College resigned their chairs, as the minutes state, in order that the trustees might fill them again with perfect freedom. The vote upon the resignations was unanimous. The names of those voting were Judd, Eames, Bowman, Park, and Chase. On June 20th of the same year the following faculty were elected to fill vacancies caused by the resignations: H. S. Chase, professor of the institutes of dental science; J. T. Hodgen, professor of anatomy; A. Litton, professor of chemistry; C. Baumgarten, professor of physiology; J. S. B. Alleyne, professor of materia medica; E. H. Gregory, professor of principles and practice of surgery; C. W. Rivers, professor of operative dentistry; A. H. Fuller, professor of mechanical dentistry; Homer Judd, lecturer on pathology; W. H. Eames, lecturer on metallurgy; J. H. McDowell, demonstrator of anatomy; R. H. Mace, demonstrator of operative dentistry; Frederick Kempff, demonstrator of mechanical dentistry; C. W. Rivers, dean of the faculty.

In 1875 W. H. Eames was elected professor of the institutes of dental science and dean of the faculty, and Isaiah Forbes was made professor of surgical and operative dentistry; M. A. Bartelson,

professor of mechanical dentistry; H. H. Mudd, demonstrator of anatomy; H. H. Keith, demonstrator of mechanical dentistry. The board of trustees for this year consisted of Isaiah Forbes, president, and A. H. Fuller, secretary. The following members composed the board: E. H. Gregory, H. Judd, E. Park, W. H. Eames, J. C. Goodrich, J. A. Price, G. V. Black, Geo. A. Bowman, W. N. Morrison, H. Newington, and C. W. Rivers.

The only change that was made in the faculty for the term of 1876-77 was the election of H. H. Keith as professor of mechanical dentistry, N. Stark as demonstrator of operative dentistry, and H. C. Macey as demonstrator of mechanical dentistry.

In 1877 Isaiah Forbes was made emeritus professor of the institutes of dental science; G. V. Black, lecturer on histology and microscopy.

In 1878 J. Ward Hall was made professor of surgical and operative dentistry and A. H. Fuller professor of the institutes of dental science. On September 16, 1878, H. H. Mudd was elected dean of the Missouri Dental College and served as such from that time until the day of his death, which occurred on November 20, 1899. It might be well to say in this connection that Dr. Mudd served as demonstrator of anatomy from 1875 to 1883, although he had been made professor of anatomy in 1880. In 1886 he was made professor of surgical anatomy and clinical surgery.

In 1879 A. H. Fuller succeeded J. Ward Hall as professor of operative dentistry, a position which he filled for twenty-two years. Among the special lecturers of this year appear the names of G. V. Black, H. Judd, I. P. Wilson, and John J. R. Patrick.

The only change made in the faculty

in the year 1881 was caused by the resignation of H. H. Keith as professor of mechanical dentistry and the election of W. N. Morrison to fill the same.

In 1885, on the list of special lecturers for this year appear the names of Homer Judd, lecturer on the histology of the dental tissues; John J. R. Patrick, lecturer on mechanism of the jaws, progressive and retrogressive metamorphosis of the jaws and teeth, and special description of the regular set of teeth; H. H. Keith, lecturer on soft-foil fillings and continuous gum; W. N. Morrison, lecturer on root-fillings, transplantation, and replantation.

In 1886 H. H. Mudd was made professor of surgical anatomy and clinical surgery, B. J. Prim being made professor of descriptive anatomy, the position formerly filled by Dr. Mudd.

There were no changes made in the faculty for the season of 1887-88, but at this time was added a list of clinical instructors, the list being composed of Drs. Bowman, Whipple, Wick, Newby, Holmes, Conrad, Prosser, and Fisher.

In 1893 the Missouri Dental College became the Dental Department of Washington University, and the term opened in the new building, 1814 Locust street, on September 27th.

In 1893 W. H. Eames was made superintendent of the infirmary and remained in this position until his death, the following year.

In 1894 J. B. Vernon was made superintendent of the infirmary; O. W. Bedell, lecturer on dental embryology and diseases of the teeth; M. R. Windhorst, lecturer on operative dentistry; J. B. Kimbrough, demonstrator of operative dentistry.

In 1895 O. W. Bedell was made professor of mechanical dentistry.

In 1897 O. W. Bedell was made professor of the institutes of dental science; R. R. Vaughn, assistant professor of mechanical dentistry and superintendent of infirmary; C. W. Richardson, demonstrator of dental technics.

The following year, 1898, E. H. Angle was made professor of orthodontia; C. W. Richardson, professor of dental technic, and R. R. Vaughn, professor of mechanical dentistry.

In 1899 A. H. Fuller was made dean to fill the vacancy caused by the death of Henry Mudd. O. W. Bedell was made secretary to fill the vacancy caused by the election of Dr. Fuller to the office of dean. R. J. Terry was made assistant professor of anatomy; W. H. Warren, assistant professor of chemistry; H. F. Cassell, professor of mechanical dentistry; A. E. Matteson, professor of orthodontia.

In 1900 J. H. Kennerly was made professor of mechanical dentistry and secretary of the faculty; H. F. Cassell, assist. professor of mechanical dentistry.

In 1891 A. H. Fuller resigned from the faculty and was made emeritus professor of operative dentistry; J. H. Kennerly was elected dean of the faculty, to succeed Dr. Fuller.

In 1902 R. J. Terry and Wm. H. Warren were elected to a full professorship of the chairs of anatomy and chemistry; Willard Bartlett was made lecturer on oral surgery.

The Kansas City Dental College, Kansas City, Mo.

The Kansas City Dental College organized in 1881 as the Dental Department of the Kansas City Medical College, with the following faculty:

J. K. Stark, dean of the faculty; A. H. Thompson, D.D.S., professor of operative dentistry; J. D. Griffith, M.D., professor of anatomy; R. P. Loring, M.D., professor of physiology; T. J. Eaton, M.D., professor of materia medica; George Halley, M. D., professor of surgery; A. Lester Charles, M.D., professor of chemistry; W. T. Stark, D.D.S., professor of mechanical dentistry; J. D. Patterson and C. L. Hungerford, associates to the chair of operative dentistry; L. C. Wasson and A. C. Schell, assistants to the chair of mechanical dentistry; C. B. Hewitt, E. N. LaVeine, J. K. Stark, R. I. Pearson, and J. K. Boyd, demonstrators in operative dentistry; H. S. Thompson, W. A. Drowne, and W. H. Buckley, demonstrators in mechanical dentistry; L. P. Meredith, W. H. Shulze, and R. Wood Brown, clinical lecturers.

Foremost in the establishment of this school was Dr. R. I. Pearson, a zealous man who had retired from practice. Dr. Pearson, with Drs. Stark, Hungerford, Hewitt, Patterson, and others, realizing that in the future Kansas City was destined to yield an increasing influence in professional fields and that eventually it would be the center for a wide area in educational efforts, determined to organize a dental college upon the best standards, with the best men of the West, and to vigorously sustain the very highest reputation. At that time it seemed wise to ally the college with the Kansas City Medical College, which was the medical college *par excellence* of the West, and this was accordingly accomplished. In 1890 the officers, deeming it best that dental education should be followed independent of affiliation with a medical college, purchased the franchise of the Kansas City Dental College and since that time the college has taught dental science strictly, and has secured an enviable reputation for the preparation of young men for the practice of their profession. During the twenty-three years of its existence there have been of necessity changes in the faculty; notwithstanding this, the year 1904 finds five of the original faculty still active as teachers, viz, W. T. Stark, C. L. Hungerford, J. D. Patterson, A. H. Thompson, and J. D. Griffith.

The college owns its building on the corner of Troost avenue and Tenth street, and in the near future will erect a new building to accommodate the growth of the institution. Its graduates number 460 and are scattered over the entire world.

The college is an original member of the National Association of Dental Faculties and has always been active in furthering the interests of dental education.

The present officers of the association controlling the Kansas City Dental College are J. D. Patterson, president; J. G. Hollingsworth, vice-president; C. C. Allen, secretary; W. T. Stark, treasurer.

____

Dental Department, University of California, San Francisco.

On recommendation of the medical faculty of California the dental department of the university was established by the regents, May 28, 1881. S. W. Dennis, professor of principles and practice of operative dentistry, was the first dean of the faculty. The present faculty are Benjamin Ide Wheeler, Ph.D., president of the university and *ex officio* president of the faculty; L. L. Dunbar, D.D.S., emeritus professor of operative dentistry and dental histology; C. L. Goddard, A.M., D.D.S., emeritus professor of orthodontia; H. P. Carlton, D.D.S., professor of operative dentistry and dean, and Morris J. Sullivan, D.D.S., professor of dental pathology, therapeutics, and materia medica; A. A. d'Ancona, A.B., M.D., professor of physiology and histology; J. M. Williamson, M.D., professor of anatomy; W. F. Sharp, D.D.S., D.M.D., professor of prosthetic dentistry; J. D. Hodgen, D.D.S., professor of chemistry and metallurgy; J. G. Sharp, M.D., D.D.S., professor of principles and practice of surgery; C. A. Litton, D.D.S., professor of orthodontia. Besides the faculty the college has a large staff of demonstrators and lecturers. The course of studies is arranged as follows: Freshman year—anatomy, with dissection; physiology; chemistry, with laboratory work; prosthetic dentistry; operative technic; prosthetic technic; microscopic technic. Examinations will be held at the end of the year in all of the above branches. Junior year—anatomy, with dissection; physiology, with laboratory work; chemistry; prosthetic dentistry; operative dentistry; pathology; therapeutics, and materia medica; orthodontia technic; histology; general and dental bacteriology. Examinations will be held at the end of the year in all of the above branches and will be final in anatomy, physiology, and chemistry. Senior year—operative dentistry; prosthetic dentistry; orthodontia, with practical cases; comparative anatomy of the teeth; metallurgy, with laboratory work; pathology, therapeutics, and materia medica; surgery, general and oral.

The Dental Department of the University of California occupies one of the buildings of the affiliated college on Parnassus avenue, San Francisco, where all the lectures and laboratory courses in chemistry, metallurgy, histology, opera-

tive and prosthetic technic are given. The operative work is done in the infirmary in the Donohoe Building on Market street, where a large clinic is held daily. The number of students has increased from 26 in 1882 to 112 in 1903-04.

Chicago College of Dental Surgery, Chicago.

During the summer of 1882 a movement to organize an independent dental college took definite form, and in October of that year application was made to the Secretary of State of Illinois for a license to organize such an institution. A license was issued to Gorton W. Nichols, Truman W. Brophy, Frank H. Gardiner, A. W. Harlan, and Eugene S. Talbot, as commissioners to open books and transact the business of the corporation. On February 20, 1883, in the office of the Secretary of State, the commissioners filed their report of their proceedings under the license, upon which date a charter was granted legalizing the corporation under the name of the Collegiate Department of the Chicago Dental Infirmary. On June 30, 1884, the name of the institution was changed to that by which it is now known.

The first regular course of instruction to students in the Chicago Dental Infirmary opened on March 12, 1883, continuing twenty weeks, or until July 31st. This was the beginning of the college which has since developed into the largest institution of its kind in the world.

At its origin the college was a postgraduate school, known as the Collegiate Department of the Chicago Dental Infirmary. Its students were first required to obtain the degree of Doctor of Medicine or its equivalent from some college recognized by the Illinois State Board of Health, and to take two courses of lectures in dentistry before receiving the degree of Doctor of Dental Surgery. Such a system of education for dentists was urged because the prime movers of the establishment of the institution held that dentistry was but a department of medicine, believing that dentists should be educated in medicine before beginning the study of this specialty. The organization was effected under the most favorable auspices. Six of the medical colleges then in Chicago were represented on its board of directors.

During the first session there were three professors and eight lecturers in the institution. The professors taught the principles and practice of dental surgery, operative dentistry, and prosthetic dentistry, and the lecturers devoted themselves to dental anatomy, dental pathology, and other special branches not followed minutely in medical colleges. Eighteen students were enrolled for the first course and at its close there were no candidates for the degree. Two, however, entered the examinations for a special certificate, both of whom failed. During the following course eleven names were entered in the matriculation book, two candidates entered the final examinations, and, after successfully passing them, received the degree of Doctor of Dental Surgery. It was in the middle of the second course that a new charter was obtained for organization of the Chicago College of Dental Surgery, which from that date, June 30, 1884, supplanted the Collegiate Department of the Chicago Dental Infirmary. The number of teachers was increased from nine to seventeen, and the college during the session of 1884-85 showed an increased attendance.

During the first two sessions, as infirmary and college, it was located in two small rooms on the third floor of Nos. 22 and 24 Adams street.

At the beginning of its existence as the Chicago College of Dental Surgery it was moved to and occupied the fourth and fifth stories of Nos. 4 and 6 Washington street. In 1886, owing to the rapid growth of the college, it was moved to the building at the northeast corner of Madison street and Wabash avenue. After remaining at this location for five years its removal to more commodious quarters again became necessary. The management secured the three upper floors of the building situated at the northeast corner of Michigan avenue and Randolph street.

Realizing in 1888 the necessity of securing a permanent location for the college, the lot was purchased upon which the building now stands. The first section of the structure, covering half of the lot —85 by 120 feet—was erected in 1893, and the first course of instruction began in it the first of November of that year.

The faculty believed at the opening of that session that they had provided sufficient room for the accommodation of classes for many years; but the increase in the number of students made it absolutely necessary to enlarge the building for their accommodation. Beginning with the year 1897 plans were perfected and the building of 1893 was doubled in capacity, so that it is now a six-story structure. Each floor contains an area of 10,080 square feet, or a total of 60,480 square feet, divided in accordance with suggestions and plans made after having carefully examined the best regulated dental schools in the United States, thus enabling the incorporation of the most modern features in its construction.

As illustrating the growth of the college, it may be set forth in tabular form as follows: During the first course of the

summer of 1883, the faculty consisted of
3; matriculates, 18; no graduates. Summer of 1884, faculty, 3 (other teachers,
5); matriculates, 11; 2 graduates. In
1884-85, after reorganization was effected, the faculty was increased to 17;
matriculates, 50; graduates, 22.

Thus, year by year the teaching force
and the number of students in attendance
has increased, until in the term ending
May 1, 1903, the faculty numbers 75;
matriculates 570, and 170 graduates,
while the alumni number 2106.

The first faculty of the session of 1883
consisted of W. W. Allport, M.D., D.D.S.,
professor of dental pathology and therapeutics; Geo. H. Cushing, D.D.S., professor of principles and practice of dental surgery; L. P. Haskell, professor of
prosthetic dentistry and oral deformities.

Lecturers: John S. Marshall, M.D.,
adjunct professor of dental pathology
and therapeutics; Edmund Noyes, materia medica; A. W. Hoyt, D.D.S., dental
histology and physiology; P. J. Kester,
D.D.S., chemistry; R. H. Kimball,
D.D.S., dental anatomy; J. N. Crouse,
D.D.S., oral deformities; E. D. Swain,
D.D.S., demonstrator of the minute anatomy of the tissues of the mouth; A. W.
Hoyt, D.D.S., demonstrator of operative
dentistry; Professor Haskell, demonstrator of prosthetic dentistry (giving special
attention to continuous-gum work).

Assistants to operative department: C.
P. Pruyn; Geo. T. Carpenter, M.D.,
D.D.S.; T. B. Wheeler.

Assistants to prosthetic department:
O. D. Swain; H. A. Armitage.

Clinical Instructors: W. W. Allport,
M.D., D.D.S.; R. F. Ludwig, D.D.S.;
C. H. Thayer, D.D.S.; Geo. Cushing,
D.D.S.; G. A. Christman, D.D.S.; Jos.
Marshall, M.D.; W. C. Dyer; James A.
Swasey; W. A. Stevens; P. J. Kester,

D.D.S.; J. W. Wassell, D.D.S.; T. W.
Brophy, M.D., D.D.S.; Edgar D. Swain,
D.D.S.; A. W. Harlan, D.D.S.; E. Honsinger, D.D.S.; J. A. Swartley; R. H.
Kimball, D.D.S.; A. B. Clark; W. B.
Ames, D.D.S.; G. W. Nichols, M.D.;
Frank H. Gardiner, M.D., D.D.S.; Eugene S. Talbot, M.D., D.D.S.; A. E.
Brown, D.D.S.

Northwestern University Dental School, Chicago.

The University Dental College, which
preceded the Northwestern University
Dental School, was organized under a
charter from the state of Illinois in 1887.
The first session was held in the winter
of 1887-88 with six students, the
dental faculty consisting of W. W. Allport (emeritus), L. P. Haskell, R. F.
Ludwig, John S. Marshall (dean), A. E.
Baldwin, Charles P. Pruyn, C. R. Baker,
and Arthur B. Freeman. An agreement
was effected between President Cummings of Northwestern University,
Nathan S. Davis, dean of the Chicago
Medical College, and the faculty of the
new dental college, by which its students
should take lectures in anatomy, physiology, histology, materia medica, pathology,
and surgery with the medical classes; but
this agreement involved no further connection with the medical college. Also,
the connection with Northwestern University was nominal and prospective, the
university assuming no responsibility for
the dental college.

The new college was located on Twenty-sixth street, near the medical college.
The students were required to take a
course of three years of seven months
each before graduation; at this time other
dental schools required two years of six

months. This was the first dental college to make this requirement, and this fact operated very much against its success in obtaining students, so that its classes remained very small, there being only eleven students at the end of the second year. With the beginning of the third year the three year course was made optional, and the students were allowed to elect to take a two years' course. At the end of the fourth year the class numbered nineteen. The college could not continue to meet its expenses on the income derived from this number of students, and at the end of the year the faculty resigned. This was in the spring of 1891.

In the winter of 1890-91 there were a number of men who had obtained some prominence as teachers in dentistry in Chicago who were not then engaged in teaching. Thomas L. Gilmer gave a dinner at the Leland Hotel, to which George H. Cushing, Edgar D. Swain, Edmund Noyes, and W. V-B. Ames were invited, and to whom he opened the subject of the formation of a dental school. There were at the time two or three dental schools in the city that were not succeeding well and the question of the reorganization of some of these was discussed, with the result that Dr. Gilmer was authorized to investigate the advisability of the purchase of the American College of Dental Surgery, then under the control of Dr. Clendenen. At a subsequent meeting Dr. Gilmer reported adversely to the purchase of that plant. Chicago University was then in process of organization, and an interview was held with President Harper with reference to the organization of a dental school as a department of that university, but at that time they were not ready for such an undertaking. The discussion of various schemes continued

from time to time until the resignation of the faculty of the University Dental College seemed to create an opening in that direction. Dr. Henry Wade Rogers had recently become president of Northwestern University and was actively engaged in bringing the professional schools, which had previously but a nominal connection with the university at Evanston, into a closer relationship. He was seen with regard to the reorganization of this college, which he actively favored. After a number of conferences between the parties interested, which included the outgoing members of the old faculty and the officers of Chicago Medical College, an organization was effected under the charter of Northwestern University, and the charter of the University Dental College from the state allowed to lapse. In making this change the word college was dropped and the word school substituted, in accord with the policy of the university, in which the teaching organizations under its jurisdiction are called schools rather than colleges. The new school took the name Northwestern University Dental School. Chicago Medical College also came into a closer relationship with the university and took the name Northwestern University Medical School.

The new faculty was composed of Edgar D. Swain (dean), Edmund Noyes (secretary), G. V. Black, George H. Cushing, J. S. Marshall, Charles P. Pruyn, Isaac A. Freeman, Thomas L. Gilmer, Arthur B. Freeman, B. S. Palmer, W. V-B. Ames, Arthur E. Matteson, E. L. Clifford, G. W. Haskins, G. W. Whitfield, D. M. Cattell, and H. P. Smith. Arrangements were made with the medical school by which the dental students took the lectures in anatomy, physiology, histology, chemistry, materia

27

medica and therapeutics, medical juris-prudence, and general surgery with the medical classes. The school was removed to more commodious quarters on Twenty-second street, but near enough to be convenient to the medical school, which was also removed to new quarters on Dearborn street near Twenty-fourth. In the summer of 1889 the National Association of Dental Faculties passed an order which required all schools affiliated with it to extend the course of study to three terms of not less than six months each in separate years before graduation. Beginning with the session of 1891-92, the order was complied with at once and the new organization began its first session with a class of fifty-three students, only six of whom came from the old school.

After two years in this location the school was moved into new buildings erected on Dearborn street between Twenty-fourth and Twenty-fifth streets, and was housed with the medical school, each, however, having its own rooms, clinical outfits, and laboratories. In this location, and with these arrangements, the school was fairly prosperous and the number of students more than doubled, so that in the fall of 1895 there were a hundred and twenty-eight. With this number in the dental school, and the continued increase in the medical school, the space was overcrowded, so that it became necessary to procure additional buildings outside for a portion of the laboratories of the dental school. This arrangement was very unsatisfactory, as it required much running to and fro. It was clear that something else must be done in order to accommodate the increasing demands.

In the meantime the American College of Dental Surgery had been purchased by Theodore Menges and others. Its equipment had been improved, it was being put in a better condition for giving instruction, and its classes were rapidly increasing in numbers. Dr. Menges, who was showing much energy and tact, especially in gaining students, proposed in the winter of 1895-96 a consolidation of these two schools. After numerous conferences usual to such proceedings, this was effected during the following spring on terms which for the time left the principal immediate management of the school in the hands of Dr. Menges, but provided for its ultimate complete ownership by the university. The faculty was again reorganized, a part of each of the old faculties being retained. The new faculty at the beginning of 1896-97 was composed of Edgar D. Swain (dean), G. V. Black, George H. Cushing, Thomas L. Gilmer, J. S. Marshall (emeritus), B. J. Cigrand, A. H. Peck, E. H. Angle, Edmund Noyes, I. B. Crissman, W. E. Harper, G. W. Haskins, James H. Prothero, G. W. Schwartz, William Stearns, Charles B. Reed, F. B. Noyes, T. B. Wiggin, W. T. Eckley, L. B. Haymen, George Leininger, C. E. Sayre, V. J. Hall, and Theodore Menges (secretary and business manager). The dental school was removed to the building that had been occupied by the American College of Dental Surgery, on the corner of Franklin and Madison streets, where it remained until the summer of 1902. In this building additional space could be had from time to time for indefinite expansion. In this arrangement the American College went out of existence, and as its students would have no alma mater it was agreed that those students who graduated from that college in 1890 and since should be made alumni of Northwestern University Dental School.

Northwestern University Dental School now undertook to teach all of the departments, including the fundamental branches, by its own professors and instructors, thus separating them entirely from the medical school. The work was now with much larger classes than had before been assembled in dental schools, and as the year passed it was seen that while the general methods of instruction in vogue were well adapted, much improvement in the systematizing of the work of the teaching force was desirable. At the end of the year the dean, Edgar D. Swain, resigned. G. V. Black was then appointed dean, and was charged especially with the systematizing of the methods of instruction. Each of the departments of instruction was gradually brought under the control of a single responsible professor, who controlled the methods of presentation of the subjects in his field of work by those associated with him, and the courses of study so graded that the classes of each year remained separate in the classroom. Personal teaching was provided for by the separation of classes into sections, and the arrangement of quiz masters and demonstrators for special duties, so that the individual student could at any time obtain a personal answer to his questions or the demonstration of a technical procedure.

In 1898 the Northwestern Dental College was purchased, the college closed and its plant added to Northwestern University Dental School. This arrangement included the recognition of the recent graduates of the Northwestern Dental College as alumni of Northwestern University Dental School.

The school prospered and the classes increased in numbers steadily until, in 1899-1900, there were six hundred students. Additional space in the building was obtained from time to time for additional laboratories and classrooms. In 1899 an entire additional floor was added to gain additional space for necessary classrooms, lecture rooms, and laboratories, and also to provide space for a library, museum, and reading room. It had been found particularly desirable that students be provided with well-arranged space in the school building, to which they could go during any leisure hour for the purpose of reading and study, or which they could occupy at regular hours and find books upon any topics in dentistry. The work of assembling a library and museum of comparative dental anatomy and dental pathology was actively undertaken, and the material has been rapidly brought together, so that at the present time these may be justly regarded as excellent, and as quite fully supplying the needs of a dental school. To these, members of the profession have contributed books, journals, and specimens liberally, and have in this way very materially aided in the gathering of the collection. This work is still in progress. Members of the profession may make use of this library.

On June 1, 1900, Theodore Menges, secretary and business manager of Northwestern University Dental School, died of appendicitis, after an illness of a little less than one week. He was thus cut off seemingly before his time, in the midst of robust manhood and mental vigor, while in the active prosecution of the work that seemed to have been allotted to him to do. His sudden death threw a wave of grief over all connected with the school, to its alumni, the dental profession, and to all who knew him and the work he was doing. He was an active, energetic, and resistless worker, devoting his life to the upbuilding of the dental profession.

After the death of Dr. Menges a settlement was made between the university and the Menges estate which left Northwestern University Dental School the property of the university. William E. Harper was appointed secretary, and the school proceeded with its work without other change. At the end of the year A. H. Peck resigned and Elgin MaWhinney succeeded him.

Very soon after the death of Dr. Menges a movement was made by the university to obtain a building of its own for its professional schools that were not provided for. These comprised the School of Law, the Pharmacy School, and the Dental School. The Tremont House, an old-established hotel of excellent construction, was purchased and the internal parts torn out and rebuilt in form adapting it to the purposes of these schools, at a cost approximating eight hundred thousand dollars ($800,000). This made the building a new one to all practical purposes, and it is now known as the Northwestern University Building. It is situated on the southeast corner of Lake and Dearborn streets, in the business center of Chicago.

This building was completed and occupied by the university in the fall of 1902 and the above mentioned schools moved in. In the arrangement of the space the Dental School was allotted the two upper floors, the fifth and sixth, and space for its chemical laboratories on the second floor. The sixth floor is twenty-four feet from floor to ceiling, and those parts not devoted to the great clinic and lecture rooms are divided, making an additional or seventh floor, creating additional space for the use of the Dental School. These floors, with the space occupied by the chemical laboratories on the second floor, gives the Dental School a net floor space of 57,000 square feet. The building is substantial, and very neatly finished. The rooms are well lighted and thoroughly adapted to their various purposes. They are ample for the accommodation of two hundred students in each class, and by a little crowding will accommodate two hundred and thirty-five, or six hundred to seven hundred and fifty in the three classes of a three-year course, or eight hundred in a four-year course. The great clinic room, lighted upon two sides and by skylight its full length and accommodating a hundred and thirty operating chairs provided with fountain cuspidors, brackets, and tables, is the best yet provided for the clinical teaching of dental students, and its central position in the great city of Chicago gives it an abundant clinic. The lecture rooms are especially well arranged. The lighting is entirely from the ceiling, and the walls are so constructed as to eliminate all noises from the streets of this busy down-town district. So completely is this accomplished that the lecture rooms are as free from noise as if the city were eliminated.

The oral surgery clinic room, with its waiting room, preparation room, and recovery room for the temporary care of patients needing hospital advantages, is very compact and convenient for the preparation and care of surgical patients, and the seating capacity is sufficient for two hundred and twenty-five students. This space is reserved strictly for surgical work. The different laboratories are on a similar scale, so that each class finds its accommodations ample in each separate part of the work in which it is engaged.

In the method of teaching employed

no two classes attend the same lectures or laboratory exercises. For instance, in operative dentistry the student is engaged in study every year of his course, but the subject is strictly divided into the freshman, junior, and senior courses in the three-year course, each taking up a different part of the work. The same is true in prosthetic dentistry and any other subject of study. In this division of work the professor in the particular department has especial control of the plans of presentation of his subject in each separate year, no matter what his number of assistants.

———

Colorado College of Dental Surgery, Denver, Col.

The Denver School of Dentistry was organized in 1887, and during the seventeen years of its existence has steadily grown in favor with the dental profession and people of Colorado, and has won its place among the dental colleges of our country.

It has been a member of the National Association of Dental Faculties since 1891, and is also recognized by the National Association of Dental Examiners.

Its first dean was A. B. Robbins, in 1888-89. He was re-elected in 1889-90. The second dean, 1890-91, was P. T. Smith. Thomas Gaddes was dean in 1891-92.

The following deans and secretaries were elected in the succeeding order:

1892-1893. Geo. J. Hartung.
1893-1894. Geo. J. Hartung.
1894-1895. R. B. Weiser; A. H. Sawins, secretary;

1895-1896. R. B. Weiser; A. H. Sawins, secretary;
1896-1897. J. M. Porter; W. E. Griswold, secretary;
1897-1898. A. H. Sawins; A. C. Watson, secretary;
1898-1899. A. H. Sawins; A. C. Watson, secretary;
1899-1900. A. H. Sawins; A. C. Watson. secretary;
1900-1901. L. S. Gilbert; A. L. Whitney, secretary;
1901-1902. L. S. Gilbert; A. L. Whitney, secretary.

The real history of the Colorado College of Dental Surgery dates back to April 1896, at which time the board of regents of the University of Colorado organized a department of dentistry with the following as a board of directors, viz:

W. T. Chambers, D.D.S.;
M. S. Fraser, D.D.S.;
J. S. Jackson, D.D.S.;
H. A. Fynn, D. D. S.;
A. L. Whitney, D.D.S.

The school opened November 2, 1896, with seven students.

The officers of the dental department were:

J. H. Baker, LL.D., president.
W. T. Chambers, D.D.S., dean.
M. S. Fraser, D.D.S., secretary.
A. L. Whitney, D.D.S., superintendent of infirmary.

In all there was a teaching faculty of nine professors and nine special lecturers with a clinical staff of six dentists.

The infirmary was located at Eighteenth and Stout streets, in connection with the medical department of the state university.

Application was made for admission into the National Association of Dental

Faculties, and a committee from that association examined the school during the winter session and reported favorably upon it.

In June 1897 a decision of the Supreme Court, in a long-pending suit, declared that it was impossible for the state university to conduct any of its departments outside of Boulder, the seat of the university.

Recognizing the impossibility of conducting a dental college in a small city, and wishing to continue the work so well begun, the Colorado College of Dental Surgery Corporation was organized from the faculty of the Dental Department of the University of Colorado, and incorporated under the laws of the state of Colorado in July 1897.

The first officers of the Colorado College of Dental Surgery comprised the stockholders, viz:

H. A. Fynn, D.D.S., president.
W. T. Chambers, D.D.S., vice-president.
A. L. Whitney, D.D.S., secretary.
J. S. Jackson, D.D.S., treasurer.
M. S. Fraser, D.D.S., auditor.

The dental faculty consisted of twelve professors, eleven special lecturers, and a clinical staff of six.

The officers of the faculty were as follows:

W. T. Chambers, D.D.S., dean.
M. S. Fraser, D.D.S., secretary.
J. S. Jackson, D.D.S., treasurer.

The school opened on October 4, 1897, at Eighteenth and Larimer streets, with thirty matriculates.

Application was made for admission into the National Association of Dental Faculties under the new name of Colorado College of Dental Surgery, and during the session of 1897-98 a committee from that association visited the school and reported favorably upon it.

At the next meeting of the National Association of Dental Faculties, held in Omaha in July 1899, the school was admitted to membership. Early in the year 1900 the Colorado College of Dental Surgery secured suitable quarters at Champa and Eighteenth streets and moved to that location.

On March 29, 1901, a union was effected between the Denver School of Dentistry and the Colorado College of Dental Surgery, and an agreement entered into with the Colorado Seminary and the University of Denver, whereby the Colorado College of Dental Surgery contracted to become the Dental Department of the University of Denver, and to conduct said department for a term of years.

The faculty of the united schools was composed of eighteen professors, eleven special lecturers, and thirty-eight demonstrators and assistants.

The officers of the faculty were:

H. A. Buchtel, D.D., LL.D., chancellor.
L. S. Gilbert, D.D.S., dean.
A. L. Whitney, D.D.S., secretary.
J. S. Jackson, D.D.S., treasurer.

The college occupies desirable quarters, centrally located at Fourteenth and Arapahoe streets. The school year opened October 7, 1901. Ninety students matriculated with the school that year.

During the session of 1901-02 the resignation of L. S. Gilbert, dean of the school, was received, and W. T. Chambers was elected to fill the vacancy, which position he has since retained.

The school is now thoroughly equipped with every modern convenience for imparting dental knowledge. Its prosthetic laboratories are furnished with electric lathes, electric furnaces, compressed air, and every necessary appliance. The anatomical laboratory is completely furnished with the most approved appliances. The histological, pathological, and bacteriological laboratories are equipped with the Bausch & Lomb and Zulauf microscopes, incubators, sterilizers, etc. An up-to-date electric arc lantern with projecting microscopic attachment is used for viewing specimens direct from the laboratory. The chemical laboratory has every facility for the practical study of chemistry and metallurgy. The infirmary is equipped with S. S. White, Columbia, and Morrison chairs, fountain cuspidors, and compressed air is at each chair.

Gas is administered in the extracting room, and students are admitted to the various hospitals to view operations under ether and chloroform.

The matriculates for the year 1903-04 number 58.

—

University of Minnesota College of Dentistry, Minneapolis, Minn.

The first step toward the establishment of a dental college in Minnesota was taken in 1883, at which time the Board of Directors of the Minnesota College Hospital organized a dental department with a two years' course of five months each. With the session of 1884-85 the College Hospital closed, but was organized again as the Minnesota Hospital College and removed to a new and more commodious building. The dental department was continued in practically the

same relation to the medical school as before. The office of dean was created this year, and W. F. Giddings, D.D.S., was appointed to the position. His removal from the city early in the session left the office as well as the chair of operative dentistry vacant. W. A. Spaulding, D.D.S., filled the deanship from this time until the surrender of the charter in 1888.

For the session of 1886-87 the term was lengthened to six months. At the close of the session of 1887-88 the Hospital College with the St. Paul Medical College and the Minnesota Homeopathic Medical College surrendered their charters. The State University then established a department of medicine which comprised a "college of medicine and surgery," a "homeopathic college of medcine and surgery," and a "college of dentistry." The course in dentistry was extended to three years, with terms of six months each. Students in these colleges received instruction in anatomy, physiology, and chemistry, and were subjected to the same examinations, and the course of instruction in the college of dentistry was more systematically graded than heretofore.

The formation of a College of Dentistry under the auspices of the state university marked an epoch in the history of dental teaching in the Northwest, and by it the dentists interested in teaching accomplished much for which they had labored since the small beginning as a department of the College Hospital. The school became in fact as well as in name an integral part of one of the departments of the State University. The school, too, was one of the first to require a three-year course for graduation. It exacted and adhered rigidly to the highest standard for admission, and required its students to pass examinations in the primary branches, in common with the students in medicine, before they could come up for examination in the dental studies, and did much toward establishing dentistry as a specialty in medicine.

In 1890 W. X. Sudduth, A.M., M.D., D.D.S., of Philadelphia, was elected by the Board of Regents to the position of secretary of the faculty, and the affairs of the college were given into his charge. At the close of the year the title of dean was conferred upon him. The length of the school term was again extended, this time to eight months. A new building being completed on the campus in 1892 for the department of medicine, the College of Dentistry (with the medical schools) was removed to it for the session of 1892-93. The faculty was augmented by several new professors and instructors and the school at once took high rank among those engaged in modern dental teaching. Professor Sudduth remained with the school until the close of the session of 1894-95, when he removed to Chicago. Thomas E. Weeks, D.D.S., succeeded Professor Sudduth, and was dean until the close of the session of 1896-97, when he resigned from the office, but continued work in the school until 1901. At the beginning of the session of 1901-02, W. P. Dickinson, D.D.S., was called by the Board of Regents to assume the duties of the position, and holds the place at the present time.* Beginning with 1897 the term was again lengthened, this time to nine months.

The college has always stood for that which was highest and best, and was one

---

* [Succeeded, 1905, by Alfred Owre, D.D.S.]

of the very first to advocate and put into effective practice courses of graded and systematic technic instruction.

Western Dental College of Kansas City, Mo.

The Western Dental College of Kansas City was chartered June 24, 1890, and organized by the following gentlemen: D. J. McMillen, president (first year); J. S. Letord, vice-president; H. S. Lowry, secretary; E. E. Shattuck, treasurer.

Board of directors: W. G. Price, H. S. Thompson, E. E. Shattuck, I. D. Pierce, J. S. Letord, H. S. Lowry, D. J. McMillen, S. C. Wheat, J. W. Heckler, J. H. Kinley, J. M. Gross, T. J. Beattie.

First faculty: H. S. Douglas, M.D., professor of oral surgery; J. T. Eggers, M.D., T. J. Beattie, M.D., professors of anatomy; J. S. Sharp, M.D., professor of materia medica and general pathology; Claude C. Hamilton, M.D., Ph.G., professor of chemistry; H. O. Haniwalt, M.D., professor of physiology; H. S. Lowry, D.D.S., professor of prosthetic dentistry and metallurgy; D. J. McMillen, D.D.S., professor of operative dentistry and dean; J. M. Gross, M.D., D.D.S., professor of dental pathology and therapeutics.

Sixty students were enrolled the first year; eighty students the second year; one hundred and twenty-six students the third year, and two hundred and forty for the session of 1903-04.

Dental Department of Milwaukee Medical College, Milwaukee, Wis.

This school was organized September 26, 1894. The founders of the school were W. H. Neilson, M.D., president; W. H. Earles, B.S., M.D., treasurer; B. G. Maercklein, D.D.S., M.D., dean and vice-president, and W. B. Hill, M.D., secretary.

The following branches were taught: anatomy, physiology, chemistry, oral surgery, dental pathology and comparative dental anatomy, operative technics, bacteriology, operative dentistry, prosthetic dentistry, orthodontia, infirmary practice, dental hygiene and jurisprudence, histology, materia medica, metallurgy, oral deformities, dental anatomy.

Dental Department of the College of Physicians and Surgeons of San Francisco.

The Dental Department of the College of Physicians and Surgeons of San Francisco was incorporated June 18, 1896. It was framed in connection with the medical department, and the original Board of Trustees was composed of S. M. Mouser, M.D.; J. R. Laine, M.D.; Samuel O. L. Potter, M.D.; Winslow Anderson, M.D.; W. F. Southard, M.D.; Thomas Morffew, D.D.S., and Charles Boxton, D.D.S.

A faculty was organized consisting of Chas. Boxton, D.D.S., professor of prosthetic dentistry and metallurgy; J. R. Laine, M.D., professor of principles and practice of surgery and clinical surgery; Winslow Anderson, M.D., acting professor of chemistry; Silas M. Mouser, M.D., professor of pathology and bacteriology; Elmer E. Kelly, M.D., professor of anatomy; William S. Whitwell, M.D., professor of materia medica, pharmacology, and therapeutics; Frank Donaldson, M.D.,

professor of physiology and histology, and Thomas Morffew, D.D.S., professor of operative dentistry.

Instruction began January 1, 1897, and the first class was graduated in July of that year.

The Dental Department succeeded from the beginning. Students came in large numbers from all portions of the Pacific Coast, and the school boasted that in the first year of its existence it had the largest classes of any dental school ever organized west of Chicago. They established a high standard and the instruction was efficient and practical. These things were appreciated by the dental profession of the Pacific Coast and as a result the college received the support of a large portion of the dental practitioners.

Soon after its organization the college made application for membership in the National Association of Dental Faculties. The usual routine of examination and investigation was gone through with, and the college became a full-fledged member of this select organization in the summer of 1898.

Its curriculum of study covers the entire field embraced by dental schools generally in America.

University of Southern California College of Dentistry, Los Angeles, California.

The history is similar to that of many young institutions that have grown from small beginnings. It was organized 1897 under the auspices of the College of Medicine of the University of Southern California. For one year the dean of the medical college, H. G. Brainerd, was also dean of the dental school.

Then the latter assumed a more independent position with a dean of its own. Edgar Palmer was dean three years. He was succeeded in 1901 by the present incumbent, Garrett Newkirk.*

It may be said from the start the growth of the school has been steady, both in the number of students and measure of influence. Thus far each year has seen a gain in attendance of about twenty per cent., so that for the year 1903-04 the enrollment is seventy. The freshman class is as large with the prospective four-year course as for the year previous—an exceptional fact in the history of the four-year movement.

The College of Medicine, located near the dental school, has excellent facilities for teaching anatomy, chemistry, general pathology, histology, and bacteriology, and it is there that the dental students receive instruction in these branches.

A list of those who have assisted in building up the school includes the following:

Medical—H. G. Brainerd, George L. Cole, George W. Lasher, Stanley P. Black, Claire W. Murphy, L. J. Stabler, E. L. Leonard, E. M. Pallette, T. C. Myers, and John L. Kirkpatrick.

Dental—L. E. Ford, J. D. Moody, M. Evangeline Jordan, W. C. Smith, H. Gale Atwater, J. A. Cronkhite, F. M. Parker, E. Allin, C. A. Kitchen, Wm. Bebb, R. H. Shoemaker, E. L. Townsend, B. W. Harper, U. D. Reed, and E. C. Baily, attorney. Also the president of the University of Southern California, George F. Bovard, D.D.

---

*[Succeeded, 1905, by Lewis E. Ford, D.D.S.]

The Illinois School of Dentistry, Chicago.

The Illinois School of Dentistry, Chicago, was organized in 1899. The first faculty consisted of Frank N. Brown, D.D.S., dean, prosthesis and technics; David M. Cattell, D.D.S., professor of operative dentistry and operative technics; Geo. T. Carpenter, M.D., D.D.S., professor of oral surgery; Elgin MaWhinney, D.D.S., professor of materia medica and therapeutics; Geo. W. Cook, D.D.S., professor of pathology and bacteriology; B. J. Cigrand, B.S., D.D.S., professor of dental history and special prosthesis; J. A. McKinley, M.D., professor of anatomy; Charles J. Drueck, M.D., professor of physiology and histology; George E. Rollins, M.D., professor of chemistry and anesthesia; Edson B. Jacobs, D.D.S., professor of orthodontia; Elmer DeWitt Brothers, B.S., LL.B., professor of dental jurisprudence; U. C. Windell, M.D., adjunct professor of anatomy and demonstrator on the cadaver; G. Walter Dittmar, D.D.S., adjunct professor of operative technics and superintendent of infirmary.

Lecturers—R. H. Jenning, M.D., special lecturer on hygiene; Oscar Dodd, M.D., special lecturer on the care of the eyes.

In 1901 this institution became the dental department of the State University, working under the title of the College of Dentistry of the University of Illinois, with the following officers and faculty:

Officers of Faculty—Andrew Sloan Draper, LL.D., president; Oscar A. King, M.D., chairman committee of organization; Adelbert Henry Peck, M.D., D.D.S., dean; Bernard John Cigrand,

B.S., D.D.S., secretary; Daniel Atkinson King Steele, M.D., actuary.

Faculty—Adelbert Henry Peck, M.D., D.D.S., professor of materia medica, special pathology, and therapeutics; David Mahlon Cattell, D.D.S., professor of operative dentistry and operative technics; Bernard John Cigrand, M.S., D.D.S., professor of prosthetic dentistry, technics, and history; George Washington Cook, D.D.S., professor of bacteriology and general pathology; Daniel Atkinson King Steele, M.D., professor of oral surgery; James Nelson McDowell, D.D.S., professor of orthodontia; William Thomas Eckley, M.D., professor of anatomy; Jacob F. Burkholder, M.D., professor of physiology; Fred. Carl Zapffe, M.D., professor of dental histology; J. Alfonzo Wesener, Ph.C., M.D., professor of chemistry; Seth Eugene Meek, M.S., Ph.D., professor of comparative anatomy; Oscar A. King, M.D., professor of neurology; Elmer DeWitt Brothers, B.S., LL.B., professor of dental jurisprudence; Joseph McIntyre Patton, M.D., professor of general anesthesia and physical diagnosis; George Walter Dittmar, D.D.S., associate professor of operative technics and superintendent of infirmary; Charles Orville Bechtol, M.D., adjunct professor of chemistry.

The session of 1903-04, Dr. Peck retired as dean and Dr. Cigrand assumed his duties. Dr. Cattell also retired from the faculty and Donald MacKay Gallie, D.D.S., was elected professor of operative dentistry and operative technic in his stead. John P. Buckley, Ph.G., D.D.S., was elected professor of materia medica and therapeutics; George Thomas Carpenter, M.D., D.D.S., professor of oral surgery; Frank Ewing Roach, D.D.S., professor of porcelain work; T. Elhanan

Powell, D.D.S., professor of comparative anatomy; Levitt E. Custer, D.D.S., professor of radiography; Charles Erwin Jones, B.S., D.D.S., associate professor of prosthetic technic; James C. Bishop, M.S., professor of chemistry; Clayton M. McCauley, B.S., D.D.S., adjunct professor of operative technic; Ashley Hewitt, D.D.S., professor of electricity; Corinne B. Eckley, associate professor of general and regional anatomy.

———

The Barnes Dental College,

DENTAL DEPARTMENT OF THE BARNES UNIVERSITY, ST. LOUIS.

This college was organized August 25, 1903, with the following officers and faculty:

Burton Lee Thorpe, D.D.S., dean, professor of operative dentistry and dental history; D. O. M. LeCron, D.D.S., vice-dean, professor of crown and bridge work and porcelain dental art; Samuel Taylor Bassett, D.D.S., secretary, professor of prosthetic dentistry and metallurgy; Richard Summa, D.D.S., professor of orthodontia and fractures of the maxillæ; Russell H. Mace, D.D.S., professor of oral hygiene and prophylaxis; George Haritt Owen, B.D.S., D.M.D., professor of clinical operative dentistry and dental surgery; George Henry Gibson, D.D.S., professor of dental pathology and embryology; Clarence Oliver Simpson, D.D.S., professor of dental anatomy, histology, and operative technics; Wm. F. A. Schultz, LL.B., M.D., D.M.D., professor of oral surgery; Willis Bertram Arthur, M.D., D.D.S., professor of prosthetic technics; Charles H. Hughes, M.D., and Marc Ray Hughes, M.D., professors of neurological dentistry; Pinckney French, M.D., professor of principles and practice of surgery; C. M. Riley, M.D., professor of chemistry, toxicology, and director of laboratories; Z. L. Dickerson, M.D., professor of therapeutics, materia medica, and director of therapeutic laboratory; Jas. A. Close, M.B., L.R.C.S., Edin.; professor of general pathology, clinical microscopy, and director of pathological laboratory; A. R. Kieffer, M.D., professor of anatomy; R. C. Blackmer, C.M., M.D., professor of dental jurisprudence; J. J. Johnson, B.S., M.D., professor of physiology, chemistry, and director of physiologic laboratory; M. Dwight Jennings, M.D., professor of bacteriology and director of bacterical laboratory; L. C. Stocking, M.D., professor of physical diagnosis; Olney A. Ambrose, A.M., M.D., Ph.C., professor of histology, analytical chemistry and anestheria; M. E. Bradley, M.D., professor of histology and director of histological laboratory; Harold C. Herrick, Ph.B., professor of physics.

Nineteen students were enrolled the first session; at the close of the session May 4, 1904, one student who had attended two full courses at another college was graduated.

————

After the reading of the foregoing report of the Historical Committee, the session adjourned, at 5.30 P.M., until 3 P.M. Friday.

SECTION IX—Continued.

FIFTH DAY—Friday, September 2d.

THE meeting was called to order by the chairman at 3 P.M.

Dr. José J. Rojo, City of Mexico, Mexico, read his paper, "Historical Annotations and the Present Condition of Dental Education in the Capital of the Republic of Mexico."

The paper here follows:

Historical Annotations and the Present Condition of Dental Education in the Capital of the Republic of Mexico.

By Dr. JOSÉ J. ROJO, City of Mexico.

I MUST begin by making public my profound obligation to the members of the Committee of Organization of this illustrious Fourth International Dental Congress, for the esteemed honor they have conferred on me and the great satisfaction they have afforded me by appointing me a member of the Section on Education, Nomenclature, Literature, and History.

When I consider that the gentlemen on whom the progress of the profession is most directly dependent will be gathered in this section, that it will be here that educational matters, which form the basis of all progress, will be discussed, my satisfaction is still further enhanced by the hope of seeing the problems solved which at present occupy the mind of the educator, thus supplying him with additional knowledge for the more efficient discharge of the duties of his difficult post.

The firm belief that on returning to my country I shall find my ideas on dental education, history, and literature vastly improved, impels me to repeat my thanks to the respected organizers of the Fourth International Dental Congress, and to my esteemed friends who furnished me with the means of increasing my limited knowledge.

At the meeting of the Faculty of the Mexican Dental School, held in June 1904, it was resolved to confer upon me the honorable commission of representing the professors of my country at this congress, and I bear you a sincere and hearty greeting from each and every one of the professors of dentistry in the neighboring republic.

The work I am bringing you is one of

great effort, but little fruit. It is divided into two parts. The first part consists of historical annotations on dental instruction in Mexico before and after the discovery of the new world, and the second part deals with the present condition of dental education in my country.

ANNOTATIONS ON DENTAL INSTRUCTION AMONG THE TRIBES THAT POPULATED THE WESTERN CONTINENT BEFORE ITS DISCOVERY.

Innumerable were the cities founded here, and varying the degrees of civilization reached by them up to the last days of their prosperity. However, archæological discoveries and the few trustworthy data we possess enable us to state that they all practiced the arts and sciences in some form or other.

A great many of the data given in this paper have been taken from the work of the eminent Professor Flores, entitled "History of Medicine in Mexico," 1881.

Diseases of the mouth of man, no matter how hardy his constitution, exist and have always existed among all races, perhaps from their very beginning, as is proved to us by reading history, and these diseases vary in magnitude according to the factors involved.

The Aztec race, owing to its iron-like constitution, suffered from very few affections of the mouth, but notwithstanding this fact its physicians performed numerous dental operations.

As to dental instruction among the Aztecs, the law of induction leads us to suppose that for the sake of convenience, or owing to their lack of great legislators, or to the knowledge they possessed of the natural laws of heredity, professions were in those remote ages transmitted from father to son.

Ixtlilxochitl, a direct descendant of

Netzahualcoyotl, in his historical writings says: "The wise men were charged with the painting of all the sciences they knew and the teaching by heart of all the songs that had any reference to their wars and histories."

This leads us to infer that those who were ambitious of knowledge in those days, and had no means of acquiring it at home, could find the information at certain centers.

Nowadays we are becoming day by day more forcibly convinced of the fact that subdivision of labor is the most powerful lever of all progress, but the probabilities are that in those days the physicians undertook the practice of medicine, surgery inclusive of dental surgery, and perhaps also pharmacy. Only obstetrics constituted a separate profession, which was intrusted to women and transmitted from mother to daughter.

Corresponding to the gods Apis, Apollo, and Æsculapius, the deities of medicine of the old world, the Mayas also had their god of medicine, Sitbolutim and his companion the goddess Yxchel, and the Aztecs their goddess Tzapotlatenan, which proves beyond all doubt that they cultivated medicine.

The Aztecs were familiar with dental pathology and therapeutics, for they knew the properties of a multitude of herbs and prepared them in different ways for the treatment of their ailments. Señor Flores cites the names of a vast number of medicinal plants* in his works. It is certain beyond all doubt that they treated stomatitis, bad breath, toothache, caries, and other affections.

With regard to surgery, there is a fact

---

* Mecaxotitl, quimchpatli, chicomecatl, ytzcuinpatli, flanquizpepetla, flanchinchinoaxohuitl, yamancapatli, flepatli, flancacaoatl. and many others.

the importance of which can never be adequately expressed to the dentist who is at all interested in the history of his profession; that fact is the following:

Professor Batres has in the course of his archæological explorations encountered very many specimens of human teeth which reveal the degree of culture in dental surgery attained by some

The first specimen is an upper left incisor with an incision in the form of a right angle at the approximal and distal angles of the tooth, thus forming a surface which is the exact reverse of that of nature, there being two right-angled incisions extending throughout the entire thickness of the tooth instead of a round and more or less acute edge. These in-

PLATE I.

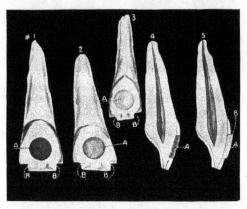

Fig. 1. Front view of incisor of Zapoteca Indian, showing inlay of iron pyrite and mutilated angles. A, Inlay. B, B, Mutilated angles.

Figs. 2 AND 3. Upper central and lateral incisors of Maya Indian, showing inlays of jade. A, Inlay. B, B, Mutilated angles.

Fig. 4. Vertical section of Fig. 1, showing inlay on a level with the labial surface of the tooth. A, Inlay.

Fig. 5. Vertical section of tooth shown in Fig. 2. A, Inlay. B, Portion of inlay projecting beyond the margin of the cavity.

of the Aztec tribes. These specimens form a collection of upper human incisors which Professor Batres classifies according to the place of their discovery, as follows: Zapotecas, teeth with inlays of iron pyrites; Mayas, inlays of jade; Taracos, with a groove in the center of the cutting edge; Totonacos, with two grooves in the cutting edge. Professor Batres states that he also found an example of interstitial metallic filling between the molars of one of these crania.

cisions are not only symmetrical but also present a perfectly polished surface.

In the center of the labial face of the tooth there is an inlay of iron pyrite three millimeters in diameter, symmetrically placed, perfectly circular, and marvelously well fitted; the edges of the inlay are in perfect adaptation to those of the cavity and no adhesive substance can be detected.

It is wonderful that after such an immense lapse of time the tooth and inlay

PLATE II.

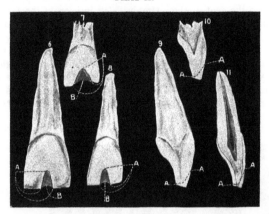

FIGS. 6, 7, 8. Front view of central and lateral incisors of a Trasco Indian, showing a groove in the cutting edge. A, Contour of the groove. B, Greatest depth of groove.

FIGS. 9 AND 10. Lateral view of teeth shown in Figs. 6 and 7. A, A, Dotted line indicating the contour of the bottom of the groove.

FIG. 11. Vertical section of tooth shown in Fig. 8. A, A, Contour of groove.

PLATE III.

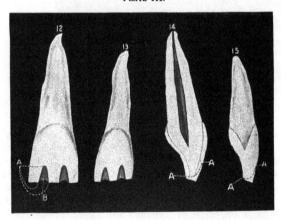

FIGS. 12 AND 13. Labial surfaces of central and lateral incisors of Totonaco Indian, with double grooves in the cutting edge. A, Contour of grooves. B, Greatest depth.

FIG. 14. Vertical section of tooth shown in Fig. 12. A, A, Line showing contour of grooves.

FIG. 15. Lateral view of tooth shown in Fig. 13. A, A, Line showing contour of grooves.

still hold together, owing to either the perfect adjustment or to the presence of some intervening substance.

The inlay is of a dark brown color, resembling that of iron oxid (perhaps this color is the result of age); the body of the tooth is of a normal color, from which we are led to suppose that the substance of the inlay is of such a nature as to render it proof against the action of the saliva. The state of the root shows us that the pulp of the tooth preserved itself in a sound condition, notwithstanding the operation. (See Plate I, Figs. 1 and 4.)

The second specimen is a central upper incisor, the two angles of which have been cut; this example like the previous one has an incision of about a millimeter and a half on each of its angles, the surface is perfectly smooth, and the vertex of the angle points toward the neck of the tooth.

The difference observed on comparing this specimen with the previous one is that the substance used for the inlay is jade, which the ancients used so much for making beads, amulets, and other ornaments. (See Plate I, Figs. 2, 3, 5.)

Some of the inlays are flush with the surface of the enamel, while others protrude about a millimeter above its level; in all the specimens the inlay has a perfectly polished surface.

The third and fourth specimens are central and lateral upper incisors with perfectly symmetrical incisions or grooves; the third specimen has one groove in the center of the cutting edge, and the fourth has two. The bed of these grooves is semilunar in form, and their surface is perfectly smooth. Their approximate dimensions are—A millimeter and a half in width; a millimeter and a half in depth; one and a half or two and a

half millimeters in length. The place they occupy is the cutting edge of the tooth; they begin at the lingual face of the enamel, deepen as they approach the labial face of the enamel, and are continued on the labial face of the tooth to a length of from one to two millimeters. (See Plates II, III.)

A coating of a vivid red color, like

PLATE IV.

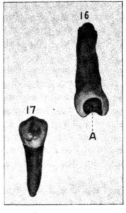

FIG. 16. View of upper canine of the same source of that of teeth with inlays of iron pyrite. A, Cavity from which inlay came out.

FIG. 17. View of a small lower grinding tooth (from same skull as canine shown in Fig. 16), showing the difference between its healthy root and the diseased one of the canine.

cinnabar, is observed on the surface of the majority of these teeth.

I shall make one of the inlaid specimens the subject of a few essential observations. It is a canine tooth from the same source as those already described. It also had an inlay, which has fallen out; it has no incisions on its cutting edge. The cavity, which is circular and perfectly cut, occupies over half the crown of the tooth; its exterior diameter is exactly five millimeters, that of its interior is slightly greater, and it has a general depth of about a millimeter and a half.

The cusp is worn away by natural use, this wear extending to the lower border of the cavity made for the inlay. The root of this tooth is porous, its vertex truncated, and its surface rough. A comparison of this tooth with the sound and compact root of another tooth from the same cranium indicates that its root was affected by some morbid process, perhaps caused by the falling out of the inlay and the death of the pulp. (See Plate IV.)

The natural wearing away of the cusp and the loss of the inlay clearly demonstrate that the operation was performed during the man's life, between the ages of twenty-five and thirty, and the state of the root also warrants the supposition that the death, decay, etc., of the pulp set in some time after the inlay fell out.

The fact that these remains were found in earthen vessels, that the crania and other bones contained in the latter are painted red, and the places in which they were found, seem to demonstrate that it was an infrequent operation, perhaps only performed on rulers or priests, or that it was a religious emblem. It may also be taken for granted that it was an operation only performed in the last years of the zenith of progress and prosperity of these races, as the specimens encountered are not numerous.

We can assert after a close study of these specimens that some of the aboriginal races of this continent practiced operations of a most delicate nature upon the teeth, attaining a very high degree of perfection in their execution, which shows that they were acquainted with the ana-tomical structure of the teeth, and possessed instruments and the other necessary means for making these inlays, which are a wonderful surprise to those who see them.

Consequently, we can affirm that the Aztecs knew and practiced pathology, therapeutics, and something like dental surgery.

DENTISTRY AFTER THE CONQUEST.

Shortly after the conquest the corporation of the city of Mexico, on January 13, 1523, agreed upon the following resolution: "This day the said gentlemen acting on the petition of Francisco de Soto, barber and surgeon, ordered that as long as it were the pleasure of the said council the salary of fifty dollars in gold a year be assigned to him, and paid to him in three instalments, in consideration whereof the said Soto shall reside in this city and here practice his trades." According to Dr. Flores this was the first decree regarding medical studies in Mexico ever issued by the authorities.

Following the example of the Roman College of Physicians (a licensing and examining board), the city council on January 11, 1527, decreed the formation of a Mexican College of Physicians, of an official character, its object being the supervision of examinations and of the practice of the medical sciences; it also kept a close lookout for quacks, punishing all those who attempted to practice a profession without possessing the necessary qualifications.

Between the years 1551 and 1553 of the viceroyalty the Spanish government issued a decree ordering the foundation of a university in Mexico. During the early years of its existence this institution devoted all its efforts and resources to the teaching of theology, and it was not until the year 1580 that the first professorship of medicine was founded. However, a long period elapsed before medicine was properly taught; a perusal of historical data tells us that it was only in 1816, or six years after the declaration of independence, that there were four professorships of medicine, and it is only after that date that medicine can be said to have had a special course devoted to it.

The first text-books used in this university were based on the doctrines of Hippocrates, Galen, and Güido, from which it is evident that the mouth was studied in the classes of anatomy and surgery, although but little attention was given to that organ.

At that time the study and practice of medicine were divided among the following: physicians, surgeons, pharmacists, phlebotomists, bone-setters, and midwives. Physicians and surgeons were obliged to study and graduate at the university; the others were required to possess the rudimentary knowledge necessary for their trade, and had to give a practical demonstration before the College of Physicians to be able to obtain a license or diploma authorizing them to practice their trade.

The above regulation, with very slight modifications, existed during a great many years. In 1833 one of the first presidents of the republic ordered the university to be closed.

The closing of the university that had existed so many years must have caused great agitation at the time, but the president, Doctor Gomez Faríaz, thoroughly convinced of the wisdom of his orders, shortly afterward—that very same year, in fact—ordered an Institution of Medical Sciences to be founded. This was without question the beginning of the era of progress of medicine in Mexico.

After the foundation of the new school the study of medicine and general surgery made remarkable progress in Mexico notwithstanding the fact that the constantly recurring dissensions and revolutions of that epoch obliged the school to close its doors for some time on different occasions.

The professions of pharmacy, obstetrics, and phlebotomy did not receive any great benefit during that early period, and continued subject to the regulations of the epoch of the university, with very slight modifications.

In 1870 the study of pharmacy and obstetrics received the attention of our legislators, and new chairs for the teaching of these two professions were founded at the School of Medicine.

The studies of the phlebotomists and dentists, formerly called barber-surgeons, were but slightly changed during that period.

In the course of the years 1841 to 1866 the profession of phlebotomy became gradually substituted by that of dental surgery; the records of that period show that there were examinations for both those professions, but after 1866 there were no more candidates for the examinations in phlebotomy, while the applicants for dentistry increased considerably.

The instruction in dentistry continued to improve during the last stages of this period, for although there were no special courses for the study of that profession, the candidates could acquire the necessary knowledge, as a group of physicians (nearly all being professors of the School of Medicine) gave private classes of descriptive anatomy, dissection, histology, bacteriology, therapeutics, and dental surgery; besides this, the candidates had to present to the secretary of the school, together with their application for an examination, a certificate sworn before a notary testifying that they had practiced all the surgical and prosthetic operations in the surgery of a qualified dentist. If this application was admitted the candidate was examined in order to test his proficiency, and in the event of his being successful the department of public instruction gave him a diploma. The last diploma of a dentist and surgeon obtained by this procedure was issued in 1900.

The latest stage in the evolution of the dental profession in Mexico began in 1896. At about that time several corporations and some private persons approached the president of the republic and the minister of justice and public instruction with petitions asking for the establishment of a special school for the teaching of dentistry. Three different schemes were proposed: The establishment of a private institution which the government would aid pecuniarily and invest with an official standing; the next proposed that the government should found a national dental school entirely independent of the National School of Medicine; the third and last was that a school of dentistry should be established as an annex of the National School of Medicine.

The government, realizing the necessity of the proposed institution, appointed a commission, formed by the eminent doctors of medicine Don Manuel Carmona y Valle, Don Rafael Lavista, and Eduardo Liceaga, to reform the plan of studies of the School of Medicine, and at the same time consider the best manner of regulating the study of dental surgery.

The consideration of such a complex matter naturally required some time, but in the end the decision proved favorable to the dental profession.

During this period there was considerable activity among the dentists. In 1896 the well-known engineer, Don Sebastian Camacho, aided the efforts of a group of dentists by furnishing the necessary funds for the establishment of a private school of dentistry. The school was not properly organized and was closed after an ephemeral existence of four or five months.

About two years later Dr. Soriano, a dentist, established a private dental college; but it did not flourish, and shared the same fate as the other.

EFFORTS OF THE MEXICAN DENTAL SOCIETY.

In the very first year of its foundation one of its members, Juan Falero, was the first to advance the idea of forming a dental school, during the session of August 3, 1898. On September 7, 1898, Drs. Carmona and Engberg made a motion that a petition be addressed to the president of the republic, protesting against the existing regulations affecting the study of dental surgery and the examinations. At the next session the proposal was discussed, approved, and carried into effect.

On November 25, 1898, all the members being in attendance, the project of founding a dental dispensary was discussed. The idea was to afford students of dentistry opportunities for practice, and at the same time to provide a suitable place in which the poor could be treated and the society also hold clinics and sessions. In the session of December 7, 1898, the plan of founding a dispensary was read, discussed, amended, and approved, Dr. Carmona being elected its director and Dr. Reguera its secretary and treasurer.

Session held December 5, 1900. Dr. F. Pastor, one of its members, returned after having attended the International Dental Congress in Paris as an official delegate. Dr. Pastor sent a report to the president of the republic on the result of his mission, and acting on the suggestion of the Mexican Dental Society, particularly that of Dr. Ricardo Crombe, explained to him the imperative necessity of a dental college in Mexico.

Session held November 28, 1901. The president of the society informed the assembly that Dr. Liceaga, the director of the National School of Medicine, had asked the society to appoint a commission of its members to formulate a plan of studies and regulations for the profession of dental surgery, and to make out a list of the equipment required for the future school. Several members discussed the matter at this session without reaching any definite decision, whereupon the chairman called for another meeting, and requested the members to give the matter their full attention and consideration, so that this most commendable project might be decided upon at the next session.

Session held December 11, 1901. The president of the society announced that he had already delivered to Dr. Liceaga the proposed plan of instruction for the profession of dental surgery.

Session held February 12, 1902. It was announced to the assembly that Dr. Liceaga had informed the Mexican Dental Society that the plan of studies presented by them had been officially adopted and incorporated into the laws of the country and duly promulgated in the official gazette (*Diario Oficial*).

September 24, 1902, the government commissioned the writer of this paper to visit and study the dental colleges of the United States of America. He was most courteously and kindly received at all the great institutions he visited, and on his return presented a detailed report. This report was officially published in the *Bulletin of Public Instruction* of March 10, 1903.

As soon as the secretary of justice and public instruction, Lic. Don Justino Fernandez, understood the necessity of establishing a school of dentistry, he took great pains to accomplish the realization of the project. Accordingly, when toward the end of 1901 Dr. Liceaga presented his plan of studies and regulations for the National School of Medicine, he ordered the study of dentistry to be included in it, as he favored the idea of making the proposed school a branch of the School of Medicine. On January 11, 1902, the president of the republic, in the law referring to the course of study to be followed in the National School of Medicine, and acting in conjunction with the secretary of justice and public instruction, ordered the courses for the study of dentistry to be included in the plan, and that the necessary professorships be established.

After this the rules to be observed in the new department were formulated, the arrangement and equipment of the premises decided upon, and the professors appointed.

As an honor deservedly due to them, I shall enumerate the founders of the dental school whose advent marks the beginning of a new era in the annals of Mexican dentistry: The president of the republic, who as a lover of all that tends to progress and improvement, cordially greets and esteems all that redounds to the benefit of the nation. The secretary of justice and public instruction, Lic. Don Justino Fernandez, who, zealous in the discharge of his high mission and recognizing the benefits that would accrue from the founding of a school of dentistry, facilitated the necessary appropriations and personally inaugurated the new institution. The sub-secretary of justice and public instruction, Lic. Don Justo Sierra, who realizing the importance of the new school, exerted all his efforts in behalf of its foundation. Dr. Don Eduardo Liceaga, the director of the National School of Medicine, who lent his vast scientific knowledge toward the creation of the new school.

To conclude I must express a kind remembrance of the faithful members of the Mexican Dental Society who witnessed the realization of their ideal.

THE SCHOOL OF DENTISTRY ANNEXED TO THE NATIONAL SCHOOL OF MEDICINE.

This institution, called the "Consultorio Nacional de Enseñanza Dental," and inaugurated April 16, 1904, is a branch of the National School of Medicine, and with it forms a part of the general scheme of professional schools, owing to which fact it is closely related to the Superior Board of Public Education and the National Preparatory School.

The Superior Board of Public Education is an advisory body formed of the directors of all the higher educational institutions.

THE NATIONAL PREPARATORY SCHOOL.

As can be readily understood, this is a preparatory institution for the professional schools. No students are admitted unless they have completed their primary or elementary education. All applicants for admission into the professional schools must present a certificate testifying that they have studied and passed an examination of all the courses of the preparatory school.

The curriculum extends over a period of six years and is as follows:

First year. Elementary algebra; plane and solid geometry; first course of French; first course of Spanish; first course of freehand drawing; gymnastics.

Second year. Plane trigonometry and the elements of spherical trigonometry; analytical geometry and the elements of infinitesimal calculus; second course of French; second course of Spanish; second course of freehand drawing; gymnastics.

Third year. Elements of mechanics and cosmography; physics; first course of English; third course of Spanish; Greek roots; third course of freehand drawing; gymnastics.

Fourth year. Chemistry; elements of mineralogy and geology; elements of meteorology; general geography and climatology; second course of English; fourth course of Spanish; fourth course of freehand drawing; gymnastics.

Fifth year. Botany; elements of anatomy and physiology of the human body; American and national geography; universal history; third course of English; general literature; first course of mechanical drawing; fencing and target-practice.

Sixth year. Psychology; logic; sociology and ethics; national history; fourth course of English; Spanish and Mexican literature; second course of mechanical drawing, and the elements of topographical drawing; fencing and target-practice.

BUILDING AND EQUIPMENT OF THE SCHOOL OF DENTISTRY.

The building is divided into twelve compartments conveniently arranged: The director's and secretary's offices; a well-furnished reception room; a hall for surgical operations and clinics (14 x 8 meters) with six windows facing the north, provided with six Wilkerson chairs, dental engines with their respective brackets and spittoons, apparatus for disinfecting, a complete supply of instruments for the professors, electric power, etc.; a room (6 x 6 meters) for operations with general anesthesia, with two windows facing the north, equipped with the latest pattern S. S. White Dental Mfg. Co.'s chair, a gasometer for nitrous oxid, and all necessary instruments and apparatus for performing surgical operations on the mouth; a general storeroom, well stocked with materials, utensils, etc.; cloak and toilet rooms for the professors; a lecture room with accommodations for eighty students; a laboratory for gold and metal work, with the necessary tables and apparatus; a laboratory for rubber and celluloid work; a laboratory for fire and acid work; cloakroom and toilet room for the students; museum and library.

Methods of Instruction. In all subjects oral, objective, and experimental or practical methods are employed.

SUBJECTS STUDIED BY DENTAL STUDENTS AT THE SCHOOL OF MEDICINE.

First year. Descriptive anatomy and dissection, three classes a week; histology, especially that of the elements of the mouth, three classes a week.

Second year. Topographical anatomy, that which refers to dental surgery; physiology, three classes a week; morbose processes, three classes a week.

Third year. Bacteriology and microscopy, three classes a week.

STUDIES AT THE NATIONAL SCHOOL OF DENTISTRY.

The methods of instruction are essentially practical and are divided into two parts. The oral methods consist of lectures amplified by the use of text-books and always illustrated by the objective system. The practical methods consist of clinics and the execution of all the surgical and prosthetic operations under the supervision of the professors.

First year. First course of dental surgery, with daily attendance at the clinics from 8 to 10 A.M., and three lectures a week. First course of prosthetic dentistry, daily attendance at the clinics and laboratories from 2.30 to 4.30 P.M., two oral lessons a week; dental metallurgy, one lesson a week.

Second year. Dental materia medica, two lessons a week; second course of operative dentistry, daily attendance at the clinics from 8 to 10 A.M., and three oral lessons a week; second course of prosthetic dentistry, daily attendance at the laboratories from 2.30 to 4.30 P.M., and three lectures a week.

Third year. Dental pathology, three lessons a week; dental surgery, third course, with daily attendance at the clinic from 8 to 10 A.M., and three oral lessons a week; third course of dental prosthesis, daily attendance at the laboratory from 2.30 to 4.30 P.M., three lectures a week; special course of orthodontia, three lessons a week, both theory and practice.

Besides the above the students go and practice at the general hospital whenever the professors and director consider it necessary.

LENGTH OF THE COURSES.

The curriculum is divided into three separate years. The classes meet on January 7th and close on September 30th; the sessions are suspended on national holidays and for a week in spring.

TEXT-BOOKS.

Descriptive Anatomy: B. Beauni. Topographical Anatomy: P. Tillaux. Normal Histology: S. Ramon y Cajal. Physiology: J. P. Langlois and Varigny. General Morbid Processes: Sanchez Ocaña. Bacteriology: Albert Besson. Dental Pathology: Frank Abbott. Dental Materia Medica: Frank Abbott. Operative Dentistry: American Text-Book of Operative Dentistry, Edward C. Kirk. Orthodontia: E. H. Angle. Prosthetic Dentistry and Dental Metallurgy: C. J. Essig. Crown-, Bridge-, and Porcelain-Work: G. Evans.

EXAMINATIONS.

The ordinary examinations of all the courses are generally held from October 15th to November 15th. The general or graduation examinations are held at any time between January 15th and September 15th.

The tests at the examinations are both theoretical and practical. The first are oral and written, and the second consist of the performance of operations.

Discussion.

A. H. THOMPSON, Topeka, Kans. I was much interested in this excellent paper and congratulate Dr. Rojo upon his careful researches, especially among Spanish archives, for he has certainly given an excellent presentation of the condition of dental education in Mexico.

I was especially interested in these archæological specimens and would like to know if any of them were set with hematite or turquoise. The nicety of the operation is quite interesting, and one cannot but wonder how they drilled these holes so symmetrically. The holes may have been made in some way similar to the manner in which these primitive people drilled holes in crystals, with a reed tool and sand and water. Yet it took a lifetime to do it, as a rule, and these holes were evidently drilled during the life of the patient, so that they probably did it with a drill. I would like to know what the cementing substance was that they used. It probably was bitumen. There are some specimens in the New York Museum of Natural History which seem to have been set with bitumen. Dr. Seville has some specimens set with hematite and jade. An interesting thing is the notches that are cut on the edges. Dr. Seville has some cut with double notches. In one skull all six of the anterior teeth are cut with double notches like a step. This evidently has some religious significance, for some of the idols have these same notches cut in their teeth. The notches probably have some relationship to the storm clouds and the rain prayer, but the mythology is so complicated it is hard to trace the connection.

Dr. V. GUERINI, Naples, Italy. I find the paper of Dr. Rojo very interesting, especially the part that speaks of the fillings. It would be still more interesting if he could establish, approximately at least, at what epoch this special work was done. I would like to know someone in this country who has made a study of this subject. I hope the photographs of these specimens will be published in the Transactions.

Dr. Rojo (closing the discussion). I have not seen specimens set with hematite or turquoise. The specimens that I have seen and mentioned were of iron pyrite of a brown color, and of jade—this of a light green color resembling turquoise. I do not know what substance was used as a cement.

Replying to Dr. Guerini's question: The time was approximately about the year 1300, and I shall be very glad to give Dr. Guerini the address of Prof. Leopoldo Batres, who is probably the best authority on the subject.

On motion, the paper by Dr. BURTON LEE THORPE of St. Louis, Mo., entitled "A Biographical Review of the Careers of Hayden and Harris," was, in the absence of the author, ordered to be read by title.

The paper here follows:

A Biographical Review of the Careers of Hayden and Harris.

By BURTON LEE THORPE, M.D., D.D.S., St. Louis, Mo.,

DEAN, PROFESSOR OF OPERATIVE DENTISTRY AND DENTAL HISTORY, BARNES DENTAL COLLEGE, DENTAL DEPARTMENT BARNES UNIVERSITY.

OF the many able men who have contributed to develop the dental profession, two men stand out pre-eminent as the progenitors of dental science.

Both were men of rare native talent and genius, possessing an inexhaustible amount of energy, enthusiasm, and resourcefulness, which, when combined, united dental surgery to science and raised it to the worth and respectability of a profession. As authors, teacher-practitioners, and organizers of the first dental college, the first dental journal, and the first dental society, their names will ever illumine the pages of dental history as the leading spirits in making dentistry rank with other learned professions. To them, Longfellow's words, "Great men stand like solitary towers in the City of God," are indeed applicable.

HORACE H. HAYDEN, M.D., D.D.S.

Horace H. Hayden was born October 13, 1769, at Windsor, Conn., of honorable and Christian parentage. He was not born of obscure or poor parents, as stated by previous biographers. His ancestor, William Hayden of Connecticut (1630), won special mention for gallantry in the official report of his captain, John Mason, whose life he saved in the Pequot War of 1637. He settled in 1642 at Windsor, Conn., where he bought land, and also received land from the colony of Connecticut for his military services in the Pequot War. That land the family still owns, having held it now for 262 years. William Hayden's eldest son Daniel was a lieutenant in the Colonial service and a member of the General Court. His commission as lieutenant is extant. Lieutenant Daniel had also an elder son Daniel, who was likewise a member of the General Court of Connecticut. His eldest son, the third Daniel, was also a lieutenant in the French and Indian War, and for his day a rich man. The house he built and lived in still stands at Hayden Station, Conn., having been erected in 1740. This Lieutenant Daniel the third had as his eldest son Thomas Hayden, father of Dr. Horace H. Hayden the subject of this sketch.

and adjutant, his service extending from 1775 to 1778 and from 1780 to 1783. When the Revolutionary War was ended Lieutenant Thomas Hayden had lost

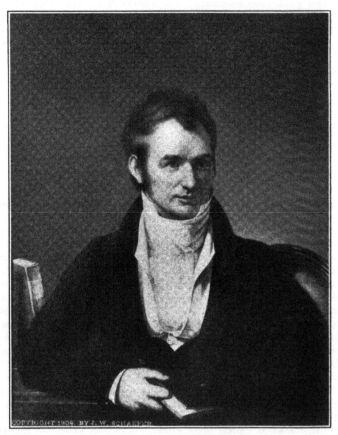

HORACE H. HAYDEN, M.D., D.D.S.

Thomas Hayden was an architect and builder, and served seven years in the Revolutionary War, as sergeant at the Lexington Alarm, 1775, and as sergeant-major, second lieutenant, first lieutenant,

much, but still held his land and business.

It was from his father that Dr. Hayden learned the business of architect and builder. He had an honored ancestry from his mother, who was Abigail Parsons, a descendant of one of the brainiest families of New England. Born 1769, he was a boy during the Revolution, when, all the men being in the army, he and his mother harvested the crops and attended to the farm. Every ancestor he had in this country was a member of the Christian Church. Rev. John Warham, the first clergyman in New England and an ancestor of the Edwards, Burr, and Parsons families, was also his ancestor, and as his mother and father were cousins the hereditary gifts of both lines united in him to some extent.

During his boyhood he exhibited a remarkable liking for natural history, often surprising his friends by his ingenuity and success in discovering objects of interest while rambling in the woods. At the age of ten he began the study of ancient languages, in which he became quite proficient. At the age of fourteen he worked his passage as a cabin boy on a brig to the West Indies, making two trips. After this he returned to school, to his books, and studies of nature, until he reached the age of sixteen, when he learned the trade of carpenter, and later became an architect.

Young Hayden was studiously inclined and whatever he undertook he worked at with a will. With characteristic ardor he diligently applied his mind to his new employment, reading such books on architecture, modern and ancient, as he could procure. He left many writings and drawings as evidence of his knowledge and skill in this art.

At the age of twenty-one he again sailed for the West Indies, seeking employment in his business, and located at Pointe à Pitre, Guadeloupe; but after a brief stay, an attack of periodic fever compelled his return to his native land, where he remained until the following year, when he returned to the West Indies, but was again forced by the pestilence to return to Connecticut.

For several years he continued to follow his vocation as architect. At the age of twenty-four he left his native home and went to New York, remaining there during the spring and summer of 1792. Meeting with little success he returned to Connecticut and taught school near Hartford during the winter. Returning to New York he called on Mr. John Greenwood, dentist, for professional service. He greatly admired Greenwood's skill and, while under treatment, concluded to adopt that calling and to devote his time and energy to dental surgery. He immediately procured from Greenwood the few books and essays on the science at that time accessible—the best being the work of John Hunter. Leaving New York, he traveled to Baltimore, arriving there in 1800 without friends or fortune and with but an imperfect acquaintance with his new calling, but possessing plenty of native ability and imbued with energy and ambition to excel in his art. He rented a room in a frame house on the corner of Fayette and Charles streets, and announced to the public that his services were at their command. His natural earnestness and aptitude quickly attracted attention and he was soon actively engaged. He used to teach a class in dentistry, and thus began the first steps toward the college which Harris and he evolved from their work. He persuaded his brothers, Anson B. Hayden of Savannah, Ga., and Dr. Chester Hayden of Windsor, Conn., to study dentistry, and both became almost as eminent as he in the profession, though neither of them engaged in other lines of study.

Horace H. Hayden was licensed to practice dentistry in Maryland by an examining board created under an act of Assembly for the State of Maryland in 1789. The board was not, strictly speaking, a dental board, but created under an act regulating the practice of medicine and surgery.

To better perfect himself in his specialty he studied anatomy and medicine, acquiring much knowledge in these sciences and thereby gaining the respect and goodwill of the medical profession, whose confidence in him was shown in later years, when, without solicitation, the honorary degree of Doctor of Medicine was conferred on him by both the Jefferson College of Medicine of Philadelphia and the University of Maryland, in 1837.

When the British attacked North Point, Maryland, in 1814, Hayden enlisted as sergeant in Captain Warner's company of militia and served through the action, when, medical men being in demand, General Samuel Smith, knowing his skill in surgery, ordered him to the hospital as assistant surgeon, where he cared for the wounded until no longer needed. He came of a martial family, every Hayden ancestor having been a soldier.

Hayden rose rapidly in public confidence. He became associated with the most celebrated physicians and medical teachers in Baltimore and his opinions were listened to with respect and his suggestions frequently adopted. He was the first to give the profession caste in Baltimore. In 1825 he accepted an invitation to deliver a course of lectures in dental surgery to the medical class of the University of Maryland, an honor never before conferred upon any practitioner of dentistry in the United States. He contributed many essays on dentistry and medicine to the medical journals.

He delved into physiological and pathological research, making new discoveries, especially investigating the use and functions of the thyroid, salivary, lacrymal, and other glands of the human system, thus showing his acuteness of mind and experimental abilities. Having attained personal success and secured a professional standing he was anxious to improve the standing of his profession in general. He first advocated a union of dental practitioners into an association for mutual improvement, in 1817, but this was not effected until August 18, 1840, when in New York city assembled L. S. Parmly, Elisha Baker, Eleazar Parmly, Patrick Houston, Enoch Noyes, Vernon Cuyler, John Lovejoy, Chapin A. Harris, Jehiel Parmly, Joseph N. Foster, A. Woodruff Brown, C. O. Baker, J. Smith Dodge, and Solyman Brown, who actively aided him in founding the American Society of Dental Surgeons, and he was chosen its first president, continuing in that office four years, until the date of his death.

At the birth of this society he remarked that the formation of a national society of dentists had long been a favorite project with him and that he had not been alone in this desire. Many years ago he had consulted the elder Hudson of Philadelphia, who was favorably inclined to such an association. On a visit to Boston and Eastern cities he consulted his professional brethren and found them ready to co-operate in any practicable scheme to elevate the profession. He said that forty-three years ago the name of dentist was a reproach and a byword, and that he had resolved to improve and exalt the profession so that it was not a disgrace to be called a dentist. From that time he had seen the science assuming more importance in the public eye—men of learning, worth, and genius being added to the ranks of its professors from year to year.

"At the present period," continued the speaker, "renewed efforts are making in England, France, and Scotland to place our profession on still higher ground than it has yet attained; and shall we of these United States of America remain inactive in this grand endeavor? If, like the Jews, we are scattered and despised, may we not, like that persecuted people, at least hope for a day of restoration to our promised land? There are indeed many obstacles still to overcome!

"A new race of Canaanites must be expelled from our borders. Many errors must be exploded and much ignorance must be dispelled before the light of truth will beam clearly upon our path; but with diligence, zeal, and perseverance we are certain of ultimate success.

"Let us, therefore, go forward in the good cause, unintimidated by the skepticism of the faithless, the fears of the timid, or the apathy of the selfish. If there are some who prefer to plod onward in the path of private enterprise, let us unite our efforts in one great social endeavor to elevate our profession from the degraded condition to which it has sunk, and in which it must ever remain until the high-minded and well-educated among practitioners shall unitedly arise and shake themselves from the dust."

At the next meeting of the society, in 1841, he was instrumental in organizing, with the aid of his confrères, the American Journal of Dental Science, the first dental journal ever published.

With the aid of his friends and co-laborers, Drs. Chapin A. Harris, Thomas E. Bond, and Willis A. Baxley, he formu-lated and founded in 1839 the first institution dedicated to special dental education in the world—the Baltimore College of Dental Surgery—of which he was, at the age of seventy years, the first president and first professor of principles of dental science and later professor of dental physiology and pathology, serving in that capacity until his death. The establishment of this college met with bitter opposition from many sources, and it was predicted by many that its success would be short-lived, but the zeal and conscientious efforts of Hayden and Harris made it the success they had hoped for. Long before 1841 Hayden said that "mechanical and operative dentistry" was "not, in strictness, the indispensable requisite qualification of a dental surgeon." He believed that the dentist to be qualified in his profession should be thoroughly educated in the science of medicine.

As a token of professional and personal merit he was created an honorary member of the Virginia Society of Surgeon Dentists, October 11, 1842.

February 11, 1842, Hayden was granted a patent, which has been entirely overlooked by his early biographers; but this he atoned for in his later years, and at the time of its issuance it was not considered unprofessional. His claim was "preventing caries of the human teeth, and the exclusive privilege of using and rendering the empyreumatic oil (tar or balsam) and acid obtained by distillation of wood, which oil or acid, when properly modified, proportioned, and applied, is used for the purpose of counteracting decay in human teeth, and the diseases consequent thereto, and to the human mouth." For this remedy Hayden claimed "an antiseptic property which counteracts caries, allays pain and irritability of the vessels of the teeth and mouth, lessens morbid sensibilities, and arouses and restores a healthy action."

Besides being a pioneer dentist, Dr. Hayden was a pioneer geologist. All through his career he was constantly examining mineral peculiarities, the result of that love for nature which was developed in his early youth when living on the banks of the Connecticut river. He was far ahead of his age in his scientific discoveries. There were then very few geologists in the United States. He collected a valuable cabinet of American minerals which in 1850 became the basis of the complete collection of Roanoke College, Virginia. So limited was the literature of geological science in English that he was compelled to master the French language to be able to read the best books on geology, from which he made many translations.

In 1821 he published an interesting work of 400 pages entitled "Geological Essays," the first general work on geology printed in the United States, and dedicated to his personal friend, Judge Thomas Cooper of Pennsylvania. He discovered a new mineral which was named Haydenite in his honor.

He was a botanist of no mean attainment, and he wrote on silkworm culture, etc. He was also a great sportsman; with gun and rod he excelled.

He married, February 23, 1805, at Baltimore, Md., Miss Maria Antoinette Robinson, daughter of Lieutenant Daniel Robinson of Baltimore, a United States revenue officer who had served in the Pennsylvania navy during the Revolution as lieutenant and quartermaster, and had succeeded John Dickinson as a member of the finance committee of Delaware in 1777. His children were Eliza Lucretia Hayden, Mandel Mozart Hayden, M.D.,

D.D.S., Edwin Parsons Hayden, lawyer; Horace William Hayden, merchant, and two others who died in infancy.

Dr. H. H. Hayden died Friday, January 26, 1844, at Baltimore, Md., aged 75 years, and was buried in Greenwood Cemetery, Baltimore, where his remains still lie in the family vault.

Hayden spent forty-four years in the active practice of his profession. He had a prophet-like mind that foresaw the result of great enterprises. His keen intellect and foresight has made him the hero of our profession. To his last breath he spoke with love and praise of his students and the profession he did so much to advance and improve. He was a diligent student, a deep and independent thinker, eminent as a scientist in Europe and America, and an excellent teacher for fifty years, far in advance of his day. He was a God-fearing and truly scientific man, loving knowledge for its own sake, and was an honor to the profession that honors him. Time may erase his fame as practitioner, author, and scientist, but his name will ever live as "father of the American Society of Dental Surgeons."

CHAPIN A. HARRIS, A.M., M.D., D.D.S.

Chapin A. Harris was born at Pompey, Onondaga co., New York, May 6, 1806. His ancestors were of English origin, of rank and position, being a branch of the Harris family in England now represented by the Earl of Malmesbury. Captain Joshua Harris, who fought bravely under Stark at Bunker Hill, was his granduncle.

His grandfather, James Harris, who was killed in a skirmish during the Revolutionary War, was a native of England, as was his father, John Harris, born

December 30, 1773, who married November 25, 1791, Elizabeth Brundage. They man; John, a physician and dentist, and Chapin Aaron.

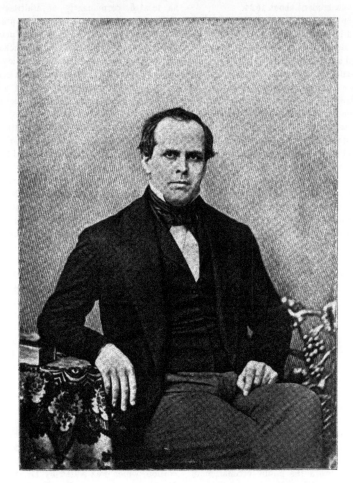

Chapin A. Harris A.M., M.D., D.D.S.

came to America and to them were born two daughters—Amanda and Eliza—and three sons—James, who became a clergy- About the age of seventeen young Harris moved to Madison, Ohio, at which place his brothers James and John had previously located, and where John was practicing medicine, and he entered his office as a student about 1824.

After pursuing the course of study prescribed by the law of the state he applied to the Board of Medical Censors, who examined and licensed him to practice medicine and surgery. He commenced the practice of this profession in Greenfield, Highland Co., Ohio, where he continued for some years, when his attention was called to the possibilities of dentistry, by his brother John, who was well skilled in medical theory and practice before he engaged in dentistry in 1827. Chapin A. Harris and his friend James Taylor, later organizer of the Ohio College of Dental Surgery, were both students of medicine and dentistry under the tutelage of John Harris.

Chapin began the practice of dental surgery in Greenfield, Ohio, in 1828 by extracting, cleaning teeth, and inserting a few fillings. Not satisfied with the meager knowledge he possessed, he secured the books of Delabarre, Fox, Hunter, and other recognized authorities, and soon acquired a thorough knowledge of the profession in which he afterward became so eminent. He remained in Greenfield about a year and then moved to Bloomfield, Ohio, where he combined the practice of dentistry, medicine, and surgery for two or three years. Leaving that place, he traveled through the South and Southwest, visiting the larger cities as an itinerant. Wherever he went, by his good work the public estimation of the profession was elevated and his own reputation established.

Tiring of travel, he located at Fredericksburg, Virginia, where he devoted his time exclusively to the practice of dental surgery, his success being such that he entirely abandoned the practice

of general medicine and surgery, but continued the study of medicine. In 1835 he located permanently at Baltimore, which offered many advantages for practice, and announced his readiness to practice his profession in all its branches. From that time until 1837 he employed a large portion of his leisure time in contributing to the pages of medical and periodical literature. In 1838, feeling his contributions were not producing the best results, he resolved that his writings should take a more compact and permanent character. This resolve induced him to prepare and publish his first book, entitled "The Dental Art: A Practical Treatise on Dental Surgery," which was issued in Baltimore in 1839 and dedicated to his medical friend Dr. Thomas E. Bond. This book consisted of 385 pages, illustrated by three lithographic plates. A second edition was issued by the firm of Lindsay & Blakiston, Philadelphia, in 1845, under the title of "Principles and Practice of Dental Surgery." This was a volume of 600 pages, containing sixty-nine wood engravings. Other editions were issued in 1847, 1850, 1852, 1855, 1858, 1863, 1866, 1871, 1885, 1889, 1898. During all these years many thousands of copies of the book have been sold, it being in all probability the most popular dental work published before or since that period. All the later editions have been edited by Dr. Ferdinand J. S. Gorgas, who has revised the book for each edition, except the tenth edition, which was edited by Dr. Philip H. Austen. His next literary effort was Harris' "Dictionary of Dental Science, a Dictionary of Dental Science, Biography, Bibliography, and Medical Terminology," published by Lindsay & Blakiston in 1849; other editions followed in 1854, 1877, 1891, 1898. The later editions of this work have also been edited by Dr. Gorgas, and it has had, considering its special character, a large sale throughout the English-speaking world.

Harris remodeled in 1846, with an introduction and numerous additions, Joseph Fox's "Diseases of the Human Teeth, Their Natural History and Functions, with Mode of Applying Artificial Teeth, etc." He also translated from the French the works of Delabarre, Lefoulon, Duval, Desirabode, and Jourdain, all republished in the *American Journal of Dental Science.* Dr. Harris was an untiring worker, and during the winter of 1838 he spent a month professionally at Littleton, N. C., where, one of his old friends writes me, he did over four thousand dollars' worth of dental work in an office room 12 by 16 feet. He had no dental chair or head-rest, but sat in a chair and put his foot on a stool, the patients sitting on the floor, resting the head on his knee. He would work hard all day operating and write on the manuscript of his book, "Dental Art," until one or two o'clock in the morning. He was a laborious student and followed this practice of writing far into the morning after days of ceaseless labor and fatigue, to the end of his life.

Feeling the need of some receptacle for treasuring the experience of the profession and its current literature, he visited New York and urged upon a few professional friends the propriety of establishing a periodical devoted especially to the interests of the dental profession.

His plan was readily embraced by a few progressive men, who promptly called a meeting composed of some of the foremost of the profession in New York, some of whom subscribed one hundred dollars and others lesser amounts toward the expense of one year's publication of a monthly journal to be known as the *American Journal of Dental Science.* The first issue appeared June 1839, published at Baltimore, under the direction of a publishing committee, namely, Eleazar Parmly, Elisha Baker, and Solyman Brown, with Chapin A. Harris and Eleazar Parmly as joint editors. This journal consisted of forty-eight pages, twenty-four of which were to be devoted to the publication of standard works on dental theory and practice. Among them were the treatises of John Hunter, Leonard Koecker, Baume, Gariot J. Nasmyth, T. Berdmore, Jobson, J. White, Blandin, R. Blake, S. Brown, and T. E. Bond. By the fourth number the circulation reached 511, with 174 subscribers. At the close of the first year the journal came into possession of the American Society of Dental Surgeons, at this society's organization in 1840, who issued it quarterly instead of monthly, and increased the price of subscription from $3.00 to $5.00 and changed the title to that of the *American Journal and Library of Dental Science.* For a period of ten years this society conducted the journal, Dr. Harris remaining continuously its chief editor, assisted by others, until 1850. After this date it was transferred to and conducted by him as a personal enterprise, until his death, which closed his editorship of twenty years' standing, during which time he was assisted by Eleazar Parmly, Solyman Brown, Edward Maynard, Amos Westcott, W. H. Dwinelle, A. A. Blandy, and A. Snowden Piggott. Dr. Harris was a voluminous and able writer, and contributed many valuable essays to the journal's pages.

Dr. Harris was the first to respond to the call of Dr. Hayden to organize the American Society of Dental Surgeons and was one of its sturdy supporters. It was on his motion the organizing convention resolved "That a national society of dentists be formed." He was chairman of the committee to prepare the society's constitution and was elected the first corresponding secretary of the society. In 1856-7 he was elected and served as second president of the American Dental Convention, which was the successor of the American Society of Dental Surgeons. Dr. Harris agreed with Dr. Hayden in the future educational needs of the profession and conceived the organization of a dental training school as an adjunct to the medical department of the University of Maryland, to whose faculty he made a proposition, but his overtures were rejected. They feared the chartering of a dental school would prove detrimental to the interests of the medical school, and strenuously opposed the movement, giving as an excuse "That the subject of dentistry was of little consequence, and thus justified their unfavorable action."

Not disheartened, Drs. Hayden and Harris went to New York city and consulted the leading men of the profession, and with their aid endeavored to establish a chair of dentistry in one of the New York medical colleges. Meeting with discouragement but stimulated with renewed energy, they returned to Baltimore, and during the winter of 1839-40, almost entirely unaided secured the signatures of representative citizens to a petition to the Legislature of Maryland for the incorporation of a college of dental surgery at Baltimore. After numerous difficulties and considerable opposition by jealous medical rivals, which they finally overcame, the charter was granted, and with the aid of Drs. Bond and Baxley they organized the Baltimore College of Dental Surgery, of which

Harris was the first dean. He was also professor of operative dentistry and dental prosthesis, and at the death of Dr. Hayden was elected president of the college. The college had the support of the members of the American Society of Dental Surgeons, which at the first meeting, New York, August 20, 1840, on motion resolved "That the society approve of the establishment of the Baltimore College of Dental Surgery, and will co-operate with the other friends of that institution in promoting its designs."

Dr. Harris received the honorary degree of Doctor of Medicine from the Washington Medical College at Baltimore, of which he was a professor in 1838. His D.D.S. was obtained from the American Society of Dental Surgeons, all of whose members were granted a diploma from the society, which entitled the holder to the title of Doctor of Dental Surgery. The honorary degree of Doctor of Dental Surgery was also conferred on him February 28, 1854, by the Philadelphia Dental College.

He had a number of honorary degrees conferred upon him by professional, literary, and historical societies. The degree of Master of Arts was conferred upon him by the Maryland University. He was an active member of the Maryland Historical Society. As a token of high esteem for distinguished professional labors and personal merit, he was made an honorary member of the Virginia Society of Surgeon Dentists, October 11, 1842. The Harris Dental Association of Lancaster, Pa., organized June 21, 1867, with Dr. John McCalla as president, was named in his honor.

He was correspondent and friend of many eminent public and professional literary men. He was a diligent reader and student and collected a large and valuable private library of many rare books, the finest in Baltimore at the time, excepting that of the Bishop of Baltimore, which was the most complete collection.

He kept up an extensive correspondence with authors and publishers in the principal cities of Europe, and had standing orders for anything old or new appertaining to dental science and art, all of which was gathered at his own expense.

Chapin Aaron Harris was married January 11, 1826, to Lucinda Heath, daughter of the Rev. Barton Downes Hawley, of White Chimneys, Loudoun Co., Va. Her mother was Katherine Heath, whose ancestor, the Roman Catholic Archbishop of York, refused to take part in Queen Elizabeth's coronation. Both families, the Heaths and Hawleys, were of high social position.

The Carmichaels of Maryland and Virginia, the Carys of North Carolina, and the Sturgis family of Kentucky were also relatives of Harris. His maternal grandmother was a Chapin, and for her brother he was named. To Dr. and Mrs. Harris nine children were born, viz, Darwin Barton, who died young; Ozella Louisa, who married Alfred Addison Blandy, M.D., D.D.S., an Englishman by birth, living at Zanesville, Ohio, and later at Baltimore, where he was associate editor, with Dr. Harris, of the *American Journal of Dental Science;* Zairah Cazilda, who married Louis Rimy Mignot, an artist of New York; Mary Caroline, who died young; Chapin Bond Harris; Alice Elizabeth; Irvan Lamer; Helen Pendleton Harris, and Anne Meredith Harris. The two latter are the only surviving children of Dr. Harris and now reside in London, England.

He loved art and literature. He was a devoted admirer of Sir Walter Scott,

and knew a great part of "Marmion" and "Lady of the Lake" by memory; he also greatly admired Byron's poetry. One of his favorite works was Napier's "History of the War in the Peninsula"; Rollin's "Ancient History" was another work he much admired; also Motley's "Dutch Republic," Macaulay's "History," and Agnes Strickland's "Queens of England." He was an enthusiastic chessplayer, devoted to young people, and the playfellow of all children. In all, he was a very lovable character, and is described by his children "as a most tender and devoted husband and father, and sincere friend; devoted to all good, public-spirited, benevolent works." He loved animals and was especially fond of horses and dogs.

He was extremely generous, and assisted his professional brothers and the poor liberally. He literally went about doing good. He brought up and educated nine children besides his own, and for years took care of and supported a sister and her son and a sister-in-law and her son. He kept "open house" and entertained many eminent men as his guests. Among his personal friends were Rufus Choate, Edward Everett, Longfellow, Lowell, and Henry Clay, with whom he corresponded for years.

At an early age he was deeply impressed by a sermon at a Methodist Episcopal church, and was induced to join it. He was a deeply religious man and a strong advocate of temperance. He was large-minded, and so free from sectarian bias that he numbered among his intimate friends Roman and Episcopal clergymen. He was especially fond of the Episcopal church, and was in the habit of attending it.

Dr. Harris is described as a remarkably handsome and intellectual looking man,

six feet two and one-half inches in height;
broad shouldered and finely proportioned,
of distinguished carriage, and with a benevolent, kindly expression; he was cour-
teous after the old school of polished gentlemen. His hair, naturally dark, became gray early in life. His eyes were
of hazel color. In politics he was an old-
fashioned Whig, and was an enthusiastic
Mason, high in the degrees. A few
years before his death he bought a small
place near Baltimore, where he spent his
leisure enjoying nature, of which he was
a great lover. Dr. Harris' death occurred
on Michaelmas Day, September 29, 1860,
and was due mainly to overwork. After
a hard day's labor with professional
duties and in the lecture room and infirmary at the college, he would write
nearly all night, revising his "Principles
and Practice of Dental Surgery" for a
new edition. This continued extra work
so overtaxed his energies that he was ill
for eight months, suffering acutely with
an obscure disease of the liver that finally
caused his death in the midst of his usefulness, a martyr to his professional
duties. He was buried in Mount Olivet
Cemetery, Baltimore. On his unpreten-
tious tombstone his Christian faith is en-
graved: "E mortuis resurgam" (I shall
rise from the dead).

In recent years bronze memorial tablets to the memory of Hayden and Harris
have been placed in both the Baltimore
College of Dental Surgery and the Dental Department of the University of
Maryland. (See page 297.)

Liberal in life to an extreme, Dr. Harris failed to leave his family well provided for after his death. Shortly after
that event a memorial meeting was called
in New York, October 8, 1860, at which
fifty prominent dentists attended, and a
public subscription—known as the "Harris Testimonial Fund"—was started for
the relief of his family. A committee
was appointed for this purpose, with Dr.
Eleazar Parmly as treasurer of the fund.
After canvassing the profession for some
months, at much expense, the committee
reported that nearly one thousand dollars
had been subscribed, but that about nine
hundred dollars had been expended in
collecting it—the balance of eighty-five
dollars was sent to Dr. Harris' widow.

He was a leading light of dentistry,
likely more highly distinguished and accomplished than any of his predecessors.
Dr. Eleazar Parmly truly said of him at
the time of his death, "He has labored
more arduously as a practitioner, more
untiringly as a writer, and more devot-
edly as a teacher of the principles and
practice of dental surgery than any person who has in any way or in any country
been connected with our professional
art."

His unwearied labor and sacrifice of
time and health for the advancement of
his profession; his industry as a writer
and editor; his untiring efforts in building up the first dental journal, the first
dental society, and the first dental college
in the world's history—the three most
important factors in our professional existence, all of which can be traced to
the energy and foresightedness of Hayden and himself—made him a martyr to the profession that he so greatly
honored.

On motion, the paper by Dr. M. CHI-
WAKI of Tokio, Japan, entitled "Dentistry in Japan," was, in the absence of the
author, read by title.

The paper here follows:

Dentistry in Japan.

By Dr. M. CHIWAKI, Tokio, Japan,

PRESIDENT OF THE TOKIO DENTAL COLLEGE.

I. GENERAL STATEMENT.

AT the opening of a statement of the status of dentistry in Japan it may not be out of place to devote a few words to the dental art practiced by the Japanese in former times. In Japan, dentistry had its origin somewhere about two hundred years ago, when it was practiced as a branch of medicine and was then known as *kochiu-kwa,* or stomatology. Our medical science at that time, though primitive in its theory and practice, was classified into eight divisions: (1) Medicines for adults; (2) Pediatrics; (3) Gynecology; (4) Stomatology; (5) Ophthalmology; (6) Surgery; (7) Acupuncturing; (8) Massage. But the medical operations of stomatologists seem to have been limited to the extraction of diseased teeth, the remedying of toothache, and somewhat simple treatment of the various diseases of the mouth by a primitive mode.

At the present day it is not an easy task, even for the Japanese, to obtain full information as to the medicines these stomatologists used, and the artistic skill exercised in the execution of their dental operations. This is due to the fact that they seldom had any written form of instruction and that they had no textbooks. After diligent research the writer has found a few of the dental tools used by these practitioners, and something about their medicines, besides some information as to their curative methods.

As in every other country at any period, the extraction of carious teeth was in Japan the most common operation for the dentist. The easiest of these cases was usually executed with the thumb and index finger instead of with dental forceps. In case these handy natural tools were ineffective a pair of nippers were used. Sometimes an instrument, similar in its construction to a sickle, only much smaller, was used to loosen a diseased tooth from the gum. This sickle-like tool corresponded to our lancet. After the edge of the gum was cut loose from the tooth, a certain quantity of mercury bichlorid was applied to free the root of the tooth from the gum. Then their ever-ready tools, the thumb and finger, usually did the rest of the work.

Not seldom, a stick and a mallet were used to remove teeth. The stick was made of a hard wood, about six inches long, and one of its ends was finished much finer than the main body. The finer end was firmly applied to a tooth, and then the mallet, which was also made of a hard wood, about twelve inches long, was used to hammer the thicker end of the stick. These devices—ingenious as they thought—were employed to remove or rather knock out diseased teeth, much to the annoyance and discomfort of the patient. For pyorrhea alveolaris, opium (*konronsan,* "mixed drug") is said to have been used.

Artificial dentures were invented by

Bunchu Sato, a famous stomatologist at that time, who had the honor of attending on Princess Fumi, a daughter of the Shogun. The denture made by this pioneer dentist was wholly of wood, carved with a knife or a chisel, so as to take the place of a natural tooth as nearly as possible on inspection, and it seems to have been intended to restore the natural appearance of the mouth. Meanwhile, teeth were carved from alabaster, white marble, or ivory, and riveted with strong glue to the base of a hard wood with metal pins. These dentures were retained by atmospheric pressure, without providing any special air chamber, independent of natural teeth—this method being invented incidentally. Afterward, a great improvement was accomplished in the making of dentures; they began to be made from a wax impression and a wax model, carving wood blocks by hand and tools, paint aiding in the adaptation. Although these dentures did not serve as well as those now made of india-rubber, yet they were practically attached, and they are known to have served the purpose of mastication tolerably well. Thenceforth they were no longer considered as mere ornaments. Strange to say, the right of making these dentures, during that time, was reserved by the stomatologist, it not being allowed to those outside the profession to make them after his method or even to use them, unless they signed an oath to keep strict secrecy even toward their parents and brothers.

It is beyond possibility to ascertain exactly how far back all of these arts and methods began to be practiced, but, as stated before, since the first part of the Tokugawa dynasty, say about two centuries and a half ago, dentistry was practiced here and there in Japan. These

practitioners were for the most part either men of means or *samurai* (knights) who had abandoned knighthood for the profession; and a few of them were respectable physicians who inherited their profession from their ancestors. Among these, Bunchu Sato, the inventor of the artificial denture, and Anchu Shimidzu, once a student of the above, who had also the honor of attending on Unemenosho Toda, the feudal lord of Ogaki, are known to us. Consequently these practitioners were regarded with respect by the public. Afterward, however, men in lower classes, or *ronin* (men expelled from knighthood for their misconduct), who were quite ignorant of everything connected with the treatment of the tooth, came to take up the dental profession. They extracted teeth by force and sold dentifrice in the streets, crying in a curious tone of voice to advertise themselves to passers-by, or attracting people around them by means of a peculiar kind of fencing with a sword four or five feet long, or a skilful art of spinning tops. As a matter of course, their dentistry was a clumsy art; and their dangerous manner of carrying out the operations gradually brought the profession into contempt, and it was no longer considered by the public as a profession worthy of a man of self-respect. Therefore, even at present, the words *iainuki* (the name of a peculiar kind of fencing) and top-spinners make one think of the profession of dentistry; and naturally some suppose that their profession includes the practice of dentistry. Owing to this circumstance, the investigation of all matters connected with dentistry was totally neglected by our countrymen, except for some families known as *matsui gensui* (a popular name of top-spinners) and *nagai hiyosuke* (a popular name of peculiar fencers) or their pupils allowed to call themselves by such names.

Such was the condition of dentistry in Japan until the flood of Western civilization poured in as the result of the advent of Commodore Perry of the United States Navy, in 1854. This, of course, brought about a many-sided change in the political, social, and educational institutions of Japan; and, in consequence, the old system of dentistry could not remain unaffected. The presence of American dentists, the late Dr. Eastlake of Shanghai, and Dr. W. St. George Elliott, of New York at present, both of whom opened their offices in Japan in the beginning of the *Meiji era*, was the first direct cause of the development of our dentistry in the true sense of the word. The former visited Yokohama early in 1868; and after having practiced one year there, he returned to Shanghai. Dr. Eastlake took with him to Shanghai the late Dr. T. Hasegawa, the first Japanese student of modern dentistry and afterward a reputable dentist at Tokio. Dr. Elliott arrived at Yokohama early in 1870, remaining there until late in 1875; and Dr. Y. Obata, who has been practicing at Tokio since 1873, was his first student. Dr. Elliott's five years' stay in Japan gave invaluable benefit to the dental profession by imparting an idea of the modern art of dentistry to some of the old-fashioned practitioners. He imported during his stay a dental engine, tools, and some of the materials, and introduced a primitive dental chair of wood, which was afterward improved and is now generally used by our dentists. From that time, as the years went by, the number of students of the new school gradually increased. Some of them began to practice, and succeeded not only in winning the admiration of the general public by their thoroughness

and skill, but also were welcomed by patients of the higher classes whose fathers and forefathers had looked down upon dentists with contempt. Many of our countrymen began gradually to realize the necessity of taking good care of their teeth with competent dentists' aid; and old-fashioned practitioners were entirely abandoned by them, being considered very dangerous and not fit to be relied upon.

It was impracticable, however, at that time to strictly prohibit these old-fashioned dentists from practicing. But, at last, a measure was adopted by the government which had the effect of gradually consigning them to oblivion. This measure was the regulation concerning medical licenses and licensing examinations for both medical and dental practitioners which was promulgated in 1883. This regulation laid down that every dental practitioner must have passed the examinations for a license in dentistry, and the old-fashioned dentists were allowed only to extract diseased teeth and to make artificial dentures, superintended under the by-law published by prefectural offices, according to their local conditions. (See Regulations, given later in this paper.) Though this was not a fatal blow, yet the occupation of these poor practitioners was henceforth, like Othello's, "gone"!

The examinations, thus ordered, consisted of two parts, written and oral. The former comprised six subjects, namely, anatomy, pathology, materia medica, physiology, prosthetic and operative dentistry, the latter being to test the candidates with regard to their practical knowledge as well as their acquaintance with the art of dentistry.

In those days, however, there was no book on dentistry in the Japanese language, neither was there any institution organized for the teaching of that important subject; so that young men who desired to become dental surgeons could find no other means of acquiring the necessary knowledge than by becoming apprentices. None but those who lived at the time and went through the experience can form any idea of the difficulty of attaining a thorough acquaintance with this art without the aid of books and school, and of properly qualifying oneself as a dentist. As a consequence of the conditions mentioned, very few candidates were fortunate enough to get the privilege of practicing; and for the first six or seven years after the date of first examination, the licensed practitioners remained very few in number. (See table, page 440.)

While the study and the practice of dentistry were in this poor condition, the progress made in all the other departments of medical science in Japan had already become very marked. Large numbers of well-qualified men were enrolled in the medical gazette published by the government, and the educational institutions for medical students were established by the government in the chief towns of the empire. It is needless to remark that the contrast was striking. Unless a more effective plan for the advancement of dental education were laid down by the government, it would of course have been entirely hopeless to bring it up to the level of that of the mother science. Yet the government could not then take any active steps in the matter, being too much occupied with more direct and pressing affairs.

Thus, at that time, the need of an institution designed to promote the specific study of dental surgery was keenly felt. Suggestions looking to the formation of a dental school were heard from time to time, but no definite step was taken.

This task was reserved for Dr. K. Takayama, Japan's most renowned dentist. He established a dental school at his own expense in November 1889, at Tokio. The institution was called the Takayama Dental College, being the first school of dentistry ever established in Japan, and the predecessor of the present Tokio Dental College. It was founded with the purpose of educating men to practice dentistry as a specialty of science. The curriculum included the fundamental departments of medicine, with prosthetic and operative dentistry. The courses of instruction, however, were very primitive at its inauguration, owing to the paucity of funds and the deficiency of good instructors. He delivered several lectures himself on dentistry, and he constantly contributed to the school a large amount of money, and his unceasing labor and services brought at last the present development and prosperity of the college (see page 432). Evidently the result of the organization of the college was important; it led the public to appreciate the importance of dentistry, and put dentists on a higher professional plane than before. Since its establishment, the college has sent out a great many well-qualified practitioners, and it is no exaggeration to say that the college has come to be recognized as the only means calculated to aid those who are desirous of specially qualifying themselves for the practice of dentistry in Japan.

In 1894, another dental school was founded by Dr. K. Watanabe, lately at Nagoya. This school, called the Aichi Dental College, is now existing, yet small in its scale compared with that of Dr. K. Takayama.

Prior to the organization of the Takayama Dental College, Messrs. K. Kanno, Y. Yoshida, and G. Sudzuki are said to have established an apprentice school of dentistry at Tokio, under the superintendence of Mr. S. Kubota, but owing to financial difficulties it did not exist later than 1889.

Besides the organization of these educational institutions, an important step toward the investigation of modern dentistry as well as enlightenment as to dental hygiene, was taken in 1890 by some of our dentists establishing an odontological society at Tokio. At that time the measure was highly appreciated, owing to the fact that almost all dental apprentices were unable to attend the dental school in the daytime, for they had to work from morn to eve in the laboratory of their preceptors. The society of this kind first established was that known as the Shikwa Kenkiu Kwai. Its first meeting was held in November 1890. From the time of its organization, meetings held once a month were always crowded by younger practitioners and dental apprentices. They read and discussed their papers, and a monthly magazine, called the *Shikwa Kenkiu Kwai Geppo*, was published. This society, presided over by Dr. S. Yenomoto, has done very much to introduce the American system of modern dentistry among our dental circle, as well as to facilitate the study of apprentices who have no reliable books to aid them. It continued to exist till late in 1900, but unfortunately, with the resignation of President Yenomoto, who, with unceasing labor maintained during his presidency had brought the career of this society to the highest point, this pioneer institution began to deteriorate, and at last it was dissolved in 1900.

At the same time with the organization of the above society, another institution, called the Shikwa Kogi Kwai, was established by Messrs. K. Kanno, S. Yoshida, and G. Sudzuki, dental practitioners of the old school. The object of this society was to start some lectures on modern dentistry for the apprentices of its members, all of whom were old-fashioned dentists previously referred to. These lectures were printed and distributed among the members. It was natural that old practitioners were refused any social intercourse by the dentists of the new system, and as a matter of course their apprentices wished among themselves to study the new lines of dental science necessary for passing the licensing examinations. Among their lecturers S. Izawa, D.M.D., and Mr. Y. Kojimahara, a translator of American dental books, are said to have incessantly labored for the prosperity of this society, while Dr. K. Takayama taught successfully in his college, which was open to any dental student who desired to be educated.

At that time the failure to restrict the practice of the old-fashioned dentists according to the regulations promulgated in 1883 was a source of constant annoyance to the new dental practitioners. The question of the domain of the license of the former has been discussed eagerly by some dentists, but without any effect. Although prohibited, yet the practitioners of the old system frequently prescribed poisonous medicines for their patients, which caused deaths here and there. This lamentable condition at last caused an association of dental licentiates to be organized in 1893, with the object of carrying out an effective plan for the amelioration of the social position occupied heretofore by the members. It was also the object of the association to protect their profession against the old-fashioned dentists, who occasionally violated the regulations. This organization, the pioneer of professional associations on this line, was named the Shikwa Ikwai and held its first meeting in June 1894 at Tokio. From that time on, many local associations with the same object were organized throughout the empire. But these associations, which had grown up without any connection between each other, gradually felt the necessity of amalgamating into one body. Thus a new organization of national character sprang up, under the name of the Nihon Shikwa Ikwai (the National Dental Association of Japan), in 1903, and the local associations united are now endeavoring to promote the professional status of dentistry, with a closer uniformity.

Prior to the union of these associations, an odontological society, called Shikwa Igaku Kwai, existed, and was attached till the end of last year to the Shikwa Ikwai; but by the dissolution of its mother association, it was reorganized as an independent society chiefly devoted to the investigation of dental science. At present the society holds a monthly meeting, in which essays are read and their merits discussed, and its transactions are issued from time to time.

In 1898, the government recognized the necessity of dental education as a department of science—which had been for a long time ignored, in spite of earnest advice given by some of our licentiates—and sent H. Ishiwara, M.D., as assistant professor in the Medical Department of the Imperial University at Tokio, to visit Europe and America with the object of investigating the educational system of dentistry. He came back in 1903, but he was unsuccessful in his ambition to find himself the founder of a dental course in the university, owing to the lack of a government subsidy, and, lately, was obliged to satisfy himself with the opening of a dental infirmary in the university hospital. The writer, therefore, feels quite hopeless of a decisive step to be taken in the near future by our government toward the furtherance of our dental education, and regrets there are no dental courses or departments provided in the universities at Tokio, Kioto, and Fukuoka.

Now for the practical side of the profession. There was another hidden power, probably more direct than those organizations above referred to, in developing both the art and operations of our dentists. I mean the introduction by our graduates of American dental schools of the new methods and discoveries of American dentistry. They have been coming back to Japan, one after another, since 1889. The first graduate was A. Katayama, D.D.S., formerly an apprentice of Dr. K. Takayama. Soon after his return, he delivered several lectures in the Takayama Dental College. Among these lectures, those on crown and bridge work gave much benefit to the dental profession; but these arts seem to have been more precisely taught by M. Ichinoi, D.D.S. The next phase to be remembered is the return of S. Izawa, D.M.D., to whom we are indebted for an improved method of operation on root-canals, especially in the scientific field. Besides these men, R. Sone, D.D.S., Dr. M. Yamamura, and Dr. H. Matsubara have also done very much since their return to Japan in introducing up-to-date knowledge of operative dentistry. Many graduates recently came back from America, and are all striving to instruct their professional friends in lately advanced system of dental prosthesis. These graduates number nearly twenty, and they are practicing their art with great success at Tokio.

As to those dental practitioners who

were once abroad to qualify themselves, it is the writer's duty to specially mention in this essay the names of two preceptors, Dr. Van Denburg and Dr. L. L. Dunbar of San Francisco, both of whom, though they never visited Japan, contributed a great deal to the advancement of dentistry in Japan by training Drs. K. Takayama, A. Katayama, M. Ichinoi, R. Sone, M. Yamamura, and H. Matsubara as first-class practitioners. The former gentleman instructed the first three, the latter the others, in their offices.

During that time, however, many of our practitioners could not rest content without rendering some service in investigating the new line of dental science. Among these, the writer recollects Drs. S. Yenomoto and S. Tomiyasu on cataphoresis and Drs. S. Tomiyasu and K. Ogawa on oral bacteriology. The latter two have been incessantly studying the oral microbes since 1888.

Before closing this essay, a few considerations on the methods of practice of our practitioners may be briefly stated, that we may appreciate fully their present standing. Twenty years ago the chief materials used in filling teeth were amalgam and gutta-percha, the roots of the teeth being filled with cotton saturated in creasote or carbolic acid; but at present, with the improved methods of root-canal operation, these materials are rarely used as temporary fillings. The gold foils made in Japan are so excellent in their quality that cohesiveness can be altered easily by heat or ammonia. Since 1889, crown and bridge work has been introduced, and this art is now very familiar to first-class practitioners of our country. To a great extent, however, vulcanized artificial dentures, with clasps or without, are welcomed by the majority of our patients, who are unable to pay so much fee

as is demanded for the former operation. For the same reason, continuous-gum work is rarely met in practice. General anesthesia is as yet quite unknown to our dentists, owing to the fact that their patients never seek to escape suffering by such means. Between 1888 and 1890, cataphoresis was highly recommended by some practitioners, but the result being unsatisfactory we find at present no apparatus of this process in any dental office. Thus the local anesthetic agent now in vogue is a mixed dose of cocain and adrenalin, and some recommend the Schleich local anesthesia. Recently, porcelain inlay work is attracting much attention. As to antiseptic arrangements, our practitioners are always paying great attention to it. It is to be attributed to the fact that our physicians have appreciated to a considerable extent the importance of asepsis; and dentists could not alone remain indifferent. The sterilizing agents now generally used are carbolic acid and formaldehyd. Many convenient sterilizing apparatus have been invented, and at least one of them is recognized as indispensable in a dental office.

Concerning the dental specialties, Japanese manufacturers have recently made rapid progress, and dealers carry a fairly good line of goods, many of them being imported and many now being made by themselves. Yet, with few exceptions, wooden chairs of old style, very clumsy in form, are seen in most operating rooms. Some time ago, a few chairs were made on the same pattern as American dentists', but being liable to get out of order, our first-class operator now prefers the Wilkerson chair, and up to the present nearly one hundred of these chairs have been imported. Electric or hydraulic dental engines have not yet been imported.

Foot-power dental engines are generally in use, most of them being made in our country; they are practically serviceable, except their sheaths. Almost all the instruments, such as drills, excavators, nerve-broaches, forceps, etc., are also made in Japan; the faults once common in most of them are no longer met, and their use is increasing day by day. Electric appliances of all kinds made in Japan are excellent, comparing with those made in America or Europe. They are clumsy in form, but not different at all in their effect. The manufacture of artificial teeth is still in a very primitive stage of evolution. Most teeth for rubber work are pinless—platinum being too expensive—having an undercut for the retention of rubber. Lately, Dr. R. Watanabe made teeth with metal pins, infusible like the platinum pin and applicable to any metal base; but they are made only for his own use.

All in all, however, the Japanese manufacturers are still in the most immature state of development, and it is no exaggeration to say that to a large extent American firms are supplying at present dental goods, especially up-to-date appliances, for Japan. The best known to us in superiority of their goods is The S. S. White Dental Mfg. Co., the first exporter of dental specialties. Recently, the Consolidated Dental Mfg. Co. exported their goods, their customers increasing day by day in our market, heretofore monopolized by the first-named company. Besides these firms, H. D. Justi & Son and Claudius Ash & Sons are exporting teeth and rubber specially.

Thus far the writer has given only a short sketch of the past and present of dentistry in Japan. Undoubtedly every reader will recognize the fairly rapid progress it has made during the past thirty years. But no one could possibly disagree with the writer in saying that it is still in a primitive state of development. There are altogether 766 dentists in the empire, some of whom were barely licensed in virtue of doubtful knowledge acquired as apprentices. Granting that all of them are capable of attending to the teeth of the nation, we must remember that Japan has fifty million inhabitants. This means only one dentist for every 65,274 persons. No wonder that so many Japanese suffer from caries, and consequently from dyspepsia. It need not be said that the present slow state of progress is far from what we can be satisfied to tolerate. Reviewing all the conditions, we realize most conscientiously that the mission of the present dental practitioner is very great, and we are sincerely hoping that the time shall speedily come when we shall be able to turn out the necessary number of dental licentiates, so that they may better meet the demand of the field before us, which is already white.

II. DENTAL SCHOOLS.

Tokio Dental College.

The Tokio Dental College, the oldest institution of dental education in Japan, was established at Tokio in November 1889, by Dr. K. Takayama. The institution was called at that time the Takayama Dental College, after its founder. The aim of the college is to furnish dentists and those desiring to engage in dentistry with every opportunity of acquiring a thorough practical education in that science.

At the first session of the college the faculty was composed of seven instructors, the majority of whom were former apprentices of the founder, and who were all reputable practicing dentists at that time. The chair of the president was occupied by the founder. In the beginning of the first session, only nine students were enrolled, but the number was increased to forty-five in July of the next year. From the inauguration of the college, financial difficulties were very considerable; consequently a certain sum of money was contributed by the founder to make good the deficit. The courses of instruction at that time were very primitive, owing to the paucity of the fund, and all the students were instructed in one classroom. The course consisted of instruction in physics, chemistry, anatomy, pathology, physiology, materia medica, operative and prosthetic dentistry, and clinical lectures were given twice a week. There being no text-book, it was a matter of pressing importance to provide them, so as to facilitate the investigation of the students. After incessant labor of four years, from 1891 to 1895, text-books on dental metallurgy, operative dentistry, prosthetic dentistry, dental surgery, materia medica, and anatomy of the fifth nerve were written by the professors, and published by the college year after year. Besides these works, notes of lectures delivered in the class room were also published monthly for the convenience of outside students who could not attend the college regularly. In January 1900, Dr. Takayama was obliged to place the college under the control of Dr. M. Chiwaki, one of the faculty, being himself too busy with his practice to look after the business of the institution. Dr. M. Chiwaki then took upon himself the sole responsibility of the college. He removed the institution to the present building at Misakicho, Kanda, which was bought at his own expense. In the beginning of the annual session Dr. Taka-

yama resigned, and the presidental chair was given to Dr. M. Chiwaki as his successor. After the removal of the college to this location its name was changed to that which it now bears, and improvements were made in the schedule and in the system of instruction so as to bring them up to the level of modern requirements and of the present standing of dentistry in Japan. Thus the courses of instruction were extended over three collegiate years, and some able professors were added to the college staff. Owing to these innovations, the prosperity of the college was considerably increased and the faculty have steadily carried out further improvements, their object being to secure a more thorough scientific training of the students. In addition to those facilities, the recent advancement of dental science in America necessitating the publication of new text-books in lieu of those hitherto used, the college has published more full and up-to-date works, written by the professors during last session. The subjects of these text-books are—Dental anatomy and histology, dental pathology, orthodontia, operative dentistry, prosthetic dentistry, materia medica, crown and bridge work, and oral bacteriology.

Since its establishment the college has sent out 138 graduates, and nearly four hundred students have passed the licensing examinations. These qualified dentists constitute over one-half of all the practitioners who have so far qualified themselves in Japan. The college therefore is recognized as the only means calculated to aid those who desire specially to qualify themselves for the licensing examinations.

The course of instruction of the college extends over three years of ten months each. Information is imparted by lectures, recitations, clinics, and practical exercises with the aid of text-books appointed by the faculty. Schedule:

Freshman — Chemistry and physics, physiology, anatomy (general and dental), materia medica.

Junior—Dental metallurgy, therapeutics, general pathology, bacteriology, operative and prosthetic dentistry, laboratory work, infirmary practice.

Senior—Surgery, bacteriology, operative and prosthetic dentistry, crown and bridge work, laboratory work, infirmary practice.

All candidates for admission must present a satisfactory evidence of moral character, and are required to pass a preliminary examination or to present a certificate of graduation from a middle school, or a first-class certificate covering the subjects enumerated: (1) History, universal and Japanese; (2) Elementary physics and chemistry; (3) Rhetoric, Japanese and English; (4) Arithmetic; (5) Algebra; (6) Geometry.

Candidates for advanced standing are admitted upon the following conditions:

(1) Candidates for the junior class are to present a freshman class certificate of a medical school, or to pass final examination of freshman class of the college.

(2) Candidates for the senior class are to present the above-mentioned certificate, and are required to be properly certified by a reputable practicing dentist, or to pass final examination of junior class of this college.

For graduation, every candidate is required to devote three years to the study of dentistry, including his collegiate course, or to have attended three full courses of lectures in separate years which must have been in this college. At the end of the third year, a student who has satisfactorily passed the final examination of this college receives a diploma. At present the college does not confer a degree.

Aichi Dental College.

The Aichi Dental College, one of the two institutions of this kind now in existence, was established at Nagoya in August 1894, by K. Watanabe, D.D.S., at his own expense. The object of the college is to furnish a complete course of instruction in the theory and practice of dentistry. The first president of the college was Dr. J. Ito. In 1898, the institution was removed to the new building at Sasajimacho, Nagoya, specially designed for that purpose. Since that time, the presidential chair has been occupied by K. Watanabe, D.D.S., the founder of the college. The number of its students at present is fourteen. The college has sent out twelve graduates and twelve licentiates since its establishment.

The courses of instruction of this college consist of the preliminary course (two years) and the dental course (two years and a half). The schedule of studies consists of the following:

Preliminary Course—Physics, chemistry, anatomy, histology, physiology, and embryology.

Dental Course—Dental anatomy, dental histology, dental pathology, materia medica, prosthetic and operative dentistry, and infirmary practice.

Candidates for admission are required to present evidence of good moral character, and to pass an examination for admission to each course respectively.

As to the present status of the college, the writer has failed to get any information.

III. DENTAL PUBLICATIONS.

(1) Books.

Since 1885, a large number of dental books have been written and many translations have been made by our licentiates, of which the writer has compiled the accompanying table (see below).

Besides these books, the Takayama Dental College published monthly during 1890-92, notes of lectures given by its professors in the form of a magazine. This magazine, entitled the *Takayama Shikwa Igakuin Kogiroku* was circulated among the outside students who could not attend college regularly. It consists of twenty-four volumes, each containing at least one hundred pages on several subjects of dentistry; but these volumes are now scarce.

The most important foreign works consulted in writing the books tabulated are: "Garretson's Oral Surgery"; "Parreidt's Compendium of Dentistry"; "Abbott's Dental Pathology"; "Fillebrown's Operative Dentistry"; "Webb's Operative Dentistry"; "Metallurgy and Dental Jurisprudence from American System of Dentistry"; "Essig's Dental Metallurgy"; "Richardson's Mechanical Dentistry"; "Gorgas' Materia Medica"; "Rymer's Dental Anatomy"; "Harris' Principles and Practice of Oral Surgery," etc.

While the works above referred to include almost all the necessary subjects of dentistry, the recent advancement of dental science in America necessitated the publication of new text-books in lieu of those hitherto used; and the writer edited the following complete and up-to-date works, written by the professors of the Tokio Dental College, after incessant labor for five years, specially taking care to avoid contradiction in their contents as well as their theories (Text-books of Dentistry, edited by Drs. M. Chiwaki and T. Okumura): (1) "Dental Anatomy and Histology," by Dr. T. Okumura; (2) "Dental Pathology," by Dr. T. Okumura; (3) "Orthodontia," by Dr. M. Chiwaki and K. Sato, D.D.S., M.D.; (4) "Operative Dentistry," by Dr. M. Chiwaki; (5) "Prosthetic Den-

Published.	Translators or Authors.	Titles.
1885	K. Otsuki	Shikwa Zensho.
1887	S. Izawa	Shikwa Mondo.
1889	Y. Kojimahara	Shikwa Teiyo.
1890	Y. Kojimahara	Shikwa Shogi.
1890	K. Takayama	Yeisei Hoshi Mondo.
1890	K. Takayama	Hoshi Shinron.
1890	R. Watanabe	Shikwagaku, Vol I.
1891	Y. Kojimahara	Shikwa Byori Kakuron.
1891	K. Takayama	Gotsui Shinkei Kaibohen.
1892	K. Takayama	Shikwa Shujitsu-ron
1892	K. Takayama	Shikwa Kikaigaku.
1892	K. Takayama	Shikwa Hanron.
1892	Y. Kojimahara	Shikwa Seirigaku.
1893	K. Takayama	Shikwa Yakubutsu.
1894	Y. Koidsumi	Shikwa Zairiogaku.
1895	K. Takayama	Shikwa Yakubutsugaku.
1897	N. Takahashi	Shikwa Byorigaku. Vols. I, II.
1897	M. Araki	Kammei Shikwa Shujitsu gaku.
1897	M. Araki	Basshishi-jutsu.
1897	M. Araki	Insho Saitokuho.
1901-02	N. Takahashi	Shikwa Byori Shinron, Vols. I, II.

tistry," by Drs. H. Uriu and T. Okumura; (6) "Dental Materia Medica," by Dr. U. Hayakawa; (7) "Crown and Bridge Work," by Drs. T. Fujishima and T. Okumura; (8) "Oral Bacteriology," by Drs. K. Nakagi and K. Ogawa.

These works are recognized at present as the standard books on dentistry. In writing these works, their authors in respect to theories and methods referred chiefly to the contents of the following books now used in American dental colleges: "Kirk's Operative Dentistry"; "Essig's Prosthetic Dentistry"; "Eckley's Anatomy of the Head and Neck"; "Gray's Anatomy"; "Miller's Micro-organisms of the Human Mouth"; "Sewill's Dental Surgery"; "Black's Descriptive Anatomy of the Human Teeth"; "Bödecker's Anatomy and Pathology of the Teeth"; "Hopewell-Smith's Dental Microscopy"; "Burchard's Dental Pathology and Therapeutics"; "George Evans' Artificial Crown- and Bridge-Work"; "Guilford's Orthodontia"; "Angle's Malocclusion of the Teeth and Fracture of the Maxillæ"; "Fillebrown's Operative Dentistry"; "Gorgas' Dental Medicine"; "Broomell's Anatomy and Histology of the Human Mouth and Teeth"; "Harris' Principles and Practice of Dentistry"; "Litch's American System of Dentistry"; "Johnson's Principles and Practice of Filling Teeth"; "Talbot's Interstitial Gingivitis"; "Cryer's Internal Anatomy of the Face"; *Dental Cosmos, Dental Review,* etc.

(2) *Periodicals.*

The periodicals in our language, directly referring to dentistry, published heretofore are—

(1) *Shikwa Kenkiu Kwai Geppo,* the monthly transactions of Shikwa Ken-
kiu Kwai, an odontological society, presided over by Dr. S. Yenomoto. First issue, January 1891; last issue, No. 132, 1900.

(2) *Shikwa Zasshi,* a journal of dentistry, an advertising medium of Messrs. Midzuhoya's Dental Depot, having some translations of foreign dental journals. First issue, September, 1891. Date of publication irregular.

(3) *Shikwa Kensan,* a dental journal edited by Dr. S. Tomiyasu, chiefly devoted to the investigation of oral bacteriology. First issue, April 1898. Date of publication irregular. The last issue (No. 23) June 1904.

(4) *Shikwa Kokiu Iho,* Dr. S. Izawa's report of the progress of dental science. Date of publication irregular. Ten volumes have been published.

(5) *Shikwa Gakuho,* previously entitled *Shikwa Igaku Sodan,* a monthly record of dental science, oral surgery, and medical miscellany in the interests of the alumni of the Tokio Dental College, edited by Dr. M. Chiwaki. First issue, October 1885. The last issue (vol. ix, No. 7) July 1904.

Among these publications, the last one is published punctually at present. Since its first issue, the journal is said to have had an unrivaled circulation of two thousand copies, distributed monthly to the alumni of the Tokio Dental College and its subscribers, as well as to many dentists and physicians throughout the empire, and it is now recognized as a leading journal of dentistry in the Orient.

IV. DENTAL ASSOCIATIONS.

As previously referred to in the first part of this paper, the pioneer association of dental practitioners, called the

Shikwa Ikwai, was organized at Tokio, in 1893, and since that time many local associations with the same object have been established, from time to time, without any connection between them. These associations, however, moved by the necessity of carrying out their plans with closer uniformity, were united into one body of a national character in 1903. The National Dental Association of Japan, thus organized, was entitled the Nihon Shikwa Ikwai; it is now doing its best to strengthen the unity of the dental profession throughout the empire.

The object of this association is to ameliorate the status of dental practitioners as well as to protect their profession. The membership consists of dental practitioners who have the licensing certificates of the Japanese government. The committee of the association is composed of one president, one vice-president, and an executive committee of three, all elected by votes of delegates who represent the local associations organized by the members. All the committee hold their offices for one year. A general meeting of all the members is held once in three years to carry out the plans of the association, and the delegates, presided over by the president, meet annually for the transaction of business. The executive committee are informed of the regulations or orders as well as of necessary affairs closely connected with dentistry, and their duty is to furnish the information above mentioned to all the members of the association. The present committee is as follows: K. Takayama, president; S. Yenomoto, vice-president; Executive Committee—M. Chiwaki, K. Sato, R. Sone.

At the same time with the organization of the above association a society chiefly devoted to the advancement of dental science was organized by the members of the Shikwa Igaku Kwai, the predecessor of this society, and belonged to the Shikwa Ikwai till the end of last year, when it was dissolved by the union of its mother association. The new scientific society—that is, the Nihon Shikwa Igaku Kwai, the Odontological Society of Japan—meets monthly. The membership consists of dental licentiates, and one president, one vice-president, and five on the executive committee constitute the officers of the society. The members of the executive committee are elected by the members, and they hold their office for one year. Besides these officers, thirty members are nominated by the president as the councilors of the society, their term of office being one year. The officers are as follows: S. Izawa, president; S. Tomiyasu, vice-president; Executive Committee—T. Fujishima, D. Tsukahara, N. Takahashi, K. Ogawa, and T. Okumura.

V. DENTAL LEGISLATION.

(1) *Regulations relating to the License of Medical Practitioners.*

Published by Notification No. 35 of October 23, 1883, and enforced from January of the next year.

ARTICLE I. Physicians must pass the examinations for practicing medicine, and must hold a license from the Home Minister. The licenses obtained before the enforcement of these regulations may continue effective.

ART. II. Those persons who desire to obtain a license for practicing medicine shall forward a request to the Home Department through the local government, with a diploma proving that they have passed the examinations for the practice of medicine.

ART. III. When the graduates of the government and local medical schools desire to obtain a license for practicing medicine, upon presentation of the diploma given at these schools, the Home Department may grant licenses without requiring further examinations.

ART. IV. When those persons who have graduated from medical colleges or schools in foreign countries, or those who had licenses for practicing medicine in foreign countries, desire to obtain a license for practicing medicine, upon the presentation of their diplomas or licenses, the Home Minister may grant licenses to them without any examination, after having carefully inspected the foreign diplomas or licenses.

ART. V. In remote and out-of-the-way places where physicians are very scarce, temporary licenses may be granted to persons without examinations, in consideration of their experience in practicing medicine, but only with the approval of the local governor.

ART. VI. Persons who desire to obtain the licenses for practicing medicine, shall pay each a fee of twenty yen at the time when they receive them.

ART. VII. The names of physicians to whom the medical licenses have been granted, shall be registered in the list of physicians of the Home Department, and shall be published occasionally.

ART. VIII. Any physicians who desire to obtain new licenses on account of having damaged or lost their previous licenses, or of having changed their names or provinces, shall make application to the Home Department through the local government, stating the reasons for such application.

ART. IX. Those who desire to exchange their license for a new one, shall pay a fee of one yen at the time when they receive the same.

ART. X. The medical licenses of those physicians who have died or have given up their profession shall be returned to the Home Department through the local government.

ART. XI. If any physician commits a crime or any fraudulent act in connection with his profession, the Home Minister, acting on the decision of the Central Board of Health, may suspend him from practicing. Even when such a crime or fraudulent act has been committed before the license was granted, he shall be treated according to this article.

ART. XII. When any physician is forbidden to practice medicine according to the preceding article, the local government shall confiscate the license and return it to the Home Department. When any physician is temporarily suspended from practicing medicine, the term of suspension must be indorsed and sealed on his license by the local government, and the license shall be given back to him.

ART. XIII. After such a physician has been suspended from the practice of medicine, the Home Department shall keep a careful watch over his future conduct, and after the decision of the Central Board of Health, special arrangement may be made in order to restore him to his profession.

(N. B.—In the above regulations. the term "physician" includes dental practitioner.)

When the above regulations were enacted, the regulations concerning the examinations for the practice of medicine as well as dentistry were promulgated as follows, and the same were enforced from January 1884:

(2) *Regulations with regard to the Examination for the Practice of Medicine.*

ARTICLE I. All persons who desire to practice medicine shall pass examinations according to the regulations.

ART. II. The examinations will be held twice a year under the direction of the Educational Minister, and the time and place shall be notified previously by the same minister.

ART. III and ART. IV annulled.

ART. V. The examinations shall be two in number: a preliminary examination and a final examination; and no one shall be allowed to take both examinations at the same time; provided that only one examination is sufficient on dentistry.

ART. VI. The subjects of the examinations shall be as follows:

For physicians: *Preliminary examination* —(1) Physics; (2) Chemistry; (3) Anatomy; (4) Physiology. *Final examination*— (1) Surgery; (2) Medicine; (3) Materia Medica; (4) Ophthalmology; (5) Obstetrics; (6) Clinical Operations. *For dentists*—(1)

Dental Anatomy and Physiology; (2) Dental Pathology and Operative Dentistry; (3) Dental Materia Medica; (4) Prosthetic Dentistry; (5) Clinical Operations.

ART. VIII. For each of the preliminary and the final examinations, a course of study of at least one year and a half is required; provided that a course of no less than two years' study is required for dentistry.

ART. IX. Candidates for the preliminary examination must present an application and also state the course of their studies; and candidates for the final examination, an application with the course of their studies and a diploma stating that the preliminary examination had been satisfactory. Such applications, with the required documents, must be presented to the local government during January or July. The local government will receive these applications and other documents before the fifteenth day of the following month, when they shall be sent to the Educational Minister. To the candidates' applications, the signatures of their preceptors or of not less than two physicians are required to be appended.

ART. X. When applicants for examinations commit a crime or any fraudulent act in connection with the medical profession, the local government shall make a report of the same to the Educational Department. In such cases, the said department may suspend them for a certain term from taking examinations according to the decision of the Central Board of Health in regard to their misconduct.

ART. XI. Questions for the examinations shall be selected by a consultation between the chairman and the members of the examining board; at the examination places, the applicants must answer the question in writing; provided that oral answers may be occasionally allowed.

ART. XII. Annulled.

ART. XIII. Candidates who fail in the examinations cannot be allowed to be examined again until six months have elapsed.

ART. XIV. The following fees must be paid by the candidates at the time when they present their applications; provided that no fees shall be returned when once paid: 5½ yen for the preliminary examination; 9 yen for the final examination, and 9 yen for the examination of dental practitioners.

ART. XV. Annulled.

In 1898, the following orders were published and enforced:

(3) Order No. 2 of the Home Department, dated February 5, 1898.

To those candidates who have passed the theoretical part of the final examination for the practice of medicine, and to those who have passed the theoretical part of the examination in dentistry may be given diplomas certifying that they have been successful in the examinations.

Candidates who obtain the diplomas above mentioned may receive the practical part, i.e. clinical operation only, of the final examination.

Candidates for the practical part of the final examination shall present an application with a diploma given by the chairman of the examining board, proving that the theoretical parts have been successfully passed, provided that 6 yen must be paid as fee for the examination.

Combined with the enforcement of these regulations, it became necessary to adopt measures to supervise the practice of old-fashioned dentists, who were allowed only to extract diseased teeth and to make artificial dentures. Accordingly, local governments each enacted several orders on the matter according to their local conditions, of which the following rules enforced at Tokio since 1884 are typical and worthy to be referred to. They were published by the Tokio Municipal Office—Order No. 58 of 1884:

(4) Rules relating to the Supervision of Makers of Artificial Dentures, Tooth-Extractors, and Bone-Setters.

ARTICLE I. Makers of artificial dentures, tooth-extractors, and bone-setters, who have heretofore obtained licenses for their practice, shall be required hereafter to hang their tablets, on which the names, professions, and addresses are precisely written, in the shop fronts, provided that they must not use any tablets resembling those of physicians or dentists.

ART. II. Those practitioners above mentioned, who desire to open a branch office, must previously forward a request to the Tokio Municipal Office, stating their addresses and office hours.

ART. III. Poisonous medicines listed in Order No. 2 of the Home Department are strictly forbidden to be used by those practitioners above mentioned.

ART. IV. When those practitioners go out to visit their patients, they must take with them their license tickets; and they are strictly prohibited from lending the tickets to others.

ART. V. The license tickets of those practitioners who have died or have given up their practice or removed their offices to other districts of the Tokio Municipality,

purpose of the regulations is carried out by some members of the medical examining board, appointed specially by the Minister of Education from among practitioners of acknowledged ability, to examine the candidates for dental licentiate. These examiners are included at large under the name of medical examiners, and they are presided over by the chairman of the said committee. The qualification of these members is quite unknown. Their office is unfixed, and their number also unlimited. Questions for the examinations are selected by a consultation of these members, each forwarding

YEAR.	Number of Practitioners licensed.	YEAR.	Number of Practitioners licensed.
1884	2	1894	42
1885	12	1895	39
1886	22	1896	38
1887	14	1897	48
1888	23	1898	98
1889	30	1899	54
1890	27	1900	42
1891	27	1901	51
1892	28	1902	73
1893	31	1903	74

shall be returned to the Tokio Municipal Office.

ART. VI. Those practitioners who desire to obtain new license tickets on account of having damaged or lost their previous ones, or of having changed their names or addresses, shall make application to the Tokio Municipal Office, stating the reasons for such applications.

ART. VII. If any practitioners above mentioned violate these rules. they shall be liable to confinement in a police station of not less than two days but not exceeding five days, or to a penalty of not less than 50 sen, but not exceeding 1½ yen.

(5) Dental Examinations.

In our country, at present, there is no special board of dental examiners, but the

a few questions on the subjects for which he has responsibility to examine their papers; and clinical operations are performed, at Tokio, in the presence of at least two members, each asking two or three questions on operative dentistry as well as prosthesis, on a patient presented. At present, theoretical or written examinations are held at the same time in every town of the empire where the local government is seated, and their questions are the same throughout the country. This board of dental examiners at present consists of three members: M. Ichinoi, D.D.S., S. Izawa, D.M.D., and H. Ishihara, M.D., presided over by Dr. H.

Adachi, the chairman of the medical examining board.

VI. Number of Dental Licentiates.

Prior to the promulgation of the regulations concerning medical licenses and licensing examinations for both medical and dental practitioners, in 1883, nineteen dentists were recognized by the evidence of many years' experience or of their practice in foreign countries. These licentiates, at that time, were enrolled in the medical gazette of the Home Department with the same certificates as physicians. Among these we find Drs. Y. Obata, K. Takayama, S. Nishimura, well-known professional men of the present time.

The table opposite shows the number of dental licentiates since the enforcement of the regulations.

The total number of dental practitioners at the end of 1903, including those licensed prior to 1883, is 766.

———

On motion, the paper by Dr. H. O. Heidé of Christiania, Norway, entitled "The Training of Dentists in Norway," was, in the absence of the author, read by title.

The paper here follows:

The Training of Dentists in Norway.

By Dr. H. O. HEIDÉ, Christiania, Norway.

The first public supervision in the training of dentists in Norway was ordained by an order in Council made November 16, 1852, when it was resolved that dentists should pass a public examination, the requirements for this examination being fixed by the regulations of September 9, 1857, which provided that practical and theoretical tests should be submitted to a committee of three members appointed by the Royal Department. New regulations for the dentist's examination, in place of the earlier ones, were made by an order in Council of March 14, 1892; and in 1893 a dental college was established consisting of two departments, one for dental surgery and one for filling teeth. A course here takes two semesters. The training in prosthesis had to be gone through as formerly with authorized dentists. The following provisions of these regulations of 1892, which are still in force, are appended:

An examination in dentistry is held in Christiania twice annually, and consists of oral, written, and practical tests. The examining committee consists of four members, namely, two doctors—as a rule two university professors of medicine—and two licensed practicing dentists. Before obtaining permission to enter for the examination in dentistry, the candidate must have passed the "middle" school examination, and have received instruction in the art of dentistry for three entire years from a licensed practicing dentist in Scandinavia, or in an officially recognized dental college that may be considered satisfactory.

Concerning the requirements of the examination, Section VI of the regulations runs as follows:

The examination consists of: I. Written; II. Theoretical oral, and III. Practical tests.

I. The written test consists in answering a paper (the same for all candidates) set by the examination committee, in dentistry or the branches of science connected with dentistry.

II. The oral examination is a test of the candidate's knowledge in—

(a) The principal anatomical divisions of the human body, their histology and physiology, and more particularly the anatomy and physiology of the teeth, jaws, cavity of the mouth, and adjacent parts.

(b) The general and particular pathology and therapeutics of the teeth, jaws, and cavity of the mouth, with the pharmacology relating to them in so far as dentistry is concerned.

(c) The various dental operations, the use of instruments, the making of general materials for filling and replacing, composition and technical manipulation, and the part of chemistry, metallurgy, and physics relating to these.

III. At the practical tests, to which each candidate must bring and display the necessary apparatus, instruments, and materials, and the patients upon whom the prescribed operations and work are to be performed, the candidate is required to give proofs of his skill in—

(a) Doing (1) contour-filling with gold, and (2) a root-filling.

(b) Extracting one of the large molars, or one or several roots.

(c) Taking an impression, and from it preparing a model and an entire set of teeth, one of the pieces being of metal, with the teeth soldered on, the other of vulcanite.

The patients must be presented for approval by the examining dentist as long before the examination as the committee shall determine.

With regard to the instruction at the dental college founded by the government, it may be mentioned that the course lasts from September 1st to December 15th, and from January 15th to May 15th. The department for dental surgery is superintended by a teacher who is a medical man and has also passed the examination in dentistry. The department for filling is under the management of a practicing dentist. The practical instruction is given from 9 to 10 A.M., and from 5 to 7 P.M.; one hour daily is devoted to theoretical instruction. The medical man gives instruction in anatomy, physiology, pathology, and pharmacology, four hours weekly; the dentist instructs in the science of operating and prothesis.

It is now proposed, however, to found a complete dental institute, in which all theoretical and practical instruction shall be given. The following paragraphs from the proposed regulations are appended:

PROPOSED REGULATIONS FOR THE ROYAL DENTAL INSTITUTE.

(A) The Institute from a general point of view.

SECTION 1. The Royal Dental Institute, at which the poor receive mainly free treatment for dental diseases, is under the immediate direction of the civil medical board.

The institute has to impart to dental students the theoretical and practical instruction necessary for the practice of dentistry.

SEC. 2. The board of the institute consists of a chairman and the regular masters, who are also the superintendents of the various departments of the institute. One of the medical faculty's professors of surgery or anatomy is appointed as chairman.

The appointment of the masters is by free competition. The department to which the medical board belongs has the appointment of the chairman and masters, with six months' notice to be given on either side.

SEC. 3. The Board of Management superintends the economy and instruction of the institute, and must see that all rules are kept.

It sends in every year to the department concerned, through the civil medical board, a proposed estimate of expenditure and receipts, and at the conclusion of the college year a report of the work of the institute. The report shall contain a list of the dental students in each year's class, and the number of patients treated in the various departments.

SEC. 4. All materials that are of no great value are found by the institute; the more expensive, on the contrary, must be paid for by the patient, as the teacher concerned shall determine. The sums received shall be entered among the receipts of the institute, and be paid in to the treasurer.

SEC. 5. The Dental Institute consists of three departments, each with its regular teacher as manager: (1) a prosthesis department; (2) a filling department, and (3) a dental surgery department.

In the first, the student does practical duty for two years, and then passes the first section of the examination.

In the last two departments the student does practical duty during the third year, after which he passes the final section of the dental examination.

(B) Chairman, Masters, and Assistants.

SEC. 6. The chairman of the board has to superintend the work of the institute.

He conducts the proceedings at the board meetings, receives all written communications, indorses all accounts, and inspects the fittings and collections.

The board elects a vice-chairman every year who acts in case of the chairman's absence. If the chairman is absent more than six weeks, further measures must, after consideration by the board, be taken by the department.

SEC. 7. The masters of the institute are as follows:

(1) The manager of the prosthesis department, who shall be an authorized Norwegian dentist; he must give theoretical and practical instruction in prosthesis, including the part of metallurgy relating thereto, and in the regulating of teeth.

(2) The manager of the filling department, who shall be an authorized Norwegian dentist, must give theoretical and practical instruction in filling.

(3) The manager of the dental surgery department, who shall have taken his medical degree and passed the Norwegian dental examination must give (a) theoretical instruction in the special pathology of the teeth and mouth with bacteriology, and therapeutics with pharmacology, especially extraction and the instruments and apparatus belonging thereto, and the employment of anesthetics; (b) practical clinical instruction in the diseases of the teeth and mouth, in extraction and in the employment of anesthetics.

Each of the above-mentioned masters must give an historical survey of his subject in each course.

(4) The master in anatomy, who shall be a certified doctor, must give instruction in anatomy, physiology, and general pathological anatomy, with the employment of anatomical preparations to a satisfactory extent.

SEC. 8. Assistants are appointed for a period of one year, a Norwegian dentist in the prosthesis department, and another Norwegian dentist in the filling department and the dental surgery department.

Assistants can be dismissed at any time by the chairman of the medical board at the proposal of the board of the institute.

The assistants must follow instructions, whenever given.

(C) The Instruction.

SEC. 9. A three-years' course of instruction is given at the Dental Institute. The yearly period of instruction is from January 10th to June 30th, and from August 25th to December 20th, during which time the examinations are also to be held.

At the beginning of each year of study, a printed plan of study is published. The lectures must be so arranged as not to interfere with one another.

SEC. 10. The theoretical instruction is given in two or three weekly lectures and trials by each of the masters, as the board may determine.

Each master, when the class is over, shall enter in a common journal the points he has touched upon in his lecture.

SEC. 11. The practical instruction is given in the various departments of the institute.

(1) In the prosthesis department, instruc-

tion is given for two hours every weekday, under the direction of the prosthesis master. The laboratory shall be open for students' work for an additional four hours daily.

(2) In the filling department, instruction is given every weekday for two consecutive hours, under the direction of the master in filling.

(3) In the dental surgery department, instruction is given for two hours every weekday, under the direction of the master in dental surgery.

SEC. 12. (1) During the first year of study, the subjects anatomy, physiology, and general pathology are taken up.

Further, during the first two years of study, the student goes through theoretical and practical prosthesis and the regulating of teeth.

(2) During the last year of study (after the first part of the dental examination has been passed) theoretical instruction is given in special dental pathology, with bacteriology, and in therapeutics with pharmacology, as also in the theory of filling; the students have, moreover, to do duty in the dental surgery department and in the filling department.

(D) Dental Students.

SEC. 13. In order to gain admission to the Dental Institute, the candidate must have passed his matriculation examination, with tests or additional tests in physics and chemistry.

Admission to the institute takes place once a year, at the beginning of the autumn semester. Application for admission must be sent in to the board before June 1st, accompanied by certificate of age and matriculation.

SEC. 14. The dental students admitted to the institute must themselves procure such instruments as the board may determine.

SEC. 15. The students must conform to all regulations issued by the board.

Should any student show insubordination, remissness, or bad conduct, the board, with the approbation of the medical director may send him away for a period or permanently.

SEC. 16. Every dental student admitted to the institute has to pay in advance 300 kroners for each year of study.

(E) Bachelors of Medicine.

SEC. 17. Bachelors of medicine who intend to pass the dental examination, may, after sending in their application accompanied by their medical diploma, obtain permission to do duty in all departments of the institute for one year, and have therefor to pay 400 kroners in advance.

Of the proposed regulations for the dental examination, the following paragraphs may be quoted:

SECTION 1. The dental examination is held at the Royal Dental Institute once a year, toward the end of the spring semester.

SEC. 2. The *viva voce* examination is held publicly; the written and practical sections are held under such supervision and in such manner as the board shall determine.

SEC. 3. Both the *viva voce* and the practical examinations are conducted by the masters of the institute. each in his own subject, and are judged by the examiner and two arbiters.

SEC. 5. Anyone may enter for the dental examination who can produce a certificate to show that he has satisfactorily gone through the necessary courses at the Royal Dental Institute.

Bachelors of medicine must produce their medical diploma and show that they have done satisfactory duty for at least one year in the department of the institute (*cf.* Sec. 17 in the Regulations for the Dental Institute).

SEC. 6. The dental examination consists of two parts. The first part cannot be passed until the end of the candidate's second year of study, and the second part is passed at the close of the third year.

Bachelors of medicine may pass both parts at the end of their year of study.

SEC. 7. At the dental examination, the candidate has to be examined in the following subjects:

(A) At the first part of the examination.

I. The theoretical *viva voce* examination in (a) General knowledge of the anatomy of the human system and the most important physiological processes, more especially the anatomy, histology, and development of the teeth, jaws, mouth, and adjacent parts, as also their special physiology. Further, the principles of general pathological anatomy. (b) Prosthesis, with the physics, chemistry, and special metallurgy belonging thereto.

II. The practical test. Preparation and fixing (a) A whole set of teeth in vulcanite. (b) (1) Part of a set of teeth in *gold* with teeth soldered on; (2) Bridge work; (3) A crown.

(B) At the last part of the examination.

I. A written paper set by the board and arbiters upon any part of the science of dentistry.

II. Theoretical *viva voce* examination: (a) The special pathology of the teeth and mouth, with bacteriology, the therapeutics of diseases of the teeth and mouth with pharmacology, extraction with the instruments connected therewith, the apparatus and employment of anesthetics; (b) Filling.

III. The practical tests: (a) The candidate has to examine and describe the condition of the mouth and teeth in patients, receive the anamnesis, determine the diagnosis, form a prognosis, and propose a treatment, and also extract some teeth. (b) (1) To perform three gold fillings, two of them being contour fillings; (2) two approximal amalgam fillings in molar teeth (one mesial and one distal); (3) one cement and one approximal porcelain filling in a front tooth; (c) two root-treatments, one of them being that of a double tooth.

Bachelors of medicine are exempt from the *viva voce* examination in anatomy, physiology, and general pathology (*A*, I, a).

SEC. 8. Six hours is the time allowed for the written paper, which is given to all the candidates at once. In each of the theoretical *viva voce* subjects, the examination may last as long as one hour.

The patients for the practical tests are chosen by the examiner and the arbiters, and are allotted by the drawing of lots.

For the practical tests in the first part (*A*, II) a time of up to twenty-four working days is allowed within the hours 9 A.M. to 2 P.M. and 4 to 7 P.M.

For the practical tests in the second part (*B*, III), one hour is allowed for that mentioned under III, a, in which the candidate has to examine and treat the patients, and for

those under III, b and c, the candidate is allowed from 1 to 3 hours as the examiner and arbiters shall determine.

The above proposal is now being considered by the Royal Department.

[Signed] THE BOARD OF TEACHING
AND EXAMINING.

The CHAIRMAN. It has been very gratifying to us to listen to these excellent papers and I feel that when the Transactions of this congress shall have been prepared that all interested in the subjects here named, history, education, literature, and nomenclature of dentistry, will find that the products of this section will be very valuable. It has been to me a very great pleasure to have listened to these papers. As to the work we have done in this section of the Fourth International Dental Congress, I am sure everyone who has been here will be proud of the work. There were fifteen papers, and the report from Manila being in three sections, that would make seventeen, and I believe this will be the banner section in the number of papers presented, every one of which has been of interest. We have brought out here the development of dental education in the United States, France, Mexico, Japan, Norway, the Philippine Islands, and Italy, and an examination of these papers showing the work that has been accomplished up to the present time in dental education will furnish most valuable information to anyone interested.

I desire to especially thank all who have been present for the earnestness exhibited here at all times. Though we have not had a large audience we have always had a very enthusiastic one, showing very great interest in the work.

The Chairman then declared Section IX of the Fourth International Dental Congress adjourned *sine die*.

Fourth International Dental Congress.

SECTION X.

SECTION X:

Legislation.

Chairman—WILLIAM CARR, New York, N. Y.
Secretary—L. ASHLEY FAUGHT, Philadelphia, Pa.

FIRST DAY—Monday, August 29th.

THE chairman, Dr. William Carr of New York, called the meeting to order. Dr. H. C. Brown of Columbus, Ohio, acted as secretary *pro tem.*

The CHAIRMAN. The first papers to be read before this section are those by Dr. Anema of Rotterdam and Dr. Patterson of Kansas City. As it is now, however, nearly half-past three o'clock, with your approval the section will adjourn until to-morrow—the time and place to be announced from the platform of the congress in general session this afternoon.

The section thereupon adjourned subject to the call of the chairman.

SECOND DAY—Tuesday, August 30th.

THE Chairman called the section to order at 2.30 P.M. Dr. H. C. Brown of Columbus, O., acted as secretary *pro tem.*

The Chairman then read his address, as follows:

Chairman's Address.

Gentlemen of Section X,—It gives me great pleasure to welcome to this section so many eminent members of our profession, and particularly to extend the hand of good fellowship to our brethren from across the sea. It is encouraging to see so many gentlemen who have traveled hundreds and thousands of miles to take part in such a congress as is assembled in St. Louis at this time, and all animated by the desire to do what we may for the good of our chosen profession. I must say without any desire to belittle the work of other sections, that ours is one of the most important in bringing our profession to its proper position as a branch of medical science. Without dental legislation dentistry would soon sink to the level which it occupied so many years ago when barbers and bloodletters generally practiced dentistry—save the mark!—and when a dentist occupied a position no higher than that of a barber of today.

Professional legislation has been the work of the last twenty-five years of my life. During that time we have made a hard fight in our state of New York to secure the enactment of laws which would govern wisely and well the study and practice of dentistry and at the same time prescribe the preliminary education requisite for those who desire to study dentistry with the view to practice. In the report which will be read to you I have attempted, as well as possible in the necessarily limited time at my disposal, to make a comparison between the laws of our country and those of foreign governments. This report will show generally that while our higher professional education may be and doubtless is equal to that of foreign countries, it is the standards of preliminary education in which our states are generally deficient, and it is our duty, in my opinion, to strive to raise the standard of our respective states in this particular, if not to that of the state of New York, at least to a degree commensurate with its requirements.

I desire to thank the eminent gentlemen who have so kindly contributed papers bearing on the subject-matter of our deliberations, and trust that our discussions of these papers as well as the report will be thorough and general, and further, if possible, that we may formulate a plan and decide upon ways and means whereby such legislation as may be necessary to unify the laws and impose parallel conditions regarding preliminary education preparatory to professional training may be enacted.

Again thanking you all, gentlemen, for your attendance, and trusting that our work may not be in vain, let us now proceed to the business for which we have assembled.

Dr. L. C. Bryan, Basel, Switzerland, was called to the chair as honorary chairman, and the chairman, Dr. WILLIAM CARR, read his report, as follows:

A Review of Interstate and International Dental Legislation.

By WILLIAM CARR, M.D., New York, N. Y.

Gentlemen,—As chairman of Section X, on Dental Legislation, I beg to report as follows: It is with considerable difficulty that we have been able to obtain copies of the laws governing the study and practice of dentistry in foreign countries, and the data at hand are far from complete, although the best procurable after months of effort.

A compilation has been made of the various laws regulating dentistry in the United States, and it is our purpose to summarize and compare these statutes separately, afterward comparing them with the laws of foreign countries in our possession.

After careful study and comparison of the laws regulating study and practice of dentistry in the United States and its territories, we have tabulated the result of our research below, in two tables, one giving an analysis of the laws in force in 1899, the other being brought up to July 1, 1904.

Examination of these tables will show at a glance the elevation of standards and general progress in dental legislation during the five years just passed.

SYNOPSIS OF REQUIREMENTS IN 1899.

In twenty-three states dental diplomas do not now confer the right to practice, an examination being required in all cases:

Alabama	New Jersey
Colorado	New York
Connecticut	North Carolina
Delaware	Oregon
Florida	Pennsylvania
Georgia	Rhode Island
Idaho	South Carolina
Maine	Vermont
Massachusetts	Virginia
Minnesota	Washington
Mississippi	West Virginia
New Hampshire	

The following require for admission to the licensing examination:

Colorado. Diploma from legally organized reputable dental school.

Connecticut. Diploma from recognized dental school, or three years' instruction, or three years' practice.

Delaware. Diploma of recognized dental school.

Florida. Diploma of reputable dental school.

Georgia. Diploma of reputable dental school.

Idaho. Three years' experience, certificate from another state board, or diploma from legally organized dental school.

Minnesota. Diploma from reputable dental school, or evidence of ten years' continuous practice previous to September 1889.

New Jersey. Common school education, diploma from recognized dental school or a written recommendation from five experienced dentists.

New York. Full high-school course, degree from registered dental school or medical degree with a special two years' dental course.

Oregon. Diploma from dental school in good standing, or study and practice in Oregon prior to this act.

Pennsylvania. A competent common school education, diploma of recognized dental school.

Virginia. A fair academic education.

Washington. Diploma from recognized dental school or evidence of ten years' practice.

The following require the licensing examination only:

Alabama	North Carolina
Maine	Rhode Island
Massachusetts	South Carolina
Mississippi	Vermont
New Hampshire	West Virginia

In the following political divisions either approval of dental diploma or examination by state or other duly qualified board is required:

Arizona	Montana
California	Nebraska
District of Columbia	Nevada
Hawaii	New Mexico
Illinois	North Dakota
Indiana	Ohio
Iowa	Oklahoma
Kansas	South Dakota
Kentucky	Tennessee
Louisiana	Texas
Maryland	Utah
Michigan	Wisconsin
Missouri	

The following requiring either approval of diploma or examination, admit to examination on conditions named:

Iowa. Satisfactory evidence of three years' study.

Missouri. Three years' study with legally registered dentist or license from another state.

Montana. Three years' practice or three years' study under licensed dentist.

North Dakota. Three years' active practice or three years' study with practitioner.

Utah. Two years' practice or two years' study under licensed dentist.

Arkansas. Requires only a diploma approved by the board.

Wyoming. Requires only presentation of diploma to unqualified local officers.

Cuba, Philippine Islands, and *Porto Rico.* The requirements are in process of transition.

Alaska and *Indian Territory* have no laws.

SYNOPSIS OF PRESENT REQUIRE-MENTS. JULY 1, 1904.

For purposes of comparison the synopsis of requirements in force in 1904 follow those in force in 1899. An interesting comparison can be instituted from these two synopses showing the advancement made in requirements for admission to dental practice in the United States during the five years, 1899 to 1904.

In thirty-four states dental diplomas do not now confer the right to practice, an examination being required in all cases:

Alabama	Mississippi
Arizona	Montana
Arkansas	New Hampshire
California	New Jersey
Colorado	New York
Connecticut	North Carolina
Delaware	Ohio
Florida	Oregon
Georgia	Pennsylvania
Hawaii	Philippines
Idaho	Rhode Island
Indiana	South Carolina
Iowa	Utah
Louisiana	Vermont
Maine	Virginia
Massachusetts	Washington
Minnesota	West Virginia

The following require for admission to the licensing examination:

Arizona. Diploma from reputable dental school, member of the National Association of Dental Faculties or four-year high-school course and three years' apprenticeship with licensed practitioner, or certificate from a state board showing five years' practice as licensed dentist.

California. Diploma of reputable dental school indorsed by state board of dental examiners, or three-year high-school course and four years' dental apprenticeship, or certificate of examining board of another state showing five years' practice.

Colorado. Diploma from legally organized reputable dental school.

Connecticut. Diploma from recognized dental school, or three years' instruction, or three years' practice.

Delaware. Diploma of recognized dental school.

Florida. Diploma of reputable dental school.

Georgia. Diploma of reputable dental school.

Hawaii. Diploma of reputable dental school.

Idaho. Three years' experience, certificate from another state board, or diploma from legally organized dental school.

Iowa. Diploma of reputable dental school.

Indiana. Diploma recognized by National Association of Dental Faculties or five years as assistant to licensed dentist.

Minnesota. Diploma from reputable dental school, or evidence of ten years' continuous practice previous to September 1889.

Montana. Diploma of reputable dental school, or five years' dental practice, or five years' study under licensed dentist.

New Jersey. Common school education, diploma from recognized dental school, or a written recommendation from five experienced dentists.

New York. Full high-school course, degree from registered dental school or medical degree with a special two-year dental course.

Ohio. Diploma from a legally chartered dental school.

Oregon. Diploma from dental school in good standing, or study and practice in Oregon prior to this act.

Pennsylvania. A competent common school education, diploma of recognized dental school.

Philippine Islands. Diploma from legally incorporated dental school.

Utah. Diploma recognized by National Association of Dental Examiners, or ten years' practice, or three years' study with licensed dentist.

Virginia. A fair academic education.

Washington. Diploma from recognized dental school, or evidence of ten years' practice.

The following require the licensing examination only:

Alabama	North Carolina
Maine	Rhode Island
Massachusetts	South Carolina
Mississippi	Vermont
New Hampshire	West Virginia

In the following political divisions either approval of dental diploma or examination by state or other duly qualified board is required:

District of Columbia	Nevada
Illinois	New Mexico
Kansas	North Dakota
Kentucky	Oklahoma
Maryland	South Dakota
Michigan	Tennessee
Missouri	Texas
Nebraska	Wisconsin

The following, requiring either approval of diploma or examination, admit to examination on conditions named:

Missouri. Three years' study with legally registered dentist or license from another state.

North Dakota. Three years' active practice, or three years' study with practitioner.

Porto Rico. Diploma approved by Superior Board of Health.

South Dakota. Three years' practice or three years' study with practitioner.

Wyoming. Requires only presentation of diploma to unqualified local officers.

As will be seen, in 1899 there were only twenty-three states in which a dental degree alone did not confer the right to practice, an examination being required in all cases. In 1904, however, we find these conditions existing in thirty-four states, a very gratifying and material increase in number.

Comparison of the requirements of the various states, however, discloses a wide divergence in the standards of preliminary education. An encouraging fact, however, is that the increase has been steady, and it is to be hoped that in the near future some concerted action may be taken by the various state authorities whereby the educational standards may be made to conform to a uniform regulation. This action is necessary not alone for the purpose of securing a higher degree of collegiate training, but also to enable us to secure recognition from foreign countries, which the low standards prevailing in many states now tend to prevent. The general raising and systematizing of standards will also enable us to secure reciprocity with foreign countries. The standards of the schools and colleges are fairly uniform today, and the bar to foreign reciprocity and recognition of our degrees is our low standard of preliminary education.

In order that the question of preliminary and professional education may be intelligently discussed, it is necessary to carefully examine the requirements of the various countries as compared with the requirements of the state of New York, which possesses the highest standard in the United States today. For this purpose we have made a comparative list of the educational requirements of England, Germany, and France, together with those of New York state, as we regard the three countries mentioned as being representative of foreign countries, which, although they vary somewhat in detail, are practically the same. (See table on next page.)

Ireland, Scotland, and Wales are governed by the same laws as England, so far as the study and practice of dentistry are concerned, and the same requirements are in force. This applies in a measure to Canada, Australia, and other English provinces, although no local statutory provision is made for preliminary education.

Japan has but one dental institution, the Tokio Dental College, which requires as a preliminary to a course of dental instruction the passage of an examination in the following subjects:

1. History, general and Japanese.
2. Elementary physics and chemistry.
3. Rhetoric, Japanese and English.
4. Arithmetic.
5. Algebra.
6. Geometry.

Every candidate for graduation must have devoted three years to the study of dentistry, including the college course,

Year.	Term.	Studies.
1	1	First year English. First year Latin, U. S. history, Physiology.
1	2	First year English, First year Latin, Civics, Physical geography.
2	1	Second year English, Cæsar, First year Greek, Algebra.
2	2	Second year English, Cæsar, First year Greek, Algebra.

EDUCATION PRELIMINARY TO DENTAL REGISTRATION.

England.	Germany.	France.	New York State.
English language, including grammar and composition; Latin, grammar and translation; arithmetic, algebra, geometry, Greek or a modern language.	Seven-class gymnasium is preliminary to the study of dentistry. (A full nine-class gymnasium is equivalent to the Freshman year in a first-class college in the United States.)	The preliminary education required is a diploma o "Bachelor," or a f certificate of the superior primary studies (equivalent to a high-school course.) These studies comprise French, geology, botany, natural history, physics, arithmetic, algebra, and geometry.	January 1, 1905. Full four-year high-school course. (See below for detailed high - school course.)

or have attended three full courses of lectures in this college. At the end of the third year, after having passed a satisfactory examination in the theoretical branches, performed an oral operation in the dental infirmary of the college, and satisfactorily completed an operation in mechanical dentistry, the candidate receives a degree and is thereafter entitled to practice in the empire of Japan.

In order that we may understand the comparisons which follow, we give below the curriculum of a representative high school in New York state:

Year.	Term.	Studies.
3	1	Third year English, Cicero, Anabasis, Plane geometry.
3	2	Third year English, Latin composition, Anabasis, Plane geometry.
4	1	English reading, Virgil's Æneid, Homer's Iliad, Greek history.
4	2	English reading, Virgil's Æneid, Mathematics or science. Roman history.

A regents' diploma is required for graduation. This is granted to any candidate who successfully passes an examination in the following subjects:

English,	8 counts.
Science,	8 "
Mathematics,	8 "
History and social science,	8 "
Optional,	16
	48 "

The term "count" represents ten weeks' work in one of these studies.

It is difficult to give a representative course in an English secondary school, as the courses differ widely; but the English base their standards so fully upon examination tests that the curriculum of the school itself has little weight. The regents of the University of the State of New York regard the credentials earned in the English "preliminary" examination as equivalent to two years' high-school course, and the "first professional" examination as equivalent to the requirements for a dental student's certificate in this state.

In New York, the certificate of a nine-class German gymnasium is equivalent to the freshman year in a registered college of the first class, and the "maturity certificate" of a "real-schule" fully equal to a four years' high-school course.

REQUIREMENTS IN ENGLAND.

The "first professional" examination in England is identical with part one of the first examination of the examining board in England. Before admission to this examination the candidate must produce a certificate.

Of his having received instruction (which may be taken prior to the date of registration as a dental student) at a regularly recognized institution in chemistry, physics, and practical chemistry.

Of having been engaged during a period of not less than three years in acquiring a practical familiarity with the details of mechanical dentistry under the instruction of a competent practitioner or under the direction of a superintendent of the mechanical department of a recognized dental hospital. Qualified surgeons afford evidence of two instead of three years' instruction.

Of registration as a dental student by the General Medical Council.

Of having attended at a recognized dental hospital and school, (a) a course of practical dental metallurgy; (b) a course of lectures on dental metallurgy; (c) a course of lectures on dental mechanics; (d) a course of practical dental mechanics, including the manufacture and adjustment of six dentures and six crowns.

Candidates may present themselves for the first professional examination after six months' attendance at a recognized dental hospital and school. The examination in dental metallurgy will be by written paper.

The second professional examination: A candidate must possess the following certificates:

Of having been engaged during four years in the acquirement of professional knowledge subsequent to the date of registration as a dental student.

Of having attended at a recognized dental hospital and school: (a) a course of dental anatomy and physiology; (b) a separate course of dental histology, including preparation of microscopic sections; (c) a course of dental surgery; (d) a separate course of practical dental surgery; (e) a course of not less than five lectures on the surgery of the mouth; (f) a course of dental materia medica; (g) a course of dental bacteriology.

Of having attended a recognized dental hospital or in the dental department of a recognized general hospital, the practice of dental surgery during two years.

Of having attended at a recognized medical school: (a) a course of lectures on anatomy; (b) a course of lectures on physiology; (c) a separate practical course of physiology; (d) a course of lectures on surgery; (e) a course of lectures on medicine.

Of having performed dissections at a recognized medical school during not less than twelve months.

Of having attended at a recognized hospital the practice of surgery and clinical lectures on surgery during two winter sessions.

Of being twenty-one years of age.

Certificates of professional study must show that the students have attended the course of professional study to the satisfaction of their teachers. Candidates may present themselves for the second professional examination after the completion of four years' professional study from the date of registration as a dental student and after the lapse of not less than six months from the date of passing the first professional examination.

The second professional examination consists of two parts: (1) General anatomy and physiology, general surgery and pathology; (2) Dental anatomy and physiology, dental pathology and surgery, and practical dental surgery.

As stated, the first professional examination is registered by the University of the State of New York as meeting the full requirements for the dental student's certificate; evidence of the successful completion of all the dental courses with the requirements in mechanical dentistry is registered by the University as meeting the requirements for admission to the third year of a registered dental school of the United States. The degree of licentiate in dental surgery (L.D.S.) is registered by the University as meeting the professional requirements for admission to the dental licensing examination of the state of New York.

This recognition of the English degree of L.D.S. is not reciprocated. It is manifest that the discrimination shown is due to the fact that there is no uniform standard in the United States similar to their own.

At first glance it may seem that the law of the state of New York is harsh and arbitrary, and to work an injustice to candidates of limited means, or who may not have had the time or opportunity to procure a high-school certificate. This is not the case, however, as the law will accept forty-eight regents' academic counts as equivalent to a four years' high-school course, these counts being obtained by examination held by the regents simultaneously in four of the largest cities of New York state four times a year. These examinations may extend over an indefinite period, the candidate receiving credit and a regents' pass card for each subject which he passes successfully, and, upon the completion of his examinations and his return to the regents of the cards representing his forty-eight academic counts, he receives a dental student's certificate, exactly the same as that granted to the holder of a high-school certificate or diploma. The dental student's certificate, however, must be obtained two years prior to graduation and the granting of a degree.

REQUIREMENTS IN DENMARK AND OTHER
EUROPEAN COUNTRIES.

Denmark has no statutory requirement as to preliminary education. The student desiring to commence the study of dentistry must show two years' apprenticeship in the workroom or laboratory of one or more dentists. He cannot complete his examinations for graduation until he is twenty-one years of age, and cannot practice until he is twenty-five years of age and has worked two years after graduation as an assistant. The course in dentistry is two years. Every Danish surgeon, if licensed, is allowed to practice dentistry.

Regarding license and the rules governing the examination of candidates in European countries, the licensing boards are usually composed of medical men, generally including one or two dentists in their number. This does not seem just, in our opinion, as a board of dental examiners should consist entirely of dentists, who are naturally better qualified to examine candidates for admission to license, knowing what is required by the needs of their profession, and understanding more thoroughly than it is possible for medical men to do, just what knowledge the candidate possesses or should possess in order to obtain a license.

Dr. BRYAN. Gentlemen, you have heard the report of Dr. Carr, which was exceedingly interesting, and I would ask any of those interested in the discussion of this subject to let us hear their voices.

Dr. CARR (having resumed the chair). If it be the pleasure of those present, we might listen to Dr. Anema's paper, and then discuss both papers together.

The suggestion having been approved, Dr. RENÉ ANEMA, Rotterdam, Holland, then read the following paper:

The Value of Dental Legislation.

By Dr. RENÉ ANEMA, Rotterdam, Holland.

A LITTLE prologue is given to point toward the common troubles in the discussion of sociological problems.

As my essay touches upon sociology and the relation of dentistry to the commonwealth, it may be remembered that sociology often gets mixed with politics. Talleyrand, the famous French statesman and diplomat, used speech to conceal thoughts. Many a dental diplomat and lawmaker apparently does the same. This is a source of difficulty when one comes to the treatment of dental sociological questions.

Next to the diplomat, and even more dangerous, stands the preacher, the man with ideals too high for utility, whose enthusiasm allows his heart to go astray with his head. May we be both open-hearted and open-minded by freely uttering our thoughts and trusting to fraternal feeling to prevent any misunderstanding.

The interests of one individual are often opposed to the interests of another. The interests of a number of individuals belonging to the same class can, to some extent, be opposed to the interests of the rest. According to the well-recognized principle, "The greatest happiness of the greatest number," the interest of the class must be subordinate to that of the mass, i.e. the general public; yet it has sometimes happened that the power of a class was so well organized that for a long time the interests of the minority predominated those of the majority.

We find this condition where a certain class has been long enough in power to make the laws of the country. Laws are the crystallization of customs. Laws become obsolete when the customs to which they owe their existence are changed. Laws are "mummies" when they are not in accord with customs and with what is right. Bloody revolutions were often necessary to change laws. Therefore, the particular kind of laws called dental legislation is a serious matter. In my opinion, state dental laws should only be made under the inspiration of the desire for public welfare and not under the influence of class interests.

This is something not to be forgotten at a time when dental legislation endeavors to keep up with the advance in dental science; and with the above in mind, allow me to ask you the following question: What do you consider the true value of dental legislation, and what may the public expect from it? This question, to my mind, has yet to be satisfactorily answered, which is my excuse for presenting a paper before you.

In the case before us of the public interest vs. dental legislation, allow me to introduce as the principal factor making for ill "professional egotism," a spirit related to self-preservation of the class on one side and professional jealousy on the other.

Permit me to diverge for a moment to make myself here better understood by quoting from my paper, "The Interest of the Dentist vs. the Interest of the Public," delivered before the Pennsylvania State Dental Society, Wilkes-Barre, Pa., July 13, 1904:

In my language—the language of the Netherlands—there are two words for the English word "profession," both Netherlands words being in almost equally common use. The one gives the concrete signification of profession, meaning the number or class of men that practice the same art, the other gives the abstract signification and means vocation or calling.

With these two words in mind, it is easier to make one's self understood than with one. Because class differences are not as distinct as in older countries, the concrete word "class" for dental profession is a less familiar word in American society. It is a more familiar word, or at least the idea representing the word is more familiar to men in older parts of the world. When one keeps in mind only the abstract signification of the word "profession," professional egotism is a contradiction of terms, but when one thinks of the concrete form the new term becomes more familiar.

To my mind there is no more doubt of the existence of professional egotism than there is of a certain kind of patriotism, called "jingoism," that preaches "My country, right or wrong," or of that egotism which, by instinct and brute force, extinguishes weaker races. Of the latter we have in the history of mankind many instances. Of the former I hope to give you an instance later on. All these forms of egotism are brought about by instincts of the individual becoming active in the mass at certain times and intervals of its existence.

In giving the genesis of professional egotism, something must be said of the instinct of self-preservation and of self-preservation of the class to which professional egotism is closely related. In our day, when the effects of learning and education are, in my opinion, overestimated, it needs some courage to make the statement that a dentist and even a high professional man is a being belonging to the mammalia, with instincts given for a great amount of active power to his mind and body. However, it has been said by one of the best American authors that of all animals man possesses the most instincts.

Among the strongest instincts of man is that of self-preservation. It is a common truth that instincts are hard to deal with, if indeed they can be dealt with at all. They may become concealed to the inexperienced eye, covered by today's civilization, which ofttimes is not much more than a social veneer, or by an amiable self-deceit of good-natured and well-to-do people who believe that, at least among their class, instincts, and especially the instinct of self-preservation, are rudimentary. If, however, those less critical believe that the better classes look out mainly for the interests of others, then to my mind they are mistaken. The lesson given nearly two thousand years ago, "Love thy neighbor as thou lovest thyself," is still generally applicable, which implies its reverse, that as a rule man looks out more for his own interests than for the interests of others. I will not say, however, that there are no exceptions to this rule, inasmuch as there are such people as martyrs, for example, in whom the instinct of self-preservation seems almost lost; but this specimen is very rare. This exception shows up more clearly the rule that says the instinct of self-preservation is stronger than the instinct of altruism.

When a man joins a profession he brings his instinct of self-preservation with him. This instinct brings him often in closer contact with the profession, as he hopes that the profession may after a time be of some use to him.

Notwithstanding man's idealistic feelings and the almost overwhelming influence of them, as can be the case after long solitary contemplation, or by transferring thought to others in enthusiastic gatherings of men with the same interests, it cannot be denied that the average professional man not only possesses this instinct of self-preservation, but that he needs it wherewith to earn his daily bread. When we take the dental profession as a class, each member making a living through dentistry, to protect himself from starvation, should it be at all surprising that there exists such a thing as professional self-preservation?

The following is a direct proof of the existence of such an instinct: In a certain country a society of dentists, forming the editorial staff of a dental journal, desired to change the rules. One of the members proposed the following as the principle on which the new structure should be erected: "The society intends to serve the public by promoting dentistry in the most remote sense of art and science." His obvious reason, as he explained at the time, was to have as the leading motive the "interest of the public." After having been carefully considered, the proposition was rejected almost unanimously. So far as the thoughts of the opposition could be understood, the men who voted against the public-interest proposition, feeling themselves representatives of their profession, considered it their duty not to look out—at least, not in the first place—for interests other than those of the body of men represented. The new rules are now based upon a foundation which can easily be laid bare and understood by looking upon the flag and emblem of some of our best dental journals, which say, "Devoted to the interests of the profession."

As dental journals are leaders and at the same time the voice of the profession, I consider these facts as valuable ones and as a proof that the dental profession needs devotion to its own interests. And as devotion to one (the profession) excludes devotion to another (the public)—otherwise it is no devotion—what else can be the cause of the demand for this highest form of affection than the instinctive self-preservation of the class, namely *professional* self-preservation.

So far about the genesis; now following is an instance of the existence and action of professional egotism at the present time.

In France a body of over two hundred and fifty dentists, the Syndicat des Chirurgiens-Dentistes de France, use their power to bring before court respectable foreign dentists for using legally acquired but foreign degrees of 'doctor." As their country does not furnish a dental doctor's degree, the dentists claim that the foreigners gain an undue reputation by the use of that title, thus doing harm to the interests of the local dentists.

That this feeling is more or less common to all lands was illustrated in a conversation bearing on educational matters I lately had with a dental professor in Europe. In replying to a doubt expressed by me as to the advisability of the bachelor's degree and the official medical studies, and the detriment they might work in debarring many from entering the school and in denying the blessings of dentistry to the masses, he remarked, jokingly, "Oh, we don't need any more dentists here."

After this I hope to be understood if I repeat that professional egotism is an ill-natured feeling related on one side to the self-preservation of the class and on the other to professional jealousy. This potent inner prompting becomes highly active in times and places where attacks are to be feared by competition, in the same way as wars are brought about by collision of the interests of nations.

Now, some of you may ask, "Why all this talk about self-preservation and professional egotism where only a few of the better dentists are interested in legislation and men who are subject to the instincts mentioned have no influence whatever upon the laws?

In my opinion, however, every dentist, even the dental-parlor man, has his influence upon legislatures, simply by feeling public opinion, without the sanction of which no legislation is possible. The man in the street has more influence, indirect though it may be, on legislation than the legislator himself, who depends upon his constituents for information.

Self-aggrandizement, among the many factors affecting dental legislation, is the most subtle and delicate and the more dangerous because it appeals to men of the highest type. In dentistry possibly more than in other professional life there exists the desire to reach the unobtainable. Many of us have "arrived" and have all that money can buy, only to feel keen disappointment at the lack of public recognition granted so freely to medical men. Therefore the hue and cry, "Raise the profession!"

Human nature is very complex; "Know thyself" is an axiom portentous to all who think—and who is to judge as between those who place self-aggrandizement or the public welfare first? But of one thing we are assured; no other individual motive is acceptable and no other growth will more truly raise the profession than that fixed in the solid groundwork of the public weal. When the appeal of self-aggrandizement is heard in the forming of dental statutes it is well for the legislators to be hypocritical.

If it occurs that the profession as a body, limited in motive power and handicapped on the way to a high ideal by its class instincts, "fathers" all dental legislation, the question What may the public expect from such legislation? becomes a very serious one. For this statement and to show that it is not exaggerated, I bring forward the following proofs—one from the new world and one from the old world:

"Much of our (American) legislation owes its existence to the effort of those who make the protection of the dental practitioner against the competition of his unqualified neighbor the primary and leading motive."*

In France there exists the condition of affairs that debars any foreigner from practicing his art, no matter from what reputable school he comes or how many years of reputable practice he may have, but compels him to pass through all the preliminaries and to spend at least two years in the local dental school, after which he may appear before the state dental examiners.

Nietche, the German philosopher, in his "Die Wille zur Macht" tells us that the main desire of man is power, and we have an illustration of this in the damage done by high-handed class legislation found in a bit of history of the healing art in Germany. When the all-powerful guilds or trade corporations of which the surgeons were one, passed regulations, limitations, and laws unbearable, there resulted a healthy reaction, and the "Gewerbefreiheit," or trade freedom, in Bismarck's time, was established, granting freedom in the healing art, which of course includes dentistry.

---

* E. C. Kirk. "The Unification of State Dental Legislation."—*Items of Interest*, vol. xxi. p. 109.

Is it merely accidental that about the time when this law originated the fore-mentioned philosophical thought came also to the surface again? Possibly not. And I am well informed that not only the German, but many men of today still preach to the "Almighty" and not to the "Alrighty."

In this modest effort, seeking first and always the truth, if I have been rather hard on our profession and its youthful progeny, dental legislation, I must be for-given, in the desire that many may rise in its defense; otherwise I shall do so my-self.

The CHAIRMAN (Dr. Bryan). You have heard the philosophical thesis of Dr. Anema in connection with Dr. Carr's practical consideration of the subject of legislation. Are any remarks to be made on either?

We have with us our late consul-general at Munich, who has probably given more thought, and care, and study to the sub-ject of dental legislation and interna-tional dental affairs than anyone. He is recognized by German writers and law-makers as the greatest authority on American conditions and American schools. He is quoted by the authors of German books on legislation and on the qualifications required in America for dentists. We would be pleased to hear from Consul-General Worman, late of Munich.

Consul-General J. H. WORMAN. I hardly know to what I owe this laudatory introduction. I grant, however, that on the question under discussion, viz, legis-lation, I am, in as far as competent, most ready to speak. The time allotted to the subject this afternoon in the essays which I have had the honor to listen to, gave us a most careful presentation of the subject; but the last essay dwelt especially on a selfish protection. I stand here as the advocate of its antithesis—the represen-tative of pure altruism. I have for the last five years fought unselfishly for the interests of dentistry—American and in-ternational—and I presume for that rea-son you wish to hear me on this topic.

When I went to Germany five years ago I found that the name of American den-tistry was being traduced by a traffic in diplomas, and that the legislation of America was exceedingly deficient in its provisions for protecting not only the home but the foreign element in the pro-fession. Legislation is needed in Amer-ica and elsewhere to protect dentistry from the imposition of quacks and from unjust discrimination. It is particularly a question whether a man shall be allowed to come to America and practice dentistry because he has the stamp of approbation from Germany, and an American go abroad with our best attestations and not have the same privileges there. That is a question for us in national legislation. The congress, as such, however, has the greater and more welcome mission to work for international reciprocity. The feeling of brotherhood in the nineteenth century was great. In the twentieth cen-tury it will be greater, and only he will live in the memory of his fellows who fights for his brother man, and not he who is selfish enough to think and care only for personal interests. We have passed the day when we can say anywhere in the civilized world that there is no room for others than those native to the soil. America is the best example of this spirit of generosity. Every breast here swells with the spirit of universal brotherhood. I am proud to be called an American be-cause of the knowledge that that spirit lives in all of us. It shall never die with me as long as my life lasts.

What shall be our work—the work of Americans on behalf of the cause of this great congress? That is the practical question. Five years ago there were swindling institutions in this land. Now we have crushed them out. We must legislate in justice for our self-protection, but we must have generous consideration for all others. We must, first of all, have a law that shall be universally applicable and acceptable. And what shall that law be? That no man may belong to the profession of dentistry in the twentieth century who has not had the requisite preparation for that profession. How will you obtain that preparation? By demanding of the schools such general culture as shall fit a man to stand abreast with his profession in the entire world, not on our continent alone. There was a time when American dentistry was looked up to in Europe and everywhere else.

Here sits one of the noble representatives of Europe, Dr. Godon of Paris. He and I are the antipodes so far as the existing laws make us representatives of diverse laws, but we are both fighting on this question for the same end, and fighting it out honorably. We shake hands. Why? Because we wish to have for France and America one common law—the law of universal competition. I know you and I will have his hand and heart. I know you and I will have the hand and heart of every honest man; that of the dishonest man I do not want, you do not want him, and none of us have use for him. We seek no frauds. We want a profession that shall be looked up to the world over and recognized as second to none.

I am not of you, but for you. I have suffered more in spirit and body for you than you ever have or will yourself, and I can speak with authority, because in this city, only two blocks from here sits the wife who has been separated from her babes for three years because I had announced three years ago that I would go back to Germany for one more year and finish your work there. I have been busy these five years and have not finished it yet. I have now come here as the honored representative of the German graduates of American dental colleges. Why? Because they believe I shall help you do the work that you have to do. Mine is the task of a spirit of pure altruism, not base selfishness. Do you wonder then that I am an enthusiast on this subject? —that I am more in earnest than any one of you? For the principle of international comity and professional parity and purity I have fought, and for this principle I am willing to die; that is the kind of American spirit that will never die as long as America lives. When it shall die our institutions will die with it, and our country will be no more.

Now to the point. What is the practical work to be done by those of us in the congress representing American dentistry? We must have perfect unity between the National Association of Dental Examiners, the National Association of Dental Faculties, and the National Dental Association. There must be no littleness of spirit between you—no political divisions. There must be the one ambition to frame a law that shall become general in the United States. Every state must carry through what we want, not what they want. What are legislatures for? What am I for? I am the servant of my country. What are legislators? They are your servants. Dictate to them what shall be done and do not fail to see that it is done. Let this Section on Legislation formulate such

resolutions as shall embody the spirit of
the good laws of each state, and let these
be made the laws of each respective state
from which you come, and when this has
been done we shall have a unified code
of laws which although emanating from
each state in particular, will be recognized as the universal expression of our
country. Then the central government
will be able to express for you that which
each state in its dignity has expressed.

Don't tell me this is impossible. Nothing is impossible. When three years ago
I stood before the leaders of your profession in the city of Chicago they told
me that it was impossible to suppress
Huxmann. I said that I would fight
him; and today the German-American
Dental College is no more, and Huxmann is no longer its pretentious head.
The swindling college is closed. What
did it? Who did it? Let the records
speak for me. Shame on the state of Illinois—and there sits one of its worthy
representatives, Dr. J. N. Crouse—that
up to this hour the man whom I caused
to be indicted for the crime of falsifying
the records of the state of Illinois, and
deluging Germany with fraudulent licenses, and false certifications is not yet
behind the bars! Shame upon a state
which for three years will allow a crime
of that kind to go unpunished! No re-
vengeful spirit moves me. Let the law
be avenged; then pardon if you please.·
We do not sufficiently influence our legislators, and we do not carry out our
obligations, each of us, as we should.
Do not say your neighbor's duty is not
your duty. Duty begins at home. We
want to go to the state of Illinois, to the
state of Michigan, to the state of Kansas,
to the state of Nebraska, no matter where,
how near or how far, and see that the
same good laws that prevail in one state,

as for instance in New York, shall prevail in all the other states.

What shall that law be? The right
of any man to practice provided he have
the qualifications. What shall these
qualifications be? First, a good general
education; second, a thorough academic
training in the profession. Do not let
it go out that in the state of Kansas something can be done that cannot be done
in the state of Illinois. Do not let it be
thrown in my face over in Europe that in
the colleges of Wisconsin the work is not
as well done as in the colleges of Chicago.
There are fifty-two colleges united for the
purpose of uniformity of study and mutual protection. There must be the noble
spirit of unity in these colleges saying
that in that fraternity no college shall do
what the other does not do and enjoy
membership. In the very membership
there must be the absolute guarantee that
when a man comes from the smallest and
weakest of our colleges his work has been
as honestly performed as in the largest
college the country holds. When Gar-
field was running for President, he made
a speech at Chautauqua that I shall never
forget. He said, "Give me Mark Hopkins in a country schoolhouse with one
single bench, he sitting at one end and I
at the other, and I will have the greatest
college the world has ever seen." Such
is the spirit that makes a college and
makes men that are worth turning out.
The character of the head of the school is
the soul of the young man that goes into
the profession; and it should make him
an honor not only to the teacher whose
spirit has been breathed into him, but the
nation of which he is a part and the age
in which he lives.

I want to remind you that the work
you have to do at this congress is first,
last, and always, to give these foreign rep-

resentatives who have come so far to meet
you—to bring you greetings and to extend their hand of fellowship to you—the
assurance that American dentistry is and
shall remain in the vanguard of the profession as much as in 1839 when you
founded your first college in Baltimore,
and that it shall ever partake of the same
spirit and be the product of the same
character of excellence as long as America
lives, and that you will not suffer any
country to stand ahead of you in theory
or in practice. How are you going to
do it? Not by talk. I have not come
for that purpose four thousand miles and
after parting with my youngest child two
hours after a separation of three years,
which means since its birth. I gave up
my place in Munich and asked to be
transferred to Canada, all simply to be
near my family; but I shall not be happy
in my new station until I see the work
which I began five years ago carried to
success.

I want a committee appointed by this
body that shall formulate a law based
upon an intelligent knowledge of the subject nationally and internationally. I
have studied not only the German
laws affecting dentistry, but also those
of France and Italy, England and
Spain. I have studied them carefully
and I feel that the little I know, although my friend Dr. Bryan said I
knew it all, should be made available for
the task proposed. It will please you to
know that I have been recognized as an
authority by the chief justice of a German state who is the highest authority
on the subject of dental laws. Here lies
on the table a copy of a letter from the
highest judicial authority of Germany,
saying to me, "You have not only done
noble work to help suppress the swindling
colleges and the issuance of bogus di-

plomas in Germany, but you have done
most noble work in bringing to recognition the reputable colleges of America,"
which means the recognition by the German courts of the reputability of American college work in dentistry. There is
more to me in that recognition than in
anything else. And why do I prize this
testimony so highly? Because it would
settle once and for all the question of
international comity in the profession so
far as Germany is concerned; and settled
there, it would not be long before the
same spirit would prevail everywhere.

It has been publicly stated, and widely
printed, that on the 24th of January
1904, and on the 24th of April 1904, decisions were rendered against us by the
Imperial German Supreme Court. Why?
Because we have enemies all around us,
men who like to belittle, who like to tra-
duce us—men who are mainly imbued
with the spirit of selfishness and oppose
honest competition. It is those men who
have fought me and had me indicted
for bribery and false swearing. There
sits Dr. Crouse; let him say how many
dollars, if any, he has passed over to me
to repay even what I have expended for
your interests. He is the chairman of
the prosecuting committee through whose
hands passed four thousand dollars
raised three years ago when I was
in Milwaukee. He will no doubt account
·for the money to your satisfaction; but
think of me, who have never thought of
compensation, indicted for bribery, indicted for false swearing. I swore that
certain institutions in Chicago were
fraudulent, and their titles and diplomas
illegally conferred. I passed through the
ordeal as any honest man would. I didn't
have very much worry over the outcome,
but a great deal of work, for I had to
make a defense, being a stranger and in

a foreign country. All attacks against my honor failed, of course, because my testimony was given in the interest of highest justice, but as a result of this prosecution there came to me the reports our enemies had made and those employed by other governments regarding our institutions. They said of us, that in America anything and everything was possible, that the political institutions of America are so peculiar that today men are in power who tomorrow are removed, and there can be no guarantee that the work in America will be lasting or permanently reliable. What a slur upon the grand institutions under which we Americans live! We have and use our political influence, but thank Heaven! we have enough honest men to combat and suppress any fraud attempted in this country, and the guarantee we give to any people we can make good. It is but too true that by our works shall we be known. *Our* work must be immediate and well-considered legislation that will bring us in accord with the requisites of Europe, in accord with the wants of the world, so that American dentistry may be in accord with every man in the profession anywhere and everywhere, so that we may be able to exchange with Germany, France, Italy, Spain, at any moment when it may be our pleasure to do so.

The day has gone when you can say "We cannot afford to have reciprocal legislation for Missouri and New Jersey, because a man can go to the schools in Illinois and come home to us and get in easier than if he had stayed at home and studied." That is one of the arguments that is used. I want to destroy that feeling here; for that am I here. You must rise above this question of possible injury, to the higher question of what is desirable

for us not in one particular state but for us as a nation. Though you may suffer today in the profession in New York state or other Eastern states by the operation of such defective laws in some of the Western states, the ultimate outcome will be such as to work out everywhere the salvation of the profession. We need further the possibility of exchange between other nations and ourselves, and we therefore demand that what we grant shall be granted to us. Those are the three essential points that must be considered in all legislation that shall be framed by the agency of this body for the good of the profession everywhere, and then we shall have in the dental profession perfect altruism.

At this point the chairman of the section, Dr. William Carr, resumed the chair.

The CHAIRMAN. Gentlemen, we have been honored also with the presence of Dr. Godon of Paris, and it gives me great pleasure to introduce to you Dr. Godon at this time. He will speak for France.

Dr. CH. GODON, Paris, France. Excuse me if I do not reply to all that the speakers have said, because I did not understand all of it. I was much pleased that Dr. Anema raised the question in his paper, because you know I am president of the International Dental Federation. One of the questions in Dr. Anema's paper was the protection of practitioners in different countries from the encroachments of foreigners. I believe in the liberty of the profession and that equal privileges should be accorded to all. I am not one who would prosecute a dentist. I would not prosecute any dentist in any country, because I am a friend of liberty. When I attended the congress in Chicago in 1893 I was a victim of the law, and we were obliged to give up professorships in the dental schools of Paris because we were against the law. At that time I declined to join the society whose object was to prosecute dentists. Sometimes it is wrong to prosecute dentists; I have given my support and protection to many of those who were prosecuted. I have heard, I think, that in your country many societies prosecute dentists who are not in perfect accord with the laws of the country. Again, we must treat this question from its international aspect. There must be reciprocity between each country; it is what we may call the doctrine of free trade or protection in dental education. This phase can only be handled by the International Federation. We have appointed a committee of which your president, our honored and esteemed *confrère*, is a member. This committee will urge reciprocity upon the dental faculties of each nation, and perhaps it will be possible to prevent unjust discrimination. The committee will study the question from an international point of view, and I am ready to give it my hearty support. (Applause.) I must say that we have some unjust laws in my own country, but it is not I who made the laws, as you know. I have fought for twenty-five years to obtain reforms in dentistry.

Consul-General WORMAN. The French are truly the friends of all. But for this spirit of generosity in the breast of the French, the American revolution would never have been carried to success, and with the help of generous France we shall accomplish much on the continent of Europe for American dentistry and international comity. Let me say also that that same spirit of generosity prevails not only in France but in Germany and elsewhere on the continent. On this floor this afternoon, in another portion of this house, sits Dr. Jenkins, one of the most illustrious of American dentists in Germany. He was with me when I was at the ministry in Prussia, in Saxony, and in the Foreign Office of Germany, and he will tell you that I never had more cordial words spoken to me of approbation for the work that I have done in Germany or a warmer tender to second my efforts than from the Cultus Minister of Prussia, who is in this particular instance the highest authority in the land. He put his two hands over mine and said, "Mr. Worman, I am glad to have given you half an hour, and I am grateful that you came. We never understood the question as you present it, and we see no difficulties in the way of international exchange." I tell you if we will do what is right at home and unite for that purpose, we can get what we want, and we will get it not only for ourselves but we will have the satisfaction of having cleared away the prejudices of ages, and will make many nations act as one.

The CHAIRMAN. After listening to Mr. Worman and Dr. Godon we can only feel very much encouraged on this great subject of reciprocity. I would like to ask Dr. Grevers to speak a word on the laws of Holland as related to the question of reciprocity.

Dr. JOHN GREVERS, Amsterdam, Holland. I would rather speak on the paper of Dr. Anema. Of course, I have something to say about this question of reciprocity, because the law of Holland is fairly strict in regard to admitting foreign dentists. Foreigners can practice, but they must comply with the first requirement, and that is to speak the language of the country. Now as far as reciprocity is concerned, permit me to say that I have been a member of the board of examiners for over thirteen years, and have found it not only very difficult but unfair to examine in their own language, foreigners who come there to practice. Now although I speak English, French, and German fairly, yet I do not think it is fair to compel a native examiner to examine in a foreign language. It is very difficult to speak on this subject of reciprocity in a country where the Dingley and McKinley tariff laws are in force. With us it is the language that bars a great many foreigners from coming to my country. My government has done something in this by recognizing a few reputable colleges. It has recognized Harvard and also the University of Pennsylvania, but no private schools. We are brought up in the belief that universities and not private schools are the places for scientific studies. I think it would tend to bring about a universal recognition if private schools were abolished and universities only were to take up the teaching of dentistry. I do not mean to say by this that we want the dental student to be a medical man, but that each university should have a dental department and educate a dentist for the profession of dentistry. That is what I mean by a university course.

Now, bearing upon that question of reciprocity, Holland gives the students of different countries advanced standing, but they all have to comply with the requirement for a practical examination.

I still want to say a few words on the paper of Dr. Anema, as I am afraid I have not understood my friend and countryman in what he said. Dr. Anema said that in a certain country they were about to publish a dental journal, and it was proposed that it be made broad enough to include the public interest in

general, for the benefit of the public, and it was voted against unanimously. I think my friend misstates the case. I believe that a dental journal is for the dentist and not for the public. I do not believe the *Dental Cosmos* or any other dental journal is read by the public at large. You don't find newsboys on the street selling a dental journal for five cents. The dental journal my friend alluded to is published for and by dentists. I take it the dental journal is published for the dentist and not for the public at large; so I do not see that this example that Dr. Anema gave of class interest was a fortunate one.

Dr. Godon has spoken on this subject for France, and I want to add that before 1892 there was no dental law in France. Dentistry was free—they overlooked it before that time, in the year 1892, when a new medical law was introduced. There was a law pertaining to dentistry from 1699 and 1768, but by a mistake dentistry was forgotten, and after that time everybody could practice dentistry. Even the village blacksmith could practice dentistry without having any knowledge of dentistry; he could practice in Paris and there was nobody to hinder him. Then in 1892 the present law was passed, and I am very glad that the law was passed, because ever since 1892 dentistry in France has risen and is taking the place again that it had before this omission occurred. Ever since that law was omitted our art, which had its birthplace in France, went to the dogs in France. Now see what this law has done in this short time for the profession in France. Notwithstanding Dr. Anema, I think we must have a law; it is called for in the public interest; the public is protected by a law that regulates the practice of dentistry.

Consul-General J. H. WORMAN. To explain the differences between these gentlemen and myself, we are all in perfect accord. There is still freedom of trade in Germany, but you cannot take up medical, dental, or veterinary practice, and call yourself a doctor, because by that title you convey to the public the impression that you are academically fitted for the profession and legitimately entitled to practice, while the other may or may not have academic training, does not possess the status or approbation, and is in short simply a free trader. Now, in France and in Holland, also in some other countries, this species of free trade has fortunately been done away with, and I am the last man to protest. I am for a law for Germany that shall do away with free trade and make the profession a recognized profession whose duly licensed and authorized practitioners shall perform the service to which their life study entitles them. I am for that and nothing else; but we must recognize the fact that in seeking these laws we must at the same time regard each other's interests and work together so that our laws shall be applicable to all countries. When I said that I want American dentistry to stand at the head, I meant that these gentlemen themselves will have to acknowledge that by so achieving we do not take from them the opportunity of equaling us or surpassing us if they can. They are to join us so that we may be welded together as one profession the world over. Then dentistry will be like medicine—respected the world over as a profession of which it is an integral part in the gentility of the nations.

The CHAIRMAN. It gives me great pleasure to call upon the honorable member from Switzerland, Dr. Bryan.

Dr. L. C. BRYAN, Basel, Switzerland. As a delegate to this meeting from the National Association of Dentists in Switzerland, composed of about 120 members (of which fifty are American graduates), and as the representative of the D.D.S. Society in Switzerland, and also of the German D.D.S. Association, I think I can speak pretty generally for the feeling all over Europe—in Germany and Switzerland at least, and through the center of Europe and the adjoining countries, which are very similar in their legislation.

I will speak first in regard to Switzerland. There the last law that was framed was evidently framed to keep out foreigners—Germans and French, and first and last, Americans. I had the former president of the dental and medical examining board of Switzerland with me one day, and thought I could impress him with the necessity of allowing some advantages to those who had qualified themselves in America, giving them a chance to pass the examinations in Switzerland. It now takes about seven years for a man to get through who is a graduate from a high school in America and the dental department of a university in America. They make him pass everything, from his high-school studies right down to the examination time, and then they put him to work on dissecting, and everything in the universities there for dentists. Well, I thought I would get a good word in for the American degree; so, with this gentleman I invited to dine with me an influential friend of the president. I thought we could make the president see he was doing an injustice to America. After dinner I said, "Now, don't you think, Professor, that you are doing an injustice to America? Our young men came over here in former days and practiced dentistry when there was no modern dentistry in Switzerland, when there was no means of getting a dental education except with another dentist. Your young men have gone to America, secured a degree and have come back to establish themselves. Practitioners from America have started here and educated the people; one or two in every city of Switzerland have educated a high class of practice—a high class of patients—up to an appreciation of good dentistry, and they have taught them to pay for it, and your young men are profiting by that. You have every reason to be grateful to America, and I don't see that we have ever done you any harm. Where one American dentist has started a practice here, ten of your native men who are graduated in America settled down and prospered. There is leaven in this American element which has raised the whole, and made it a prolific field for the native practitioner." I thought I was impressing him seriously, and asked, "Don't you think you have done an injustice to America in your exclusion laws?" "Why," said he, "That is our McKinley bill" (laughter)—and I could not get a single concession out of him in any way or manner whatever. Said he, "You have built up a Chinese wall around your country in the matter of protection; with your economic bill you have shut out our ribbons and St. Gall embroidery, and we are doing this as a kind of retaliation." (Laughter.) Now it may be a feeling of retaliation or it may be simply a desire to hold the country in the interests of the native practitioner, which is noticeable in every European state.

If we can bring to the authorities of Switzerland some reciprocal proposition which they can accept, and will have to accept, we will do something toward progress, and I hope that something in that direction may be done at this meet-

ing. I interviewed the present president of the examining board just before leaving Switzerland. The medical faculty have charge of dental affairs. There are no dentists on it. The dentists this year have applied for a representative on that board. The president said, "Yes, we are doing something here in educating dentists. We are giving a good medical education and we have one professor at the university who gives lectures on dentistry. We know very well that we do not educate our young men up to the standard in America, so we send them to America to get their finishing touches as dentists." Our work is recognized over there; our schools are recognized and I hope that at this great congress with 2000 representatives from all countries of the world—from Japan to Norway—we will come to a mutual understanding by which there will be made at least a first step toward reciprocity.

The CHAIRMAN. I will now call upon Dr. Barrett of Massachusetts.

Dr. T. J. BARRETT, Worcester, Mass. The instructive, well written, and very intelligent papers of Dr. Carr and Dr. Anema have interested and enlightened me, and have held the close attention of this great number of gentlemen present. The discussion of the papers has brought to light much that is new to me. It has revealed to us all a condition of things that most of us never knew existed in Europe. This is a subject that I have given little thought to. To be perfectly candid, it is new matter to me, but I have heard so much of it both on my way to St. Louis and since arriving here that I now feel fairly well informed on it. I believe it is one of the most important subjects that this congress could deal with. The gentleman from Munich, who has sacrificed so much of his energy

32

and time in his five years of untiring
labor in the interests of American dentistry, has described to us eloquently the
condition of affairs abroad, and is deserving of our deepest gratitude. He has
also outlined a method to change all that
is now inimical both in this country
and the old. He has concluded by describing a condition of affairs that would
be ideal, and result in the adoption of a
universal standard of dental qualification,
should it be brought about. I should
like nothing better than to have a voice
and a vote in adopting resolutions on a
line with his remarks. But, gentlemen,
that condition is so far ahead of us that I
doubt if any of us here will ever live to
see it enacted. We have been striving in
this country for a number of years for
the unification of our various state laws,
but we have not reached it and it will be
years, if ever, before we do. Our friend
from Munich has told us how all this
can be brought about, and that too very
shortly. I hope that if all this state, national, and international dental legislation that will bring about this ideal condition can be so readily and easily accomplished, I may live to see it.

Permit me to say a word about dental
legislation in this country. In all the
states of this Union where we have dental
laws we have never enacted a law that
was unfair toward any man. The laws
of this country have ever been fair and
just toward all men, no matter from what
state or country they hailed. Dental politicians did not create or enact the laws,
nor do the laws offer or afford them any
protection. The laws in this country are
solely for the protection of the people
against incompetents. No clique of dentists, no organization of dentists, can inspire or enact legislation in this country
to keep out competent men from other

countries. Legislation that strongly sa-
vors of that has been enacted in other
countries whose representatives are within hearing of my voice. We allow any
man in this free country who comes up
to the standard of the state in which he
seeks registration, to come before the
board and take his examination, and that
examination is alike for all men. If he
comes up to the standard of that state's
requirements he is then and there allowed
to take his place among us as a registered
practitioner of dentistry, entitled to all
the protection of the laws regulating its
practice.

But what are the requirements from
Americans seeking registration abroad?
I submitted this question to the representative of one of the European countries
last night, viz, "What would you require
of a man from this country seeking registration before your national board of examiners, the applicant being a graduate
of a high school with a four-year course,
a graduate of a reputable dental college,
and with eighteen years of successful dental practice to his credit?" A man with
that knowledge and experience I claim can
practice in any community without doing
harm to its people, and should be able
to pass any reasonable examination that
is intended to deal with all that is required of a dentist in general practice to
know. The answer was, "The applicant
is first required to take his preliminaries
in our language, no matter what diploma
or degree he holds, as we give no recognition to any of your schools, colleges, or
universities. If he pass the preliminaries successfully he will then be admitted
to our dental colleges, where he must then
take a two-year course, no matter what
his experience or skill. He will at the
end of his two-year course be examined,
and if found qualified, he is registered."

Have we in this country ever enacted a law like that? No, gentlemen, never. A law like that could not find a place in our statute books. The people of this country would not allow a law so unfair as that ever to be enacted.

At the meeting of the National Association of Dental Examiners, just closed, we have adopted resolutions that tend in a degree to meet the conditions here described. Dr. Carr gave us the benefit of his study and research in this subject, and much credit is due him for his work as well as for the advice given us as to the wisdom of adopting the resolutions.

Let me say one thing more, as a member of the Massachusetts state board. What has been the action of our board toward foreigners coming before us seeking registration in our state? A young man would come and say, or have it said for him, "I do not speak your language, and I certainly cannot write it intelligently, but if you will give me an oral examination perhaps I can satisfy you that I know my business." We have been so kind to him that we have made an exception of him, given him an oral examination, and exacted a written one from our own boys. Under the resolution adopted by the National Association of Dental Examiners, we now demand, and it is not unfair, that the candidates seeking registration in this country be able to read, write, and speak intelligently the English language. We also request that any candidate seeking matriculation at a dental college in this country be able to do the same before he is matriculated. We have never exacted that from young men from foreign countries. We have allowed them to come here, done the best we could for them, and have given them recognition when they were on a par with our own young men.

Dr. GODON. May I tell you that I wish for reciprocity to permit a dentist to exercise his profession in any country. The laws of each country are different. This is an international congress, and we have appointed a committee to examine into that question and try to remedy it.

Dr. BRYAN. I hope that Dr. Godon will not feel worried about the way we are discussing these things here in America. You know we are just on the eve of a presidential election, and you must remember that there is nothing personal in this to him or to his country.

The CHAIRMAN. I would like to call upon a gentleman from New York, Dr. Wm. Jarvie, who served for nearly thirty years on our state board, and he is thoroughly qualified to speak upon this subject. I know Dr. Jarvie has given a great deal of thought to the matter.

Dr. WM. JARVIE, New York, N. Y. This subject is one of much interest to me. I may differ somewhat from some of the gentlemen who have preceded me, inasmuch as I consider that the address of the president of the section, the papers presented, and also most of the remarks which have been made are in harmony, and in a line which is leading up to something practical, which I hope may be the outcome of the afternoon's meeting.

There has been, and very properly, I think, great freedom in the discussions, and reference has especially been made to the conditions existing in France. I am sure the speaker did not for one moment think of criticizing the laws of France or the officials of the French government. He might just as well have referred to conditions existing in England or Germany in instancing conditions which must be considered in any effort to be made to procure universal recognition of dental licenses issued by any one of the countries represented at this congress. I sincerely hope that our respected member, Dr. Godon of Paris, will not be offended at anything which has been said. It has all been intended with the utmost courtesy and free from any fault-finding or captious spirit, and we all have the utmost respect for the government and the laws of France.

I deem it most fortunate that in the opening address Dr. Carr presented the subject of dental legislation in a paper which was largely statistical—a paper which set forth very fully the particulars of the laws of the various states in this country and in the countries throughout the world. The paper which followed claimed that many of the laws regulating the practice of dentistry had been conceived in a selfish spirit and had been created in the interest of the members of the dental profession alone rather than in the interest and for the protection of the people. I am not prepared to indorse all the statements contained in that paper, for I know that much of the legislation concerning dentistry has been conceived for the protection of the people against the impositions of incompetent quacks, and only incidentally has such legislation benefited the dental profession. Any law which requires that dental services shall be performed by intelligent and competent practitioners cannot but help to raise the standard of dental attainment.

Consul-General Worman very ably and strongly urged that laws of such a character be framed and enacted in the different countries that those licensed under them could have their licenses recognized in England, France. Germany, Holland, Italy, Spain, and America—and in fact throughout the world.

If we can bring about such a condition of affairs it will be highly desirable, and while there are difficulties in the way, as has been stated by the gentleman from Massachusetts, I think they are not insurmountable, and if they cannot be surmounted today, I feel confident that they will be in the near future, and that it will not be long ere licenses granted in this country and by the universities of France, Germany, England, and the other countries, will all confer the right to practice in any one of the civilized countries.

To bring about such a greatly desired consummation is a very proper work for an international dental congress and an international federation, and I should like to see some measures taken for its commencement.

Consul-General WORMAN. I assure you that the day, the millennial day, is here. Right here in this congress we are able to do it if we will. "The way to resume," as Horace Greeley said, "is to resume," and so it is with us. We must not sit idly by. It is a conception in which the great minds of Europe are fully in harmony with us, in perfect accord with the ambition of the members here for a law that shall consider and adjust the rights of all. The great difficulty, gentlemen, is this—we do not quite understand each other's institutions; we must learn to understand each other. In Germany they do not recognize our colleges because they say they are private institutions. They do not understand that in America state and church have nothing in common, and that the school is a private foundation for public good. Make that plain to them, and they will work with us. They say that the seal of the state must give its approval to the act of the individual. How is that to be accomplished? By just such legislation as I have suggested, making our laws uniform in the different states, so that the central government can put its seal of approval upon it and the foreign nations recognize us as working in unity. You say it is not possible today. I will prove to you the contrary by a single fact, and all discussion will cease in an instant. The United States government owns a little territory called the Philippines. You had yesterday a representative on the stage who helped frame a law that carries with it the right to exercise the profession of dentistry in that country, the right to use the academic title of a reputable alma mater, and precludes the use of fraudulent diplomas and worthless titles. Here is a law of the United States government establishing certain privileges. For the first time in the history of the United States, the national government has indorsed and put its seal upon a law of the kind we need for universal practice—for international exchanges. That law is just as possible of enactment in one state as in another state of the Union. Study that law and you will see that the millennial day is near, if not already here.

The CHAIRMAN. It gives me great pleasure to call upon Dr. Roussel of Paris.

Dr. GEORGE A. ROUSSEL, Paris, France. After the speech just delivered by Dr. Godon I do not have anything to add, as he expressed his regrets for the non-observance of professional courtesy toward the American practitioners in our country. If a certain group of French dentists have acted contrary to the laws of any code of ethics, though this body claims by their constitution and by-laws that they follow the rules of the code of ethics adopted by all the professional so-

cieties in America, there are others, Mr. President, who give the right credit and are full of admiration for your countrymen on our side. My appointment to your section is the proof of what I set forth, and the best-qualified men in our country have not to bear the responsibility for what has happened, as Dr. Godon pleaded, and no doubt he will do his utmost to carry out the wishes of the dental profession in that respect.

It was indeed too bad in the cases alluded to and that have been so much talked about, that men who had devoted their time, their energy, and had given material support for the benefit of French students should be treated in this way. Let us hope it was a misunderstanding, as the body which has taken such steps is mostly composed of the pupils of these gentlemen so worthy of consideration, and also that in the future reputable men in the different countries will be treated in accordance with the rules of the code of ethics.

Dr. JARVIE. I do not suppose that as a section we should take any action which might in any way embarrass the main body of the congress, but that something practical may result from the discussions of the afternoon I move that it be—

RESOLVED, That it be the sense of this section that a committee be appointed by the congress to be composed of one member from each country represented at the congress, to formulate and report a plan by which licenses to practice dentistry issued by the authorities of one country shall be of such a character as to permit the licensees to practice in any other country.

The CHAIRMAN. I will state for Dr. Jarvie's information that the Fédération Dentaire Internationale has already established a new commission that will unquestionably take that topic up, and I am looking for assistance—for fortunately or unfortunately I have been appointed chairman of that committee, and it is my duty to look it up.

Dr. GODON. Excuse me one minute, and I will say that the committee exists now, yet I think that this section can pass a resolution which would be submitted to the Committee on Resolutions of the congress.

The CHAIRMAN. If there be no objection the plan embodied in the motion suggested by Dr. Jarvie of New York will be carried out and submitted to the congress.

Dr. S. W. WHERRY, Ogden, Utah. I would like to offer an amendment to that, that it is the sense of this meeting that the subject of legislation be recommended as a subject for proper discussion in the congress. I will put my motion in this form:

RESOLVED, That it be the sense of this meeting that the subject of legislation be recommended for proper discussion in the congress.

The CHAIRMAN. I do not believe it would be possible, in view of the work that has been laid out, and I doubt if it would be possible to have an open discussion of this subject before the congress. The time of the congress is limited; there are many papers of a scientific character, and these will occupy every moment of the three days yet remaining. In addition to this, we have a large clinic. I can assure you, however, that the committee that has been appointed by the Federation, with the resolution of Dr. Jarvie, will have all the weight necessary to carry the matter through in accordance with the wishes of this meeting.

Consul-General WORMAN. I would second that motion, as I believe it is of the highest importance at this time, when we have so much difficulty in Europe, and I recognize it as the question of the hour.

The CHAIRMAN. You must remember that the committee has already been appointed, and you must also recognize the fact that as this congress has met for specific purposes, which have been advertised, it would be impossible to do this subject justice before the full congress. However, your chairman will see that it is brought before the Committee on Resolutions or the Committee of Arrangements, if possible.

Dr. J. N. CROUSE, Chicago, Ill. There is one point in this question of legislation and of the qualification of the practitioner of dentistry in this country that has not been touched upon, and that is, that the courts have already ruled that a man is entitled to an examination before any board. No matter whether he has a diploma or where he got his education that board will be bound to grant him the required papers to practice in whatever state he wants to if he can stand that examination. That is the ruling of the courts already in this country. And one other point we have lost sight of in this discussion, and because I have denounced it I am called the enemy of the college: the trouble in this country has been that the boards of examiners have been the tools of a lot of peculiar guides, and their influence is such that the boards of education are the power behind the throne to decide who shall practice dentistry.

Dr. JARVIE. Examiners, you mean.

Dr. CROUSE. Yes, boards of examiners, according to the court's ruling in this country, are the power behind the throne. Now in regard to the college faculties' association, they have passed a lot of legislation and changed it two or three months afterward, and they don't know where they are. On the other hand, the boards of examiners are not competent; in some states the laws are not what they ought to be. Now what is necessary is for the members of the dental profession to band themselves together, and then it becomes a political power. We have the political power if we band together. The medical men are doing that now and they would be glad to unite with us. We have started the movement in Illinois.

My friend Consul-General Worman talks about the shame of the state of Illinois in not putting a man in the penitentiary who has lost his health and who has a family depending on him. He is entirely out of the way of any mischief. When the Hon. Mr. Worman came with his mass of evidence, and we got it into the state attorney's office, they threw it out.

I think the dental profession should take an interest in politics so that politicians will recognize that we are a power in politics. We have had the hardest kind of a time with our last governor until a few months ago. He was going to appoint on the commission a fellow that ran horses—a horse-racer—who had contributed to his campaign fund, and we had a great time to keep him from putting him on. So that politics has got to come into play.

The CHAIRMAN. It gives me great pleasure to call on Dr. Aguilar of Spain, who has recently come into the room.

Dr. FLORESTAN AGUILAR, Madrid, Spain. Mr. President and gentlemen, I am very sorry that I did not hear the papers read, as it is a matter of great interest to me, but if reciprocity is the question treated in the paper, I understand you wish to know the legislation in Spain regarding that question.

Legislation is such in Spain that the teaching of all the professions is controlled by the government. It is not as in America, where the teaching of medicine, law, history, etc., is given by private institutions, which though of very high educational standard are not controlled by the government. In most of the European countries the teaching of all professional studies is given by the state, and the state provides for the fees of the professors, expenses, etc., and receives all the matriculation fees from the students. Now the question, I will not say of reciprocity, but of allowing students from foreign colleges of high standing to practice in Spanish territory, was brought up not very long ago, and raised a great deal of discussion in the educational centers of the medical and the dental professions; and it was decided that Spain could not recognize the medical or dental degrees coming from American countries because it had been demonstrated that some private institutions in America gave, sold, or distributed medical or dental degrees to persons who had no instruction. It is very easy for you gentlemen here in America to distinguish between good and bad diplomas, but for an official department in a country far away like Spain, it is not easy to distinguish if that parchment comes from a real university or from some bogus institution, or was written by some person who has sold it for twenty dollars, perhaps. For that reason, means have to be adopted in order, first, to prevent the issuing of false diplomas, and the prosecution of all those who issue them; and when that has been accomplished—when there has been an agreement as to the requisite education for the admission of dental students—the question of reciprocity could then be approached, and perhaps it would be right to establish reciprocity between all reputable institutions in different parts of the world. Reciprocity exists today in Spain for the German medical diplomas. A Spaniard may go to Germany, and he is allowed to practice; or a German physician may come to Spain and he is allowed to practice in Spain on the strength of his German diploma exclusively. Reciprocity exists also for medical and dental degrees between Spain and Portugal, and when a Portuguese comes to Spain, or a Spanish physician goes to Portugal, he may practice without any requirement whatever. Reciprocity exists also with Nicaragua and with the United States of Colombia. Each one of those dispensations has been made by a special treaty like the treaties of commerce which have been entered into by the representatives of both nations.

I say that while reciprocity already exists between some countries, it would be difficult for European countries to establish reciprocity with dental institutions in America until the American authorities demonstrate that it is impossible that any diploma coming from America be a spurious one—until they demonstrate that in America they are not issuing any bogus diplomas.

The CHAIRMAN. May I ask the gentleman who has just spoken whether the basis of this suggested reciprocity would be placed largely upon primary education, and will you kindly state (because Spain is the only country from which I have not already succeeded in getting reports) what you require as a preliminary education, as a prerequisite for dental education.

Dr. AGUILAR. The system of dental study in Spain has been very recently reorganized. Five years ago the requirements for practice in Spain were only that the candidate should come up before the board of examiners at the medical department of the University of Madrid, and there prove proficiency in anatomy, physiology, and the elements of medicine, and of course in dentistry. We made a movement in Spain toward establishing dental teaching in the University, because there was only an examining board but not a teaching body; and five years ago the congress provided sufficient funds for the establishment of a dental department in the University of Madrid, and created the chairs of operative dentistry, prosthetic dentistry, and assistant professors of these chairs, and the requirements are exactly the same as for medical studies—that is to say the student before commencing university studies must be a Bachelor of Arts. For this six years of study are required, which comprise the elements of science and literature, French and German, or English, geography, history (history of Spain), chemistry, etc. Then when the student has this preliminary education, which is the same as is required for entering upon the studies of law, of medicine, or any other university profession, he enters the medical school, where he studies during three years before passing into the dental department; and in those three years he studies the same courses, the same subjects, as the medical student. At the end of the three years the dental student goes from the medical class to the dental department, and there his studies are confined exclusively to dental subjects. Before that he takes the medical studies—physiology, histology, microscopy, dissection, and general pathology; and when those have been passed, he enters the dental department. Therefore, from five years ago until the present time all the students of dentistry have been practically medical students.

Consul-General WORMAN. I would like to reply to the address of the gentleman from Spain who has so admirably detailed to us the laws and conditions of Spain, regarding our swindling institutions: They are things of the past!—and I hope the members from foreign countries will go away convinced that they are things of the past, and that new legislation—and that is why I talk again —will be of a character to prevent the possibility of a fraudulent college in America.

Dr. Crouse—who, I am sorry to say, is not here—made a statement that is not true. The fact is, the American courts have not thrown out the evidence regarding the case in question, and the conviction should be carried out, even if the man were on a dying bed, in order to have justice prevail—and then let mercy speak a word, as loud as she pleases. We want to convince the world that legislation in America is just as good as legislation elsewhere. I furnished the evidence upon which that man can be convicted. I have it in my possession, and it is in the possession of the courts. The courts ruled that it would not only be accepted, but it was a strong point in his own defense and he had to acknowledge on the stand that he had committed the forgery. This evidence I myself furnished, and no one else, not the committee on prosecution. I furnished it—and I am glad I did so—because I came to wipe the stain from our American institutions.

Dr. M. F. FINLEY, Washington, D. C. Mr. Chairman, I would like to ask just one question of these foreign delegates, and that is, When Congress shall establish commissioned rank for dentists in both the army and the navy of the United States, will the standing thus given to the American dental degree have any effect upon foreign countries in creating a standard that could possibly be accepted as approaching their own—their institutions all being national institutions, while ours are state and private?

Consul-General WORMAN. It would not satisfy the European governments, I am sorry to say, so far as I have been in touch with them, and for this reason, that you cannot get the stamp of the state, not only for these particular branches, but for the institution as such, and they desire to get such knowledge from the states and then from the nation.

Dr. AGUILAR. Answering Dr. Finley's question, I will say that no reciprocity could be obtained until a national diploma existed. If the national diploma existed, it would be sufficient. The national diploma does not exist in America. Till a national diploma exists in America there would be no reciprocity. In the army, it would represent a national recognition of the capacity of the dentist; the army is not the affair of one state or of another, but it is a national affair. If that would constitute a national recognition of a dentist's capacity, it would be a step toward establishing reciprocity, because it is a national title; but I think that until a national diploma exists in the United States the question of reciprocity would be a very difficult one to deal with.

Dr. C. R. TAYLOR, Streator, Ill. I believe the first thing necessary for reciprocity is the *spirit* of the desire for it; then everyone from every country will work for the consummation of that spirit and that desire. My own judgment is— and, belonging to a board, the National Association of Dental Examiners, I introduced a resolution which they thought was premature, to work through the State Department of the United States to further this plan of action—and I believe that we must reach this through the arm of diplomacy and by the reciprocal action of the government of the United States with other governments. I believe that we have to act in the *spirit* of fair interchange, be honest in it, show to the governments of the world that we are glad to have any honest and necessary restriction in reference to this professional education, and show that it is for the best interests of the people of the country, and not simply for the benefit of the dental profession, and get the men who have the interest of the United States, as well as of the world at heart, thoroughly imbued with the idea that we are honest, that we are sincere, and that we want the best for all the world and for our profession—and we will get it.

The CHAIRMAN. Dr. Anema will please close the discussion.

Dr. ANEMA (closing the discussion). On the question of reciprocity, in my personal opinion I do not think it is so very idealistic. Take Holland, for instance; we have no real reciprocity with different countries, but we recognize the diplomas from Germany, from France, from Switzerland, and also from four American colleges; men coming from those colleges may come up for the last and practical examination. Yet, of course, this may be extended farther. I think this is a practical starting-point in reciprocity, and if other nations could follow the example of Holland in this direction, that might be the first step to an extended international reciprocity.

Gentlemen, I thank you very much for the attention you have given to my paper.

The subject was then passed.

The CHAIRMAN. Gentlemen, I feel that we must all be encouraged at the interest which has been displayed in the discussion this afternoon, and I trust it may be possible for you to attend tomorrow, when we shall listen to papers by Dr. Finley, Dr. Coyle, and Dr. Dubeau. I trust that you will give the matter some thought, so that we may enter into the discussion with the same earnestness that characterized the meeting and discussion today. I thank you for your presence, and declare the meeting adjourned.

SECTION X—Continued.

THIRD DAY—Wednesday, August 31st.

THE Chairman called the section to order at 2.30 P.M., and called upon Dr. M. F. FINLEY, Washington, D. C., for his paper, entitled "Some Thoughts on Legislation."

The paper was as follows:

Some Thoughts on Legislation.

By M. F. FINLEY, D.D.S., Washington, D. C.

LEGISLATION is as necessary in the control of professions as in the control of society. There are dishonest and evil-minded individuals who, gaining access through a little learning to the threshold of a profession, work incalculable injury to the progress of ethical or honest procedures, and make dark spots on the shield of honor of those callings. Honesty, in its most comprehensive meaning, is the prerequisite to a proper fulfilment of the career of an individual hoping to enter the profession of dentistry, if he desires to escape the pressure of some legal restraint upon the boundaries of his desires. Honesty—take its synonyms integrity, probity, uprightness, trustiness, faithfulness, honor, justice, fairness, candor, plain dealing, veracity, each of these adds a shade of meaning to honesty, which should enter into the make-up of the character of an ideal dentist. Why should we speak of ideals? They are necessary to a proper working out of standards in the make-up of what shall eventually control men in their relations with their fellow-men. The function of colleges is to disseminate knowledge, but with that knowledge should be imparted as much wisdom as possible. "A little learning is a dangerous thing," "And with all thy getting get understanding," were never more genuinely true and applicable than in our own professional work. Dr. Angell, president of the University of Michigan, in his recent baccalaureate address to the classes going out from that institution, differentiated between knowledge and wisdom as follows: "By knowledge, I mean the possession by the mind of facts and principles, scientific, historical, philosophical, literary—an acquaintance with ideas, the perception of truths. By wisdom, I mean the power and the disposi-

tion to make a right and effective use of
our faculties and our knowledge, a happy
adaptation of ourselves and our resources
to our circumstances. Knowledge may
be regarded as the sum of our intellectual
attainments. Wisdom has an intellectual, but also a moral element. It not
only measures our relations to our environment, but with a high purpose and
pure spirit and discreet temper adjusts
our personality to our surroundings to
secure the largest result."

The test of the impartation, reception,
and assimilation of knowledge by examination conducted by others than those
who give instruction is the wisest control
of the fitness of the individual for entrance upon professional work.

Open and clear manifestation that
knowledge has been acquired should be
given. For instance, evidence of proper
preliminary qualifications to enter upon
the study of dentistry should be shown in
the use of proper words, properly spelled,
when the candidate for practice answers
questions in an examination. A lack of
that ability should be a disqualifying
point in such examination. The test of
acquisition of knowledge upon the subject of sterilization, which is but cleanliness carried to its finality, should be manifest in the appearance of the individual
as he presents himself ready for operation
in the mouths of patients. Unclean linen
and, far worse, hands and finger-nails
indicating the failure to use soap and
water and nail-cleaners, show a disqualifying point to be seriously considered.
Instruments, however carefully sterilized,
in such hands are dangerous, for the infection is quickly transferred to them.
More illustrations might be given, but I
hope you grasp my meaning in this effort
to establish a principle that is essential
for those who expect to make a success in

the practice of this profession, that each
step should be thoroughly and honestly
taken, that at no time carelessness or lax-
ity may be charged or that any departure
may be taken from the straight and narrow path. Make each operation an ideal
one. Get into the habit at the threshold
of the profession of being honest and
faithful.

The aim of associated effort, such as
we are gathered here for this week, is to
elevate the profession by elevating the
individual, but how slow almost to stagnation will be that upward progress unless more care be exercised than is used
today in receiving material into schools
for the purpose of molding it into professional character and ability! This
condition of affairs is clearly manifest
in the work of examining boards whose
efforts are conscientious. Having been
engaged in such service, these lamentable
conditions have been forcibly presented to
me.

Again, the effort now being made by
the National Dental Association through
its committee, supported by educational
institutions, to secure dental positions in
the army and navy on a basis of commissioned rank, is about to be consummated,
in that the authorities of those two departments have agreed to this demand,
which gives us an ideal basis upon which
to stand. This gives us an opportunity
of placing our men beside the men of
other professions under government control and inspection on an equal foundation, and that they will not suffer in comparison is the hope and belief of us all.

Quoting from the remarks of a distinguished professor, "We hear much in our
day about selfishness or self-seeking *versus* altruism; of individualism *versus* so-
cialism—as if these words stood for opposing tendencies between which it was

necessary to make a choice. Our moralists preach the duty of self-sacrifice, and while they mean the right thing, they sometimes seem to imply that it is a man's duty to sacrifice his real self, his happiness and welfare to the demands of a mysterious but terribly insistent corporation called Society, as if we were somehow required by the eternal power that makes for righteousness to be continually taking bitter pills for the good of mankind at large. But this is not so. The work that we do as social beings, the work that we will do in the conscientious pursuit of our chosen vocation, or in the furtherance of any good cause that may commend itself to our judgment, does not come under the head of self-sacrifice, but of self-realization. And just in proportion as we do it reluctantly, and with a feeling that we are really sacrificing ourselves, will it be apt to be ineffectual as social service. What is called self-sacrifice is taking sides with the wider social self against the narrower material self.

When a gentleman gives his seat to a lady, he does not sacrifice himself—let us hope—but takes the part of his chivalrous social self against the old Adam. He does not do the thing for her sake, but for his own, though he probably has an illusion to the contrary. His act makes him "feel better"—feel more of a man; and if it did not, he would not do it.

Now, ethical merit is the progressive realization of the social self, the substitution of the higher, that is, wider tribunal for those of petty jurisdiction.

To bring about a consummation such as is desired and such as I have tried to indicate, would be somewhat more easy if the colleges engaged in giving instruction were upon a financial foundation which would place them beyond the necessity of depending upon the fees of matriculates. If our philanthropists in and out of the profession will lend their efforts to this millennial ideal, we may hope to see such a consummation within our generation. Failing in this makes the necessity for such broad laws in every state as are now on the statute-books of the state of New York, and the conscientious carrying out of the spirit of those laws by those entrusted with their enforcement, not for the purpose of crushing the weak necessarily, but by letting it be thoroughly known what are the requirements, what is expected, so that those who have any doubt of their ability or determination to succeed will be deterred from making the attempt lest they cannot fulfill the ultimate purpose of approaching near enough to an ideal to become good practitioners.

Dr. H. C. BROWN, Columbus, O. Mr. Chairman, I move you that the discussion of Dr. Finley's paper be dispensed with until Dr. Keefe presents his paper, and that the two be discussed together.

Dr. M. S. MERCHANT, Giddings, Texas. I second the motion.

The CHAIRMAN. That method will be followed. Dr. Keefe's paper is a short paper on "Reciprocity," and I now take pleasure in introducing Dr. Keefe.

Dr. D. F. KEEFE, Providence, R. I., then read his paper, as follows:

Reciprocity.

By D. F. KEEFE, D.D.S., Providence, R. I.

So much has been talked about the subject of interstate reciprocity and the benefits that will be bestowed on the members of the dental profession when such a condition shall have been brought about, that it is almost impossible to present to you any new phase of the situation.

I trust some day we shall have unification of state dental laws, but how soon depends entirely on the energy displayed by dental examiners, deans of the dental colleges, and the members of the dental profession as a whole.

In the past, while many attempts have been made to bring about this state of affairs, our efforts have been in vain and to my mind the chief cause is our lack of energy.

Interstate reciprocity will tend to harmonize the members of the dental profession and place our science on a much broader and higher plane.

If, as some say, the time has not yet come when we can do this in our country, state laws being so different, then let us make a beginning and take sections made up of a half-dozen states where the standard is about equal, apply to the legislature for a reciprocal clause, get these states started in the right direction, and in a few years with hard work we will attain the end desired. A few years ago we came together in New England with the idea that we could have a modified form of reciprocity, but after several meetings I believe that is impossible, as in all the

New England laws (with the exception of New Hampshire) you *must* examine the candidate for registration; but with a reciprocal clause, I think the desired end could be accomplished, and it seems to me that with very little difficulty such a clause could be added to our laws.

Then let us make a beginning, and when our legislatures meet make an effort at least to see what we can do in this direction.

Discussion.

The CHAIRMAN. This subject of reciprocity is an extremely interesting and important one, and I trust that you will discuss the matter with the enthusiasm which it deserves. We shall be pleased to hear from Dr. Sanger on this subject.

Dr. R. M. SANGER, East Orange, N. J. This subject is a very broad one, and the desirability of interchange is not questioned, yet the difficulties in the way seem at first glance to be insurmountable. It is possible, however, and I believe the time is coming when reciprocity will be an accomplished fact between most of the states of the Union and the foreign countries having a standing equal to their own. This must come by progression, as Dr. Keefe has suggested. The battle, I believe, is being fought along proper lines, as indicated in the papers read before us. That is, interchange must be brought about by a proper and uniform preliminary standard, as I think we will agree that the collegiate standard is practically uniform today. This will be purely interstate interchange, however, and must be completed before international interchange can be considered seriously. Meanwhile, I believe it is the duty of every man to place himself in line and endeavor to secure the adoption of the proper standard by his state—this standard to be determined by his own opinion of that adopted by the state which he considers to be a model in this respect. To this end, it appears to me that papers along the lines of those heard today, read before such bodies as this, will do much to educate us to our duty in the matter.

Dr. Louis Ottofy, Manila, P. I. I listened with great interest to the papers of Dr. Finley and Dr. Keefe. As far as we are concerned in the Philippine Islands, we naturally will reciprocate with you at any time, and hope that you will do likewise with us. When our law was passed, which by the way, was the result of considerable work, extending over two and one-half years, I included in the original draft the recognition of the National Association of Dental Faculties and the National Association of Dental Examiners of the United States, and as this was allowed to stand it is so embodied in the law.

The Chairman. That is the status now, is it?

Dr. Ottofy. That is the status at the present time. In the preliminary discussion of the bill, the question arose whether we should accept diplomas of recognized schools or examine. In the draft I had put in the word "or," so as not to create too much opposition; some wanted examination, though others thought that a diploma would be suffi-

cient. While it seemed that we could not agree, I suggested that the word "or" be stricken out and replaced by the word "and," which was done, so that on that point our law is as good as that of any of the states, and now it requires diploma and examination to engage in dental practice in the Philippine Islands.

Our standard, in some respects, is not as high as yours; but that is purely a local matter. Thus, our law has a provision that anyone who has received the title of "Cirujano Ministrante" (ministering surgeon) from the University of St. Thomas of Manila, which is granted at the end of a course extending over two years, covering the fundamentals of medicine and surgery, and makes of the recipient a first-class nurse, is entitled to practice as a dentist after four months' study of dentistry, although only in provinces where no other dentists are located; and inasmuch as there are no dentists located anywhere outside of the city of Manila and three or four towns, the provinces are open to men of this class, their certificates specifying the locality to which they must confine their practice. The masses know nothing of dentistry, and we shall have to send these men out at first with a limited education, to educate the people, and create a demand for dental services. As rapidly as consistent the standard will be raised.

The Chairman. I would like to call upon Dr. Grossman of Hawaii, and ask him in discussing this question to please give some attention to the preliminary requirements necessary as a prerequisite to dental education.

Dr. M. E. Grossman, Honolulu, Hawaii. In speaking of dental legislation and reciprocity I will state that prior to 1893 there was no law in the Hawaiian Islands regulating the practice of dentistry. At that time Hawaii was a monarchy. As early as 1885 myself and others endeavored to procure some proper legislation, but our efforts were of no avail until about 1892, when we were successful in having a law passed, or rather an apology for a law, which simply required a diploma from a college, and compelled us to issue licenses to practice to anyone holding a diploma irrespective of where it came from. Those not holding a diploma were required to pass an examination before our examining board, and if successful were issued licenses to practice. Our examining board at the time was composed of two dentists and one physician and we had a hard fight to procure even this concession. What they wanted was two physicians and only one dentist. We finally compromised on two dentists and one physician. We considered that a fair start from which we could build, and after over ten years' effort on the part of our profession in legislature after legislature, we have managed to have a law enacted that I think is a good one, a law that protects the masses as well as our profession.

One of our principal stumbling-blocks in endeavoring to procure dental legislation was with the Hawaiian or native legislators. They were very clannish and imagined that such a law would work a great hardship upon their own race. At that time there were several native youths at work in different offices and one who was in practice; his experience had been gained in the office of one of our old practitioners. The cry went up among our native legislators that such a law would work a great hardship to their own boys, as we had no dental colleges in Hawaii, and those who were then working in offices and others who may come later would be denied an opportunity of mak-

ing a living at their chosen profession, but must go to America and there attend universities for years before being able to practice; that would cost money and therefore was only for the rich. Such a law would shut out a poor boy entirely.

Notwithstanding this opposition we managed to have a form of law passed. I do not wish you to infer from my remarks that out in our part of this great United States that we are a lot of uneducated people. Far from this, we are a cosmopolitan territory, and our people are broadminded and well educated. There is hardly a university of any prominence in the states, from the Pacific to the Atlantic, that has not upon its rolls representatives from Hawaii and graduates from our high school and Oahu College, and I do not know of one who has ever failed to gain admission into any university. We have our boys at Harvard, Yale, Princeton, Williams, Cornell, University of California, Stanford, and Ann Arbor, and I know from reports and records that they manage to pass through their college lives very creditably to themselves and to the country they represent.

The Hawaiian people as a race are well educated, and from an educational point of view will compare more than favorably with any race of people. I know that I am safe in asserting that there are not ten per cent. of the Hawaiian people who cannot read and write the English language, and not more than two per cent. who cannot read and write their own language. So you can see that there is very little illiteracy among our people, and I doubt if such a record can be claimed for any other state or territory, to say nothing of other nations.

On the 25th of last April, after over ten years of effort upon our part, we managed to procure a law which is upon proper lines and one that will compare favorably with any. It is not perfect, but we hope to make it so. The requirements now are that one must be a graduate of a reputable and recognized dental college and pass a satisfactory examination before our board of dental examiners before he can receive his certificate of license to practice, and our board is now composed of three dentists appointed by the governor upon the recommendation of our dental society. I am sorry that we were unable to manage to have "only diplomas accepted from such colleges as are recognized by the National Board of Dental Examiners," but we will manage to get that in at some future time.

There is nothing particularly original about our law. It is made up of parts of the different laws in the states adapted to our conditions. I drafted it myself after reading every dental law on our statute books, and afterward took the draft to a lawyer to be put in shape. And after that, to make certain I took it to another lawyer, one of the leaders of our bar, to put the finishing touches to it, and I think we now have a law that will stand the test of courts. It is not perfect, but it is a step in advance, and in a short time we will have it equal to any.

Another thing that we have to contend with in our territory that I do not think any other board has had to contend with, is the examination of candidates in their own languages. I think our board has had more applications and been asked to examine more people in more languages than any other board. We have had them in Chinese, Japanese, Portuguese, German, Spanish, French, and English. I do understand a little of the English language, but hardly a word of the others, and just imagine how we were handicapped! Our law virtually compelled us to examine them in any language. We had to resort to interpreters; sometimes they were horse doctors, once a professional coach, and at others we were fortunate in having the services of a graduate of medicine who kindly assisted us, but we could never tell who answered or passed the examination, the applicant, the horse doctor, or the coach. We then decided in future not to examine except in the English language, and so notified foreign consuls, as did also the medical board. That drew a hornet's nest about us and there were numerous protests, but in conversations with several of the foreign consuls, who were patients of mine, and in asking if upon my going to their country they would extend to me the same courtesy and examine me in the English language, they saw the right of it and the matter was dropped. But in our new law we specifically mentioned that all examinations must take place in the English language, which created a howl—so much so, through outside influence, that the law was endangered, and we then transposed the wording and through a little scheming managed to pass it, worded differently but meaning the same.

In regard to reciprocity I trust that we will soon see the time when it will be universal. I will state here, as president of our examining board, that I am willing to accord all the courtesy possible to everyone—all the courtesy that will be extended to me or to any American if we go to a foreign country, and not one iota more, and I trust that every other board will do the same—examine applicants in the language of our country just as we are compelled to pass in the language of the country if we go to France, Germany, Spain, South America, or anywhere else. Be we ever so able in our profession they throw every obstacle in our way. They

33

compel us to pass examination in their language, which is impossible for many of us to do without remaining several years in their country to perfect ourselves in the language. No liberal allowances are made to us; why, then, to them?

I think we are working along the proper lines, and a move was taken in the right direction when the National Board of Dental Examiners the other day adopted as a prerequisite to admission into a dental college, a high-school preliminary education. This is along the lines we must work—higher standard for our educational institutions, and that will bring us to our goal. Through a few freak advertising bodies guaranteeing the D.D.S. degree at so much per head, for foreign use (these, I am happy to say, have been wiped out of existence), and also through the kindly action of many of our colleges toward foreigners holding foreign degrees, in admitting them as advanced students in our senior classes, these returning to their own country in a short time with the D.D.S. degree, the latter has come into ill-repute.

Now in regard to young men coming from foreign institutions, I think our honored *confrère* from Paris, in his remarks yesterday, is correct. Let every person be put on the same footing, the same as is done with American boys in our colleges. Show neither more nor less courtesy, and compel them to pass the same examination in the same language as our own boys, and they will graduate with honor to the American dental college.

We cannot entirely blame foreign countries for not paying the respect that is due the degree of D.D.S. when we accept a young foreigner who probably is a graduate of some college at home of absolutely no standing; he comes here, cannot speak two dozen words of our language, and is graduated. This has been done in my own alma mater, and how they did it is a mystery to me when American boys had a hard time to pass. This should cease, and I think this body should place itself on record in a way that will be understood. I think the suggestion of Dr. Finley of Washington, D. C., a very good one and one to be followed up. Let us insist and work for such legislation as will place our profession in the army and navy not as contract dental surgeons, but on the same footing as the M.D. Then our country places her official seal on our profession and officially recognizes it and the world must follow suit.

For general reciprocity at home my remarks are equally applicable. Raise our standard of education, raise our preliminary requirements, and see that our colleges have a proper curriculum and that they live up to it, or drop them from the indorsement of the National Board of Dental Examiners. Endeavor to have the standards in every state as nearly similar as conditions will allow. Then we are working along the proper lines. This cannot be done in a day, but if we hope to accomplish anything we must all put our shoulders to the wheel and work. We will meet stumbling-blocks, but the object is worth the price.

I am happy to see that several of the states have extended reciprocity, and hope to see more in the near future. In my territory our law, as it now stands, does not permit us to do so, but upon my return home I shall bring this matter before our board and we shall endeavor to change our law so that it will admit of our board extending reciprocity. But I assure you as a member of the board from Hawaii, that if any reputable practitioner comes to Hawaii with the recommendation and indorsement of his board, provided that his state board is composed of men qualified and appointed for their qualifications and not through politics, he will meet all the consideration that any man wants. As I have stated, our law does not allow us to extend reciprocity; but let him come with the proper credentials and I will agree that it will not take him more than a month or two to qualify himself, just so long as I am a member of the board, or my present associates.

The CHAIRMAN. We are indeed glad to have with us today a gentleman from Spain; I will call upon Dr. Losada of Madrid, to speak to us upon the subject of reciprocity and preliminary education.

Dr. JAIME D. LOSADA, Madrid, Spain. I was very much pleased to hear my *confrère* from Hawaii give his thoughts on the subject. I agree with him in everything he has said; especially about speaking the language. I think that is one of the first requirements for a man who desires to practice in a foreign country. He may not speak the language well—he may have a foreign accent—that has nothing to do with it; but he must be able to read, and write, and speak fluently in the country where he is going to practice, or wants to be able to practice, because I don't know how a dentist can get along in his profession without understanding what the patient wants, what he feels; still some men seem to be able to do it.

And about the examinations, I think it is quite right that they should be passed in the language of the country, and a man should not come for examination until he knows the language thoroughly. That is one thing. The second thing is to establish practical reciprocity upon a basis of equivalents, because we are not going to admit in Spain anybody whose standard of education is much lower than we require from the Spanish. I think that would not be fair. We will treat foreigners the best we can, but we must not treat them better than we treat our own people. Charity begins at home. Now, unfortunately, there have been Americans who went to Spain whose diplomas were procured I don't know how, because we knew very little about most of them; some of them learned after arriving there, but most of them didn't know much about dentistry. I suppose they could not apply in their own country and they tried to impose upon us as if we were a half-savage race. Against that practice I would strongly protest, because they could benefit nobody but themselves, and it lowers the standing of the American dentist all over the world. In Europe they have a very poor idea of most of the American dentists, because, as the gentleman said, those that have gone to Europe are not the best of your people. Of course, I quite agree that the best dentists as a rule are in America. I know that very well, but those good dentists do not go over there; they stay here, and because we want to protect ourselves against that, the law of Spain is that to be a dentist you must be an A.B. in one of the universities. To be an A.B. requires you to pass examinations in about fifteen, or sixteen, or seventeen matters—I don't know how many now, because when I passed mine there were fourteen or fifteen; that was many years ago, but now they have changed it, and have made the examination harder. I think in no country are the requirements for entrance higher or even equivalent. Besides, when you get your A.B. you must pass an entrance examination before the Faculty of Medicine, which is the same as though you were going to be a medical man. That takes on an average one year. Then you have to put in two years studying anatomy, histology, physiology, and chemistry with the students of medicine, and you pass your examinations the same as if you were going to be a medical man, intending to get through that board. Then you have to take at least one year or two in the special branches of dentistry. I know that one year is not enough to learn dentistry. The law stands that way in Spain. We are doing our best, and we hope we will make it at least two years, so then we will be able to train men almost as well as they do in other countries, though perhaps it is not so good as you get in America; the theory is as good as you can get anywhere in the world, because every one of the professors we have is well known here. Dr. Aguilar tries his very best to teach his students American theories, and we have some of the American books translated into Spanish. We have three journals, giving monthly everything new and good in dentistry all over the world, and especially in America, so that the student has chances to get along all right, perhaps not so well as if he were here, but as I said the other day, each man must stand on his own merit. I can only say about myself, that I received an average of 97 out of 100 at the University of Pennsylvania, and that I am a fair sample of what a Spaniard can do if he wants to. We want equivalents because it would be very sad for us to have men going to another country, say Morocco, or Turkey, or India, in that way securing a diploma —and on the strength of that diploma to try to practice his profession. We do not want that. We will allow a man to practice in Spain if he has a diploma that is equivalent to ours. I have very little

use for a Spaniard ignorant of dentistry undertaking to go to your country, get a diploma in about six months, and come back to Spain. We want to protect ourselves.

The CHAIRMAN. That is, doctor, you will not recognize his diploma, but you will grant him a license for examination?

Dr. LOSADA. He has to be able to practice legally—for we have two ways of practicing. You may practice without any diploma whatever until you are caught—

The CHAIRMAN. Oh, yes.

Dr. LOSADA. And then you have the right to proceed to pass an examination equivalent to your state board here; but to pass that examination you must have a diploma—foreign diploma of a reputable school—and you must have been in legal practice six years any way, six years in actual practice after leaving college. That is, now; unfortunately it was not so at that time, nor until these Americans I am talking about came. I understand that the feeling all over Europe is what I am telling you gentlemen. There is a gentleman here from France; I am sure he will say just the same. It is a pity that you have had schools in America that will give a diploma for $30 or $50, I don't know which, and then those people come back to Europe, styling themselves "American dentists," and do more harm to dentistry and to the American people than can be told.

The CHAIRMAN. We have a distinguished member of the section present from Canada—from Montreal—who will kindly read us a paper entitled "Dental Laws and Educational Methods in Canada." With your permission, we will ask the gentleman to read his paper, and as it is practically along the same lines as those of Drs. Finley and Keefe, we will discuss the three together. I take great pleasure in introducing to you Dr. Dubeau of Montreal, who will now read his paper, entitled "Dental Laws and Education in Canada."

Dr. EUDORE DUBEAU, Montreal, Canada, then read his paper, as follows:

Dental Laws and Education in Canada.

By EUDORE DUBEAU, D.D.S., Montreal, Canada.

CANADA, with a population of five millions consists of seven provinces, each having its dental law, viz, Ontario, Quebec, New Brunswick, Nova Scotia, British Columbia, Prince Edward Island, Manitoba, and the Northwest Territories. Only two provinces have dental colleges, Ontario and Quebec.

Ontario has a fine college, well equipped, giving a dental education to one hundred and fifty students annually. It is affiliated with Toronto University, and is known as the Royal College of Dental Surgeons of Ontario. Trinity University also gives a dental degree to students presenting credentials showing that they have completed a dental course in a reputable college.

The province of Quebec has two dental colleges, the Laval University Dental School, where the tuition is given in French, and the Dental Department of McGill University, where the course is given in English. Those two schools, though established this year, have practically existed for eleven years, as they are the continuation of the Dental College of the Province of Quebec, which was established in 1893, giving lectures both in French and English.

The course in the Province of Quebec extends over a period of four years, and we are going to keep it as it is, notwithstanding the action of other colleges. Moreover, a student unsuccessful in his final examination at the Laval School is obliged to take a fifth year in order to present himself for the degree of D.D.S.

McGill University gives the degree of M.D.S. at the end of the course, and the degree of D.D.S. on presentation of a thesis after a year's practice or more. As to the length of the course in Toronto, I am not in a position to say whether the course will remain at four years or be reduced to three.

As I have said before, the other provinces have no dental colleges. British Columbia, Prince Edward Island, Manitoba, and the Northwest Territories accept for examination to practice graduates from reputable dental colleges. New Brunswick and Nova Scotia do the same, but in addition require a matriculation examination.

In the province of Quebec, a student who intends to practice there must previously pass the matriculation examination, which is very high, and subsequently take the whole course.

Two years ago the Canadian Dental Association was established. It comprises the dentists of the whole Dominion of Canada, and its object is to create a council which would issue a license giving the right to its owner to practice all over Canada. The second meeting of this association will be held in Toronto next week.

As far as discipline is concerned Quebec and Ontario have the best two laws. In the province of Quebec a law was passed four years ago to prevent a dentist from advertising more than his name, address, and profession, the space for such advertisement being limited to twenty lines. A dentist who does not pay his annual tax to the dental association, after a sixty days' notice, is suspended from practice, and sued for illegal practice if he disregards his suspension. We have had much trouble in obtaining such a law and in putting it into effect, but we have succeeded. Until yesterday I thought we were the only province prohibiting advertisements, but I was informed that Ontario has the same power, and is actually gradually enforcing it.

I wish that all the other provinces, states, and countries of the world would follow this example, and then quackery would have seen its good days.

I should have liked to go more into details, but lack of time has not permitted me to do so.

Now as to reciprocity, if you will allow me to say a few words. Personally, my *confrères,* I am disposed to exchange with any province, state or country which has privileges as large as we have. Our examination is pretty good. Our examination is one in science and letters, and in order to pass the applicant must obtain sixty per cent. on each subject. Personally I would like to see my country meet with other countries with high standards.

Discussion.

Dr. A. E. WEBSTER, Toronto, Canada. I wish to say a few words on the question of reciprocity in Canada. An effort has been made for the past thirty years to harmonize the dental laws of Canada so

that we could have but one licensing body. These efforts have met with but meager results until recently and I believe now that all the provinces have the power, or soon will have it, of accepting candidates to practice without further examination. The candidate of course must present the proper credentials. I mean such credentials as may be acceptable. The several boards having agreed upon a standard and all complying with that standard will have all the rights granted no matter from what province or county the applicant may come.

In Canada there are greater difficulties in organizing a single national diploma than in the United States, because of the treaty of Paris of 1763, by which the religion and education of the French were to be under their own control. In 1867 when all the provinces were united into one Dominion, each province was given control of its own educational and religious affairs. Thus you see there can be no power given the Dominion Parliament to pass a national dental act unless the British North America act is changed, and this cannot be changed without the consent of the French government with whom the treaty was made in 1763. Though this is a great obstacle, there is still a possibility of working out an interchange of licenses by voluntary agreement. Very shortly this will be carried into effect.

There is another aspect of dental law in Canada which is worthy of notice in this connection. The dental acts as passed by the legislatures give the profession some control over their members. Most of the acts state that the board or council may discipline its members. Until recently no by-laws had been passed defining what is meant by discipline. In most of the provinces at the present time members cannot do anything that will tend to lower the dignity or professional standing of dentistry without incurring the risk of losing their license. In Ontario there have been a few prosecutions under the new by-laws resulting in a rather wholesome effect on many others. The main object is to protect the public against dishonest practices.

The CHAIRMAN. In this connection I would like to call upon a gentleman from France, Dr. Roussel of Paris, who will speak to us on reciprocity.

Dr. GEORGE A. ROUSSEL, Paris, France. Before coming to the subject of reciprocity I would like to explain in a few words the condition of the dental laws in France. I am going to read to you a paragraph from our body which we sent to the Association of Dental Faculties in 1901: "One entitled to practice dentistry in France must have a diploma of French M.D. or a diploma of Surgeon-Dentist." The degree of M.D. is required, without any special knowledge of dentistry; any doctor of medicine is entitled to practice dentistry in France. Second, we have a diploma of *Chirurgien Dentiste* given by the Faculty of Medicine. The requirements to get this diploma may be divided into three different steps. The first one is the preliminary. This preliminary examination is passed before the Sorbonne when the candidate has not a diploma of Bachelor (French Bachelor). This diploma he gets at the Sorbonne; it is called the *certificat d'études*. When a student has passed these examinations he is entitled to matriculate in a dental school; we have three. The certificate is rather difficult for a foreigner to get. The examination is composed of two parts—written and oral. The written one consists of a composition in French and a translation into

French from a foreign language. The composition of 800 to 1200 words must be on a subject announced at the time of examination. Three hours' time is allowed. The composition is graded with reference to thoughts expressed, the arrangement, the general plan and arrangement of the subject, and also correct knowledge of the common use of words and spelling, and even of paragraphing. The translation must be in correct French, and a selection of about 200 words taken from a standard author in one of the following languages, at the option of the candidate: German, English, Italian, or Spanish. For this translation about two hours' time is allowed. The oral examination embraces the following subjects: French literature, elements of arithmetic, elements of algebra, German, chemistry, zoölogy, and botany. After a student passes that examination he is entitled to matriculate in the dental college. This is the second step.

We have in France three dental colleges. They have not exactly the same standing, but legally they have the same rights. After the student has spent his three years at the college he may come up before the board of the Faculty of Medicine without having to pass any examination in the school where he has followed the three years' course. The studies consist mostly in theoretical work. Now, after having passed that time in a school, the third part of the curriculum is for the examination at the Faculty of Medicine, which is divided into three parts. No practical examination except one extraction and a clinic.

The examining board is constituted of medical men only for the first and second examinations. For the third it consists of a medical man and two dentists (two dentists connected with the hospitals). After the student has passed that examination successfully he receives a diploma of Surgeon-Dentist (which is the only diploma given in France) and a government diploma entitling him to practice dentistry, to give anesthesia, and formulate prescriptions.

Now, Mr. Chairman, to come back to the question of reciprocity. It has been our endeavor for the last six months, with two other members of the advisory board of the National Association of Dental Faculties, to study the matter of reciprocity and to compare the French examinations and the French diplomas.

In regard to the position of an American dentist in our country. The American dentist who wishes to practice is bound to go through the elementary examinations. In France, a foreigner coming into the country must speak fluently the language and have a thorough knowledge of French literature, and prove that he has a scientific knowledge sufficient to practice our profession. This cannot be avoided by any stranger coming into France. The second part of the dental requirements concerns advanced standing given in our schools to foreigners. Formerly we gave two years' credit to the foreigners who came into our country. Now we have reduced it to one year's advanced standing, and the student who comes into our country has to pass through. If he is an American dentist he must spend two years in one of these institutions. We had a few years ago a very good man from your country come to France. He was an A.B. from Williams College. No equivalents whatever were given for the preliminary examination, and he was required to go through a two years' course in the dental college. The first examination cannot be avoided, but I think the standing in the colleges

can be somewhat more liberally allowed to American practitioners, as Dr. Godon stated the other day. Of course, in our country a foreigner has to show what he can do in the professional line. A year might be sufficient to see if a man be fit to go up for the final examination before the Faculty of Medicine. The gentleman whom I just mentioned is one of those of whom we are very proud in our country. He had to waste two years of his time in an institution where no practical work is done. This, we hope, will be changed. These are points that may be altered to advantage.

As to the third examination, which is the final examination. This is generally rather easy for Americans, as they all have sufficient knowledge of medicine, surgery, and dentistry, and as the examination is passed almost entirely on the medical and surgical ground, the candidates are only examined on medicine and surgery, and only one extraction and the clinical examination is required. So this is very easy for the foreigner. The difficulty is the amount of time he has to spend in the dental school. The first part of the dental studies in France cannot be avoided in any way by the foreigner. The second part, the time the foreigner has to pass now in the dental school—it is too long when the man is well qualified. As to the final examination, the foreigner, particularly an American, is not at all afraid to pass that examination to get the final diploma, as it is in accordance with the curriculum and the studies in the American colleges.

Now, Mr. Chairman, I wish we could make it as easy as possible for Americans who may desire to come over to France; much has been done by those who are already in our country to raise the standard of the profession.

The CHAIRMAN. I will call upon a gentleman who is the chairman for the time being of one of the largest delegations to this congress and who lives in the largest state—I call upon Dr. David of Texas to give us a word on reciprocity and tell us what Texas thinks of reciprocity.

Dr. J. W. DAVID, Corsicana, Texas. I do not think there is any hope for reciprocity as long as our examining boards pass men who are undergraduates. Whenever we have laws that will require a man to be a graduate before he can come up for examination, then we may look forward to reciprocity in the true sense of the word; but as it is in our own state, we have a larger proportion of undergraduates who come up for examination than of those with diplomas, and as long as that condition exists we cannot expect reciprocity as it should be. We have only in recent years had a dental law in Texas. Our state has been a dumping-ground for the various states of the Union, and I hope in a few years that conditions will be improved.

The CHAIRMAN. Now we will hear from Dr. Merchant of Texas.

Dr. M. S. MERCHANT, Giddings, Texas. As Dr. David has told you, we have only had a law for a few years and our law is a defective one in that it does not require graduation before the candidate can come before the board of examination. Several years before this law was passed our state association drafted a bill and had it introduced in the legislature, requiring graduation from a reputable dental college as a prerequisite for examination. That bill was defeated by the opposition of the dentists of the state. When the present law, which makes the board recognize diplomas from reputable colleges went into effect, giving, however, the right to discriminate and say what colleges shall be recognized as reputable, one of the provisions of the law was that all dentists who had vested rights—that is who had been in regular practice or practicing dentistry for a certain number of years previous to the passage of the act—should be licensed by the board. So we were compelled at our first meeting to license six hundred dentists, although probably a very meager part of that number were graduates. That is the reason we have such a large percentage of undergraduates in the legal practice of dentistry in the state of Texas. Since our board has had charge of the examinations we have been making examinations harder each year. While we are required to examine any man who applies to us, regardless of the kind of training he has had, or whether he has ever been to college, we have each year made the examination harder and harder, until now not nearly 50 per cent. of even second-year students, that is, men who have attended two years at the best colleges, get by the board, and we hope, as Dr. David has said, that we will have a better law and as nearly as possible examine only graduates.

As to reciprocity, our board will be as charitable in that as the other states and will recognize as nearly as we can graduates who have passed such boards as those of Pennsylvania and New York, that is, we will recognize them as far as we can. The examination will not be so severe.

As to reciprocity of the United States with foreign countries, I think that our National Examiners have passed a wise rule directing that foreigners shall be examined in English, and requiring about the same things that those foreign states require of us. I do not think that reciprocity is practicable as yet, but hope the time will come when this body will be able to make some suggestions that will enable all countries to recognize certain standards, and finally that a degree of D.D.S. will be an honorable degree recognized in all countries of the world.

Allow me to make an announcement, Mr. Chairman. There is another committee which will have a meeting tomorrow afternoon, I believe at four o'clock, in the committee room of the Hotel Jefferson, to which all parties interested in the promotion of dental surgeons, with commissioned rank, in the armies and navies of the world. All who are interested in that question we hope will be present at that meeting. All are specially invited.

The CHAIRMAN. I will call upon Dr. Hetrick of Kansas to speak on reciprocity.

Dr. F. O. HETRICK, Ottawa, Kansas. I am glad to hear this discussion and these papers, but I hope we will bear in mind that dentistry is as yet a baby. It is in its infancy, and while I believe that desirable conditions will come about, let us be patient, hoping that in this process of evolution the best may come forth. When I studied dentistry the degree of D.D.S. did not count for very much. A man could get it by standing around in front of the dental college a few hours each day and going to a few lectures; but I recognized that the preliminary education was more desirable to me, and consequently I stayed in school. It was possible in those days to get an education in dentistry very easily. Great changes have occurred since then, and on the whole I believe that dental teachers are doing the best they can to eliminate the troubles, but they cannot overcome them in a short time.

When the dental college is as it should be, when the proper authorities, be it the government of the United States or the state governments, set their seal to the standards, it won't be necessary for the state boards to examine candidates. That is one point I want to make. Another is in the matter of reciprocity. I can speak only from hearing the gentlemen from abroad, Dr. Bryan and others, and I do not think that they have taken a very unreasonable position. It has been possible in times past for students to come from Europe to America, get diplomas, and return in a very short time. Their standards of education are very high, and I do not see that they are making an unreasonable protest. That should not concern us as much as raising the standards in the states on this side of the water. I was very much pleased with what the gentleman from Toronto said in regard to the reciprocity they have. I think they have thrown it just a little wide open. Not all of the state boards require the same standard; but I believe, gentlemen, that the keynote to the entire dental educational problem is the preliminary requirement, because when a man reaches that stage in education he is not satisfied. If he is the kind of a man he should be, he is satisfied with nothing less than the best. And as for our good friend from Texas, I disagree with him. It would be good for reciprocity with states who examine men that are not graduates, for this reason: As yet in the matter of dental education the line has not been drawn closely enough, although it is gradually being drawn closer; not as to how a man gets his knowledge, but that he has it now, basing that on the preliminary education. Gentleman, as I said the other day, you may polish, and polish, and polish, but if the finish is not complete you will have an incomplete finish; and a man without the preliminary education!—in our state board this year, I do not hesitate to say to you, gentlemen, I threw out two men absolutely because their preliminary education was so abominable that they could not spell very many words with two syllables, and their grammar and their English was simply—

Dr. MERCHANT. Fierce.

Dr. HETRICK. There was hardly a word in the English language that they could pronounce. I did not care to go any farther. I pronounced them unqualified to practice dentistry until they knew more of their mother tongue, and consequently I concede the point that this gentleman from France makes, that one who would practice dentistry in France, Switzerland, and Spain should know the language of the country. It is a perfectly reasonable request.

Now as to the point that Dr. Finley of Washington made, Would it make a difference when our government recognizes the profession? I think it would. But, gentlemen, until the government of the United States or the state government puts its seal of approval upon the product of her schools, it is unreasonable to ask European countries to accept a diploma as *prima facie* evidence of qualification. I suppose some of these men never heard of Kansas, but we have a state university, that is, the state sets its seal of approval upon a school in that state. Our friend from Switzerland might say to his government, "This has the stamp of the seal of the state of Kansas upon it, and I know that it is not below what we would require. Let them learn the language and practice dentistry." I don't believe one could ask them for any more, and it might come from the United States gov-

ernment. So that I feel heartily in sympathy with reciprocity with Canada and with our own states, and believe that in the right time, when the standards are right, we will have no trouble about reciprocity with Europe.

Dr. GEORGE A. ROUSSEL, Paris, France. Mr. Chairman, I would like to add a word. We have the obligation in France of military service, and when that question of reciprocity was put forward in France it was claimed that the Frenchman must postpone his dental studies on account of his military service. All the French people have to spend three years —at all events dentists have to spend three years in the regiment before they can practice or finish their dental studies, and I think that is one of the reasons why they have made that the law—that the Americans have to spend longer time in dental schools. It puts the French student in a less favorable position than the foreigners, who come to France and can commence practice at once while the natives are delayed for at least three years.

Dr. H. C. BROWN, Columbus, O. The question of dental legislation, reciprocity, and higher education is essentially an exceedingly live issue, and one that should receive hearty co-operation and united assistance toward its solution by the leading men of the profession of the various countries here represented. When we recognize that dentistry as a profession is in its infancy we should congratulate ourselves that the advance has been rapid, and this should act as a stimulus to increase our efforts for greater achievements in the future. However, in the face of these recent advancements such as preliminary educational requirements, the college curriculum, and last but not least, legislation, which has been a potent factor in all this, I desire to call atten-tion to the abnormal increase in our pro-fession as compared with theology, law, and medicine. Recently in reviewing statistics compiled by our government for the decade ending in 1900, I found the increase of the four professions to which I refer, as follows: Theology, 12 per cent.; law, 13 per cent.; med-icine, $20\frac{1}{2}$ per cent., and dentistry, 41 per cent. This to me is evidence of a misconception on the part of young persons desiring to prepare them-selves for a useful and remunerative future, and to some extent accounts for so many "dental parlors" and "cheap joints" whose tendency is to degrade in-stead of elevate the profession and neces-sarily to lessen the confidence of the pub-lic in our profession by gross misrepresen-tations. Recent investigations show that the various dental colleges in the United States graduated more than 2000 persons in 1903, and no doubt further evidence could be produced to show that perhaps 200 or 300 more passed various state ex-amining boards as undergraduates. Thus, it is apparent that the increase for the present decade will equal, if not surpass that of the past.

It is not a question of more dentists. but better qualified ones who will as den-tists become students and aid in any ad-vanced movement, such as is before us today. Broadly speaking, education should not be confined entirely to our profession in order to accomplish the best results for our *clientèle* and ourselves. The public have only a limited knowledge of us as a profession, and frequently less of the character of the organs which we are called upon to treat. They should not be censured, but have our sympathy. as glaring advertisements, with various claims of superior ability, painless den-tistry, and the usual twenty-year guaran-tee are frequently all that they see rela-tive to our profession. Articles prepared by men of reputation and ability, and published in the leading magazines of the day with the idea of educating the public, are within the province of education from a dental viewpoint and will accomplish much good. What percentage of parents recognize that the first molar is a perma-nent tooth? I refer to this as only one of the instances where ignorance exists. Dental hygiene should be taught in our public schools, and much accomplished there from an educational standpoint. even though this teaching be limited in its nature.

In order to obtain the full benefits of reciprocity in the United States we must first have more uniform legislation in the various states and we should work with the view of securing the highest possible standard. To secure such legislation will require strong professional support and time; but why delay the beginning of this important step? I am in full sym-pathy with any movement that will ac-complish this result, and will support it with all the energy and influence at my command.

The CHAIRMAN. Gentlemen, we have one other paper here that we would like to have read, then we will ask Dr. Worman to speak on reciprocity. We would also like to hear from Dr. Bryan still further.

This is a short paper entitled "Right Legislation a Blessing to All Mankind." Will the secretary please read the paper; it is by Dr. Patterson of Boisé City, Idaho.

The secretary here read the paper pre-pared by Dr. H. G. PATTERSON, Boisé City. Idaho, as follows:

Right Legislation a Blessing to All Mankind.

By H. G. PATTERSON, D.D.S., Boisé City, Idaho.

WE have dental legislation in every state in our Union, and as our laws now exist it works a hardship on the legal practitioners of dentistry. The hardship is worked in this way: It makes no difference how well qualified or how long A has been practicing in any one of our states, when he, by reason of poor health of himself or family must move to some other state to practice his profession of dentistry, the first thing that he must do is to appear before a board of dental examiners for an examination, to see if he is competent to practice dentistry.

Now, if A is competent to practice dentistry in one state, why is he not competent to practice in any state? When he passed the board and received his certificate, it stated that A has passed a satisfactory examination and is well qualified to practice in any state; but as our laws now exist they compel him to take an examination for each and every state in which he may desire to practice.

My idea on the subject of dental legislation is this: Pass laws in all of the states to the effect that we may interchange our certificates; also pass national laws, at the same time providing for a national board of dental examiners, the latter to be made up of one dentist from each state of the Union. The said board should charge a fee of fifty dollars, more or less, and meet once a year at any place thought proper. Then if A takes an examination and is successful, he may practice in any state he chooses without undergoing the ordeal of another examination every time he wishes to change his location.

To show the unfairness of some of our state boards, I have in mind now where twenty-one applicants (I think they were all graduates) came before the board I am thinking of for an examination, and there was just one successful out of the twenty-one. One can scarcely believe that twenty out of twenty-one of these candidates were incompetent men. This board either did not want to see any more dentists in their state or they were at outs with the college, for nearly all were graduates of their own state college.

I can easily see that if we have a national board of dental examiners all this trouble will be done away with. I believe that the right dental law is the law that will do the most good to the most people.

A number of years ago I spoke of this plan to one of the profession, who said, "That would never do, for then as soon as a man received a certificate from a national board to practice dentistry he would stop his study." This is a mistake, for never would a man stop his study under those circumstances. A man must study as long as he wishes to practice dentistry. When he does not study, then he must stop his practice, for in a short time he will become a back number, and be compelled to drop out of line, and make room for a studious, wide-awake, up-to-date man.

When we can get an international law,

and have a national board of dental examiners, it is then that we will feel that we have done a great deal of good for our profession, something that is right, just, and equitable.

Discussion.

The CHAIRMAN. We will now hear from Dr. Worman on reciprocity.

Consul-General J. H. WORMAN. Mr. Chairman, I have pretty well exhausted my subject. I might in connection with this paper take the liberty of saying that I do not believe it is possible for us ever to come to the suggested ideal standard of a national board. It is not within the scope of our institutions, and not in harmony with the spirit of our state organizations. These are absolutely independent of each other. The only thing that we can hope to do is by agreement, just as we have done on national organizations, bring together the representatives of the various state bodies, and thus create an harmonious whole. I believe that these suggestions might thus be brought into harmony with the spirit of our institutions, that is to say, into harmony with the laws under which we live. I believe that the organization of the army and navy boards will help materially, but those who believe that these bodies will ultimately establish a standard upon which the government will put its seal as an action of the states, are very much mistaken. The government of the United States will never lend itself to any such an act; it cannot give any such attestation. It can only, upon the request of the state, through the State Department as its spokesman, certify to the accuracy of the attestations and the asseverations of the various states.

Dr. HETRICK. That is what I mean, doctor.

Consul-General WORMAN. But in the paper that has just been read there are suggestions made that seem to me to be out of harmony with the whole character of our educational and state organizations. I do think we have touched this subject from almost every side, and now ought to see clearly what is possible and what is attainable.

I would like to say one word more, if agreeable to you, namely that on the line of reciprocity between the states you are at present perhaps too radical in your course, and most erratic when seen from the standpoint of the European. In Germany the approbation given in the Kingdom of Bavaria is just as forceful and just as effective in the Grand Duchy of Baden as it is in the Kingdom of Prussia, and yet their methods and their workings are altogether different. It is a principle on the soil of the Germans, of the French, and the English, that whatever is done by one authority under their rule must go everywhere in that realm. I think we can profit by a study of foreign nations, and I do hope that the banding together of the boards of dental examiners of the various states may lead to this, that you shall agree to uniformity of practice and interstate reciprocity. The next step to international reciprocity will then be an easy and I am sure a successful one.

The CHAIRMAN. Dr. Bryan, the audience is small, but the records will always be here. We would like to hear from you again.

Dr. L. C. BRYAN, Basel, Switzerland. In the line of remarks of Dr. Worman, and one other member who spoke, I should like to call attention to the fact that many of the underlying principles of the government of America were brought from Europe. We started in the formation of our constitution by a study of European constitutions. Having these precedents to follow, and having improved on them at the time, our constitution is recognized as one of the greatest state documents in the history of the world. We are constantly taking suggestions from foreign countries, and our laws are often quoted and copied in foreign countries, so that we are not going more to foreign countries to get points of law than they are coming to us.

In the matter of interstate reciprocity, or governmental supervision, or governmental recognition of the diplomas of the colleges or the acts of the examining boards of the different states, I think the cantons of Switzerland might give us a basis to work on and suggestions which we might adopt; and I will give you a little sketch of their systems. The cantons are, like our states, wholly competent and are anxious to maintain their state rights, and fully capable of doing anything they wish within their limits, but the general government has a certain control over them as in the United States. For instance, in the matter of the practice of dentistry, each canton has its laws; it can make such laws as it chooses; it can let all of us or any one practice dentistry, and some cantons of Switzerland do not require any qualification. But most cantons have accepted a recommendation by the general government in Bern to require a national or federal diploma. The national diploma is the basis for a license to practice, or may be the license, in any canton, and they have gradually given up their cantonal dental examination laws, and have simply in most cantons or states of the federation adopted this national diploma as the only qualifi-

cation to practice, and the federal diploma is accepted in all cantons. This is a law passed by the congress, making such federal diploma good in all cantons.

The national diploma is secured in the following way: The student pursues a certain course which is specified by the general government in a law of congress. This law specifies exactly what the course of study shall be and what the examination shall consist of. This course is followed out first in the medical schools of the universities, and then studies in dentistry are taken at one of the two dental schools which supplement the medical college course. With the certificates of two preliminary university examinations (1) in science (physics, chemistry, botany, zoölogy) and (2) the fundamental medical subjects (anatomy, histology, embryology, physiology) together with the certificate of attendance on the prescribed curriculum of the dental school (the practical part of which may be supplemented by a preceptor's certificate) the candidate applies for his state examination before the local boards. There are five of these in the twenty-two cantons of Switzerland, and these are situated in the university towns where dentistry is taught. Formerly, all cantons used to have state examining boards, but most of these have been dispensed with, as the five cities where the government examinations are held are so easily accessible. The Department of the Interior appoints for each of these boards a representative of the government who is a supervisor or superintendent of the medical, dental, and pharmaceutical examinations of the local boards, he being generally a local medical man. He does not examine the students, but he is there to see that the laws are carried out and that the examiners give the student a fair chance and at the same time give him a thorough examination, and they are there to see that the examinations are carried on thoroughly by the state boards and just how they are done. After the examination he reports to the Department of the Interior, at Berne, that certain candidates have passed the examination, and then they receive a license to practice dentistry, which entitles them to practice anywhere in Switzerland.

Now it seems to me that this mode of procedure could be adopted in America, thus modifying and unifying the laws of the country. It does not seem that our state boards would object to having their examinations for national diplomas receive the approval of the United States government through a local supervisor of their own state appointed through the President. If we could get some such general recognition of the state board's work through the general government at Washington, represented by such a commissioner, it would solve the great problem of harmonizing state laws. It would do more—it would give our licenses and diplomas a standing in foreign countries which they do not now have. How can we expect a foreign government to recognize our licenses and diplomas when one state does not recognize those of another in our Union? Why could not a government representative supervise the college examinations for the diploma of D.D.S.? This might be done by the state superintendent of education, and such diplomas should allow the holder to prac-

tice in any state, and it would go far to secure the recognition of his diploma in a foreign country, which is the object that we in Europe are seeking to accomplish, and any change in legislation in the states should keep in view our standing and the value of American diplomas and licenses abroad.

The CHAIRMAN. Is there any other gentleman who would like to speak?

Dr. HETRICK. We are a democratic people, each state being a government unto itself, each county a government unto itself, all governed by general laws, or local laws, and I believe the matter of reciprocity will work out. I believe that it is a good suggestion to work through the state simply. As the gentleman over here, Dr. Worman, has said, the state authorities could certify that the standard of education in a certain state is so-and-so; that is all in my judgment that would be necessary. I do not think we could have a law in which national examination of candidates would be by government officials, but it might be under government inspection.

Dr. BRYAN. Let it be under government inspection—or some government recognition.

Dr. HETRICK. It would result in recognition finally by the United States government.

A paper by Dr. GEORGE HABEEB ARBEELY of Damascus, Syria, entitled "The Need of Dental Legislation in Syria," was submitted to the section, and read by title. The paper here follows:

The Need of Dental Legislation in Syria.

By GEO. HABEEB ARBEELY, D.D.S., Damascus, Syria.

GENTLEMEN, I have the honor to address you as a member of your great body and as the first and the only Syrian dentist in the state of New York. I am glad to be given the opportunity to speak to you of the need of a law to enforce the study of dental surgery in the schools of Syria.

I take it for granted that every member of the Fourth International Dental Congress will be interested in glancing at the methods in use in the old country.

But before giving details, I would call attention to the fact that however limited may be the Syrian's knowledge of dentistry, his ignorance cannot be attributed either to lack of intellect or to lack of good-will.

These oriental people are intelligent, quick to seize ideas, and athirst for learning; and all that they need is freedom to study and to assimilate instruction. It is the Turkish Empire that alone is to blame. It alone is responsible for the fact that there is no Turkish law making the study of dental surgery compulsory.

Syria lacks American and European skill because she is absolutely ignorant of American and European methods. The medical board of Constantinople does not know that to neglect dentistry is to neglect an important branch of medicine. In countries like Turkey, where climatic conditions militate against close and active application to delicate details, a law is needed to protect the people against the charlatan. Nothing but law can enforce the study required as a precautionary measure. Thousands upon thousands of the people of the East suffer from diseases of the teeth and jaws, yet no medical man of Syria has drawn from that all-too-evident fact the inference impelling him to suggest the need of schools where would-be dentists can learn how to treat diseases of the teeth.

In Syria, the dentist *as a dentist* can do but two things; he can pull teeth and make rubber plates. Generally speaking, the Mohammedan sacrifices his teeth at the first hint of pain. His tooth may be flawless—no matter—let a nerve tingle, and out comes the tooth! In Syria the men who make a business of "dentistry" are the barbers. I call them barber-surgeons (or surgeon-barbers) because they are authorized to employ dry and wet cups for bloodletting, to vaccinate, to blister, to use means for the generation and production of an issue, or pus, by them considered useful for the accomplishment of certain results accessory to the peculiar practice of the so-called dentists of that far-off land. These barber-surgeons make use of two instruments in their treatment of teeth: a key-forceps, and a stout string or thread; but they extract teeth with the first tool that comes to hand, be it clean or unclean. If it is clean, so much the better. If it is unclean—if it engenders disease—so much the worse for the patient. Cases of blood-poisoning and cases of fractured jaws are

34

of daily occurrence. The doctors report them, and the board of health pigeon-holes the record. I need not call attention to the fact that the pigeonhole is a universal product, in evidence in Syria as in the more advanced West.

The oriental knows the uses of anesthetics; when he is to have a tooth pulled he benumbs his senses with spirituous liquor, and being drunk and incapable of indicating the afflicted tooth, he leaves it to the dentist to take his choice. The operator applies a string or forceps haphazard, now and then uprooting a good tooth, and leaving the bad tooth hard at work at the old stand. I remember such a case. A man had a pain in his upper right first molar. He went to the dentist, who extracted three lower teeth, and the patient went home. Soon after he returned, still in agony. The dentist made a search and found the tooth—but too late. Inflammation had set in, in both jaws. The dentist declared that there was but one way out of the affair. "Have them all out!" said he; "The way is simple, but it is sure! When your teeth are all out they cannot ache, or if they *do* ache, you will not know it!"

A barber's fee for extractions is from two to ten cents per tooth. In some cases barbers extract the teeth of their customers free of charge. Some of the men authorized to pull and fill teeth were watchmakers and jewelers before they became dentists. They call themselves dentists, and it is supposed in Syria that they are graduates from European colleges. These men give a tooth a summary treatment and then crowd into it either cement or amalgam. They know nothing of the anatomy or the pathological conditions of the jaws; therefore it cannot be said that they have ever properly "filled" a tooth. When a tooth aches after the cement or amalgam has been put in its cavity, the dentist's action is simple—he extracts the tooth, cement and all.

Gold as a filling is not used. Crown and bridge work are not known in Syria. Prosthetic work is limited to the making of rubber plates; plaster of Paris is not used. The only material used in taking impressions is a molding compound. In Syria, before a dentist succeeds in taking one impression the victim is forced to enter the chair from three to five different and distinct times. The plate thus acquired is rough, of oppressive weight, so sharply edged as to bruise the tongue, or so ill-fitting that its use is painful. I have known men and women who having provided themselves with such plates, carried them in their pockets, to avoid the torture attendant upon an attempt to carry them in their mouths.

In Syria, dentists' charges for extraction range from five to twenty-five cents (approximately). Fillings cost from fifty cents to one dollar (approximately). Rubber plates, upper and lower, cost from five to twenty dollars (approximately). The tools handled by the dentists are of the ancient form. Patients are treated seated in barbers' chairs, or chairs with movable head-rests. Not long ago I received a letter from a man in Damascus who wished me to buy a chair for his Syrian office. The chair was to be of the most approved and improved American pattern. He impressed it upon me that I was to buy him the best chair in the market, and he warned me not to pay more than thirty-five dollars for it. His plan was to open an office just opposite the office of the man in whose office he had learned his art. His ambition was to start out on the most advanced American plan. I answered that my time—the time required for his commission—would cost more than the amount offered by him for a chair; and I told him that the chair used by American barbers costs considerably more than the outlay that he had projected. I cite this incident to show how little the dentist of Syria knows of modern dentistry, or of the cost of modern American instruments. It is easy to become a dentist in Turkey, for in that country there is no law compelling a man to study his art before he practices it. I have known young men who having studied a short time in dentists' offices, decorated their rooms with gilded signs like those used in our dental parlors. In Syria, any man possessing physical force enough to draw a tooth out of a human jaw is free to set himself up as a dentist, and thereafter "to make or to mar" as occasion offers.

The Turkish government will forward an official authorization to practice dental surgery to any man who will pay from three to five dollars (approximately) for such "diploma."

Now, gentlemen, if you consider the points advanced in this paper, you must conclude that the dentistry of Syria demands a law enforcing the education of men who aspire to fit the Syrian jaw for the work apportioned to it by nature's laws. I believe that the medical colleges of Syria would welcome the admission of so important a branch of the science of medicine. It is beyond question that all serious thinkers would acclaim a law to enforce the study of dental surgery, as obviously important for the public good.

The Turkish government alone has power to make such a law. A year ago a Syrian paper of New York reported in "Kaukab" that his Majesty the Sultan was about to compel all dentists to show their diplomas in the county clerks' offices of the towns in which they exercised their professions; but that order, if confirmed, did not take effect.

There are one hundred and fifty thousand Syrians scattered over the United States, and there are seven Arabic newspapers in New York and Boston. All these people and all the men who represent the Arabic newspapers are in favor of the establishment of schools of dentistry in the mother country. I know that the editors of the Syrian journals would be glad to publish translations of any suggestions or instructions bearing upon this matter.

A paper by Dr. JOHN H. COYLE, Thomasville, Ga., entitled "Higher Preliminary Education," was presented to the section and read by title.

The paper here follows:

Higher Preliminary Education.

By JOHN H. COYLE D.D.S., Thomasville, Ga.

IN the operation of natural law, nothing remains stationary. There must be either progression or retrogression. This law applies to all life, whether vegetable or animal, and man is no exception to the rule. Whether engaged in commerce or any of the professions, there must be constant adjustment to the ever-changing conditions in order to reap the reward of highest success. The methods and attainments of our forefathers seem very crude in this day of progress and could cut no figure in the present fierce competition in all the vocations of life. This is specially true as to dentistry. In the early days the only requisite to a successful practice was the possession of a certain amount of mechanical skill. Educational attainments were not considered, because there was little actual need for it. The present status of the profession, however, demands a very different preparation for those entering its ranks. The question of questions with us now is, What shall be done to elevate the standard of dental education? Disclaiming any intention of being dogmatic, I will suggest that the question can only be solved in one way, and that is by the requirement of higher preliminary educational attainments as a condition of matriculation. The dental schools should do this of their own volition. If they fail to do this, then the profession should appeal to the various state examining boards to sustain this contention. It may not be generally known, but it is a fact that the state boards have the power to force this issue. When they pass upon an applicant's fitness to practice, it is final. There is no power in this country that can go behind the actions of these examining boards. So that my contention is, that if the different state boards would act in harmony, insisting on educational as well as technical attainments, the colleges would be forced to raise a higher standard for matriculants. When this is done and the profession is filled with educated men, we may expect to witness the decadence of commercialism and many other evils which now dominate the

profession in America. This seems to me to be a reasonable expectation, for my observation goes to show that educated men, as a rule, place a higher estimate on themselves and their work than do ignorant men, who, necessarily have a more restricted horizon—and with them a dollar is the biggest thing in it. On the other hand, men of liberal education are proverbially indifferent to money-getting; to them it is a necessary evil and only a means to an end. They take broad views of life in general and take pride in their profession. The truth is, that you cannot make a professional man out of an ignorant man. This being admitted, the conclusion is irresistible that if we desire to elevate our profession we must fill it with educated men. It seems to me that the direct way is to start at the beginning, by raising the requirements of preliminary education as a condition of entrance into the college. If any college or colleges choose to ignore these demands, let them take the consequences. I doubt very seriously whether they would remain a menace to the profession very long after they were blacklisted by the boards.

The CHAIRMAN. It seems to me that we have covered the ground pretty thoroughly. As there are no other papers before the section, if it is your pleasure I would suggest that we adjourn. I feel that we are working in the right direction, and really believe the work of our section will be productive of great good. I thank you for your presence and attention, and I now declare Section X of the Fourth International Dental Congress adjourned *sine die*.

Fourth International Dental Congress.

THE CLINICS.

THE CLINICS.

Porcelain.

JULES J. SARRAZIN, New Orleans, La.
"Retention of Porcelain Inlay Restorations, Including Angles of Incisors and Approximal Marginal Ridges of Bicuspids."

The retention and resistance of inlays for porcelain restoration of functional parts of teeth should require that we adopt the same fundamental principles for mechanical strength as the profession has arrived at for metal contours.

Correct principles hold as good for porcelain inlay contours as for metal ones.

The method described below, which is primarily applicable to incisors, although it may be resorted to for bicuspids in a similar manner, will give the amount of retention in a morsal direction necessary to sustain a restoration of any size, without danger of encroaching on the pulp by deepening the cavity, and without weakening the porcelain of the inlay, if the latter be properly constructed.

A groove is cut horizontally in the lingual face of an incisor hardly closer than 3/32 of an inch to the incisal edge. Into this groove is fitted iridio-platinum wire, No. 23 gage. The wire is bent in a labio-gingival direction as it emerges from the groove into the approximal portion of the cavity, without approaching the axial wall of the cavity nearer than 1/15 of an inch at any part. The extremity of the wire which is to be inside of the porcelain is well rounded, as is usual in such work. It is bent so as to offer greater porcelain thickness between itself and the axial cavity wall as it extends gingivally. The object is that sufficient thickness of porcelain will exist between the bending wire, the incisal edge, and the axial wall of the cavity to avoid weakening the porcelain, while the grip of the wire will be amply sufficient. A good cervical seat should be provided besides.

Some conditions of occlusion will indicate placing the lingual horizontal auxiliary groove a little farther than 3/32 of an inch from the edge of the toothblade, in order to avoid the impact of antagonizing incisal edges at or near a filling margin, or so as to eliminate the danger of a dislodging force by bringing occlusion in the center of the groove's filling. Circumstances alter cases.

The portion of the wire entering the groove receives no porcelain.

The inlay is cemented in the usual way. On the following or a later day the cement surface in the lingual horizontal auxiliary groove is burred off and replaced by a veneer of cohesive gold.

For obvious reasons, the incisal step-cavity preparation which would be typical in metal angle restorations is not resorted to, instead of which the horizontal lingual auxiliary groove (which latter is ordinarily indicated in weak natural incisal angle preservations) is made guo-approximo-occlusal angles, and which at the same time permits safe correct knuckling restoration. Grooves must be cut to some depth for the wire retention of bicuspid porcelain contours, so that a thickness of nearly 1/16 of an inch of porcelain, if possible, may exist between the morsal face of the filling and the point of entrance of the light wire into the inlay body, before bending the wire

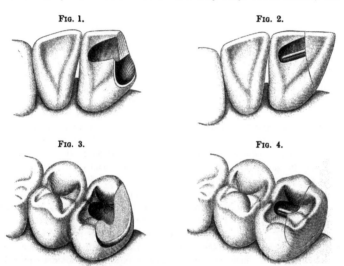

FIG. 1.   FIG. 2.

FIG. 3.   FIG. 4.

use of, because a compromise must here be reached between the resistant conditions of the filling as a whole and the strength of the porcelain material. The same pulpal inclination at the extremity of the groove's floor as in metal work should be produced.

An approximo-occlusal inlay contour, where the step may not be made of porcelain, will carry its wire into an occlusal groove cut in the central sulcus of a bicuspid, on the usual ideal plan of metal retention, which offers resistance without endangering both bucco- and lin-gingivally. Such depth of step in the pulpal wall is not objectionable, being cement-lined beneath a final gold veneer and an underlying metal wire. A good cervical seat is always necessary.

———

C. C. ALLEN, Kansas City, Mo. "Original Method of Making a Matrix for Inlay by the Aid of Gum Camphor."

Dr. Allen first takes a piece of gold or platinum foil of the desired size, places it over the cavity, and using a piece of spunk, cotton, or chamois, forces it to the bottom of the cavity in much the same manner as ordinarily followed; but he takes no particular pains to get a complete adaptation with the chamois, spunk or other substance of that kind employed.

After pushing the foil to the bottom of the cavity he immediately takes a small piece of gum camphor and presses it into the cavity with a burnisher, using as much force as is practicable to obtain. The camphor possesses sufficient flow and sufficient firmness to thoroughly adapt the foil to the walls of the cavity, swaging it to place directly.

Dr. Allen burnishes down and removes the excess of camphor until the cavity appears as though it had been intended to leave the camphor there as a permanent filling. After this he removes the camphor, matrix and all, and invests it. By setting fire to the alcohol used in the mixing of the investment, by the time the alcohol is consumed the camphor has entirely disappeared, leaving the matrix perfectly clear and clean, and ready for the baking of the inlay.

If the camphor has become contaminated with blood, he soaks the matrix and camphor in alcohol for a minute or two and removes the camphor bodily, blood and all. The camphor may also be removed direct by setting it on fire in an alcohol flame or with a match.

———

F. L. FOSSUME, New York, N. Y. "The Construction of the Porcelain Inlay Matrix with Instruments made of Ivory."

My set of ivory instruments for the construction of matrices for porcelain inlays consists of twelve burnishers, which number I believe to be sufficient for constructing the matrix in any cavity where such a filling is suggested. The advan-

tages in using these instruments are that ivory as compared with steel does not stretch or iron the metal, and consequently the matrix will adapt itself to the cavity more readily, and will be devoid of that springy and rigid condition which makes it difficult to obtain a perfect matrix, without which a well-fitting inlay cannot be constructed.

The instruments are so shaped as to facilitate the adjustment of the matrix into a cavity prepared with the walls reasonably parallel and the floor flat, and also for the various step formations.

———

F. E. ROACH, Chicago, Ill. "A New Porcelain Body and a New Automatic Furnace Attachment."

The porcelain body is a radical departure from the bodies now in use, in that it may be molded into any desired form, and after a few minutes' time hardens or crystallizes into a mass sufficiently hard to be removed from the mold without danger of breakage, and when baked forms a vitreous mass much stronger than the ordinary bodies.

In making large molar and bicuspid restorations the body is mixed to a putty-like consistence, forced to place in the cavity, and allowed to set, after which the material is removed and baked. More of the material is now added to the cavity surface of the inlay. A second impression is taken and the inlay with the refit is again baked. Usually two impressions and bakes will suffice for a perfect fit. No matrix is used at all.

By means of this material a perfect fit is easily obtained with any of the manufactured porcelain crowns. Bridges and continuous-gum cases are made without the use of platinum base-plate.

The automatic time device affords a means of uniformity in baking the porcelain without having to watch the furnace. This device differs from the ordinary clock switch in that it has a uniform starting-point, uniform increase of heat, positive automatic start and stop to clock, and cut-off on low current at first button.

L. E. CUSTER, Dayton, O.   "Management of the Inlay Matrix."

The tendency of the matrix to change shape under the contractive influence of the porcelain when melted is counteracted by having a wide unbroken rim to the matrix, and in a much better way yet by using porcelain of relatively high and low fusing-point. The matrix is first coated with a thin veneer of high-fusing porcelain, and then refitted to the cavity. The porcelain may check in places, but unless the cavity is very large the lower-fusing body can be used to finish the inlay. In large cavities a second layer of high-fusing body may be necessary. This is again fitted to the cavity and then finished with lower-fusing porcelain. In practice, Close's body was used for the first layer to retain the shape of the matrix throughout the subsequent bakings of lower-fusing, preferably Brewster's enamel. The Close body supports the matrix when the Brewster is fused, and also serves better by reason of its relative coarseness for the attachment of the cement.

He also showed his improvement in electric ovens, which consists of cutting the clay in sections whereby the contraction takes place in different centers, and the wires being wound with this in view are not mechanically broken by the contraction which gradually takes place in the clay foundation of electric ovens.

AMOS W. DANA, Burlington, Ia. "Cavity Formation for Porcelain Restoration."

The clinician demonstrated the advantage of mechanically locking the inlay to place in the cavity by the aid of grooves and prominences, as practiced by Dr. C. N. Thompson, not depending upon the adhesive properties of the cement to retain the inlay. The enamel margins are always at a right or a slightly acute angle. In bicuspids and molars porcelain is not advocated unless it be for esthetic reasons. When used in such teeth the cavity margins should be carried to safe areas by selecting the depressions on the coronal surfaces, and extending them to the axial walls, where the margins are not subjected to direct strain. Gold inlays, the clinician claimed, in bicuspids and molars, especially in approximo-occlusal cavities, are much more enduring and have all the good properties of porcelain, except, of course, the esthetic.

C. N. THOMPSON, Chicago, Ill. "Cavity Formations for Porcelain Inlays."

The object of special cavity formation for porcelain inlay restoration is to proceed with the view of obtaining the strongest possible margins to the filling, and in bicuspids and molars to secure margins between or beneath the summits of cusps to protect them from stress; the retention grooves being so aligned that the removal of the matrix is not interfered with, while the finished filling is locked and cannot be removed except from the occlusal surface.

C. M. WORK, Ottumwa, Ia. "Porcelain Restoration: Mesio-occlusal Cavity of Central Incisor."

This clinic consisted of preparing a cavity and the building of a porcelain inlay with Brewster's high-fusing body baked in a platinum matrix. The result was not altogether satisfactory, but was by no means disappointing.

———

W. II. FORDHAM, Scranton, Pa. "Porcelain Inlay on Incisal Corner."

The clinician showed the preparation and filling of two approximal cavities with porcelain, using high-fusing material. The cavities were cut out freely on the lingual surfaces so as to facilitate the removal of the matrices, thus securing a large separation. The fillings were made a shade or two lighter than the teeth to overcome the probable dark appearance caused by shadows when the teeth resume their normal positions.

———

W. A. CAPON, Philadelphia, Pa. "Restoring Incisal Edge with Loop or Staple."

The clinician demonstrated the making of a porcelain tip—the corner of an incisor—with a special wire attachment, overcoming to a great extent the difficulties of leverage, which are so peculiarly present in such cases.

———

J. Q. BYRAM, Indianapolis, Ind. "Method of Swaging Matrix from Center to Margin, and Fusing Porcelain with Pyrometer."

Demonstration showed that by use of the pyrometer, porcelain can be fused so that the same color is obtained when baking at definite temperatures.

C. W. BRUNER, Waterloo, Ia., and E. H. BALL, Tama, Ia. "Some of the Possibilities of Porcelain in a Country Practice."

———

H. M. SEAMANS, Columbus, O. "Student Technical Work and Self-Instruction in Porcelain Inlay by Means of Plaster-of-Paris Models, using No. 40 Tinfoil."

———

W. C. HERBERT, Detroit, Mich. "The Spaulding Method of Restoring the Entire Natural Enamel of a Tooth with Porcelain."

———

W. L. FICKES, Pittsburg, Pa. "Cavity Formations and Built-up Inlays."

Exhibited models showing cavity formation of some practical cases and the manner of baking inlays in layers.

———

F. E. CHEESEMAN, Chicago, Ill. "Large Molar Restoration of Lower Left Second Molar, Involving Occlusal and Buccal Surfaces: Matrix Burnished Directly to the Cavity, using High-fusing Porcelain."

———

W. T. REEVES, Chicago, Ill. "Porcelain Restorations."

JAMES O. WELLS, Minneapolis, Minn. "Cavity Preparations in the Natural Tooth, for Porcelain Restoration."

———

GEO. T. BANZET, Chicago, Ill. "Superior Right Central Distal Porcelain Restoration."

Crown and Bridge Work.

GEO. A. LOUQUE, New Orleans, La. "A New System of Crown and Bridge Work."

A side view of an artificial bicuspid porcelain tooth is here shown (see Fig. 1), provided with a concave or is slightly countersunk on the approximal surfaces, in order to afford more room for the solder to flow in and around the ends of the rod, which is placed in the tube as shown at c in Fig. 3. Platinum foil is burnished close to the tooth at the

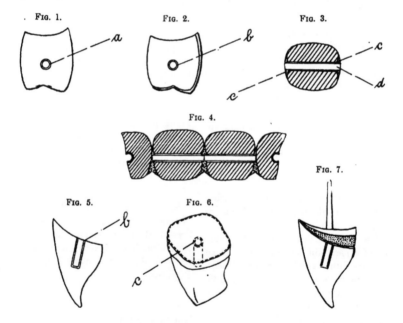

FIG. 1. FIG. 2. FIG. 3. FIG. 4. FIG. 7. FIG. 5. FIG. 6.

saddle-shape cervical end, so as to better rest on the gums and thereby conduce to the strength of the bridge and the comfort of the patient. It is also provided with a transverse aperture from one of its sides to the other, having a platinum tube baked into the bore of the tooth, as indicated by the letter a.

In putting up a bridge with these teeth, they are ground and fitted to the model in the usual manner. The tooth sides and back, leaving the front cervical end and the grinding surface open, as shown by Fig. 2. This done, holes are forced through the backing on both sides of the tooth (Fig. 2, b), and in consequence the platinum foil laps over the ends of the platinum tube—this in order to effectually prevent the borax or flux from coming into contact with and injuring the porcelain when soldering. An iridio-platinum wire is placed in the tube, *b,* so that it projects beyond the backing at the sides of the tooth, as shown at *d,* Fig. 3, and the whole is invested. Gold solder, 22-karat, is applied to the opposite sides of the metal-covered tooth so as to cover the projecting portion of the rod, as indicated by *c,* Fig. 3. The investment is made very hot prior to the application of the blaze to the solder, so that the solder will flow freely in the tube, over the rod and backing.

Fig. 4 shows a bridge of two teeth attached to two crowns. After the backing and rod are soldered, the teeth are placed on the articulator, invested, and are soldered into one piece by applying solder between each bridge tooth and the crown. After the teeth are soldered together, the platinum backing at the palatal or lingual side of each tooth is preferably removed—this in order to render the bridge smooth at the back, clear of all metal, giving the bridge a more natural appearance and having no metal exposed.

A dental bridge constructed in the manner described may be soldered or otherwise connected to abutments of different kinds, stationary or removable.

Fig. 5 shows an incisor crown, having a central aperture in its cervical end, occupied by a platinum tube, *b,* baked in the aperture. Prior to connecting the crown to the root-cap and pin the crown is ground and fitted over the cap on the articulator the same as for any facing, after which a backing of platinum foil is burnished on the cervical end of the tooth and caused to lap over the sides and back, as indicated by Fig. 6. A hole is then forced in the layer *c* coincident with the tube. This done, a rod of iridio-platinum is placed in the tube with borax upon it. The tooth is invested point down in plaster and a small amount

of 22-karat gold solder is melted over the rod so as to strongly connect the tube and rod to the backing. When cold, place and adjust the crown over the cap on the articulator, wax, invest, and solder cap and crown together as shown in Fig. 7, and finish the work as usual.

Having no pins in the way when grinding, and having no cement attachment, makes this a superior and most desirable method. It will be observed that all of the gold utilized is practically covered by the teeth.

For a close bite, these crowns can be used to great advantage over a saddle in bridge work.

———

J. C. HERTZ, Easton, Pa. "Assembling and Mounting the Platinum-Banded Porcelain Crown."

The object of his method is to produce a crown which will have no tendency to irritate the gingival margin, which will prevent the band and porcelain from causing unusual fulness at the labial margin, and which will eliminate the necessity of shading the body at the labial margin, by allowing the facing to extend under it.

To accomplish the above advantages the canal should not be enlarged toward the labial or buccal surface in order to allow for the necessary reduction of the root for the ferrule and facing.

The band should be of iridio-platinum No. 28 gage, and the cap of No. 34 gage. The dowel is made of No. 14 or 16 square iridio-platinum wire; the several parts are united with platinum solder.

Flat-back long cross-pins are preferred, but the facing may be of any tooth form which will be of the required length, as the pins are not essential in single crowns. For ordinary use plain rubber or pinless teeth may be employed, as by method of investment they are accurately retained when articulated and waxed to the metal parts in the mouth.

This method of investment consists in investing for the first biscuit in a layer of fine asbestos paste, preferably the Jenkins, which will prevent the etching

viously wiped with a thin coating of vaselin. This method proved very good in certain cases, especially where the prepared stump was not too long. In cases of molars and bicuspids where undercuts are present it is impracticable to get good impressions with cement, and modeling compound is employed, with results fully

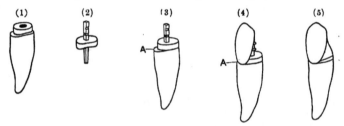

(1) Trimmed root. (2) Ferrule and dowel soldered and ready to adjust. (3) Ferrule and dowel inserted on root. (4) Crown articulated, showing symmetrical relation of crown and root at A. (5) Completed crown adjusted on root.

of the porcelain should the plaster come in contact with it. Then strengthen this by investing all the parts (except, of course, the waxed portion) in a mixture of plaster 2 parts, fire-clay 1 part. This will allow the removal of the wax and the biscuiting of the first application of high-fusing body. Then remove the investment and finish as usual.

Such investment has the following merits: It affords a wider range of selection for the crowns and facings and a more easy and artistic articulation, from the fact that pins are not indispensable.

———

F. W. PROSEUS, Rochester, N. Y. "The Land All-Enamel Jacket Crown Made from Impressions and Dies."

The first attempts were made by taking impressions of the prepared tooth. Cement thoroughly incorporated with soapstone was used, the tooth being pre-

as satisfactory and with saving of time. The tooth is prepared as described in the *Dental Cosmos* for 1903, vol. xlv, page 444. A snug-fitting German silver band is made for a Richmond crown, but extending slightly above the sides of the root. The band must be made with straight, smooth sides to avoid undercuts which would break or draw the impression material. The object of the band is to define the circumference and force the impression material about the root. With the band in place upon the root the impression is taken. If with cement, place matrices at adjoining teeth and see that the bulk of the cement does not interfere with the occlusion. The bite is then taken with modeling compound, cooled and removed. The impression should come away with sharp, clear edges; place in the compound with the band. A ring one-half inch high of unvulcanized rubber is formed about the cement and band, and a die of Melotte's or fusible metal poured into this. The rubber is then removed and a plaster cast is run. In using modeling compound the band is placed in position and a well-warmed piece of compound is used, and pressure made with the thumb and fingers to force it firmly to place until set. It is then thoroughly cooled and a bite is taken with another piece the surface of which has been heated over the flame to produce adhesiveness. After cooling and removing, amalgam, rather soft, is pressed into the space within the band and plaster model. The matrix is made and the jacket completed entirely independent of the patient. By this method a great saving of time is assured, and should the jacket become checked or broken there is no annoyance to the patient in making the second one. Also after the first baking the matrix is replaced upon the model and the body firmly pressed in, then carved to the desired shape, thus giving stronger porcelain than is produced by flowing and tapping to place.

In making the larger posterior molar jackets, first make a matrix of thin metal, not being especially particular about its accuracy, and over this on the die press the body and carve to shape and biscuit to slight glaze, strip out the matrix, then form a true-fitting matrix and into the partly formed jacket place quite wet body, and press firmly to place. This, saves time and overcomes warping, and assures a true joint.

———

J. M. THOMPSON, Detroit, Mich. "All-Porcelain Jacket Crown."

Dr. Thompson's clinic consisted in the making of a crown for a lateral incisor of the class commonly known as a "peg tooth," which was almost a perfect cone.

The preparation of the tooth was very simple, and consisted principally in the removal of the enamel upon the labial, mesial, and distal surfaces. When this had been done, a facing was ground to fit the tooth in a manner similar to a veneer. The facing and the tooth were prepared exactly as the completed case should appear, and then a cap of platinum foil was fitted to the tooth and burnished to a close adaptation. The facing was then placed in position and united to the cap by a small piece of wax and the two were removed as one piece. Pliers were then adjusted with one beak resting upon the labial surface of the facing and the other inside the cap in a manner that prevented any change of shape. The wax was then removed and a small amount of porcelain added, sufficient when properly dried to unite the facing and cap permanently. This was placed in the furnace and fused and then again placed upon the tooth for its final fitting. It was found to be correct in every way and was then removed and the entire cap covered with a layer of porcelain. After this was fused the platinum was removed and the crown cemented into place with Ames' inlay cement.

———

J. ENOS WAIT, Superior, Neb. "Method of Making Bicuspid Crowns."

Make a cope for the root of the tooth, and after taking an impression use a saddleback facing; grind to articulation; adjust to cope; invest in solder; then fill in the space with porcelain body, and bake.

———

WILLIS A. COSTON, Ft. Scott, Kans. "Porcelain Crowns."

This is the operator's original method

of making porcelain crowns. First trim
the root as ordinarily practiced. "I pay
no attention to removing the enamel, because I do not make any band. It does
not make any material difference how
badly the root is decayed. After the gum
is forced away from the root but slightly,
I take an impression of the end of the
root with base-plate gutta-percha. I then
wrap a piece of paper around it and pour
in fusible metal, thus obtaining a die.
The die only approximates perfection. I
swage a No. 36 gage platinum cap upon
this with rubber. I then carry it to the
mouth and put it on the end of the root,
putting the pins into place, and forcing
them through the platinum cap. Usually
the bur produced in forcing them will
hold them until soldered with 25 per
cent. platinum solder. After the pins are
soldered, cut them off. They will protrude into the porcelain far enough to
hold the body until fused. Then take it
to the mouth and have your assistant
mallet it around the peripheral line. It
shows very distinctly on the other side of
the cap. Then trim it almost to the
periphery and apply the porcelain. Then
build up the first body, which will be the
base color of the tooth, the color of the
dentin, and very near the color of the
enamel at the margin. Build it up,
make it as dry as possible, and then cut
it in the middle. This eliminates the
bubbles which in my opinion are always
present around a cluster of pins. I cut
it clear down until I get to the cap if I
can, and biscuit it. I then remove the
extra amount of cap with a very small
wheel or disk, cutting away from the
middle all the time, and in such a way
that the porcelain overhangs the cap and
none of the platinum cap shows. At the
final fusing the platinum is entirely
concealed. The final step consists in

packing this portion as tight as I can
and then finishing the crown in the ordinary way."

———

F. B. JAMES, Wilton Junction, Ia.
"Porcelain Crown for Badly Broken-
down Root."

The clinician showed porcelain crown
for roots so badly broken down that the
band cannot be fitted. The root is prepared in the best way possible under the
circumstances, taking an impression of
the end of the root in dental lac or any
impression material, and then swaging
thin platinum to the end of the root, No.
36 or 40 gage; finishing by swaging right
on the end of the root, to get a perfect
adaptation, nearly always using two
posts (large and small) to help the setting of the crown, so that it will go to
its proper position and will not start
down sidewise or in some other improper
way.

———

L. C. BRYAN, Basel, Switzerland.
"Exhibition of Models, Before and After
Making Bridge Work and Other Fix-
tures in the Mouth."

The clinician showed a method of retaining loose bridges or strengthening
teeth in the mouth that are loose or
liable to get loose, by a band extending
across the roof of the mouth.

He showed also models of raised bites,
saddle bridges, and teeth secured by wire
fixtures cemented on. He said: The principal object of the exhibit is to show how
we illustrate to patients what they can
expect from bridge work and what they
are likely to get. We show them the
model cases we have already finished,
and they recognize that we know what
we are talking about.

I sometimes take an impression of the

mouth and make models of the bridges with porcelain teeth and wax, trimming up and gold-plating, so that the next time the patient comes I can show him by the appearance of the model what he has to expect. Being arranged in sets in this way, and adjustable so as to be opened up or laid out flat, the patient can see the construction of the models and bridges.

———

CHAS. W. RODGERS, Dorchester, Massachusetts. "Bridge to Prevent the Grinding of Tipping Molars."

The abutments of the bridge are made as usual. The facing is backed as usual; then it is set on the model and a small line is made upon the facing in the same angle with the anterior angle of the posterior abutment. Then the backing is taken off the facing and cut into on that line and a little off each side of it, so that when the backing is replaced it will be put back in two pieces. There is then a small groove on the backing.

In the next step a piece of pure gold is taken and doubled on itself and put into the groove. Then the occluding surfaces are put on. The facing is touched with a hot instrument and taken right off. Little lead pencils are put in the places that were occupied by the pins; then the whole is invested and soldered as usual. After it is soldered and taken out of the investment, in grinding the piece of gold that was doubled on itself the two parts separate and one has it in two pieces. The anterior part is set first. The posterior abutment slides right down. The pins and the facing are threaded by means of the Bryant bridge-repair instruments. Then it is cemented on.

A modification is that the piece of pure gold that is doubled on itself can be so bent that it will form a dovetail; and then in the setting, when the anterior parts set, the little dovetail piece slides down on itself and the thing is locked in before the facing is set; then the facing is set as usual. That makes it much stronger.

———

J. G. HILDEBRAND, Waterloo, Iowa. "Method of Contouring a Gold Crown by the Use of Moldine."

Prepare the root in the ordinary way, fitting the band exactly as you would for any gold crown. Take an impression. In order to get the outlines and contour of the crown, simply take the moldine and pack it around the band and carve it just as nearly like the adjacent teeth as you can. Get your outlines cut out between the teeth at the interproximal space. Leave the points of contact at the occlusal surface, and the reproduction in the gold will be simply limited by the operator's ability to carve in the moldine.

———

S. H. VOYLES, St. Louis, Mo. "Method of Making a Saddle Bridge, using Diatoric or English Tube Teeth."

A platinum cup is made of a size to admit the tooth, and is soldered to the pier teeth and to the saddle at the same time. The teeth are removed before soldering and do not have to go through the fire. After soldering, the teeth are cemented in and the case is finished and polished.

———

CHAS. M. BORDNER, Shenandoah, Pa. "Simple Method of Making a Half-Band for a Darby Crown."

35

An iridio-platinum pin is fitted to the root. The platinum plate is soldered to the pin, and it is fitted to the root, notches are cut into the platinum plate, bent over to fit the root and then soldered.

O. V. DAVIES, Dunedin, New Zealand. "Facings for Bridges that Do Not Go Through the Fire."

The occluding surface is made in one piece and carved out, not by any system. Then, for the backing, the facing is pressed into moldine, lifted out, wiring the pins with little pieces of piano wire. Melotte's metal is poured over it. This is then struck into a piece of lead, and one gets the pinholes in their exact position; then the facings with their backings are waxed in proper position. With a small instrument the facings are pushed out and the backings left in position, waxed. In the holes where the pins come out, ordinary graphite is placed, and a piece of solder without the facings. After this the facings can be cemented in and riveted. In repairing, if it be hard to match a facing, make one with a platinum matrix and carve up in porcelain, exactly as for an inlay.

J. L. KELLY, St. Paul, Minn. "Removable Bridge."

It is possible to take advantage of the natural movements of the roots and dovetail the attachments, so that the bridge may remain in. The tubes, made in a manner so that one will fit or telescope perfectly over the other, can be made in either gold, porcelain, or rubber; easily made and easily cleaned. Cases have been worn for six years with perfect success. It is possible, where there are only two teeth left in lower or upper, to use

this attachment successfully. A most extreme case was made a success by using a canine on the right side and a second bicuspid on the left, where the second bicuspid cuts the lower gum; the right canine had been ground four times previous to operation. The bite was opened $\frac{1}{4}$ inch, and the attachments were used; the bridge has been worn for a year successfully in both upper and lower. The tubes or attachments are made from $\frac{1}{4}$ inch to $\frac{1}{2}$ inch in size to meet any condition.

C. M. WORK, Ottumwa, Ia. "Original Method of Making Gold Crowns."

This clinic consisted of the preparation of a band and the swaging of a cap in constructing a gold crown for bicuspid. The distinctive feature of this clinic was the bringing of the band down to the buccal occlusal angle and the carving of the cusps in dental lac instead of plaster. From this stage the band and its carved cusps were embedded in the plunger of a swager and the cusp swaged against the band, obviating the necessity of making a die and counter-die, and having the advantage of an absolutely accurate joint between the cap and the band, one being swaged against the other.

C. F. W. HOLBROOK, Newark, N. J. "Crown and Bridge Work."

This clinic consisted in the making of a gold bridge with teeth cemented to the bridge. This form of construction has a twofold advantage. First the teeth are removed from the bridge when the soldering is being done, there being of course no possible chance to check the porcelain in soldering. Second, the amount of gold surface showing is lessened, giving to the artificial teeth a more natural appearance. Diatoric teeth are used in this kind of work.

———

C. L. FRAME, Columbus Ohio. "Detachable Facings for Crown and Bridge Work."

———

R. C. TRAYNHAM, Pittsburg, Texas. "Diatoric Teeth in Crown and Bridge Work."

We take an impression of the base of the tooth with modeling compound, and swage a gold plate over the impression. It is then trimmed to fit and waxed up as in an ordinary case. The teeth are removed to prevent them from checking during the heating and soldering and the piece is finished as usual.

———

W. B. CONNER, Akron, Ohio. "New Method of Making Seamless Crowns."

———

FRED. A. PEESO, Philadelphia, Pa. "Crown and Bridge Work."

The demonstrator explained the technique of different styles of attachments for removable bridge work; and exhibited several pieces in situ in the mouth.

———

C. A. STEUERWALD, St. Ansgar, Iowa. "Casting Solid Gold Cusps in Cuttle-Bone."

———

L. P. DOTTERER, Charleston, S. C. "Accurate Method of Making a Gold Crown where Little Grinding Can be Endured."

———

FRANCISCO CASULLO, Montevideo, Uruguay, and PHILIP SURIANI, New York city. "Demonstration of Dr. Casullo's New Pinless Tooth for Crown and Bridge Work and Vulcanite."

———

H. F. COMBS, Chicago, Ill. "A Novel Method of Using the Davis Crown in Bridge Work."

———

R. M. SANGER, East Orange, N. J. "Method of Constructing the Sanger Half Collar Crown."

———

ROBERT N. LeCRON, St. Louis, Mo. "Porcelain Bridge: Setting with Guttapercha."

Building up bridge constructed of porcelain; seven anterior teeth on three abutments and a narrow saddle. Models were shown illustrating the work as constructed.

———

V. H. FREDERICH, St. Louis, Mo. "Construction of Porcelain Crown, Upper Central Incisor."

The framework of the crown was made in the same way as for a Richmond crown, with the facing soldered to a post and a porcelain body baked in the back.

———

C. V. VIGNES, New Orleans, La. "The Use of the Furnace in the Soldering of Facings to Posts in Porcelain Crowns."

———

F. A. GREENE, Geneva, N. Y. "Porcelain Crown Made from the S. S. White Countersunk Rubber Tooth."

———

ADAM FLICKINGER, St. Louis, Mo. "Showing Original Method of Removable Porcelain Bridge."

Gold Inlays.

H. B. TILESTON, Louisville, Ky. "Hollow Gold Inlay."

It can be made from a model of the tooth obtained from an impression taken with modeling compound, in which the tooth to be filled is made with copper amalgam and the entire model completed with plaster of Paris. Into the copper amalgam replica of the cavity 26-gage pure gold is burnished and readjusted in the cavity itself at a subsequent sitting. The inlay is completed by adding to this another piece of gold of the same fineness and thickness, completing any amount of contour necessary to produce a hollow inlay. It is filled from the back, through a hole left in the matrix piece, by fusing solder of 20 or 22-karat fineness, leaving a part of the opening at the back unfilled so as to afford a grasp for the cement. The principal features of this method are the ease with which it can be made, the perfect adaptation, and the complete protection of the cement which holds the inlay in place.

———

CLARENCE H. WRIGHT, Chicago, Ill. "Gold Inlay."

Take impression with modeling compound, using convenient shaped piece of air-chamber metal as a tray, and from this obtain a plaster model. If it be an approximal cavity, cut a slot at either side of the plaster model at a point between the cavity and the next tooth, and then break them apart. This gives access to the tooth-cavity alone, and rids the operator of the neighboring teeth. From the model thus obtained, make a fusible metal die; burnish pure gold,

No. 34 gage, to the metal die, and then to the model, and then in the mouth. Invest the matrix and build up a general framework with the necessary contour, using any gold plate such as is ordinarily used for gold crowns; flow 22-karat solder over and through these pieces. This gives the approximate shape of the inlay, which can then be dressed down roughly, and the polishing completed after the final insertion.

———

CHAS. E. PARKHURST, Somerville, Mass. "Gold Inlays."

The impression is taken in 1-1000 inch platinum. This is invested in whiting by nipping it in a pair of block tweezers; 22-karat solder is made into globules of different sizes by fluxing with borax, which aids in obtaining the contour and also avoids pitting the inlay. It is melted to contour with a blowpipe, and stoned, polished, grooved, and set.

———

W. F. WHALEN, Peoria, Ill. "Hollow Gold Inlay."

———

J. M. MURPHY, Temple Tex. "Gold Inlay in Bicuspid."

The clinician demonstrated the advantage of platinum foil over gold as a matrix.

———

C. N. THOMPSON. Chicago, Ill. "Gold Inlay: Method of Controlling Warpage Due to Shrinkage."

Fillings.

O. H. Simpson, Dodge City, Kans. "The Possibilities of Amalgamated Gold."

This material is used to set Logan crowns, repair gold plates and bridges, and to restore teeth to their original contour. Dr. Simpson demonstrated the use of amalgamated 24-karat gold, De-Trey's moss fiber, or Vernon's gold, preferred. Presumably the foil would act as well, although he has never used it.

In setting Logan crowns the root is prepared in the usual way; the crown is ground to fit the anterior surface of the root, leaving a V-shaped space on the lingual surface between the root and the crown. Then adapt a top of 24-karat gold to the prepared root by putting between the crown and the plate of gold a disk of gutta-percha, forcing it to copy the irregularities of the prepared root.

Trim the gold to the circumference of the root, and the gutta-percha to the circumference of the crown and the gold top. Now embed the Logan crown pinwise one-fourth its distance in plaster, leaving the gold top and gutta-percha in place. After the plaster of Paris has hardened, remove the crown, take out the gutta-percha and leave the gold in the bottom of the depression. Force the tooth to its original place. This can be facilitated by making a gateway for the surplus amalgam and mercury to escape. Amalgamate the gold and fill the space formerly occupied by the gutta-percha; absorb the surplus mercury with tin foil. Place the tooth, investment and all, in the center of a mass of sand and pumice, and heat over a slow fire for one hour and a half or two hours. Guard against heating too rapidly, so as to prevent the mercury from boiling. When the crown is cool, drop it in nitric acid and the gold will be restored to its original color. We now have a joint of gold that fits both crown and root.

For inlays, the matrix can be formed in any way that the operator desires, and retention by platinum pin or otherwise. After the matrix is formed, contour the proposed inlay in beeswax; remove the matrix, pins, and plates, and invest in plaster of Paris. Remove the beeswax by melting or otherwise, and fill up the space with dry amalgamated gold. Place in sand and evaporate as before. Inlays and contours should be hardened by flowing 20-karat solder on them. The amalgamated gold will take up solder as readily as blotting-paper will take up ink.

—

O. J. Fruth, St. Louis, Mo. "Mechanical Gold Filling."

This method of restoration may be used in certain cases of decalcification or faulty calcification, extensively decayed teeth and especially where the teeth are extensively worn by mechanical abrasion.

Method of Construction:

First. If any decay be present it should be thoroughly removed and all cavities and undercuts filled with cement.

Second. With a carborundum wheel grind down all frail enamel walls, and with a cuttle-fish disk slightly bevel the enamel margins.

Third. Drill two or more holes, as the case at hand demands, into the dentin, large enough to admit a No. 29 iridio-platinum wire.

Fourth.   A piece of pure gold plate, No. 34 gage, or platinum plate, No. 38 gage, is now burnished over the prepared surface, and small holes are punched to correspond to the holes previously drilled into the tooth.

Fifth.   The iridio-platinum pins are now forced through the matrix into the holes and allowed to project slightly above the matrix, care being taken that the pins are parallel.

Sixth.   The matrix is now removed with the pins in position, and the pins soldered to the matrix with 22-karat plate, after which the matrix is reburnished to the tooth, where it is again removed and more solder added until the matrix is quite stiff, and thus not easily distorted. The matrix is then again adjusted to the tooth and reburnished.

Seventh.   If an anterior tooth is being built up, the entire filling can be made of pure gold plate. A matrix is obtained and over this and around the labial and approximal surfaces of the tooth, No. 34 gage plate is adapted and tacked to the already burnished matrix with sticky wax. When the wax is sufficiently hardened the entire matrix is removed and invested in some good investment material.

Eighth.   When this is thoroughly set, the wax is boiled out and the matrix is filled by flowing 22-karat solder from the lingual surface until flush with the margin of the matrix, when it can be trimmed down roughly and set.   In cases where bicuspids and molars are to be restored, a preferable method is to take a modeling-compound bite of the teeth with a burnished matrix in position. A plaster model is then poured from this, and after shellacking and varnishing the occlusal surfaces of the teeth they are brought together after having placed a piece of soft modeling compound on the matrix. When this has hardened, the tooth-cusps are carved in the same manner as when carving a cap for a gold shell crown. When completed, a moldine impression is made, and then a Melotte's metal die is cast from that and a cap swaged of No. 30 gage 22-karat gold plate. The cusps of this swaged cap are now filled solid with 22-karat plate, and the cap is carefully trimmed and adjusted to the outlines of the matrix. After the parts are perfectly approximated they are held in position by clamp-tweezers and soldered together with 22-karat solder. The inlay or tip is now ready to set.

Method of Setting:

After cleaning and drying all surfaces of the tooth and filling, a thin mix of cement is made and filled into the holes in the tooth, when the inlay is cemented into place under pressure and is held until the cement is set. The surplus cement is carefully removed and the tooth and inlay varnished with sandarac or covered with a film of paraffin, when the patient can be dismissed until the following day or thereafter, when the filling can be ground down and polished, care being taken to run the disks from the gold toward the tooth-enamel, thus carrying the gold over the margins and producing a perfect joint.

When completed, these fillings or inlays cannot be distinguished from fillings made in the usual way.

Advantages.   The advantages claimed for this class of work are—

(1)   It does away with long tedious filling operations in the mouth, thus relieving both patient and operator of great nervous and physical strain.

(2)   It makes a stronger and more durable piece of work, and does not

weaken the tooth as would an ordinary filling of like proportions.

(3) It is cheaper to make, as scrap gold can be used instead of the pure gold foil, and at the same time it makes a denser filling which is not so readily abraded and worn down by mastication.

(4) In cases where the entire arch is to be built up, this can be effected with very little discomfort to the patient, since the tips can be made at his leisure by the operator, and when all are completed they can be set at a single sitting.

————

H. L. AMBLER, Cleveland, Ohio. "Cohesive Tin Foil."

A filling in any cavity in any tooth can be made into one solid mass from base to surface, so that if the filling were removed by breaking the tooth, it could be put on an anvil and forged out without breaking it into pieces. After partly filling the cavity, Dr. Ambler burnished the surface, then built on more tin so firmly that it could not be prized off. This foil is more tenacious, more cohesive, and makes a harder filling than any similar foil. It is used entirely for technic work in some dental colleges in place of cohesive gold, because it teaches the use of tin and cohesive gold at the same time, inasmuch as the tin is manipulated with the same instruments and hand mallet as are used for cohesive gold foil.

————

A. F. MERRIMAN, Oakland, Cal. "Combination of Cohesive with Non-cohesive Gold."

This clinic consisted of filling an approximo-occlusal cavity in a lower right second bicuspid with Abbey's non-cohe-sive gold No. 4, packed in ribbons against the cervical wall, and with Williams cylinders wedged into the center of the cavity, after having been reduced in size by rolling them between the fingers. The cylinders were annealed for the purpose of forming a cohesive foundation for the remainder of the filling. The remainder was completed with cohesive gold. The non-cohesive gold was condensed with a heavy mallet, and the surface of the filling was condensed with a light ivory mallet, final condensation being accomplished by the use of a corrugated burnisher in the handpiece.

————

B. C. HINKLEY, Keokuk, Ia. "Gold Filling in Incisor, using Iridio-Platinum Retention Posts."

The pin is extended one-tenth of an inch into the dentin at an angle so as not to encroach upon the pulp, and fitted into the center labio-lingually, leaving a space between the pin and the axial wall to admit of the adaptation of the gold at that point. The special advantages claimed for this operation consist in preserving the incisal portion of the tooth and securing the filling against displacement without making an unsightly step; fracture of the incisal angle of the tooth is prevented by leaving all of the dentin between the two enamel plates, or if wasted by caries and replaced with cement, it will leave walls well supported by a material which will be entirely free from the stress imparted to it by the filling. Experience has convinced the demonstrator that retention using the root as a base is a true and safe theory. All stress is conveyed from the incisal or occlusal surface of the tooth to the root without exerting force upon the weakened part of the crown, and in this manner renders all cutting or exertion for retention unnecessary.

———

J. W. CORMANY, Mount Carroll, Ill. "Gold Filling."

The clinician demonstrated a method of holding the rubber dam in place on lower incisors without the use of ligatures. It was done with the use of orange-wood wedges cut to fit the approximal space. A little sandarac varnish was placed at the junction of the dam with the tooth. This insures dryness of the tooth at all times.

———

W. D. JAMES, Tracy, Minn. "Gold Filling."

A simple cavity was expected, but the mesio-incisal angle was involved, necessitating its removal, and building a step in the cavity according to Black's method of cavity preparation. The tooth was reconstructed entirely with cohesive gold.

———

C. N. BOOTH, Cedar Rapids, Iowa. "Gold Filling."

A disto-occlusal cavity in an upper left first bicuspid was filled, using soft gold cylinders at the gingival seat, finishing with annealed foil.

———

W. I. BRIGHAM, South Framingham, Mass. "Gold Filling in Approximal Cavity. Burnished upon Soft Cement."

The advantage is that we place next to the tooth-substance the best filling material known—zinc oxysulfate. The filling is rendered permanent by covering it with gold, preventing thermal changes and greatly simplifying the operation. The cavity does not require undercuts, and thereby the patient is relieved of much unnecessary pain.

———

T. M. HAMPTON, Helena, Mont. "Gold Filling in Mesial Surface of Upper Incisor."

Non-cohesive gold was used at the cervical border, and heavy cohesive foil, folded for finishing.

———

J. W. S. GALLAGHER, Winona, Minn. "Combination Cohesive and Non-cohesive Gold."

———

W. R. CLACK, Clear Lake, Iowa. "Gold Filling in Mesio-Occlusal Cavity of Lower Right First Molar."

———

W. R. CLACK, Clear Lake, Iowa. "Gold Filling in Disto-Occlusal Surface of Upper Right Second Bicuspid."

———

A. C. SEARL, Owatonna, Minn. "Gold Filling."

A compound mesio-occlusal surface in a first bicuspid was filled following Dr. Black's method. Non-cohesive gold was used in the upper gingival third of the cavity, and the same gold annealed for the rest of the cavity, restoring the contour of the tooth to its original mesio-distal diameter and also restoring the interproximal space.

———

M. S. MERCHANT, Giddings, Texas. "Contour Gold Filling in Front of

Lower Left Central Incisor, Disto-Approximal Cavity."

J. V. CONZETT, Dubuque, Iowa. "Gold Filling, Wedelstaedt's Method, Disto-Incisal Surface of Upper Right Canine Involving the Angle."

W. M. SLACK, Memphis, Tenn. "Demonstration of the Use of Vernon's Crystal Gold by Hand Pressure Only, Without the Use of Mallet."

K. E. CARLSON, St. Paul, Minn. "Gold Filling in Mesial Surface of Upper Incisor."

J. B. PHERRIN, Central City, Iowa. "Filling Mesio-Occlusal Cavity of Upper Second Bicuspid."

The tooth had an amalgam filling over a capped pulp; in removing the filling the pulp was exposed and removed under cocain and adrenalin chlorid solution.

J. J. BOOTH, Marion, Iowa. "Gold Filling in Mesio-Occlusal Cavity in Upper Second Bicuspid."

A. M. LEWIS, Austin, Minn. "Gold Filling on Mesio-Occlusal Surface of Upper Right Second Bicuspid."

The cavity was prepared according to Black's method, using non-cohesive gold at the gingival seat, and cohesive gold for the finishing; one and three-quarter sheets of non-cohesive gold being used at the gingival seat, and about four sheets of cohesive gold to complete the filling.

S. BOND, Anoka, Minn. "Mesio-Occlusal Filling, Upper Left First Molar, Using Soft Foil and Rowan's Cohesive Pellets."

F. O. HETRICK, Ottawa, Kans. "Vernon's Gold."

The fillings were finished with platinum and gold.

G. A. RAWLINGS, Bismarck, N. D. "Gold Filling in Upper Right Lateral Incisor, Mesial Cavity."

D. D. SMITH, Philadelphia, Pa. "Method of Filling Front Tooth, Approximal Cavity, with Gold Without Swaging, so that the Gold Will Not Show from the Outside."

J. A. SCHLUETER, Jr., Aberdeen, S. D. "Gold Filling in Mesio-Incisal Surface of Upper Left Central Incisor."

J. V. CONZETT, Dubuque, Iowa. "Gold Filling in Mesio-Occlusal Surface of Upper Right Second Bicuspid, using Soft Foil in the Gingival Third."

A gold filling was inserted by the clinician in the mesio-occlusal surface of the upper right second bicuspid, using soft foil in the gingival third.

WM. FINN, Cedar Rapids, Iowa. "Gold Filling in Mesio-Occlusal Surface of Upper Right First Molar."

A gold filling was inserted in a mesio-occlusal cavity of an upper right first molar, using unannealed gold in the gingival seat, and annealed gold for the finishing.

The gingival seat is filled with unannealed gold, and the filling is finished with annealed gold.

———

J. G. PFAFF, St. Louis, Mo. "A Compound Gold and Platinum Filling."

The filling was on the grinding and distal surfaces of the second molar. Pure gold was used inside the cavity and platinum and gold on the outside.

———

R. B. WILSON, St. Paul, Minn. "Gold Filling in Distal Surface of Upper Left Lateral."

———

E. K. WEDELSTAEDT, St. Paul, Minn. "Gold Filling in Mesio-Occlusal Surface in Upper Right First Molar, using Partly Cohesive and Partly Non-cohesive Gold."

Surgery and Anesthesia.

OTTO J. FRUTH, St. Louis, Mo. "A Practical Case of Replantation with Porcelain Restoration of Crown and Part of Root."

Mr. L. A. S., twenty-eight years of age, presented himself at my office on February 16, 1904, with the left side of the face very badly swollen and the left eye nearly closed. Upon examination I found that the upper left second bicuspid was fractured obliquely, bucco-lingually, involving about two-thirds of this bifurcated root, and was the cause of the alveolar abscess. It was impossible to reunite the fragments, so the root was extracted and the cavity allowed to drain, there being considerable pus present. The cavity was thoroughly syringed and left open until the next day, when the cavity was packed with gauze saturated with an antiseptic solution. Edema of the face was still pronounced, but grew less after a few days. The gauze packing was renewed every other day and the edges of the wound were kept fresh until March 22, 1904, when the piece of root was re-planted after having mounted upon it a porcelain crown and a portion of root. The implanted tooth was ligated to the adjoining first molar and bicuspid, and the gums were treated with tincture of iodin. There was some soreness for about two days, i.e. whenever the patient bit on the tooth, but this disappeared altogether later. On the 27th of April the silk ligature tore and came loose, when the patient removed the entire ligature unknown to me. I again saw the patient, outside of my office, and he reported that the tooth felt comfortable, and that he could not distinguish it from the rest of his teeth, but did not tell me that he had removed the ligature.

He again called at my office on June 9th by appointment, when I found the tooth quite firm and the gums in a very healthy condition, although the tooth was slightly rotated from its original position, in which there was perfect occlusion; however, this does not interfere with mastication in the least, as he chews as well on the left side of his jaw as on the right, and today [October 20, 1905] the tooth is as firm as any tooth in his jaw.

The patient is robust and in the best of health, which naturally aided the process of repair to a very great extent.

CONSTRUCTION OF RESTORATION.

When the two fragments were extracted, great care was taken not to injure the peridental membrane. After having been extracted the pieces were put together and measurements taken of the whole tooth, and also a sketch made of the crown, which was used as a guide in building up the porcelain restoration. The root was then trimmed with carborundum stones and disks to the shape shown in Fig. 1.

The root-canals were then thoroughly cleaned and reamed out, and filled to the apices with gutta-percha. The apices of the roots were rounded off and polished.

A piece of pure platinum, gage No. 37, was then thoroughly burnished over the coronal end of the root, and two iridio-platinum posts were forced through the platinum and down into the roots. A porcelain facing of proper shade was then soldered to the post, as in Fig. 2.

Porcelain was then added and baked, and afterward more was added and contoured to conform to the original tooth.

After this was finished, the crown and root were cemented to the piece of root, and after having set the thin platinum foil was burnished over the joint of the root. When completed it had the appearance of the sketch, Fig. 3, after which it was replanted, the socket of the root having been thoroughly sterilized, as was also the root before being put in its original position.

FIG. 1.　　　FIG. 2.　　　FIG. 3.

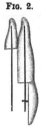
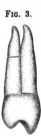

C. R. TAYLOR, Streator, Ill. "The Rubber Dam in the Mechanical and Chemical Cleaning of all Surfaces of the Teeth in the Treatment of Pyorrhea Alveolaris."

The dam is an adjunct in the exclusion of the saliva and blood, and also assists in holding the gum tissue away from the roots of the teeth, so that with the assistance of the mouth-mirror the distal surfaces of the roots can be so seen as to assist the operator in the proper direction of the root-cleaning instruments for complete removal of the deposits from the buccal and molar teeth. Pledgets of cotton can be packed between the roots of the teeth with sufficient force to more thoroughly press the detached gums from about the teeth, in this way exposing the portions of the roots which have lost their peridental membrane. In these cases the peridental membrane is very tender and painful to the touch of the instruments, and anodynes may be used, followed by a saturated solution of zinc chlorid to relieve the acute sensitivity. After the roots have been cleaned mechanically they can be polished by the usual methods and with strips of China silk covered with pumice or other polishing powders.

The rubber dam prevents the soft tissues from being injuriously affected by any of the remedies that may be used on the teeth. In preparing the dam for adjustment, the holes are punched much farther apart than when prepared for filling, in order to allow for the space between the roots of each of the teeth and for the dam to move in the direction of the apices of the roots when the pockets are being exposed. As the instruments used for the removal of the deposits are pressed against the dam, the latter is being constantly forced toward the apical end of the roots, thus clearing the field of operation.

———

GILLETTE HAYDEN, Columbus, Ohio. "The Treatment of Diseased Pulps."

The cement liquid recommended by the clinician in the treatment of diseased pulps is made according to the following formula:

Cement Liquid.

Eugenol,	ʒss;
Black's "1, 2, 3,"	ʒij;
Oil of cloves,	gtt. xx;
Oil of cinnamon,	gtt. xv;
Oil of cassia,	gtt. xv.

Cement Powder.
Zinc oxid.

The clinician claimed that when cement made with the above ingredients is placed over an exposed and aching pulp, whether the exposure be accidental or of long standing, almost immediate relief from pain is secured. Its use is indicated in all cases of acute pulpitis and of congested conditions of the dental pulp. If the cement be placed over an inflamed pulp for twenty-four hours before the application of a devitalizing agent, good results will be less painfully reached than otherwise. It is intended only for relieving pain, and not for a permanent filling material. It sets very slowly, becoming first chalky, and then growing harder as the excess of oil is dissolved out by the saliva. In mixing, use as much powder as the liquid will take up while spatulating the mass. The liquid alone, used on a pellet of cotton, will be found valuable in treating hypertrophied conditions of the gums and soft tissues.

———

H. JAMES MORRIS, Sheffield, England. "Anesthesia."

The clinician showed a simple apparatus for the administration of ethyl chlorid for general anesthesia, consisting of a face-piece and bag connected by a T-shaped tube.

To the end of the vertical arm the face-piece is attached, and the bag to one of the other arms. A third opening is for the admission of the ethyl chlorid, which is then closed by the left thumb of the operator. Three cubic centimeters of ethyl chlorid are sprayed into the bag where it evaporates.

Mr. Morris is convinced that ethyl chlorid is a safe anesthetic, statistics showing it to have a much lower death-rate than ether; also it gives a longer working time (one to two and one-half minutes) than N_2O. Two to two and one-half cubic centimeters is enough for children, but much more can be given to adults. It can be given freely and continuously, as cyanosis and other objectionable symptoms do not supervene.

The objection to the use of ethyl is that in a small percentage of cases there is some nausea and distress for a short time afterward. Patients should be prepared as for ether. The apparatus is portable. Anesthesia, with loss of reflexes, can be induced quicker than with N_2O.

———

G. D. MOYER, Montevideo, Minn. "Method of Bringing the Jaws in Apposition while a Fracture is Uniting."

The upper and lower jaw are wired together, passing a binding wire around the upper and lower teeth, making two loops to hold the jaws together.

———

M. H. CRYER, Philadelphia, Pa. "Ankylosis of the Jaws."

The patient F. H. P. is thirty years of age. When seven years old he suffered from mercurial ptyalism. Necrosed bone was exfoliated and passed out immediately under the zygomatic arch. At the age of thirteen an endeavor was made to prize the mouth open by wedges and screws. This resulted in the breaking of ten teeth.

It is more than likely that in such cases the condyloid processes have become flattened, that the glenoid fossa is the seat of bony deposits and that the inter-articulating fibro-cartilage has become ossified.

Treatment.—Take an X-ray picture of each side of the jaws to control the diagnosis. If it prove to be correct, there should then be made two false joints in the rami above and posterior to the inferior dental foramen. The making of these false joints in this position will prevent the jaw from falling farther backward. If the ordinary removal of the condyloid process was followed, there would be danger of the lower jaw falling backward and interfering with the respiratory functions.

———

A. W. HARLAN, New York, N. Y. "Pyorrhea Alveolaris."

In cases of pyorrhea alveolaris the clinician recommends the following mouth-wash:

Boro-glycerin,	ʒij;
Resorcin,	ʒij;
Beta-naphthol,	ʒss;
Alcohol,	ʒv;
Water,	ʒxxvij.

———

O. H. MANHARD, St. Louis, Mo. "Retaining Appliance to be Used in Pyorrhea Cases."

Take an impression and secure the model. Burnish thin platinum No. 38 or 40 gage over the lingual surface of the teeth required to be held in position, including one or more on either side. Reinforce platinum by soldering. Proceed in the same manner over the labial surface. Take iridio-platinum wire of tooth-pin gage and solder to either end of the lingual splint and pass through the most convenient position and through the labial splint. Use the S. S. White Bryant bridge-repair outfit and cut a thread on the pins that pass through the labial splint with the instrument supplied in the outfit for that purpose. Then proceed to apply the gold nuts furnished by the supply house and screw the appliance to position. This can be cemented or not as the requirement in the case suggests itself to the operator, and can be removed at any time in a few moments.

N. D. Edmonds, Wilmington, Ohio. "A New and Original Method of Constructing Dental Splints."

Dr. Edmonds' clinic consisted in taking an impression of the occluding surfaces of the teeth of the fractured maxillæ with modeling compound, pouring the model, and running a saw through where the fracture occurred, articulating the fragments with a cast of the antagonizing jaw, and cementing them together with plaster of Paris. All the spaces between the teeth and all undercuts are filled with wax.

A die and a counter-die are then made, and an aluminum cap of No. 28 gage is struck up. The buccal and lingual sides are trimmed to the length of the crowns and filled with a slow-setting cement. The fragments are put in place and the aluminum cap is clamped to the necks of the teeth and approximating spaces while the cement is yet soft. This is done with pliers similar to separating forceps but having oval edges and a center tongue between the beaks through which passes a set-screw, which presses upon the occluding surfaces of the cap and holds it down upon the teeth, while the beaks close in the approximal spaces and burnish the aluminum to the necks of the teeth, thus making a complete anchorage for the fracture without the use of bandages and giving the patient free use of the jaws for masticating.

———

Florestan Aguilar, Madrid, Spain. "General Anesthesia with Somnoform."

G. V. I. Brown, Milwaukee, Wis. "Surgical Operation for the Treatment of Cleft Palate."

———

E. Sauvez, Paris, France. "Local Anesthetic [Stovain] for Extractions and All Operations in the Mouth."

Dr. Sauvez gave three demonstrations of local anesthesia for the extraction of teeth with "stovain." The effects of this preparation are the same as those of cocain, but it is two or three times less toxic. Moreover it has a vaso-dilator action, and consequently the patient may be operated upon in the sitting position.

The first case consisted in the extraction of a lower bicuspid. Two injections were made, one buccally and the other lingually, and the tooth was extracted painlessly. In the second case the roots of an upper molar were extracted. After the injection was made the roots were extracted painlessly. The roots were very difficult to remove, but the patient experienced no pain whatever.

———

A. Brom Allen, Chicago, Ill. "Extracting with Nitrous Oxid."

The clinician demonstrated tooth-extraction using blunt-handled forceps. He also showed an aseptic mouth-piece for the nitrous oxid gas inhaler, and models of impacted third molars prepared by Dr. C. Edmund Kells.

———

E. C. Briggs, Boston, Mass. "Local Treatment for Pyorrhea Alveolaris."

Prosthesis.

R. M. SEIBEL, Kansas City, Mo. "Obturator."

In presenting this clinic Dr. Seibel said: My desire is to give the young practitioner a simple method for making an obturator, claiming no originality and avoiding as much as possible all of the technical details of the anatomy of the palate which have been thoroughly taught in the various schools and so ably expounded in the papers of Dr. Suersen and others.

The obturator which I wish to demonstrate, while similar to Suersen's, is different in that the obturator bulb or velum proper is hollow, and is attached to the plate in such a manner that it is freely movable in all directions and accommodates itself to all the complex movements in the many different positions of the soft palate, by this means causing much less irritation on account of its lightness and movability, and thus tending to secure a more successful piece of work.

An impression of the parts is obtained by using an impression compound, holding it in position with the fingers, spreading the compound well over the teeth and forcing it up and back into the opening. Care should be taken to remove the impression before the compound becomes too hard. The impression may be replaced to make assurance doubly sure, but it should not be allowed to become too hard. Now proceed to pour the impression as with an ordinary full denture, after the plaster has thoroughly hardened, smooth off the top of the plaster and carve guide cuts; now varnish, etc., then pour a quantity of plaster still on top of the model. Re-

move the last plaster as soon as it becomes hard; then soften the modeling compound and separate. When this is done, saw the model of the entire upper maxilla through the center lengthwise. The halves can now be replaced into the last pouring of plaster, and the parts will be in perfect apposition. Then proceed to make a wax model of the obturator to fit the cleft in soft palate; also a trial plate of the hard palate, extending it into the cleft about one-eighth of an inch. In making a hinge to connect these two parts, it should be so constructed as to have both an up and a down motion, also a free lateral movement; this can be done by making a single tongue hinge with a very loose-fitting pin. Now connect the two parts with the hinge, letting the joint come about one-eighth inch on the hard palate side, so that the projecting edge acts as a stop when the bulb is in its lowest position; also see that the hinge is so placed that it will be firmly vulcanized in position.

With the patient in the chair, proceed to fit the model, softening the bulb. Request the patient to swallow; note where the muscles impinge at the sides and back. Carve the wax at these points. Resoften and repeat as often as necessary; when satisfied that all is perfect, make the rubber plate in the usual way, with one-half the hinge in place (a straw placed in the hinge at this point will save much trouble). To make the hollow velum or bulb, flask it in such a manner as to leave only the palatal side exposed and flush; press a sheet of rubber into the holes, being careful to have it extend over the edges a little, reinforce thin places or corners if necessary, sealing with a solution of rubber and chloroform; then place two or three drops of water in the cup thus formed and seal a sheet of rubber over the top, close the flask, and vulcanize.

———

A. P. Johnston, Anderson, S. C. "New Method of Section for the Upper Plate, Plate for the Lower Jaw, and Removable Bridges; All Original Methods, Illustrated by Models."

———

T. W. Pritchett, Whitehall, Ill. "Bonwill Method of Articulating Full Dentures."

The purpose of this clinic was to show that good mastication can be made with artificial dentures when constructed upon the lines advocated by the late Dr. Bonwill. Specimen models in plaster, mounted upon the articulator, of perfectly occluding natural dentures were shown together with mounted specimens of artificial dentures. Comparison as to efficiency of mastication was made between natural and artificial teeth by the exhibition of samples of chewed beefsteak as masticated by several persons representing the models exhibited.

Geo. H. Wilson, Cleveland, O. "Vulcanite."

The clinician showed the result of double vulcanization and improper manipulation by applying too much force in packing the rubber, and that the plaster properly handled does not expand excessively or the rubber contract excessively; it is improper manipulation that warps the plates. By the use of plaster and Spence's compound non-changing plate, a good fit is obtained and the plate is not warped out of shape.

———

W. R. Smith, Pawnee City, Neb. "Method of Making a Plate with the Use of Vulcanizable Gutta-Percha Without Wax, Getting the Effect of the Pink Rubber of the Gum Without Carving, Filing, or Scraping."

———

H. F. Cassel, St. Louis, Mo. "Striking-up Partial Gold Plate with Swaged Enforcement, Using Single Thickness of Gold."

———

L. P. Haskell, Chicago, Ill. "The Insertion of Artificial Dentures."

Orthodontia.

G. D. Sitherwood, Bloomington, Ill. "Soldering, Gold-Plating, and Adjusting of Bands and Fixtures."

The clinician demonstrated a method of soldering German silver regulating bands by the use of steel binding wire, using whiting to prevent the solder from flowing where not desired. For pins or hooks, as may be desired, attach the end of an ordinary brass pin for a lug, and cut it off.

R. G. Richter, Milwaukee, Wis. "Malocclusion and Jaw-strain, or the Grating Habit as a Prime Etiological Factor of Interstitial Gingivitis and Pyorrhea Alveolaris."

It was illustrated by casts and upon a patient.

———

G. Arthur Roberts, Toronto, Canada. "Angle System of Orthodontia."

Miscellaneous.

F. H. NIES, Brooklyn, N. Y. "The Preparation of Cavities with Carborundum Stones."

The clinic was to demonstrate the larger usefulness of the carborundum stone in the preparation of cavities, especially that class of cavities known as fissure cavities. For this method is claimed greater rapidity together with thorough removal of decayed dentin with the least pain to the patient.

In the same clinic a new device for holding napkins and the rubber dam clear of the tooth while working with porcelain or otherwise was shown. The purpose of this device is to provide a simple means for holding the napkin or rubber dam in position on bicuspids and molars in order to exclude moisture from the cavities while operating. The clamp consists of two lever-like jaws pivotally connected at the fulcrum. The end of one lever is threaded, bearing a peculiar beveled nut which acts against the inclined heel of the other lever and in this way clasps the tooth. To provide for different forms and irregularities in the arch, oscillating plates are pivoted to the jaw plates, and rock about their pivot, accommodating themselves to the shape of the teeth on the slightest pressure.

The clamp used in connection with the rubber dam is placed in anterior to the ordinary bow clamp—its broad flanges keeping the rubber away from the teeth, thus permitting the operator an unobstructed view and preventing its being caught with the instruments and displaced, while its polished surface reflects the light.

When used as a napkin-holder for the exclusion of moisture on the upper jaw, the napkin is placed in the usual way and the clamp is applied to the first and second molars, where it securely holds the napkin in place without the assistance of the operator, thereby permitting the use of both hands. The mode of application on the jaw is to place the napkin in the usual position, extending slightly over the gum line. The clamp is then gently slipped over the tooth and napkin edge, pressed together against the tooth, and the beveled nut is screwed down. When it is used in this way, in conjunction with the saliva ejector, operations involving long periods of time can be successfully accomplished.

———

WILLIAM CRENSHAW, Atlanta, Ga. "Demonstrating the Improved Contour and Anterior-Teeth Matrices."

Dr. Crenshaw gave a table clinic showing the application and operation of the contour matrix in its several positions and the manner of introducing the cushions and cylinders of tin and gold. He showed also the manner of removing the device when amalgams are used, to prevent the lifting or breaking up of the filling; also the application and operation of the bow brace which aids in holding the matrix between the canine and first bicuspid.

The clinician also demonstrated the application and operation of the anterior-teeth matrix, together with instruments and the method of introducing the cushions of gold.

Dr. Crenshaw gave another clinic the second day, showing the practical appli-

36

cation and operation of the anterior-teeth matrix, in which the distal surface of the upper right central and the mesial surface of the upper right lateral incisors were filled, restoring the lost lingual portions of each. Three-fourths of each one of the cavities was filled with non-cohesive gold, and the remainder with cohesive gold.

L. A. SMITH, Port Gibson, Miss. "A System of Ordering Teeth by Measure."

This clinic consisted of a demonstration of the clinician's system of ordering teeth, facings, and crowns by measurement, and showing the instruments used in obtaining the measurements. The clinician also showed a dentimeter that measured accurately with a copper ribbon the roots of the teeth that are to be crowned, the ribbon carrier being a part of the instrument.

M. H. CRYER, Philadelphia, Pa. "Internal Anatomy of the Face."

Dr. Cryer's clinic comprised a beautiful and instructive collection of lantern slides illustrating the internal anatomy of the face. These slides, which were so arranged in a frame with reflected light that they might be readily studied in series, were made by Dr. Cryer from specimens specially prepared and dissected by him. They represented the results obtained from sections of numerous cadavers specially frozen and treated by him with a view to maintaining the true relationship of the various tissues. They are admirably adapted for teaching purposes. There were also displayed numerous specimens of dried and mace-

rated heads, many of which were used in the preparation of the slides above referred to.

Another exhibit of Dr. Cryer's which attracted much attention was a large stereoscope, a comparatively new apparatus, designed to aid in the study of radiographs, and constituting a valuable adjunct to the study of the internal anatomy of the face.

C. O. SIMPSON, St. Louis, Mo. "Demonstrating the Strength and Durability of Various Amalgams and Cements."

Amalgams from various alloys were subjected to a series of tests to determine the advantages in strength, color, shrinkage, expansion, etc. Justi's Triumph alloy showed minimum of shrinkage and expansion. Nolde's Goldine alloy showed by far the greatest strength, one specimen taking 1200 pounds pressure without fracture. Kester's alloy and Mutual alloy showed satisfactory results.

Cements were similarly treated as well as being exposed to saliva for a given period of time. Ames' inlay cement showed the greatest resistance to saliva, and Ames' crown and bridge cement showed the greatest strength. Ash's C. A. S. Ramesite and Justi's Insoluble gave good results.

W. L. ELLERBECK, Salt Lake City, Utah. "Electric Furnace Construction."

The clinician demonstrated his method of making electric furnaces so that dentists who are in remote parts of the country may very quickly and inexpensively manufacture their own muffles—as a rule, more quickly than they can repair a burn-out in manufacturers' muffles.

———

R. B. WILSON, St. Paul, Minn. "Amalgam Filling in Mesio-Occlusal Surface of a Lower Right Molar, using Alfred Owre's Alloy, and Demonstrating Wedelstaedt Method of Adjusting Matrix."

———

H. W. ARTHUR. Pittsburg, Pa. "Typodont."

This clinic consisted in showing block teeth carved from celluloid, mounted in approximal contact and occlusion.

The clinician demonstrated their applicability to the teaching of operative dentistry.

———

W. V.-B. AMES, Chicago, Ill. "Cements."

The clinician demonstrated the value of mixing pulverized porcelain with zinc oxysulfate for rendering oxysulfate fillings more permanent; also porcelain with zinc silicate for the better adhesion of the cement.

———

J. F. WALLACE, Canton, Mo. "Amalgam Filling in Mesio-Occlusal Surface of Lower First Molar, using Dr. Black's Method of Cavity Preparation and Matrix, and the Wedelstaedt Tie."

UNIVERSAL EXPOSITION, ST. LOUIS, U.S.A.

DAVID R. FRANCIS,
President of Exposition.

1904.

HOWARD J. ROGERS,
Director of Congresses.

TRANSACTIONS

OF THE

𝕱ourth International Dental Congress

HELD AT

ST. LOUIS, MO., U. S. A.,

August 29 to September 3, 1904.

*EDITED FOR THE COMMITTEE OF ORGANIZATION
BY EDWARD C. KIRK, WILBUR F. LITCH,
AND JULIO ENDELMAN.*

IN THREE VOLUMES

VOL. III.

Philadelphia:
PRESS OF THE "DENTAL COSMOS,"
The S. S. White Dental Mfg. Co.
1905.